POEM BY HILDA CONKLING · LOUISA EYRE · FECIT ·

· DEAR GOD LET ME HOLD UP
MY SILVER CUP
FOR THEM TO DRINK ·

FRONTISPIECE BY LOUISA EYRE

*The Identifying Symbol of the*
*Children's Hospital of Philadelphia*

*Courtesy of Mrs. de Lanux, Mrs. Louisa E. Norton*
*and Mr. Edwards F. Leiper, Jr., Attorney-at-Law*

# Textbook of

With 446 Illustrations
on 277 Figures

**DOROTHY R. MARLOW, R.N., Ed.D.**

*Associate Professor of Pediatric Nursing,*
*University of Pennsylvania School of Nursing*

**GLADYS SELLEW, R.N., Ph.D.**

*Formerly Professor of Nursing of Children,*
*University of Maryland School of Nursing*

# PEDIATRIC NURSING

## W. B. SAUNDERS COMPANY

PHILADELPHIA AND LONDON

# Foreword

A FOREWORD can serve a number of purposes, and it has not been an easy task to decide toward which of these this particular foreword should be directed. Much could be said which primarily would pay tribute to the authors. The pages of this book, for example, convey a warmth of feeling for children and an understanding of them seldom achieved in the printed word, and even less often in a textbook. This characteristic is so pervasive it cannot but infect the reader even to the extent of exciting like feelings. The book speaks so clearly for the authors, however, in this and in other respects that this purpose was discarded.

These introductory remarks might serve the purpose of orienting the reader to the rich and varied accumulation of knowledge and its systematic organization to be found in these pages. Undoubtedly this volume is rare among texts in the scope and completeness with which the many-faceted aspects of child life are discussed. But this fact too will quickly be self-evident, and a second purpose was rejected.

A foreword in the form of a book review offered a highly tempting, if inappropriate, possibility. The unusual features of both the content and its organization demand critical analysis and discussion. A book review would not only misuse the opportunity this foreword offers, but also would probably be of greater interest to the teacher of pediatric nursing than to the student. In any case, it must be left for the columns of the professional journals.

What, then, can this foreword provide? Precisely, because of the nature of this book, the most useful function of a foreword may be a brief guide to the student on how to get the most out of the great deal that it offers. Chapter-by-chapter reading in textbooks is not always fruitful. The student may be searching for general understanding, and specific details are offered—about procedures, about particular situations, or about a group of diseases affecting a particular organ system. Because the information needed is scattered, she may have difficulty bringing together knowledge of people, of their health problems when their defenses fail, and of the kind of nursing care required. She must, however, correlate and integrate this knowledge to give appropriate and helpful nursing care. This difficulty will not be encountered in this text.

Within three consecutive chapters of this book it is possible to acquire a comprehensive picture of the child—his growth and development, his care, and his health problems—at each developmental period. Age and developmental stage are clearly seen as important influences on the occurrence of illness and on its treatment; this fundamental basis for nursing care is obvious. The meaning and significance of illness and hospitalization to the child and to his family are also related to development and make for increased understanding of this problem. The disease conditions commonly found in a given age period become readily apparent, serving not only to sharpen observations, but also to clarify the interrelations between maturation and specific kinds of illnesses.

Read carefully, then, chapter by chapter, for a general understanding of the field of pediatric nursing, for an appreciation of its scope and complexity, for an awareness of the many factors involved in nursing care, and for comprehensive knowledge of the child and his health problems. The possibility for learning does not end here, however. Selected kinds of rereading will be effective in furthering your knowledge and understanding.

Read and study consecutively and carefully each of the chapters on growth, development, and care, in each of the developmental periods. The dynamic process of growth from birth through adolescence emerges, and a text within a text is found. In a similar fashion a text devoted to the health problems of infants and children which are acute or short-term in nature evolves; or one concerned with those problems which require long-term care can be segregated. The presence of several possible texts in one volume makes it relatively easy for you to develop and expand your knowledge of the field on a longitudinal as well as on a cross-sectional basis.

There is another facet of this book to be studied. Nursing is an applied science and of necessity draws heavily upon the basic sciences and other applied sciences for its content. This knowledge is then synthesized and extended to provide a basis for nursing practice. Nursing care practices, general and specific, and the rationale underlying these practices are discussed in some detail throughout this book. You may wish to find another text within a text by delineating those general nursing care practices, together with the supporting knowledge, which can be adapted to a number of age levels and to many disease conditions.

In the final analysis, what you gain from this textbook depends upon you. It cannot give you wisdom, but it offers a foundation for the development of wisdom. It cannot give you understanding of an individual child in the real world of nursing, but it provides the kind of knowledge through which that understanding is made possible. It cannot give you skill in the practice of pediatric nursing, but it offers you the tools with which to work. It cannot give you faith in yourself or in the patients you serve, but it can lead you to the threshold of such faith.

DOROTHY E. JOHNSON
*University of Southern California*
*School of Nursing*

# Preface

ADVANCES in the area of child care have been rapid during recent years. Research carried on by disciplines such as psychology and sociology has contributed increased understanding of the growth and development of children, the meaning of parent-child relations and the effects of their separation, and the place of the child and the adolescent in our changing world. Medical research has led to the knowledge of successful methods of therapy through the use of drugs, advanced surgical techniques and psychiatric care for children.

The role of the pediatric nurse has been influenced by both these findings and also by research carried on within the nursing profession itself. In her new role the pediatric nurse is no longer a lone practitioner; she is now a team member working with members of various professions for the welfare of the child and his family. The nurse no longer replaces the mother in the hospitalized child's life; she now helps the mother to provide nursing care for her child when he is well and when he is ill. She no longer sees the child only in a hospital bed, but recognizes him as an individual, a member of a family and of the community.

This change in role of the pediatric nurse places a broader responsibility upon her than she has known before. She must now be cognizant of the contribution she can make as a member of the team in maintaining the integrity of each family, in offering anticipatory guidance and in providing skilled nursing care for children when needed.

In considering the changing role and responsibilities of the pediatric nurse the authors became aware that the traditional internal organization of subject matter in this area might not be the best way to present these concepts to young students. After reviewing the recent trends in nursing and related fields, the concepts to be applied in the nursing of children and the basic principles of teaching and learning, an alternate organizational pattern emerged in our thinking.

In the opening chapters of the book the authors have attempted to give the student a historical perspective of the area of pediatric nursing and a broad view of the areas of knowledge which must be understood in order to provide care for children today: an overview of the concepts and principles of growth and development, a general discussion of the care of the child when ill and when hospitalized, and a review of the role of the pediatric nurse.

After this general view of content, the remainder of the book is organized into units primarily on the basis of specific growth and development and care of various age groups of children from the newborn period through adolescence. An understanding of growth and development is vital to the nurse because she is primarily nursing the child, not his disease. After the student has developed an understanding of the healthy child she is led to a consideration of the effect of illness on children in the same age group. Physical and emotional illnesses requiring short-term or immediate care and long-term care are discussed. The various conditions included in each age period have been selected either because they are related to the growth and development process, or because their incidence is greatest during that particular age span. Few conditions have been included for which there is not a discussion of the nursing care to be given in the home or in the hospital, by the mother or by the nurse. Since we have tried to present the nursing care of children so thoroughly, we have purposely not included in this book all the disorders of the pediatric years. On the other hand, we have included some conditions which were not common in the past, but which today, because of our increasing knowledge of diagnosis and therapy, are being seen with increasing frequency. In the discussion of each condition appropriate concepts such as those related to the areas of nutrition, mental health, prevention of illness, rehabilitation and public health are considered.

We found that by writing within this organizational framework more than pure subject matter could be included. By emphasizing the growth and development of children in the family constellation and in various social settings, and by helping students to view parent-child-nurse relations not only through their own eyes, but through the eyes of parent and child as well, we have tried to help students develop understandings and attitudes which should be beneficial in their work.

The material in the text was submitted to physicians, to nurses and to members of other disciplines for their opinions and suggestions. Their appraisals and contributions have helped the authors to clarify or expand important areas of content.

A selected list of teaching aids and sources of information is included at the ends of most of the chapters. Students should find these of significant value if studied and then used in their guidance of parents and children.

The references given at the end of each chapter have been selected on the basis of their scope of content and their timeliness. For the most part they present, in greater depth than was possible in this text, recent trends and newer knowledge in the medical, nursing and related disciplines. Articles in which original research findings are presented are included because the authors believe that the beginning student should become acquainted with the value of such investigations.

The study questions at the end of each unit have been included for the purpose of helping the student bring together the material presented on the care of children in each age group. Some of these questions involve the understanding of factual material, while others require the student to use judgment in answering situational questions.

It has been our hope to make this textbook representative of the current thought in the area of pediatric nursing. The authors will welcome all comments and suggestions from reviewers, teachers and students so that this text can be of increasing value to the nursing student in helping her to contribute her best efforts to the care of children and to find deep personal satisfaction in working with them and their parents.

DOROTHY R. MARLOW
GLADYS SELLEW

# Acknowledgments

MANY professional persons; physicians, nurses and members of other disciplines have contributed their knowledge and support to make the creation of this book possible.

A special tribute should be accorded to those who by their faith in the worthiness of our task encouraged us in our efforts: Dr. Theresa I. Lynch, Dean of the School of Nursing, University of Pennsylvania; Dr. Mildred L. Montag, Professor of Nursing Education, Teachers College, Columbia University; and Dr. Marcia A. Dake, Dean of the College of Nursing, University of Kentucky.

It is impossible to express adequately the appreciation of the authors for the generous assistance of several physicians who contributed to this text:

Sydney M. Borowsky, M.D., Associate in Pediatrics, Albert Einstein Medical Center and Instructor in Pediatrics, School of Nursing, Hospital of the University of Pennsylvania

Donald A. Cornely, M.D., Chief, Section of Maternal and Child Health, Community Health Services, Philadelphia Department of Health

Sidney Friedman, M.D., Cardiologist, Children's Hospital of Philadelphia

Peter Knowlton, M.D., Senior Psychiatrist, Philadelphia Child Guidance Clinic

C. Everett Koop, M.D., Professor of Pediatric Surgery, School of Medicine, University of Pennsylvania, and Surgeon-in-Chief, Children's Hospital of Philadelphia

Pierre LeRoy, M.D., Resident, Neurosurgery, Children's Hospital of Philadelphia

William J. Rashkind, M.D., Associate Cardiologist, Children's Hospital of Philadelphia

Eugene B. Spitz, M.D., Associate Professor of Neurosurgery in Charge of Pediatrics, School of Medicine, University of Pennsylvania, and Director of the Division of Neurosurgery, Children's Hospital of Philadelphia

Irving J. Wolman, M.D., Professor of Pediatrics and Head of the Department of Pediatrics, Graduate School of Medicine, University of Pennsylvania, and Hematologist, Children's Hospital of Philadelphia


Several members of other professions as well as nurses not primarily concerned with the care of hospitalized children have made significant contributions to this book:

Mary Beam, R.N., Assistant Professor of Rehabilitation and Public Health Nursing, School of Nursing, University of Pennsylvania

Mary M. Brooks, Director of the Children's Activities Program, Children's Hospital of Philadelphia

Doris Harr, R.N., Public Health Nursing Consultant in Mental Retardation, St. Christopher's Hospital for Children

Polly Hochgelerent, Hospital School Teacher, Philadelphia Board of Education

Martha Hunscher, Assistant Professor in Nutrition, School of Nursing, University of Pennsylvania

Mary M. Lang, Lecturer, School of Education, University of Pennsylvania

Barbara M. Modic, R.N., Supervisor, Graduate Hospital of the University of Pennsylvania

Marian Morris, Social Worker, Children's Hospital of Philadelphia


The authors are indeed grateful to the many members of the nursing staff of the Children's Hospital of Philadelphia who offered excellent suggestions which have been incorporated in this textbook. We would like especially to express our appreciation to the following:

Eloise Auer, R.N., Neurosurgical Nurse

Erna Goulding, R.N., Associate Director of Nursing Education

Brenda E. Ramsey, R.N., Supervisor of Private Floor

E. Cleves Rothrock, R.N., Director of Nursing Service and Nursing Education

Mary Wislosky, R.N., Supervisor of Medical Unit


We should like to express our appreciation also to the authors, publishers and companies who have granted us permission to use their illustrations in this text. We should like to thank the personnel of H. Armstrong Roberts and Gilbert and Ring, Medical Photographers, for their excellent photographs of children. A special word of appreciation should be extended to Dr. and Mrs. Robert Gens, to Mr. and Mrs. John Haffly and their daughter, Kim, and to the many parents who granted permission for pictures of their children to appear in this book. Although these parents were anxious about the health of their children, they were eager to contribute in this way to the education of nursing students.

The authors wish to express warm appreciation to the staff of the W. B. Saunders Company for their fine cooperation.

We should also like to express our personal appreciation to Mrs. L. Neffi and to Mr. and Mrs. W. Marlow for their patience and understanding during the preparation of this book.

DOROTHY R. MARLOW
GLADYS SELLEW

# Contents

# Unit III.   The Infant

CHAPTER 13

## Conditions of Infants Requiring Immediate or Short-Term Care ........ 296

CHAPTER 14

## Conditions of Infants Requiring Long-Term Care ................... 341

# Unit IV.   The Toddler

CHAPTER 15

## The Normal Toddler: His Growth, Development and Care ........... 393

# Unit V.  The Preschool Child

# Unit VI.    The School Child

## Unit VII.   The Pubescent and the Adolescent

# Introduction

# Chapter 1

# Child Care through the Ages

## HISTORY AND PRESENT CONCEPTS OF CHILD CARE

### HISTORY

LITTLE is known about the life of children in prehistoric times, but child care is believed to have been somewhat like that among primitive tribes living today in remote areas hardly touched by civilization. Primitive people tend to value a child not for himself, but as a future adult. For this reason his social development according to the customs of the group is of great importance.

Child care varies among primitive people, so that little can be said about their customs which would apply to all groups. A child, like a helpless little animal, must receive at least a minimum of care or he will die. Some primitive people give only this essential physical care and show little or no affection for a baby. An infant may be left to die because his parents do not want him, or the tribe may reject him because he is deformed or because some ill omen was associated with his birth. Among other primitive tribes both parents may love the child. A mother may keep her infant with her wherever she goes, carrying him on her hip or in a sling over her shoulder.

### Child Care in Ancient Civilizations

In ancient India and Egypt child care was based on tradition handed on from mother to daughter and on the everyday experiences of a mother with her own children. Also, the learned men of the time applied what they knew of sanitation and hygiene to the care of pregnant women and of little children. Among the ancient Jews the hygienic measures prescribed in the Mosaic Law had a great influence on maternal and child care. Parenthood was honored, and a large family was considered a sign of God's blessing upon the man and his wife.

Christianity taught the value of the child as an individual, not merely as a son or daughter who would cherish the parents in their old age and give them grandchildren so that the family might

3

extend for generations to come. Further-more, since Christianity also taught the protection of the weak by the strong, the helpless child became the object of special consideration. Early in the history of the Christian church Christians founded orphan asylums for dependent children.

As Christianity was carried to the countries that now comprise Europe, the Christian concept of child care became the basic pattern, varying, however, with the general culture of the different nations.

### Child Care in Europe

Before the nineteenth century the life expectancy of human beings was short. Many did not live long enough to rear their children in the home. Severe epidemics of contagious diseases often swept over Europe; the death rate was highest in the cities and among the poor who were crowded in slum areas. Young men died in war or from injuries sustained while at work. Women married early and had large families; the maternal death rate was high. The result of all these conditions was that there were many orphaned children among the poor of the growing cities— Paris and London, for instance. Although asylums were founded for their care, such institutions were over-crowded. It is estimated that half of the infants of the urban poor died before the age of five years.

Probably the darkest period in child care in western Europe was the early years of the Industrial Revolution. Children as young as six years of age worked in cotton mills for ten or more hours a day. They often fell asleep at their work, and accidents were common. But their small hands were nearly as skillful as adult hands in tying broken threads, and the cost of their maintenance (if they were apprenticed orphans) and their wages were so low that mill owners employed them in large numbers. Not until the nineteenth century was legislation passed that prohibited the worst evils of this form of child labor.

### Child Care in the United States

Until the early decades of the twentieth century the great majority of children in the United States lived on farms or in small villages. In general this was a healthy life, although children in such areas lacked the medical care and hospital facilities that urban parents could provide. Child labor was never the problem in the United States that it was in Europe; nevertheless the children of the poor were employed in factories and stores where working conditions were unhealthy and hours far too long. Federal legislation now prohibits child labor in industries producing goods sent across state lines, and most states limit child labor within their boundaries. If there is a child labor problem today, it is in the age group between sixteen and eighteen years and among the younger children of migratory workers in agriculture.

By the middle of the nineteenth century there were large slums in New York and other eastern cities. The people living there were generally immigrants from foreign countries, many of them from rural areas and not accustomed to city life. Tenements were overcrowded, unsanitary and in bad repair. Morbidity and mortality rates among infants and little children were exceedingly high. Accidents in the tenements and in the streets where the children played were common.

Contaminated milk led to serious intestinal disorders among infants and children. (Dairies and stores which handled milk were not inspected as they are today, and milk was not pasteurized.) Milk from tuberculous cows caused many cases of tuberculosis among children.

The condition of these neglected children aroused public sympathy. The Children's Aid Society of New York was founded in 1853. Two years later (1855) the first children's hospital in the United States was founded in Philadelphia, and in 1860 Dr. Jacobi established in New York the first children's clinic, where he lectured to medical students on the diseases of childhood.

It was not until the twentieth century, however, that measures to conserve children's health through the application of scientific knowledge were undertaken on a national scale. In 1909 President Theodore Roosevelt called the first White House Conference on Children and Youth; a similar conference has been held every 10 years since then. As a result of the first conference the United States Children's Bureau was founded. The Bureau was put under the jurisdiction of the Department of Labor, since at that time child labor was thought to be the greatest problem of childhood. In the 1930 White House Conference on Child Health and Protection the famous Children's Charter, *The Rights of the Child as an Individual in the State*, was drawn up. This is one of the most important documents in the history of child care. In 1950 the Mid-Century White House Conference in Washington, D.C., was attended by 5000 delegates from all professions and groups concerned with children, and 500 young people were invited to join the conference. The theme of the conference was *A Fair Chance to Achieve a Healthy Personality.*

The sixth, or Golden Anniversary, White House Conference on Children and Youth was held in 1960. Many thousands of adults and youths in the nation prepared for this conference. The reports of the conference reflect the general prosperity of the 1950's. Topics discussed included basic family income for buying the essentials for living, family life, values and religion, minority groups in society, juvenile delinquency, education, children in special need, health and health services, and the use of leisure time. One of the greatest needs for the future, highlighted in all the state reports from the conference, was that of coordination of efforts between public and private agencies in all aspects of programs which affect children and youth.

In addition to the efforts of individual countries such as the United States to improve the lives of children and youth, the 14th General Assembly of the United Nations (November 20,

1959) approved the *Declaration of the Rights of the Child.* This document is based on the idea that mankind everywhere owes to children the best it can give (see p. 6).

Today the over-all child care program of the Federal Government, the states, counties and cities operates through a number of institutions, such as schools, hospitals, clinics, aid societies, and institutes for handicapped children (the blind, the deaf, the crippled, the mentally defective, the neurotic and the psychotic) and for dependent and delinquent children.

The nursing care of children comes under this vast program, and nurses share with other professional persons the care of the child in all these institutions and agencies. The trend in pediatrics and in the nursing care of children has been away from focus on *illness* and toward consideration of the *well* and the *ill child.* This trend has been accompanied by the integration of all branches of science in planning the care of the child and by a team approach (a team made up of members of many professions and of nonprofessional workers) in execution of the plan. Hospitalization is no longer an isolated incident in the child's health history. Hospital care is not only a curative measure, but is also a part of continuous health care, and health care is part of a total care program in which both home and community share.

## PRESENT CONCEPTS

It is said that the twentieth century is the century of the child. The value of the child to society is not only his potential worth as an adult—a parent, a worker in the economy of the nation, a participant in the arts and sciences and in war—but also as a child with all the lovable traits of children and the maturing experiences which children, and children alone, provide for parents and all others who care for them. Without such a maturing experience life is incomplete.

The child is not a miniature adult. His body differs in quality as well as in

# DECLARATION OF THE RIGHTS OF THE CHILD

### as approved unanimously by the 14th General Assembly of the United Nations, November 20, 1959

WHEREAS the peoples of the United Nations have, in the Charter, reaffirmed their faith in fundamental human rights, and in the dignity and worth of the human person, and have determined to promote social progress and better standards of life in larger freedom,

WHEREAS the United Nations has, in the Universal Declaration of Human Rights, proclaimed that everyone is entitled to all the rights and freedoms set forth therein, without distinction of any kind, such as race, colour, sex, language, religion, political or other opinion, national or social origin, property, birth or other status,

WHEREAS the child, by reason of his physical and mental immaturity, needs special safeguards and care, including appropriate legal protection, before as well as after birth,

WHEREAS the need for such special safeguards has been stated in the Geneva Declaration of the Rights of the Child of 1924, and recognized in the Universal Declaration of Human Rights and in the statutes of specialized agencies and international organizations concerned with the welfare of children,

WHEREAS mankind owes to the child the best it has to give,

NOW THEREFORE

*The General Assembly proclaims this Declaration of the Rights of the Child* to the end that he may have a happy childhood and enjoy for his own good and for the good of society the rights and freedoms herein set forth, and calls upon parents, upon men and women as individuals and upon voluntary organizations, local authorities and national governments to recognize and strive for the observance of these rights by legislative and other measures progressively taken in accordance with the following principles:

I. The child shall enjoy all the rights set forth in this Declaration. All children, without any exception whatsoever, shall be entitled to these rights, without distinction or discrimination on account of race, colour, sex, language, religion, political or other opinion, national or social origin, property, birth or other status, whether of himself or of his family.

II. The child shall enjoy special protection, and shall be given opportunities and facilities, by law and by other means, to enable him to develop physically, mentally, morally, spiritually and socially in a healthy and normal manner and in conditions of freedom and dignity. In the enactment of laws for this purpose the best interests of the child shall be the paramount consideration.

III. The child shall be entitled from his birth to a name and a nationality.

IV. The child shall enjoy the benefits of social security. He shall be entitled to grow and develop in health; to this end special care and protection shall be provided both to him and to his mother, including adequate prenatal and postnatal care. The child shall have the right to adequate nutrition, housing, recreation and medical services.

V. The child who is physically, mentally, or socially handicapped shall be given the special treatment, education and care required by his particular condition.

VI. The child, for the full and harmonious development of his personality, needs love and understanding. He shall, wherever possible, grow up in the care and under the responsibility of his parents, and in any case in an atmosphere of affection and of moral and material security; a child of tender years shall not, save in exceptional circumstances, be separated from his mother. Society and the public authorities shall have the duty to extend particular care to children without a family and those without adequate means of support. Payment of state and other assistance towards the maintenance of children of large families is desirable.

VII. The child is entitled to receive education, which shall be free and compulsory at least in the elementary stages. He shall be given an education which will promote his general culture, and enable him on a basis of equal opportunity to develop his abilities, his individual judgment and his sense of moral and social responsibility, and to become a useful member of society.

The best interests of the child shall be the guiding principle of those responsible for his education and upbringing; that responsibility lies in the first place with his parents.

The child shall have full opportunity for play and recreation, which should be directed to the same purposes as education; society and the public authorities shall endeavour to promote the enjoyment of this right.

VIII. The child shall in all circumstances be among the first to receive protection and relief.

IX. The child shall be protected against all forms of neglect, cruelty and exploitation. He shall not be the subject of traffic in any form.

The child shall not be admitted to employment before an appropriate minimum age; he shall in no case be caused or permitted to engage in any occupation or employment which would prejudice his health or education or interfere with his physical, mental or moral development.

X. The child shall be protected from practices which may foster racial, religious and any other form of discrimination. He shall be brought up in a spirit of understanding, tolerance, friendship among peoples, peace and universal brotherhood and in full consciousness that his energy and talents should be devoted to the service of his fellowmen.

---

Courtesy of the 14th General Assembly of the United Nations and of *Children*, Vol. 7. United States Department of Health, Education, and Welfare, Social Security Administration, Children's Bureau.

size from that of an adult. His emotional and intellectual processes are different. These differences make child study a separate discipline in which modern scientific knowledge in many branches of learning is applied to the care of the child. Child care is taught in colleges, in adult education programs and in high schools and is a fundamental course in many professional schools.

Caring for children is a maturing process for the adult. An adult is not mature in the fullest sense of the word until he is a parent. One characteristic of full maturity is an unselfish love which finds satisfaction in the happiness of the loved one. Children develop in adults this form of love.

On the other hand, the care of children day and night can impose too great a strain upon the parents and hamper, if not spoil, parent-child relations. There are many institutions, however, which relieve a mother of the child's care for part of the day, e.g. the nursery school. Summer camp provides the older child with happy weeks out of doors in a different milieu. The sick child can be sent to a hospital for care which the mother cannot give and which formerly wore her out in her vain efforts to try to provide it. A good mother-child relationship is based not on the amount of time they spend together, but rather on the quality of the relationship while they are together.

One relatively new concept in child care is that the young adult who has known a happy home life and looks forward to marriage, who rates home making as of equal value to professional success, is more likely to be successful in caring for children than is the young adult who regards child care only from a professional standpoint. Today there are more parents in professions who care for children and more mothers who are professional women than there were a generation ago. Girls today look forward not to the choice between marriage and a profession, but to a combination of marriage and a profession.

A happy childhood is fundamental in the development of a fine personality.

Few adults are successful in making a child happy unless they themselves find happiness in being with the child. Children reflect an adult's emotional reactions. For this reason it is essential that the environment be pleasant to both the child and the adult and that the adult and the child not be together so long that both weary of each other's company. A child of two or three years of age is likely to find great pleasure in a nursery school where his happy home life is supplemented by friends outside the family circle. The nursery school teacher is not a substitute mother, but a friend who provides the sense of happy security which comes from being with an adult and who, like mother, does for the child what he cannot do for himself and comforts him when things go wrong.

*One result of the better and more widespread understanding of the emotional life of children is a fuller appreciation of the importance of parent-child-professional woman relations.* This, in relation to the nurse, is shown throughout this book.

## TEACHING AIDS AND OTHER INFORMATION*

Interdepartmental Committee on Children and Youth: Children in a Changing World (A Book of Charts). Golden Anniversary White House Conference on Children and Youth, 1960.

*Public Affairs Pamphlets*

Deutsch, A.: W.H.O.—Its Global Battle against Disease.

*Science Research Associates*

Jenkins, G. G.: Guide for Family Living

*U.S. Department of Health, Education, and Welfare*

Bradbury, D. E., and Eliot, M. M.: Four Decades of Action for Children, a Short History of the Children's Bureau, 1956.
Child Welfare Services, How They Help Children and Their Parents, 1957.
Children and Youth, Their Health and Welfare, 1958.
Davis, A. L.: Children Living in Their Own Homes, Social Services Provided through Child Welfare Programs, 1953.

* Complete addresses are given in the Appendix.

Gula, M.: Child-Caring Institutions, 1958. Your Children's Bureau, Its Current Program, 1956.

## REFERENCES

Apt, I. A.: History of Pediatrics; in Brennemann, J.: Practice in Pediatrics. Hagerstown, Md., W. F. Prior Co., Inc., 1945, Vol. I, Chap. 1.

Bakwin, H.: Child Care in Russia. J. Pediat., 51:313, 1957.

Barton, B., and Pringle, K. D.: Today's Children and Youth. I. As Viewed from the States. Children, 7:50, 1960.

Craig, M.: Child Care in the Outback. Am. J. Nursing, 58:1696, 1958.

Dybwad, G.: Family Life in a Changing World. Children, 6:3, 1959.

Eliot, M. M.: A Twenty-Year Perspective on Services to Children. Children, 2:123, 1955.

Ellis, R. W. B.: Social Change and Child Health. Pediatrics, 20:1041, 1957.

General Assembly of the United Nations: Declaration of the Rights of the Child. Children, 7:74, 1960.

Ginzberg, E. (editor): The Nation's Children. 1. The Family and Social Change. New York, Columbia University Press, 1960.

Idem: The Nation's Children. 2. Development and Education. New York, Columbia University Press, 1960.

Idem: The Nation's Children. 3. Problems and Prospects. New York, Columbia University Press, 1960.

Golden Anniversary White House Conference on Children and Youth. Am. J. Nursing, 60:990, 1960.

Golden Anniversary White House Conference on Children and Youth, March 27-April 2, 1960: Conference Proceedings. Washington, D.C., Golden Anniversary White House Conference on Children and Youth, Inc., 1960.

Hyde, H. V.: The World Health Organisation, Ten Years of Progress. Lancet, 78:226, 1958.

Jelliffe, D. B.: Cultural Variation and the Practical Pediatrician. J. Pediat., 49:661, 1956.

Kidneigh, J. C.: A Look to the Future in Child Welfare Services. Children, 7:66, 1960.

Lipset, S. M.: Constant Values in American Society. Children, 6:219, 1959.

Maccoby, E. E.: Children and Working Mothers. Children, 5:83, 1958.

Mead, M.: Nursing—Primitive and Civilized. Am. J. Nursing, 56:1001, 1956.

Idem: Understanding Cultural Patterns. Nursing Outlook, 4:260, 1956.

Midcentury White House Conference on Children and Youth: A Healthy Personality for Every Child. Fact Finding Report. Raleigh, N. C., Health Publications Institute, Inc., 1951.

Oettinger, K. B.: The Growth and Meaning of White House Conferences on Children and Youth. Children, 7:3, 1960.

Roney, J. L., and Wiltse, K. T.: New Approaches to Aid to Dependent Children. Children, 6:163, 1959.

Sandusky, A. L.: Services to Neglected Children. Children, 7:23, 1960.

Schlesinger, E. R.: Child Health Services since 1935. Children, 2:127, 1955.

Idem: Health Services for the Child. New York, McGraw-Hill Book Company, Inc., 1953.

Witmer, H. L., and Kotinsky, R.: Personality in the Making: The Fact-Finding Report of the Midcentury White House Conference on Children and Youth. New York, Harper and Brothers, 1952.

World Health Organization: Administration of Maternal and Child Health Services, Technical Report Series No. 115, Feb. 1957. Geneva, Switzerland, WHO Palais des Nations, 1957.

# Chapter 2

# Growth and

# Development of Children

THIS chapter presents facts and concepts of growth and development which the student should know in order to adapt her nursing care to the needs of children in different age groups.

## CHARACTERISTICS OF GROWTH AND DEVELOPMENT

A glance at a child in an adult's lap shows the great difference in bodily shape between them and, equally striking, the difference in their behavior.

In relation to the life span the developmental period is much longer in children than in animals. This gives adults a greater opportunity to influence the mental and physical development of children. A child may play with several generations of pets while he is still in school, sexually immature, not full grown, and unable to pass the mental tests designed for the average adult.

This relatively slow development of the child in comparison with animals is shown in the study of a little ape named Gua which (or shall we regard it as human and say "whom"?) the Kellogs raised with their baby boy. Chronologically the child and Gua were about the same age, but she was far ahead of the boy in physical development. She could run before he could creep. In every way she proceeded more rapidly than he toward full development. But the boy's mind continued to develop as hers did not. He spoke words at one year and showed a toddler's capacity for reasoning in his social contacts. Yet he still had twenty years before he would be considered old enough to vote.

Each child is an individual and should never be considered a typical boy or girl, one unit of a group who are all alike. Each child has his own *rate of growth,* but the *pattern of growth* shows less variability. Figure 1 illustrates the pattern of general physical growth and types of organic growth. Certain char-

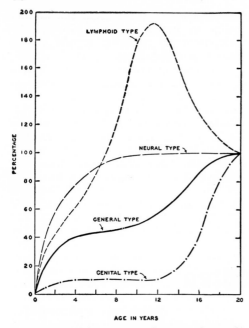

**Figure 1.** Main patterns of postnatal growth of the various parts and organs of the body. (After Scammon: The Measurement of the Body in Childhood, The Measurement of Man. Minneapolis, University of Minnesota Press.)

acteristics of emotional, social and mental growth are also typical of age and sex groups. In order to instruct students, nonprofessional workers, parents and the children themselves in good hygiene and the plan for total care which the physician has outlined for each child, the nurse must know what to expect of different age groups and must know their place in the developmental sequence which occurs throughout childhood.

The nurse must also know what to expect of a particular child at any given age and at what age certain types of behavior are likely to emerge in more mature forms. She uses this knowledge to judge each child in terms of norms for specific levels of development. A child may be guided into more mature behavior if the sequence of developmental behavior is understood.

A knowledge of growth and development is important to the nurse so that she may better understand the reason for particular conditions and illnesses which occur in various age groups. When the nurse has gained experience in applying her study of growth and development in child care, she can teach mothers how to use such knowledge in order that they may help their own children to achieve optimal growth and development.

Growth and development are terms often used interchangeably. Each depends upon the other, and in a normal child they parallel each other. But they are not the same. *Growth* refers to an increase in physical size of the whole or any of its parts and can be measured in inches or centimeters and in pounds or kilograms. *Development* refers to progressive increase in skill and capacity of function. The term "maturation" is often used as a synonym for development. If a distinction, however, is made between the two words, *maturation* has the more limited application of referring to the development of traits carried through the genes. Development is orderly, not haphazard; there is a direct relation between each of its stages and the next.

## PATTERNS OF GROWTH AND DEVELOPMENT

The relatively typical physical pattern of growth and behavior is influenced by heredity, environment and the child's state of health. The *heredity* of a man and a woman who unite in marriage determines the heredity of their children. For this reason the health history of several generations and of great-aunts and great-uncles, as well as the brothers and sisters of the child's parents, should be studied to determine the hereditary traits which are likely to exist in the child.

*Eugenics* is the science that deals with influences that improve inborn or hereditary qualities of the race. Through applied eugenics this knowledge would influence men and women in the selection of marriage partners, helping them to avoid those unions which presumably would produce children below a socially accepted standard and encouraging those unions which would be likely to produce children above this standard. A few diseases are hereditary, and a tendency to a number of diseases is genetically determined. As has been pointed out, it is the family history rather than the condition of the child's parents which must be studied to determine the probability of a tendency toward a specific disease. Such a study is difficult among the lower income group, whose health histories are carried by word of mouth and altered with each repetition. With the extension of health work in schools, clinics and work and industrial health programs, family health histories may become more reliable than they are at present.

Obviously, men and women cannot marry simply because their union would produce fine, healthy children. On the other hand, if a man and a woman are likely to pass on to their offspring such genetically determined traits as may result in lowered mentality, one of the few definitely inherited diseases or a strong tendency to any defect, they should seriously consider just what this will mean in married life, before they become engaged.

*Euthenics,* in contrast to eugenics, deals with measures to promote health. It concerns itself with healthy intra-uterine conditions for the developing fetus and with a wholesome environment not only for children, but also for all age groups.

In hospitals, clinics and public health nursing, mothers as well as students are taught the general principles of child growth and development. They are taught that each child has a different genetic potentiality for growth and that this potentiality cannot be exceeded, but may be hampered at any stage. Forcing a child to meet a standard may result in permanent damage to him. Those who work with children should remember that growth is not an even increase in size, nor a steady approach to adult behavior. There are spurts, lags and deviations. Nevertheless a child

who deviates too far from the normal range of height, weight, physical development or behavior should be referred to a physician.

The most common cause for concern about a child is a sudden slowing up in any area of his development—a slowing up which is not typical for his age. Mothers should be taught what changes in the rate of development, particularly of height and weight, to expect at certain ages. They often worry when the toddler's gain in weight slows down and he loses his chubby baby look. Yet this is normal, and were he to retain the enormous appetite of his babyhood and continue to gain a pound or more per month, he would soon become a monstrosity. Nurses working with mothers must themselves feel secure in their knowledge; otherwise what they teach is not likely to be convincing.

Although growth and development—physical, mental, social, emotional and spiritual—proceed at different rates, they are so *interrelated* in the majority of children that the result is a progressive development of the whole child, from infancy to adulthood. Only when growth in any area is unusually slow or advanced is this interrelation disturbed so that the child appears abnormal. Our attitude toward an uneven development should not be overfearful for the child's future. Conditions tend to right themselves. On the other hand, the child should have expert medical care, counseling or psychiatric aid whenever it is needed.

The concept of interrelations in growth is also true for the hospitalized child or one under medical supervision. This is one reason why professional teamwork is important in the hospital. The whole team is needed to foster progressive development in all areas of development in the hospitalized child. Thus there is the school teacher to encourage mental development, and the child care worker (the Play Lady) to create situations in which there may be pleasant social interaction. The psychologist and the psychiatrist help the nurses with the emotional problems of sick children. The dietitian, the physical therapist and all the other members of the team work together, each focusing on a different facet of growth, toward the full development of the whole child.

A child of average mental, emotional and social development for his age may yet be so small and underdeveloped that it is necessary to create opportunities for his all-round physical development. Or a child may be well developed physically, yet so dull or bright that he requires help in adjusting emotionally and socially to his mental level and its social repercussions. Some children who are socially more or less adept than their contemporaries will need help in entering into the social life of their play group and even in their relations with adults who do not understand unusual children. Whatever the cause, if a child is notably different from others of his age, he is likely to need help in order to make a good adjustment to home and community life. The child with a long-term illness or a handicap of body or mind also differs from his peers and will need help. Throughout this book we shall often speak of such a child.

### STAGES OF GROWTH AND DEVELOPMENT

*All children go through a normal sequence of growth, but not at the same rate.* Nor is the rate the same in all areas. In general, there is a positive correlation between maturation in the areas of physical development, mentality and emotional life. This may not be true in individual children, of course, and we have learned the danger of attempting to force a child into a standard pattern of growth. There are far too many variations in genetic traits and in the environment of different children to make this possible. The strain upon the child may react upon his personality and even his physical health.

Adults should have a clear understanding of the stages of growth and development commonly referred to so that they can apply their knowledge when caring for children. These stages, listed here, are considered in detail in

the chapters on the nursing care of various age groups.

1. Fetal or embryonic—from conception to birth
2. Newborn (neonatal)—from birth to two weeks
3. Infancy—from two weeks to one year
4. Toddler—from one year to three years
5. Early childhood (preschool)—from three to six years
6. Late childhood (school)—from six to twelve years or puberty
7. Adolescence—from puberty to the beginning of adult life

### NORMS OF GROWTH

In order to find norms of growth we may study age groups by the *cross-sectional technique* and make a comparison of their average weight, height or other evidence of growth. Consider, for instance, the average height of five-year-olds and of six-year-olds. The difference between these averages is taken as the average growth of a child during his sixth year. In a *longitudinal study* of growth, height and weight of individual children are followed from birth throughout childhood. Such studies show periods of accelerated growth which correlate with the individual child's stage of maturation. Spurts of growth are related to pubescence, which occurs earlier in some children than in others. This accelerated growth rate may begin in girls as early as ten years and in others as late as fourteen years; corresponding ages for boys are twelve and sixteen years. An early acceleration in growth is indicative of early puberty. Since the rate of growth slows down a year or two after the onset of puberty, a boy who is late in maturing and ashamed of his small stature and plumpness at thirteen years of age can be told that he is more likely to continue growing than his friend who matured early and is inches taller than he. But a boy who matures early and is shorter than the average for his age is likely to remain short.

The mental, emotional and social aspects of development show the same variations, but are much more influenced by environmental factors than is physical growth. Under conditions of great deprivation, however, as in wartime starvation, physical growth might be more influenced by environmental factors than mental or emotional development.

Norms or averages of growth must be used with caution, for not only do some children mature early and others late, and thus achieve early or late acceleration in the rate of growth, but also body build and potential height are inherited traits. Some children are by nature short and fat, others of muscular build or medium height, and still others may be tall and slender. Separate norms for each of these three types of body build are of more value than single tables for all children in general.

### STUDY OF GROWTH PATTERNS

The cross-sectional study of age groups antedated the longitudinal type of study. From these studies averages were readily compiled. There are disadvantages, however, in their use: (1) These studies did not take into account body build or early and late maturation. At best, in using these schedules, a decision of normality is based on only two gross characteristics: weight and height. These are poor criteria for measuring a child's potential development under his existing environmental conditions.

2. In any consideration of a child's growth the *expected rate of gain* is of greater value than a single measurement taken at any one time. In order to measure graphically a child's growth in height and weight, and to record changes in body contours as well, the Wetzel grid was devised. It is based on the assumption that physical development proceeds along regular channels for different body types. Thus each child's progress may be predicted from his own previous standards, and the physician quickly becomes aware that something is amiss when the individual growth pattern is distorted. The disadvantage of the Wetzel grid is that it is too complicated for general use.

The newer tables show more than physical growth and development. These tables include height, weight, number of teeth erupted, carpal bone age, mental age and social age. These different criteria can be plotted on a common scale. They show the correlation in measurements of physical and mental growth, i.e. the interrelatedness of growth. In normal growth there is an underlying unity, the presence or lack of which is shown on these graphs.

An adequate clinical history, in addition to the composite individual chart, is necessary for the proper interpretation of somatic and mental growth. Deviations from the average have no meaning unless factors such as dentition, illness, emotional health and interaction of the social and physical environments are used in interpreting the data.

## FACTORS IN GROWTH AND DEVELOPMENT

Growth and development are due not to one factor, but to a combination of many factors, all interdependent.

### HEREDITY AND CONSTITUTIONAL MAKE-UP

Embryonic life begins with the cytoplasm and the nucleus of the fertilized ovum, genetically formulated by both parents.

Members of families bear physical resemblances, and there is a high degree of correlation of stature with weight among siblings. The rate of growth is more alike among siblings than among unrelated persons. Some children are small not because of endocrine or nutritional disturbances, but because of their genetic constitution.

### RACIAL AND NATIONAL CHARACTERISTICS

#### Race

Distinguishing characteristics which we call racial or subracial characteristics developed in prehistoric man. As to height, there are tall and short examples among all races and subraces. Among civilized racial groups intermarriage has produced mixed racial types.

In the United States there are many examples of subraces. Of the white race there are people of Nordic, Alpine or Mediterranean descent. The Nordics are characteristically large and blond; those of Alpine stock are of medium height, with typically brown hair and hazel eyes; the Mediterranean people are dark and tend to be short in stature.

### Nationality

We think of physical characteristics of national groups because the inhabitants of the various nations of Europe tend to be made up of homogeneous subracial groups with specific characteristics. Thus we expect children whose forebears came from the Scandinavian countries to be larger, and those from Sicily to be smaller, than the average American. Yet in the melting pot of America there has been so much intermingling of subracial groups that children with all the typical physical characteristics of any national group are seldom seen.

In studying the changing characteristics of the American people one must consider the influence of immigration. This is particularly true if characteristics of economic groups are to be examined and if correlation of the influence of poverty with height and weight is sought. Infants of the lower income group are likely to be smaller than those of middle- and upper-class parents. But this is not entirely due to the influence of diet and poor hygiene. The last heavy immigration wave after World War I came from southern and eastern Europe, regions where the people are characteristically smaller than those of the north and west.

Immigrants frequently established themselves in the United States under conditions of extreme poverty. Their descendants of the second and third generations make up the majority of the middle and upper classes, and the lower-income group is now made up of more recent immigrants.

People from southern and eastern Europe and from Mexico predominate among the relatively recent immigrants of the white race. The short Puerto Ricans are recent arrivals, and the majority of them hold low-paying jobs. The shortness of stature among these representatives of the white race is a factor in the below-average height of the children of the low-income group as compared with the children of the middle- and upper-income groups. The latter, as we have noted, came from stock characterized by relatively greater height than the stock from which these more recent immigrants have come. This is not to deny the influence of good diet and of sanitation on children's height, but merely points out that different ethnic groups are likely to have different growth potentials.

### SEX

Sex is a factor determined at conception. The male infant is both longer and heavier than the female infant. He maintains this superiority until about eleven years of age, when the female, who matures earlier and so reaches the period of accelerated growth earlier than the male, is on the average taller than he. The male, during the prepuberal spurt of growth and thereafter, is again taller than the female. Bone development is more advanced in girls than in boys, as shown in roentgenograms of the wrists of infants and young children. Advance in osseous development is also demonstrated by the earlier eruption of the permanent teeth in the female.

### ENVIRONMENT

There are many interesting examples of the influence of environment upon potential height. One example is found among the first and second generations of Japanese in this country. The children are generally taller than their parents because they have had the advantage of better living conditions than their parents, who came in poverty to the United States as young men and women. A more recent example is that of children whose growth and development were stunted in concentration camps and in poverty-stricken areas in Europe during World War II and who have exhibited remarkable improvement upon being removed to better conditions.

### Prenatal Environment

Prenatal conditions are part of the environmental climate in which the child develops and should not be forgotten in considering actual development in relation to probable optimal development.

The influence of the intrauterine environment on the child's future development is believed to be great, particularly since the uterus shields the fetus from the full impact of external adverse conditions. On the other hand, the intrauterine environment itself may be substandard. In such a case, if the fetus has reached the stage of viability, early delivery may make it possible to place the infant in a better environment than that of the uterus.

The whole maternal and child care program is changing for the better the environmental influences on the fetus and the young child in the low-income group.

**Harmful Prenatal Factors.** The prenatal environment is influenced by many factors. The fetus may suffer from nutritional deficiencies when the mother's diet is insufficient in quantity or quality. There may be mechanical problems due to malposition in utero. The mother may suffer from metabolic endocrine disturbances, e.g. diabetes mellitus, which affect the fetus. If it is necessary for the mother to undergo radiation for cancer or other conditions, the infant may be blighted by the treatment. The mother may suffer from an infectious disease during gestation. Rubella (German measles) during the first trimester of pregnancy may lead to abnormal development of the fetus. Other infectious diseases may also affect the fetus in the same way, but there is less scientific proof of this. Toxoplasmosis and syphilis during the second and third trimesters adversely influence the fetus. Erythroblastosis fetalis due to Rh incompatibility of the blood types of the mother and the fetus may have a serious influence upon the developing fetus. Commonly, faulty placental implantation or malfunction may lead to nutritional impairment or anoxia.

### Postnatal Environment

A strong, healthy child can make better use of his environment, whether good or poor, than can a weak and sickly child. Likewise the child with a fine mind can learn more from his environment, be it rich or poor in learning experiences, than can the child with subnormal mentality. The child's temperament and emotional state are important. An anxious, unhappy child is likely to interpret his environment in terms of his own fears and so derives little satisfaction from even a good environment; he does not learn from it because he does not perceive it as it is. A happy child, on the other hand, will overlook defects in his environment and seize upon the beneficial factors which he can utilize.

An environment which provides satisfying experiences promotes growth. Since growth and development in all areas of the child's life are interrelated, growth in any one area influences and in turn is influenced by growth in all other areas.

Factors which influence the infant's development are more likely to be of environmental origin than genetic. Among the most important environmental factors are the following.

**External Environment.** *Socio-economic Status of the Family.* The environment in the lower socio-economic groups is apt to be less favorable than in the middle or upper groups. Lower-class parents are less likely to understand the principles of modern scientific child care, they lack money to buy the essentials of health and diet, and often they are unable to obtain medical care and hospitalization.

*Nutrition.* Nutrition is related to

**Figure 2.** Children grow up in families which differ as to socio-economic status. *A,* The middle-class family. *B,* The lower-class family. (H. Armstrong Roberts.)

both the quantitative and qualitative supply of food elements—proteins, fats, carbohydrates, minerals and vitamins. But the infant's or child's use of a good diet may be impaired by faulty absorption or assimilation of food substances.

*Climate and Season.* Climatic variations influence the infant's health. This is not an important factor in the United States, since the entire area lies within the temperate zone.

The seasons of the year influence growth rates in height and weight, especially in older children. Gains in weight are lowest in spring and early summer and greatest in late summer and autumn. The greatest gains in height among children in the United States occur in the spring.

*Illness and Injury.* Illness and injury, with their accompanying debility and nutritional impairment, have a great influence on weight and some influence on growth.

*Exercise.* Exercise promotes physiologic activity and stimulates muscular development, and fresh air and sunshine favor health and growth.

*Ordinal Position in the Family.* The child's position in the family is a factor in development for several reasons, among them the following: (1) Children learn from older siblings, and this is an advantage which an only child or the oldest child lacks. (2) The youngest child may be relatively slow in certain areas of development because he is given little encouragement to express himself. He is the baby and is petted by the whole family. (3) The only child is likely to develop more rapidly along intellectual lines than the average child because he is constantly with adults and is mentally stimulated by their companionship. Like the youngest child of a family, he may be slow in motor development, however, because he has so much done for him. When he is old enough to do things for himself, his parents and other relatives do not permit him to do so.

**Internal Environment.** *Intelligence.* Intelligence is correlated to some degree with physical development; i.e. the child of high intelligence is more likely to be better developed than is the less gifted child. Intelligence naturally influences mental and social development.

*Hormonal Balance*. Hormonal balance in the young child is important. Normal secretions of the endocrine glands tend to promote normal growth of the body.

*Emotions*. Emotional disturbances influence growth, since the disturbed child neither sleeps nor eats as well as one who is happy and contented.

## TYPES OF GROWTH AND DEVELOPMENT

### PHYSICAL GROWTH

Physical growth includes many things, among them the following.

**Changes in General Body Configuration.** Such changes result from different rates of growth in different parts of the body during the consecutive stages of development. For example, the infant's head size is one fourth of the entire length of the body at birth, whereas the adult's head size is only one eighth of his length. Growth during childhood is primarily linear; growth in adolescence is both linear and in the nature of a filling-out process until the adult proportions are reached.

**Head Circumference.** The circumference of the head is important, since it is related to intracranial volume. An increase in circumference permits an estimation of the rate of brain growth. This measurement has a relatively narrow normal range for a particular age group of children.

**Thoracic Diameter.** Chest measurements increase as the child grows and the shape of his chest changes. At birth the transverse and anteroposterior diameters are nearly equal. The transverse diameter increases more rapidly than the anteroposterior diameter; i.e. the round chest of the baby becomes wider than its depth.

**Abdominal and Pelvic Measurements.** The abdominal circumference is not fixed by the bony cage as is the chest and consequently is affected by the infant's nutritional state, by muscle tone, by gaseous distention and even the phase of respiration. The pelvic bicristal diameter (the maximal distance between the external margins of the iliac crests) is not affected by variations in posture and musculature. The pelvic bicristal diameter is a good index of the slenderness or stockiness of the child.

**Weight.** Weight is influenced by all the increments in size and is probably the best gross index of nutrition and growth. There is a wide variation within normal limits for each year of childhood. Excess weight in relation to the height and pelvic diameter is as abnormal as underweight. It may be the result of a glandular deficiency, but is more likely to be due to overeating or to a diet containing too much starch and fat and too little protein.

**Height.** Yearly increments in height diminish from birth to maturity. The pubescent spurt in growth is the only exception to this downward trend in the rate of growth. There is great variation in the yearly increases in stature among children of the same age. Some children reach adult height while still in their early teens, but others continue to grow throughout late adolescence. The periods of most rapid growth are infancy and puberty.

### Development of Muscular Control

The development of muscular control does not take place evenly throughout the body. In quadrupeds it proceeds from head to tail—along the *cephalocaudal* axis. In human beings it follows the spine downward—also termed cephalocaudal—and in addition proceeds from the *center of the body to the periphery*. The result is that the child holds up his head before he sits. The large muscles of the arms and legs are subject to voluntary control sooner than are the fine muscles of the hands and feet. As the child matures, *general movements become specific*. For example, he can use the whole hand before he can pick up a small object with the pincer grasp, i.e. between the thumb and forefinger.

**Figure 3 a.** Body proportions change during the period of growth. The head size, trunk length and extremity length differ in (A) the newborn, (B) 18-month-old, (C) 3-year-old, (D) 11-year-old, and (E) 18-year-old. (H. Armstrong Roberts.)

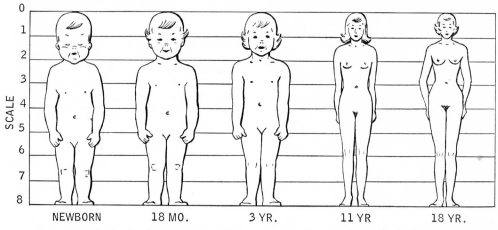

**Figure 3 b.** Scale showing changes in body proportion from birth to physical maturity.

There is a normal sequence in the development of manual dexterity and for the stage of locomotion, just as there is for mental development and for emotional and social adequacy. A child should be given the opportunity for learning—by either experience or instruction—whenever he is ready to acquire the skill or learn by indirect experience through instruction from others. If these opportunities are presented prematurely and the child is urged to make use of them, he is apt to learn slowly; if too late, he is apt to learn rapidly, but may never acquire the same skill or proficiency he might have had if the opportunity for learning had occurred at a more auspicious time. Coincidental acquisition of a skill along with others of his age group is probably more important to a child's personality development than his ultimate proficiency in that particular skill. For example, the child who is physically unable to walk until six years of age has been an atypical child among other children and in his relations with adults. This influence on his personality may be more important than its final effect on his ability to walk, run, dance and perform other activities.

On the other hand, disability during the preschool years may have no permanent effect upon a child. Children often have a remarkable resilience in regard to factors which theoretically would hinder their normal personality development. This sort of thing is often seen in children who have been denied learning opportunities because of sickness or the stultifying regime of institutional life.

### MENTAL DEVELOPMENT

Tests of intelligence and mental development have been standardized much like the standards for growth and development derived from longitudinal and cross-sectional studies in the areas of height and weight for children of different ages. There is no foolproof way of measuring the potential development of the genetically carried trait of intelligence, but among a group of children with comparable environmental backgrounds the standardized intelligence tests are valuable in predicting a child's capacity for intellectual development. Such tests are used in the school system. They are useful in determining whether achievement is comparable to innate ability.

Mental development depends on factors too numerous to mention here. It is demonstrated in problem solving and in a general understanding of what to do in a given situation. Even the best cared-for baby has problems of self-help which the most helpful of adults cannot solve completely for him.

It is important in child care to let the child solve those problems which he is able to solve by himself and to teach him how to solve problems that are

**Figure 4.** The development of muscular control proceeds from head to tail (cephalocaudal) and from the center of the body to the periphery.

within his ability, but in which he lacks the necessary experience and practice. It is also important to solve for him those problems which are either too difficult for him or are such that a wrong decision on his part might result in physical harm, damage to property or distress to others, so that the patience of even the best-intentioned adult would be stretched to the breaking point. By the time a child is one year old he should have learned to accept the decisions of those adults in whose love he feels secure. He has learned by experience that his mother is likely to be right, and moreover he wants to please her, for then pleasant things happen to him.

The first problems with which a baby is confronted are physical ones, and he is helped in their solution by the normal reflex actions of his body. The first problem is ingestion of milk. Sucking at the mother's breast and swallowing the milk are processes which require little or no practice to perform successfully. The newborn at the breast for the first time may have difficulty in getting hold of the nipple and may sputter and choke as the colostrum or milk begins to flow. But he soon learns, for he has many opportunities to practice sucking. Furthermore, he likes to suck his fingers or fist. (According to some scientists, he apparently learns in utero how to get his fingers into his mouth, but the newborn is so clumsy that he is likely to bring his fist to his face and then make several unsuccessful attempts before he makes connection with his mouth.)

An infant soon learns to want a smiling mother because she does pleasant things for him. An early problem, then, is to make mother smile. He learns not to do those things which make her say in a decisive voice, "No, no," and frown at him. He may learn that she always comes when he cries and therefore cries whenever she leaves him alone.

A small baby is more adept at solving his problems than we are likely to realize, and the behavior which gets him what he wants becomes habitual. Habits can be broken, of course, but the process is difficult for both the infant and the adults about him. He should be helped to the correct solution of a problem, a solution in which he finds pleasure not only in the behavior itself, but also in the social reward of having others pleased with him. No child is more to be pitied than the spoiled child whom nobody but his doting parents wants to have about; he is robbed of the birthright of children, that of being loved by an increasingly wide circle of adults and accepted in the play groups of his peers.

Thus, although potential mental ability is inherited and fixed at birth, the rate and extent of its development, as measured by any one of the many mental tests, are very much influenced by a child's environment.

### Determination of Level of Mental Development

As the structure of the nervous system grows during the prenatal period, rudimentary beginnings of the mind grow with it. As the child develops after birth changes occur in his mental reactions that show progress from the ability to respond to the simplest stimuli toward functioning in more complex ways. Although mental development is continuous, it may be more rapid in one age period than in another.

*Intelligence* can be defined as the ability to adjust to new situations, to think abstractly or to profit from experience. Tests of intelligence are of many types. During infancy and early childhood such tests are likely to be of the performance type. The child is asked to manipulate testing materials or to demonstrate his motor ability. Such tests show the general level of intelligence, but should not be considered accurate in predicting the child's later intellectual attainment.

When the child is able to communicate verbally, verbal intelligence tests may be given; when he is able to write (i.e. in the school age and adolescent groups), individual or group written tests may be used. There is a higher degree of consistency in intelligence test results from year to year from the age of five onward than for tests given during the preschool period.

### Meaning of the Intelligence Quotient

The intelligence quotient (I.Q.) can be defined as the ratio between the child's chronologic age and his mental age as gained from an intelligence test. The formula for computing the intelligence quotient is as follows:

$$\frac{\text{Mental age}}{\text{Chronologic age}} \times 100 = \text{I.Q.}$$

Since mental maturation is usually reached some time between the ages of sixteen and twenty-one years, the mental age of the adult cannot be computed in this way. The age of sixteen years has been arbitrarily chosen as the adult's chronologic age. For example, if an adult passed all the questions in the test designed for a 12-year-old child, his I.Q. would be 75. In the event of a perfect score in the 16-year test, his I.Q. would be 100, or normal.

An I.Q. between 90 and 109 is usually considered to be normal or average. The I.Q. of individual children may range above or below this point. Children with an I.Q. of 140 or over are called gifted children, and those with an I.Q. of less than average represent retardation of varying degrees and will be discussed in a later chapter.

### EMOTIONAL DEVELOPMENT

*Personality* is not a specific attribute, but the quality of any person's total behavior (Woodworth, 1947). Two attributes of a healthy personality in adult life are the ability to love and the ability to work.

### Stages of Personality Development

Emotional or personality development may be thought of as a continuous process. In each stage of a child's emotional development there is a central problem which must be solved. These problems are never completely solved, however. If each problem is fairly well solved at each child's particular stage of development, the basis for progress to the next stage is firmly laid. Proper training and the solution of the sequence of problems are necessary at each stage of development if eventual functional harmony is to be secured in adult life.

At no stage in personality development does a child succeed or fail completely in attainment of the goal to be reached at that particular point in his development. For example, the child does not learn to trust completely or never to mistrust. Every child leaves the period of infancy with habits of both trust and mistrust. Health of personality is determined by the preponderance of the favorable attitudes and by the kinds of compensations a child develops to take care of his disabilities.

A general, over-all view of the stages in emotional or personality development according to Erik H. Erikson, a psychologist and trained psychoanalyst, is given here. Further discussion will follow in later chapters.

**Infancy (Birth to One Year): Sense of Trust.** A baby learns to trust the adults who care for him, the mother first, for it is she who is sensitive to his needs and shows her trust in him.

**One Year to Three Years (The Toddler): Sense of Autonomy.** In this period the infant develops from a clinging, dependent little creature into a human being with a mind and a will of his own. If a child succeeds in the developmental task of this stage in his maturing process, he will have a degree of self-control not caused by fear, but by his feeling of self-esteem. If he does not succeed, he will doubt his own worth and that of others, and will have a sense of shyness and shame.

**Four to Five Years (The Preschool Child): Sense of Initiative.** The child at this age wants to learn what he can do for himself. He has an active imagination. He imitates adult behavior and wants to share in their activities. He wants the experience of following his will to the extreme limit, with the accompanying heavy sense of guilt. The positive, maturing outcome of this force within him is a sense of initiative, delineated by conscience. The negative outcome is a personality overwhelmed by guilt.

**Six to Eleven or Twelve Years (School Age): Sense of Industry.**   Children in this age group have a strong sense of duty; they want to engage in tasks of use in their social world which they can carry out successfully and want their success to be recognized by adults and by their peers. It is a calm period in which the basis is laid for later responsible citizenship. Society reaches the child directly through the school system and educates him not only in the three R's, but also in the fundamental skills of living in modern society. Children learn skills of workmanship and the ability to cooperate and to play fairly according to the rules. The danger of this period is the development of a sense of inferiority if the parents or the school expects a level of achievement from the child which he is unable to attain.

**Thirteen Years (Beginning of Adolescence): Sense of Identity.**   The sense of identity develops during adolescence. The adolescent wants to clarify who he is and what his role in society is to be. His attitude toward life is, "What will this mean to me?" Success in this period brings self-esteem, an attitude toward the self that is essential to the normal breaking away from dependency upon his parents and to planning for his future. The danger of this period is self-diffusion, for he faces at the time and in his dreams of the future a life full of conflicting desires, possibilities and chances. The childhood sense of belonging because "he always has belonged" is lost in the necessity of changing from his childhood status of dependency to adult responsibility for his own actions and those of others who are dependent upon him. He may, under adverse circumstances, develop a sense of "not-belonging."

**Late Adolescence: Sense of Intimacy.** After puberty youths outgrow the "gang age," that age when they find it essential to belong to a group of their own sex and age. Boys are likely to lose interest in scouting, and girls in cliques of

their own sex. In adolescence youth develops a sense of intimacy with individuals of his own sex or of the opposite sex, or with himself. If a youth is not certain of his identity, he is afraid to have interpersonal relations with others. Success in this period means union with the essence of others and a communion with their own resources. Failure to establish such intimacy results in psychological isolation—keeping relations with others on a formal basis which lacks warmth. This is likely to result in failure in all the steps in intimacy which lead to selection of a marriage partner ("dating," courtship and engagement) and to satisfaction in marriage.

### Evaluation of Emotional Development

Tests of emotional and social development are less concrete than those dealing with physical or mental development. They are more likely to be used in therapy than elsewhere, although they are useful in planning the physical environment and the activities and qualifications of the personnel in all types of institutions dealing with children.

Professional people working with children should be as familiar with these tests as they are with tests of physical growth and development, for a child's environment must be planned to meet all his interrelated needs, physical, mental, emotional and social.

Evaluation devices for measuring emotional or personality development are of several types. Such tests attempt to compare an individual child's stage of development with that of children of the same age and to show whether he is suffering from some type of personality maladjustment. The results of such tests are not too accurate, since personality is complex and cannot be easily evaluated.

Specific examples of such devices are rating scales, self-appraisal questionnaires, projective techniques such as finger or easel painting, play activities, the Rorschach test, and others. The *Thematic Apperception Test* is one of the most inclusive tests and is frequently used in the diagnosis of the causes of generalized anxiety or behavior problems in children.

## SOCIAL DEVELOPMENT

Socialization, or social development, means training a child in the culture of the group. Personality traits can be divided into two classes: those which are social and those which are cultural. Social traits are those found in the well adjusted members of every group; they are traits which are necessary to group survival, such as willingness to sacrifice present comfort for future benefit, and, even more important, individual cooperation with group efforts for group benefit. This social characteristic is altruism. Love and consistency in training are necessary in child care in order to socialize a child. Obviously, there are varying degrees of socialization.

Cultural traits are those which vary with the culture of different groups. Child care is a cultural trait in all groups, but the particular way in which a child is cared for is a social trait and is not the same in any two cultures.

A newborn infant is not a social being. This fact may be illustrated by the few authenticated cases of children either carried off by wild animals—presumably lactating and capable of carrying a child and keeping it alive—or lost in a forest. None of these children when found showed the personality characteristics of socialized human beings; they were not socialized according to the definition given above, nor did they behave according to any human culture pattern. To a limited degree lack of socialization is evidenced in children deprived of normal human contacts, such as illegitimate children who have been hidden shamefully in some isolated room or relinquished to an unfeeling stranger paid to house them.

### Factors in Social Development

Through broad, overlapping generalizations about contemporary American culture we shall redefine the cultural patterns of our society.

**The Home.** *Cultural Patterns: Ethnic Group, Locality, Class, Occupation.* There are ethnic groups represented by the few remaining Chinatowns of our large cities and by the Puerto Rican and Mexican communities in New York, Chicago and other metropolitan centers, as well as French-Canadian villages in the New England states. The cultural patterns of the middle, southern, eastern and western states differ. Large cities, towns, villages, crossroads neighborhoods and the open country with scattered farms all have characteristic culture patterns. In the democratic United States we do not like to speak of people as belonging to an upper, middle or lower class, although there is general recognition that there are class cultures. In general, traits found among college-educated millionaires are not those of the sons of criminals born and reared on the New York East Side or in Chicago's disorganized South Side Negro area. The culture of the ethnic group, the geographic area, urban or rural location—whether metropolis, city, town, village, crossroads hamlet or open farm country—and social class all influence the home, but are redefined by the *family* itself, that small, closely knit unit of society into which the child is born and in which he is brought up. It is the home culture that is influential in forming the child's personality. As he grows older and leaves the home and play group for school and the gang, team, club or clique, home culture is increasingly modified by that of the community.

Parental characteristics and behavior in general are modeled on those of their group. For instance, physical punishment was characteristically inflicted by immigrants from many countries of Europe, but seldom used among the Chinese or Japanese in places where they retained their native culture. The position of the father in the family varies with the customs of the group. The authoritarian father is still characteristic in the rural areas of the Appalachian Mountains. The matriarch —the oldest woman in the family regarded as the authoritarian and protective figure of the extended family—is most likely to be found in groups among whom common-law marriage is customary, recognized by law and accepted by both the group and the larger society of which they are a part. Matriarchy was common in this country among the Negroes during the years of slavery, since a child belonged to the mother's owner. In modified form matriarchy still exists among the southern Negroes in rural districts and among recent immigrants to cities in both the North and the South. We nurses know the matriarch as the grandmother who assumes full responsibility for the illegitimate children of her daughters, many of whom are sixteen or even younger when they become pregnant. Young girls who are married to or living in a common-law relation with one man after another are frequently deserted by the fathers of their children, and the matriarch assumes responsibility for the infants and little children of the temporary union. Many of these children are eligible for Federal Aid to Dependent Children, which is given to the grandmother for their support if she is able to make a suitable home for them. Frequently the children call the grandmother "Mother" and their biological mother by her first name; they appear to think of their natural mother as an older sister who has little or no control over them.

*New Types of Middle-Class Families.* In families in which the father is away from home for long periods—e.g. men in the military or maritime service and traveling salesmen—or working in remote areas where it would be impracticable to have their families with them, the mother is likely to be the head of the household. In a modified form the mother as decision maker is found in new settlements on the fringes of large cities. The father must leave early in the morning to reach his place of work, and little children may be in bed by the time he returns. On Saturdays and Sundays when he is home he is more likely to fall into the pattern of family life than to assume the control which his wife exercises from Monday morning through Friday evening.

The democratic family, in which both parents, and children when they are old enough, participate in making decisions, is the modern type. In this type, common in the middle class, both parents work to support the family on a higher level of living than would be possible on the father's salary alone. In an increasing number of youthful marriages the wife works to support or help in the support of the family while her husband finishes his professional training. She is not likely to provide full support, since certain federal legislation, large foundations and, in some cases, colleges or universities extend financial aid to students to complete their college education or study some essential profession. In former generations a man whose wife worked while he did not was blamed for his behavior, and she was pitied by her friends. Today it is understood that his education is part of his work—a job which in the long run will provide a standard of living he could not achieve without further preparation. The girl is no longer pitied, but has, in anticipation, the social standing of the wife of a professional man. This type of family is familiar to nurses and may be the type in which they begin their married life.

This new type of family life developed after World War II and the fighting in Korea, probably as the result of veterans' assistance funds for education in universities, colleges and professional schools. Later, qualified men and women were granted traineeships in order to prepare for certain socially useful professions, such as teaching, medicine and nursing. Both the husband and his wife may be studying, but the wife is more likely to be doing secretarial work in the institution in which her husband is studying or, if she is a nurse, in the hospital connected with the medical school of his university. Communities of family life such as this are found about all the large universities.

Another community of young married people has sprung up around military bases. The length of stay at any base is so uncertain that these homes have none of the stability found in civilian life. But common interests are strong, and such communities are closely knit, often in a town which seldom welcomes them to full participation in its social life. The children of military personnel may not be welcome in the crowded town schools or the local hospital. The base has no school, but the base hospital is likely to have a pediatric unit and immunization clinics. Although these military communities in many ways are like those about the large universities and colleges, the wives of service men are less likely to be employed, since their husbands receive pay and are entitled to certain benefits which, taken all in all, raise the family level of living.

Young married couples in college or on military bases want children and are willing to make many sacrifices in order to start their families early in marriage. Pregnant women in the college sections often work—with the obstetrician's approval—until one month before delivery and return to work when the baby is six weeks to two months old. Both parents help in the housekeeping and in the care of the child, fitting their hours of work or study into a schedule which provides for one or the other to be home with the baby throughout the twenty-four hours of the day. When the baby is old enough, he may be placed in a day nursery while his mother is working.

Finally, there are families with a common source of support. Such families are dependent upon some industry and are found in certain sections of many cities. An outstanding example is the area in Chicago near the great stockyards. Mill towns of New England were extreme examples, and now the mill towns of the South are likely to become one-industry towns. There, however, part-time farming creates some diversity of interest. Groups with a strong central interest are found in mining towns and in fishing villages.

Members of groups with common economic interests are likely to have many similar social traits. Houses erected and owned by an industry are apt to be similar, and their physical arrangement sets a pattern of family life. In mining and industrial communities all the men are likely to belong to the same union and may be of the same ethnic group and belong to the same church. In Catholic communities many of the schools and the hospital are likely to be under the direction of a religious community of Sisters. In the soft coal mining area of the Allegheny Mountains the United Mine Workers of America, with support from the mining companies, have built a chain of hospitals in which the wives and children of the miners are cared for, as well as the injured and sick men.

**The Community.** The general community pattern of child rearing undoubtedly influences the personality of the child. He is likely to rate his home and the way his parents treat him by group standards, and if the home differs widely from the general pattern, he knows it. If all parents inflict physical punishment, the child is apt to accept it as part of the usual child-parent relations. But if he is whipped and yet none of his friends are physically punished, he is likely to blame his parents and feel that they do not love him and that he is abused.

It is in warm home life that the child first learns the meaning of love, of giving up his pleasure because he wants the approval of loving parents. He learns to obey those who are better able than he to understand what should be done in different situations. He transfers this attitude toward authority to his baby sitter, to neighbors, nursery school workers, nurses and teachers. He adjusts to the adult-child relation in a constantly broadening area of social contacts.

**The Play Group.** Learning to live happily with adults is a quite different matter from making friends with children of his own age. In general the adult-child relation is one in which the child learns to live within certain restrictions set by loving adults. Adults are not always consistent in enforcing these restrictions. When they are tired and cross, they are likely to correct a child for doing the very thing they let him do the day before and perhaps thought cunning and amusing. A child as tired and cross as an adult is far more exasperating than when he is rested. Or a child may be feeling more exuberant than usual and may break rules he never broke before, again trying the patience of the surprised adult. Both children and adults learn to accept these reactions from each other. It is probably a good thing that children do not have perfect parents, nor parents perfect children; family life would be too unrealistic.

A child who adjusts well with adults may be unable to get along with other children. When children and adults disagree, it is usually a matter of the adult telling the child to do or not to do something the child does not want to do or is determined to do. Adults do not compete with a child on his own level for the things he wants; they do not snatch his toys, knock over his tower of blocks or brag that they can run faster than he. An only child who has no playmates finds it particularly difficult to learn the give and take of childish play. The teachers in nursery school will help him acquire the technique of getting along with other children. It may be a slow process. The adult who feels that it is easy to make the transition from being the only child in the home to being one among fifteen or twenty others in the nursery school is mistaken. Many nursery school teachers suggest that the child's mother stay with him for the first few days until he has made friends among the other children and thinks of the school as a pleasant place to be in. Eventually he learns to be one of his group, either a leader or a follower, depending on what he can contribute to the group's success in the particular activity in which it is engaged. In the middle-class play group or team and even in the gang, leadership springs less from physical superiority—fighting, running, playing ball—than from thinking up interesting activities when the group does not know what to do with itself. It is the child who can think up activities agreeable to the group, "sell" his ideas to them and lead them to a successful culmination of the project who is likely to become their leader.

As a child becomes engrossed in activities with his age group he does not love his parents less, but is less dependent on them for physical care, emotional support and a system of values. He becomes more self-reliant and learns how to use the resources of his group and community resources organized by adults for youth or for all age groups. He is preparing to take the responsibility of marriage and founding a home. Parents become dependent upon him as he matures and they grow older. He slowly learns to take his place in the economic life of the country and fulfill his role as a citizen.

## Summary

Heredity places limits upon development. But as we learn more about a child's needs, we are able to increase the influence of environment. A child needs an environment which provides satisfying experiences—for instance, splashing in the bath water, shaking a rattle or, for an older child, climbing the Jungle Gym, dressing himself and playing with toys which he can use imaginatively and "do something with." A child desires to repeat happy experiences in which he exercises his growing ability to secure the things he wants and to do the things he strives to perform. Happiness may come only from the satisfaction of having and doing, but even at an early age happiness is likely to be influenced by the approval of other people, as shown in the smiling face, the pleasant sound of the voice and physical caresses.

The child learns most of his fears as he connects unpleasant direct experience with people and things, or fear is communicated to him as he grows older by adults or other children who are themselves afraid. Adults may condition him to fear this or that in order to secure obedience. Common examples of this are such warnings as "The policeman will get you if you do that," or "You'll get sick and have to go to the doctor or, worse, the hospital if you go without your coat," and the injunction, "You will hurt yourself," often uttered to secure obedience rather than to help the child to learn prudence in his play and to exercise good judgment in new situations.

As far as possible, little children should be shielded from sources of anger. They should be taught the social consequences of anger and how to express it in socially approved ways.

A baby learns at a surprisingly early age the consequences of his behavior in a sequence of acts within a social situation in which he may be the center of attention of both father and mother. When he wants his feeding, he cries for it, and his mother comes and gives it to him. Hunger is a physical need, but its relief is social in the sense that someone must give the baby his feeding. These social experiences are fully as important as experiences with the physical world about him—e.g. that his rattle is fun to lap and that it makes a nice sound when shaken. Both types of experience help a baby to mature mentally, emotionally and socially. Since they involve physical activity and other needs for growth, they serve to further the whole process of maturation.

In her contacts with children the nurse sees the result of all these factors which we have considered under physical, mental, emotional and social growth and development. Every child is an individual; no two children are exactly alike. General statements of growth and development must be modified in the light of a child's individual characteristics. But until the nurse knows the child well enough to adapt her care to his individual needs, concepts of growth and development typical of his age group will help her to meet his needs.

Throughout this book general concepts are developed in relation to the various age groups—from the newborn through the adolescent period—whose nursing care in health and in disease is under consideration.

## PARENTAL ATTITUDES TOWARD GROWTH AND DEVELOPMENT

The old idea of child care was to bring up the child on a strict regimen of food, sleep and play. He was overprotected. The strict routine protected him from accidents and health hazards, but prevented him from acquiring the ability to adapt to life outside of the area controlled by his parents. He could not build up resistance to infection, though infection was prevalent in the society in which he was to take an increasingly active part as he grew out of babyhood into childhood and then adolescence. The overprotected child whose mother claimed that he had never had a cold or sore throat was likely to suffer from a series of severe respiratory infections when he entered school. He did not use good judgment when crossing the street or in climbing or in games which taxed his physical skills. He was apt to be accident-prone when removed from the shelter of his home. He had rigid likes and dislikes for foods and was reluctant to try new dishes. Unless he was in his own bed he could not go to sleep easily or adapt to hours of sleeping other than his accustomed periods. He was indeed geared to a strict regimen which was possible only at home, and was not prepared for even a gradual entry into community life.

Parents were likely to demand that such a child, whom they had allowed little self-direction, should direct himself successfully in school and on the playground. This was particularly true with boys. They were expected to fight their own battles, become leaders in their age group, never come home crying to mother and in general suddenly change from overprotected, overdirected, obedient little boys in the home to schoolboys who showed ability to get along, if not to lead, in their own age group.

This era of the authoritative, overprotective parent was followed by the trend toward permissiveness. The infant was to be placed on a self-demand schedule of feedings; he was to be offered an unlimited amount of his feeding whenever he was hungry and was to take as little or as much as he desired. The toddler was to choose his own diet from wholesome foods and was never urged to eat. Naps were to be taken when he was sleepy; he was never led, rebelling, to bed. He was never punished. The adult as far as possible permitted him to do what he wanted to do and trusted to the natural consequences of his behavior to show him what was the logical thing to do in problem situations. This attitude was likely to create an inconsiderate child, making heavy demands on the time and patience of his parents. Such a child may be so unaccustomed to discipline of any sort that he is resentful of the necessary restrictions of hospital life.

The newer idea is that the child must be prepared to take his place in the world and to live in a state of workable adjustment with his physical and social environment. He is to be treated as an individual, but as one who has not yet developed to the point at which he can decide what is best for him or recognize the rights of others, and therefore must be subject to parental control or that of the parents' substitute: nurse, school teacher or any adult responsible for his care.

## TEACHING AIDS AND OTHER INFORMATION*

*Bureau of Publications, Teachers College, Columbia University*

Hymes, J. L.: Being a Good Parent.
Mayer, J.: Getting Along in the Family.
Redl, F.: Understanding Children's Behavior.

*Child Study Association of America*

Wolf, A. W. M., and Dawson, M. C.: What Makes a Good Home.

*John Hancock Mutual Life Insurance Company*

Your Child Grows Up, 1957.

*National Association for Mental Health*

Frank, L. K.: Fundamental Needs of the Child.
Ridenour, N.: Keystones in Psychological Thinking about Young Children.

*Public Affairs Pamphlets*

Neisser, E., and Neisser, W.: Making the Grade as Dad.
Wolf, A. W. M.: Your Child's Emotional Health.

*Science Research Associates*

English, O. S., and Finch, S. M.: Emotional Problems of Growing Up.
* Complete addresses are given in the Appendix.

English, O. S., and Foster, C.: A Guide to Successful Fatherhood.
Olson, W. C., and Lewellen, J.: How Children Grow and Develop.
Weitzman, E.: Guiding Children's Social Growth.

*U.S. Department of Health, Education, and Welfare*

Heights and Weights of Children and Youth in the United States, 1957.
Hymes, J. L.: A Healthy Personality for Your Child, 1952.
Nutrition and Healthy Growth, 1955.

## REFERENCES

Almy, M.: Child Development. New York, Henry Holt and Co., 1955.
American Public Health Association: Health Supervision of Young Children. New York, American Public Health Association, 1955.
Berlien, I. C.: Growth as Related to Mental Health. Am. J. Nursing, 56:1142, 1956.
Bossard, J. H. S., and Boll, E. S.: The Sociology of Child Development. 3rd ed. New York, Harper and Brothers, 1960.
Bowlby, J.: Maternal Care and Mental Health. Geneva, World Health Organization, 1952.
Breckenridge, M. E., and Murphy, M. N.: Rand, Sweeney and Vincent's Growth and Development of the Young Child. 6th ed. Philadelphia, W. B. Saunders Company, 1958.
Breckenridge, M. E., and Vincent, E. L.: Child Development. 3rd ed. Philadelphia, W. B. Saunders Company, 1955.
Cooper, L. F., Barber, E. M., Mitchell, H. S., and Rynbergen, H. J.: Nutrition in Health and Disease. 13th ed. Philadelphia, J. B. Lippincott Company, 1958.
DeGeorge, F. V., and Osborne, R. H.: The Nature of Inheritance. Am. J. Nursing, 58:824, 1958.
Duvall, E. M.: Family Development. Philadelphia, J. B. Lippincott Company, 1957.
Dybwad, G.: Family Life in a Changing World. Children, 6:3, 1959.
Erikson, E. H.: Childhood and Society. New York, W. W. Norton and Co., 1950.
Idem: Youth and the Life Cycle. Children, 7:43, 1960.
Gesell, A., and Ilg, F. L.: Child Development. New York, Harper and Brothers, 1949.
Ginzberg, E. (editor): The Nation's Children. 2. Development and Education. New York, Columbia University Press, 1960.
Heider, G. M.: What Makes a Good Parent? Children, 7:207, 1960.
Hurlock, E. B.: Child Development. 3rd ed. New York, McGraw-Hill Book Company, Inc., 1956.
Josselyn, I. M.: The Happy Child. New York, Random House, 1955.
Nelson, W. E. (editor): Textbook of Pediatrics. 7th ed. Philadelphia, W. B. Saunders Company, 1959.
Osborne, R. H., and DeGeorge, F. V.: Sex Deter-

mination and Development. Am. J. Nursing, 59:213, 1959.

Pollak, O.: Family Situations and Child Development. Children, 4:169, 1957.

Rose, J. A.: Child Development and the Part-Time Mother. Children, 6:213, 1959.

Schwarz, B. E., and Ruggieri, B. A.: Parent-Child Tensions. Philadelphia, J. B. Lippincott Company, 1958.

Sigel, I.: Are Parents Changing? Children, 6:105, 1959.

Watson, E. H., and Lowrey, G. H.: Growth and Development of Children. 3rd ed. Chicago, Year Book Publishers, Inc., 1958.

Witmer, H. L., and Kotinsky, R.: Personality in the Making, The Fact-Finding Report of the Midcentury White House Conference on Children and Youth. New York, Harper and Brothers, 1952.

Woodworth, R. S., and Marquis, D. G.: Psychology. 5th ed. New York, Henry Holt & Company, Inc., 1947.

# Chapter 3

# Illness and the Child

## PHYSICAL RESPONSE OF CHILDREN TO ILLNESS

THE CHILD lacks the reserve forces which the adult has. Such lack is shown in an easily upset electrolyte balance, sudden elevation or depression of temperature, rapid spread of infection and destruction of body tissue. On the other hand, the child's body is building up to maximum development rather than being at a plateau of physical fitness or in the stages of decline.

We do not know precisely at what age the peak of the process of bodily repair occurs, but we do know that repair decreases after eighteen to twenty years of age. This phenomenon is shown in statistics of the recovery rate of men wounded in the military service and in the records of industrial disease and accidents. If we accept the statement that adolescence ends with the eruption of the wisdom teeth, we have a concrete example of the last of the building-up process of the teeth; we know from experience, however, that decay commonly occurs long before this time.

The sudden changes in the condition of a sick or injured child, coupled with his inability to express how he feels, mean that the nurse must be constantly on the alert for signs and symptoms of aggravation of or improvement in his condition. She must also be alert for symptoms which may be important to the physician in making a diagnosis or altering a tentative diagnosis.

Appreciation of the psychosomatic influence on diseases peculiar to or occurring in childhood is relatively new. It ties in with advances in the study of child psychology and child psychiatry. In these circumstances the child's emotional state interacts with his physical state to a greater degree than is commonly the case. Charting of physical symptoms means little to the physician in judging the implications of a sudden change in a child's condition unless the nurse also charts his *behavior*. Description of behavior enables the physician to draw conclusions as to the cause of symptoms which may be due to emotional rather than physical factors. The physician, viewing both behavior and symptoms charted by the nurse, has a clearer concept of change in the child's condition. Adults verbalize an emotional state as a child does not. Nurses are apt to chart behavior which causes trouble, but not that of a quiet child who has retreated within himself. The latter may be more important than the former, however, in determining the true meaning of a change in symptoms.

Children live more in the present than do adults, and the future means less to children. They are likely to interpret the past in the light of the present (yesterday's painful treatment in relation to its repetition today). Some children, like some adults, do suffer generalized states of anxiety in which a troubled past appears to be ever-present in their consciousness and present pleasures as only a prelude to unpleasant things to come. Such children need psychiatric help, in which the nurse plays an important role.

As far as possible the child's environment should be freed from threatening stimuli. Although the child should be allowed to verbalize his anxiety, the nurse should concur only in realistic fears, which should be realistically allayed. A realistic view of fears gives a logical basis for considering what can be done about them and admits that all causes of fear have a social as well as a psychologic aspect. Only rarely does a child or an adult meet alone whatever he fears, and if he does, his attitude toward it has been socially conditioned.

A child may face certain critical situations physically alone with no one to protect him. He may fall and hurt himself when no one is about. A child whose clothing has caught fire may be badly burned while he himself puts out the flames and waits, suffering, for help. He may be threatened or actually punished by an adult in authority. A child may receive rough treatment from his entire play group or gang. He may be captured by a rival gang or be taken in hand by the police. But even these crises are relatively temporary and evolve out of and merge into other less fearful situations. Even the injured child cries for his mother and appears to think that with her coming he will feel much better. Even the most anxious

child knows that pleasant things sometimes happen. A realistic view includes factors which mitigate the severity of any experience; it can place the experience in its social setting.

The child's attention span is short but intense. It can be shifted from his bodily discomfort to something pleasant in the environment. Naturally his attention is soon shifted again to his physical condition, and fresh pleasant stimuli should be provided. Yet care must be taken not to create an environment so stimulating that it wears the child out and at the same time arouses in him a demand for overstimulation. A happy atmosphere in which there is slow change of interests suited to his needs is best for him. Above all, he must not be allowed to feel that he is alone in his difficulties. One advantage of hospitalization, care in an institution for convalescent or chronically ill children, or a school for handicapped children is that he sees others who have problems not too different from his own.

Not to leave a child alone in his difficulties does not mean that someone must be constantly with him, but rather that he must learn from experience that someone is thinking of him and will come now and then or whenever he cries or calls for help. He likes to feel that his nurses like to be with him and come for that reason as much as because he needs them.

Children, like adults, are apt to plead a physical excuse for not doing things they do not want to do. When a child says that he has a "tummy ache" at school time, but is all right as soon as it is too late to go, he should not be scolded, but should be shown that such behavior is ridiculous. If he is allowed to "get away with it," his childish excuse may develop into adult neurotic behavior, and he will sincerely believe in his imaginary ailments. The influence upon his personality is more important than the fact that he has missed a day at school. Children under five or six seldom invent excuses of this kind. With them the problem is to get them to tell when they do feel sick or have a pain.

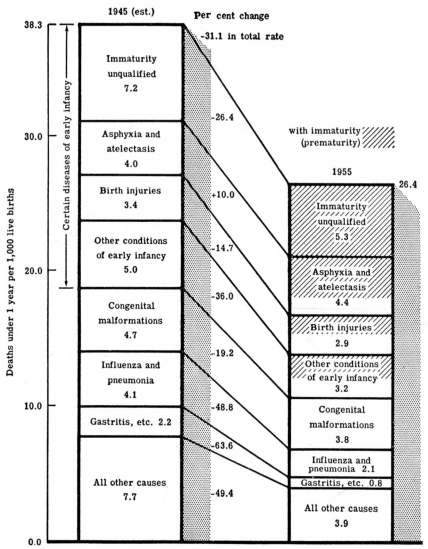

**Figure 5.** Infant mortality. Main causes by Sixth Revision of the International Lists, United States, 1945 and 1955. (From Children's Bureau Statistical Series, No. 50.)

## MORTALITY AND MORBIDITY

There is a class differential in the morbidity and mortality among children. The unhygienic environment of children in the low-income groups is reflected in the higher death rate among them as compared with that of children in the middle- or upper-income group in the same age brackets. This is due both to the parents' lack of education in mat-

ters pertaining to health and also to their inability to pay for the things that make for good health: adequate diet, good housing, clothing, recreation and adequate medical attention. Medical care and hospitalization are usually provided without charge to those who are unable to pay for them. Many people on restricted incomes can pay for medical care and hospitalization, but weigh the cost against what the money will buy when used for some other purpose. It is generally said that this group actually receives less attention when sick than those in a lower income bracket who are eligible for free care.

Each age group among children is particularly affected by certain factors of a bad environment, is more or less susceptible to certain diseases and is exposed to varying accident hazards. Figure 5 shows the causes of death during infancy, and Figure 6, during the remainder of childhood and adolescence. As science, welfare programs and even customary ways of doing things limit these specific factors, there is a spectacular drop in the mortality and morbidity rates among the age group for whom those factors were most dangerous. A case in point is the steady drop in the infant mortality rate.

Years ago the leading cause of death among infants was intestinal disturbances due to bacteria in milk and food. In hot summer weather babies from congested city slums suffering from these infectious diarrheas filled the pediatric units. Many were not brought into the hospital until they were moribund because mothers tried home remedies, thinking that loose stools were a condition that any woman who had had children could handle without help from clinics or hospitals. Strict control of the production and handling of milk sold by dairies and stores, inspection of food and places in which food was sold or served and the availability of iceless refrigeration resulted in a lessening of this once leading cause of infant morbidity and mortality.

Another great killer of infants was and still is respiratory infection. Morbidity and mortality from respiratory diseases following contagious disease (secondary pneumonia) have been reduced through immunization programs, which have greatly decreased the incidence and severity of contagious diseases of childhood. Antibiotics are avail-

**LEADING CAUSES OF DEATH**

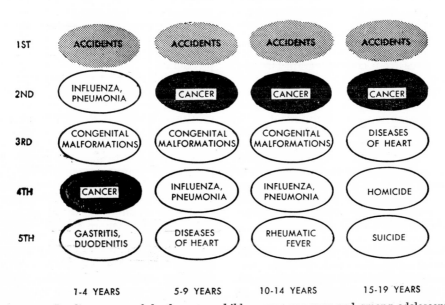

**Figure 6.** Leading causes of death among children over one year and among adolescents. Accidents cause the greatest number of deaths of children and adolescents after the first year of life. Cancer is the second most important cause of death among children after the age of 4 years. The most common form of cancer found in children is leukemia. (Interdepartmental Committee on Children and Youth, Golden Anniversary White House Conference on Children and Youth. Children in a Changing World. 1960.)

able against the bacteria causing the characteristic pathologic picture of pneumonia, whether it be a primary or secondary infection.

Overcrowding obviously leads to the spread of infection, particularly of the respiratory type. Housing conditions in slums and blighted areas are bad, though not so bad as formerly. The same is true of institutions for orphans and other dependent children, in which better hygiene and more adequate nursing and medical care have been introduced.

Broadly speaking, anomalies of the newborn are today one of the leading causes of morbidity and mortality in infancy. Many anomalies can be corrected by surgery or orthopedic procedures. A great new field of surgery has opened up in which the nurse has a singularly prominent role. She must not only be skilled in the physical care she gives the infants, but must also know when to alert the physician. She must understand the meaning of what she observes in an infant's condition in order to aid the physician by her observations, thus predicting changes which may require immediate corrective measures to preserve his life.

The drop in the mortality and morbidity rates from contagious diseases in infancy, the preschool age group and childhood is magnificent proof of the value of research in medicine. In those diseases against which immunization is being given by private physicians, and free in Child Health Conferences and clinics, the old differential between children of different income groups is not seen. The old differential was due partly to the higher incidence among very young children who, in the large families living in crowded tenements, were likely to be exposed to contagious disease at an earlier age than in the middle-class home. But a more important factor was the lack of adequate care given the child. The contagious diseases of childhood were so commonplace that mothers were likely to pay little attention to the gravity of the child's condition. Parents today know

better. They want their children immunized and given care at home under the supervision of a Public Health or visiting nurse, or in selected instances want them hospitalized. Immunization of hospitalized children is common today, since contagious disease among them was and is likely to be of epidemic nature.

One type of infection whose incidence is seemingly on the increase is that caused by *Staphylococcus aureus*. At first it was seen chiefly in hospitals, but it soon spread to the community at large. No immunization procedure has yet been found to prevent the spread of infection caused by this organism.

On the whole, with the control of disease-producing milk and foods, the use of antibiotics, improved surgical treatment of anomalies and immunization against contagious disease the mortality and morbidity rates among infants have dropped more than in any other age group. The rates rise among the adolescent group, partly because of the physical changes in the body, but more because of the social pressure which our culture brings to bear upon the adolescent, who is beyond the care of the pediatrician, but not old enough to establish a relation with his own physician.

An adolescent of the class that commonly weds at sixteen or seventeen years of age may have sexual urges gratified within the socially accepted roles of husband and wife.

The incidence of syphilis and gonorrhea contracted in marriage is less than it formerly was, for a certificate showing that the man and the woman are free from these diseases is required in most states before the marriage license is issued. Even where such a certificate is not compulsory by law, it is customary among all but the most ignorant groups. Although the incidence of these diseases, which are now cured within a few days, is probably not decreasing, the advanced stages of syphilis and the pathologic lesions of the reproductive organs caused by gonorrhea are seldom seen in young or middle-aged people.

They usually seek medical attention in the early stage of venereal disease. Among the old, who contracted the disease in the days when effective treatment was less common, advanced stages of both diseases are still found.

Since the early stages of most venereal diseases are not incapacitating, the adolescent in a disorganized neighborhood is slow to pay attention to incipient signs. Health education and physical examinations in school and in industry have lowered the rate of venereal disease among adolescents.

Evidence of syphilis in the child of a syphilitic mother is seldom seen today. Women in prenatal clinics or under the care of their private physicians receive treatment from which the fetus as well as the patient benefits. If the infant at birth shows evidence of syphilis, he is given prompt treatment.

Boys and girls of sixteen to eighteen are old enough to work in industry, at farming and mining (if this work is above ground) and to fill many service positions. Work of this sort is likely to be a kind of blind alley, and the wages are low. Federal legislation and many state laws limit the employment of young people in dangerous industries. The accident rate among boys and girls is higher than that for adults employed at the same type of work.*

The adolescent of the social class that does not marry, on the average, until

* The recovery rate of young people is more favorable than that of older people, and permanent impairment is less likely to occur. From the point of view of income through life, however, they are at a great disadvantage, since workmen's compensation is based on the wages received at the time of injury and the wage which the injured person is capable of earning after recovery, whether partial or complete. Young people naturally begin in the lowest-paying jobs within the type of occupation they have chosen, and compensation based on their wages before and after injury is less than that for a worker who has advanced up the economic ladder or reached his peak of natural earning power. In unskilled labor, in which physical strength is the chief asset, this age is about twenty-four for women and twenty-eight for men. A severe injury in adolescence, one which leaves a permanent handicap, has greater social significance for the young worker than for the older one.

the early twenties, who continues his education and is sexually mature has no legitimate outlet for his sexual urge and is dependent for support upon his parents. This situation is probably an important factor in the psychosomatic ailments of adolescence. Guidance clinics integrated with medical clinics have proved helpful.

The student nurse herself is so close to this age group that she is likely to experience in some measure these very problems. (Many senior students are engaged or married; some have maternity leaves and face the question of who is to care for the baby.) It is doubtful whether the student nurse can be objective in helping the sick adolescent, and a boy may resent having a girl in her late teens or early twenties give him physical care. Nevertheless, concepts of the role of the nurse are changing from that of "the greatest mother in the world" toward that of a competent sister or "pal" to a patient of her own age, a professional woman to those older than she, and "Mother's friend" to the children.

We might summarize these class factors in morbidity and mortality rates in childhood as follows: the class differential in mortality and morbidity rates still exists and in general has a positive correlation with income when the size of the family is also considered. Yet the rates show the greatest reduction in the low-income group. Among them practice is slowly catching up with advances in technology, and they are receiving more nearly the care given the child whose parents are in the middle income brackets than was true even a decade ago. Welfare legislation has raised the standard of living of the low-income group both through a direct increase in wages or financial benefits of some sort and through community aid in services needed by the child which his family cannot provide for him. Medical, nursing or hospital care is important in this latter class of services given free or at less than cost. The middle class has profited by insurance plans for medical and hospital care.

## ROLE OF THE PROFESSIONAL NURSE IN THE CARE OF CHILDREN

### PARENT, CHILD AND NURSE RELATIONS

No two of these relations can be considered without the third. In the first place, the child has been trained by his mother, whose immediate influence upon him is evident at the first meeting of the child and his nurse. Today's child is accustomed to care by women other than his mother. That fathers also give intimate care such as changing diapers, taking him to the toilet, bathing and dressing him, as well as cooking and serving meals and washing dishes, means to the child that men handle him in the direct-care manner, and he is likely to accept the physician's examination as the child of a generation ago did not.

The child who has known only a friendly world is most likely to accept new friends and a new environment. The modern mother provides opportunity for her child to make friends outside the home in a constantly widening circle of people whom he likes and who like him. But the child of the overprotective mother who has kept him from making adult friends is apt to be afraid in the hospital. Some mothers so need the child's dependency upon them that they are unable to help him during the separation in his unit in the pediatric area. During visiting hours they often exhibit their need of some demonstration of dependency from him by touching him, although simultaneously asserting that they do not wish to wake him from sound and peaceful slumber. At the end of visiting hours also they seem to derive a certain comfort in having to leave while he stands crying in his crib, reaching out after "Mama."

An increasing number of mothers are remarkably able to control their own emotions, however, and to interest the child in amusements provided for him by the hospital—television, for instance, or a ride in a stroller. Many fathers do the same and, in the experience of the authors, are more ready than the mothers to sponsor group play with their own child and his hospital companions.

Parents who want to help their child in his anxiety at being left with hospital personnel in a strange environment can, better than anyone else, convince him that they will come to visit him and that home is waiting for his return and recovery.

Children between birth and four years appear to suffer most from the emotional trauma of separation from a mother figure. Younger children show more signs of distress when their mothers leave them. Older children who have been to nursery school, kindergarten or grade school are accustomed to new and pleasant surroundings. Maternal deprivation is probably a smaller element in their fear of hospitalization than it is among younger children.

Children two to four years old are the ones most likely to cry when mother goes home after visiting hours. They are very much influenced by their mother's reaction to the separation. If she makes a tragedy of parting, so will they; if she treats it as a normal termination of her visit, as if she were leaving the child with friendly neighbors or a baby sitter, they are likely to accept the situation, with tears perhaps, but little emotional trauma. It would be most unfortunate, of course, for a child to be indifferent to his mother's leaving after an emotionally satisfying visit. A nurse should not be disturbed at a few tears after visiting hours, but should introduce some pleasant activity. If the mother sees preparations for this, she is more likely to leave well satisfied with the care given her child, and her attitude will be imparted to him.

### Nurse-Child Relations

**The Child's View.**   The child perceives this relation as one in which he receives from the nurse (1) physical care formerly given by his mother or some other member of the family, (2) new types of care which may be painful and frightening, (3) a sense of security in an adult's affection, and (4) the link with home and mother.

An older child realizes that in addition to the foregoing the nurse teaches him good hygiene and, for girls, is a model of one of the many things they can emulate when grown up. The child may sense, but not clearly perceive, that she teaches him to adapt to his condition, physically and emotionally. He soon learns her relation with his parents and with the physicians and makes use of her contacts with both.

The extent to which nursing care can be given in a homelike setting is a question which each hospital decides in the light of physical resources and available personnel. By homelike physical environment is meant sunlight, color, pictures, music and television, small tables and chairs, toys, wagons, tricycles, and so on. For instance, pink or blue plastic individual bathtubs, floating toys and colored towels and washcloths make the bath more homelike.

The use of a stroller instead of a wheelchair or stretcher to transport the child is another example of the introduction into the hospital setting of compatible equipment and techniques which will connect what of necessity must be strange and cause anxiety in the child with the care he received at home from his mother. Permitting a child to take a doll or other toy to the operating room or to a place where he is to be subjected to diagnostic tests is an evidence of the understanding attitude of nurses and physicians toward his fear.

More important than equipment or methods adapted to children is the rapport between the nurse and the child she cares for. Ideally, one nurse should give the child all the care he needs during her hours on duty as long as he is in the hospital. Her observations of the child would mean much to the physician, her relations with the child would be on a firmer emotional basis, she would learn his particular emotional and physical needs, and would adapt

**Figure 7.** The child receives from the nurse affection and a sense of security as well as physical care. (H. Armstrong Roberts.)

her care to him. The child would then feel that he had three nurses (one day, one afternoon and one night) who were *his* nurses and would also feel that he was their little boy. He would also be cared for by relief nurses, but they would not all relieve "his" nurses in the same twenty-four hours; there would be sufficient stability in his friendship with his three nurses to permit him to accept the relief nurses without feeling that the situation had become new and strange. That nurses wear uniforms and caps which in his view are similar and that they do things for him in much the same way helps him to accept new nurses among those who routinely care for him. A new friend may be pleasant when he knows that the old ones are still there.

**The Nurse's View.** (1) *The nurse perceives her role very much as the child perceives it* because she has defined her role to meet his needs. There are some negligent nurses who do not live up to the professional role of the nurse, and their influence is soon reflected in a change in the child's definition of the nurse-child relation. His idea that nurses are good to little children may change, and he may think nurses mean, whose role is an authoritative, punitive one, in spite of the physical care they give him according to the best technique.

But to his limited concept of their relations the nurse may add much that the child does not realize. To this we shall now turn.

2. *The nurse guides the hospitalized child to better ways of living.* The child should leave the hospital with better habits of hygiene than when he entered. As far as is possible new ways of caring for him, new equipment, new foods in his diet and new concepts of cleanliness should be introduced gradually. Helping the patient to substitute better habits for current ones or harmful ones is so much a part of comprehensive nursing that in this book such habits are taken up in connection with the nursing care of the children.

Unfortunately a child may lose good habits while he is in the hospital and regress to baby ways, or an older child may acquire undesirable habits. A case in point is that of control of urine and stool. A child's physical condition and nervousness due to his strange surroundings may make control difficult for him. But often this is not the cause of a wet and soiled bed. He has cried for a nurse to put him on the "potty" or take him to the toilet. When no one came, he stood holding on to the bars of his crib, crying more loudly, and in the end relieved himself in bed. Nurses know better than to punish or shame a child when this happens; they also realize that he is sick and still almost a baby, but often they do not understand that his emotional state and physical exertion are harmful for him. If they are too busy with some important duty, they may think that his needs are not urgent enough. They may consider that it takes less time to change his clothing and his bed when it is convenient than to come at once when he calls. In fact, they may put diapers on a child who has worn pants for months. In consequence, when he wets himself day after day, he ceases to call the nurse and returns to his infantile habit of relieving himself whenever and wherever he feels inclined to do so. He has thus lost a good habit and acquired a retrogressive, unhygienic one.

### Nurse-Parent Relations

It is a truism that the nurse's relation with the child's parents is based on the fact that they are the parents of the child in her charge. He is the focal point of their relations. Yet the mother of an acutely ill child may be more in need of the nurse's sympathetic, understanding, permissive guidance than the child is of her emotional support. The influence of the mother's attitude upon the child is so great that it is not only for the mother's sake, but also for the child's, that the nurse has a serious responsibility to help the mother. In order to understand how to help mothers the student should be willing to learn from them. She needs to know not only their weaknesses, but also their strengths, and make the most of them in the care the child receives. The nurse is more likely to have had experience solely with children deprived of their mothers' company. But in most cases separation from the mother took place under pleasant auspices, so that neither child nor mother was seriously disturbed. (One or both might have had a moment of concern over what to do without the other. No child likes to be left behind when mother goes out for the evening, and mother may have some doubts as to Johnny's being old enough to go to camp. But such partings are chosen, and no great fear is involved.) If the student comes from a large family or has younger nieces and nephews, if she has been a baby sitter or camp counselor or has otherwise come in contact with children, she is better able to establish rapport with the mother because they have a common basis of knowledge of children. On this she builds her instruction, drawing from her professional knowledge of sick children.

The mother knows her child far better than does the nurse. The mother may be so intent upon him alone that she accepts him as the prototype of all children and does not see him against a background of other typical children; she does not see wherein he is like them or differs from them—his limitations and assets, his potentiality. But even a mother who has a distorted view of her child can teach the nurse many things about him which will help her to understand his behavior. Reliance on the mother as a real help in the adjustment of the child with a chronic condition or severe handicap helps the nurse in her acceptance of his condition. If the mother is able to give the child physical care, it is usually an emotional relief to her and reassures the child in his strange surroundings. The nurse can teach the mother many procedures and ways of caring for the child which she will need to know when she eventually takes him home.

The student knows more about pathology and treatment than does the mother, but what little the mother of a child with a chronic disease or a handicap knows is in direct relation to her child and the care she has given him. Until the nurses have had time to map out a plan of comprehensive nursing for him, the mother may be better able to lift and turn him so that it does not hurt, to feed him most comfortably or to create a play situation adapted to his likes and limitations. When the student has had time to apply her knowledge to the individual child, she is able to teach the mother better ways of caring for him. Both the mother and the nurse, then, have much to contribute to each other in applying the principle of quality nursing to the child patient.

The value of a child psychologist with whom nurses can talk over the problems they meet in the human relations component of nursing is generally recognized, since these relations are so complex that the guidance of a specialist is often necessary. (This also applies to the nurse's handling of her own emotional problems in the involved social situations which constantly occur in the pediatric area.)

It should always be remembered that the child eventually goes home to his family. To bring about changes in habits, however beneficial in themselves, which cause a strained relation between the child and his parents or friends when he leaves the hospital is of doubtful value. To teach a child that he should not use indecent words when these same words are part of the neighborhood daily speech is a case in point. To teach a boy not to fight, if his father would punish him if he did not show this ability to care for himself among other boys, would be folly.

Certain undesirable behaviorisms cannot be allowed in the hospital, but the nurse must be careful not to condemn them. It is common knowledge that one factor in the neurotic disorders of American children stems from the fact that the majority in the low-income group are taught in schools, hospitals and other institutions where the culture of the middle class is held to be the goal of socialization, that their parents' attitudes, beliefs and ways of doing things are not up to standard. Many of the older immigrants and some of the migrants and immigrants of today have come to our large cities because they want their children to have advantages they themselves did not have; they want their children to move into a social class above their own. For a son or daughter to maintain the economic and social position of the parents is not the American philosophy. If their children do not surpass them, parents are likely to feel that they did not give their offspring the advantages they should have received.

In spite of this, clashes in the home often arise between parental attitudes and behavior characteristic of a lower class and those middle-class attitudes and characteristics which professional workers are teaching lower-class children, not only because they believe in the superiority of middle-class culture, but also because they are preparing the children to move up into the middle class. It is not the child's evidence of his preparation for social mobility which parents resent, but rather the lack of respect for his elders which such teaching is likely to engender. The nurse should help the child to draw a distinction between superficial cultural traits in which he differs from his parents and the fundamental traits which are recognized in all classes as fine and highly desirable. Examples are courage, honesty, fidelity, truthfulness, and self-sacrifice for those one loves.

**Parent Education.**  The discussion of nurse-parent relations leads directly into the matter of parent education. In a broad sense parent education begins in childhood, when the personality of the prospective parent is formed in the home. That is, a child from a stable home in which he participates in good parent-child-sibling relations is being educated for creating such a home when he himself marries and founds a family. In instances of juvenile delinquency or warped personality we constantly hear that the parents are to blame for their children's behavior, but we seldom stop to consider the logic of that conclusion: the parents, too, were once children and therefore were

influenced by their own home environment. This is not an acceptance of the fatalistic view whereby the blame for the faults of one generation rests upon the preceding one, and so on back indefinitely. Although personality is strongly set in childhood, it can be altered, albeit with greater difficulty, at any age up to senescence. The nurse, then, must accept the parents' personalities and their attitude toward the child for whom she is caring while she guides them to a better understanding of how to help him grow up.

The content of what the nurse teaches the parent is given her in her course in Child Development or Nursing of Children, and she has seen the application of concepts and principles both within and without the hospital. She must have a general background of knowledge which she draws upon in carrying out her role in the professional team's plan for educating parents.

The nurse in any shared nurse-parent learning situation must also remember certain basic principles. She must learn first of all what the mother already knows about what she is to learn. In other words, the nurse must know the level of the mother's understanding and her background of experience. The nurse must know the mother's resources at home. Does the mother have the equipment she will need or the financial resources to obtain this equipment? The nurse, realizing the mother's problems, must be willing to proceed slowly, allowing time for the mother to absorb what is to be learned. In order to make certain that the mother understands fully, the nurse should either write down what she has said or have the mother repeat what she has learned.

Because a nurse is in the pediatric area with children and parents, her role includes a *demonstration* of physical care and child guidance. That is why it is important that she be prepared to teach the mother. But the nurse's influence on the mother does not always center on physical care and its psychological components. She demonstrates to the mother how to help the child handle his emotions and also to create or remove stimuli, increasing those which promote a beneficial response and decreasing those which do not.

Although the nurse has a general background of knowledge and experience, she must recognize her role in her interaction with other professional personnel who give service to the child and his parents. That is, the physician and the child psychiatrist direct the medical and socio-psychological components of what is demonstrated and taught the parent. The nurse is likely to be the most effective member of the professional group working with the child in the constant application of the plan for parental education; she demonstrates, while giving physical care, how to meet the child's emotional needs. She teaches procedures which the parents will have to continue for the child when he returns home—both what to do and its psychological component.

The nurse helps the mother both physically and emotionally. She guides the mother in her attitude towards the child's condition and in her own concept of herself. Parents often blame themselves too much for the afflictions of their children. They should realize that they cannot expect perfection of themselves or of anyone else. They must also realize that child care, like all rationally directed action, is based on a weighing of pros and cons as to what is to be done for the child. Their decision must be based on the probability of the outcome. We can give statistics as to automobile accidents, certain diets and the chances of recovery from specific diseases or injuries, but no one can predict with certainty about a particular child. We often hear a parent say, "We wish we had not consented to the operation." They should be encouraged to believe that they made a wise decision even if, in their particular case, it proved to be wrong.

### SUMMARY

The nurse who cares for children sees her role in terms of her relations with various groups. In her relations with the mother, the child and with the family group as a whole the nurse may be described broadly as not a mother-substitute, but as "Mother's kind friend." In this role the nurse may individually plan for and actually give comprehensive care to children or she may function as a member of a nursing team.

The nurse who is a member of a nursing team works closely with one or more professional nurses, nursing students, licensed practical nurses, nurse attendants and others in a joint effort. In order to function as a leader or a member of this team, the nurse must understand the comprehensive care of patients assigned to her team and be willing to contribute to their optimum care.

The role of the nurse who cares for children involves not only working with the individual child, his family unit and her nursing team, but also cooperating with members of the broader health team: physician, social worker, nutritionist, school teacher, Play Lady, public health nurse, religious counselor and others as the need arises. She fulfills her responsibility as an active participating member of this team, contributing her skills and knowledge to the total effort of the group.

In order to fulfill her complex role, the nurse must understand the normal physical, emotional, social, mental and spiritual aspects of growth and development of children, and the parent-child relationship as background for her care of both the well child and the sick child of varying ages. It is to this end that the content of the remainder of this book is devoted.

### TEACHING AIDS AND OTHER INFORMATION*

Interdepartmental Committee on Children and Youth: Children in a Changing World (A Book of Charts). Golden Anniversary White House Conference on Children and Youth, 1960.

* Complete addresses are given in the Appendix.

*Science Research Associates*

Menninger, W. C.: Self-Understanding: A First Step to Understanding Children, 1951.

## REFERENCES

Aufhauser, T.: Some Trends in Pediatric Nursing. Nursing World, *127*:9, 1953.

Badgeley, E. W.: Making Friends with Children. Am. J. Nursing, 57:1558, 1957.

Baty, J. M., and Tisza, V. E. B.: The Impact of Illness on the Child and His Family. Child Study, *34*:No. 1, 15, 1956.

Caplan, G.: The Mental Hygiene Role of the Nurse in Maternal and Child Care. Nursing Outlook, 2:14, 1954.

Chenoweth, A. D., and Hunt, E. P.: Current Trends in Infant Mortality. Children, 7:213, 1960.

Frank, L. K.: Is Parent Education Necessary?, Child Study, *33*:No. 4, 10, 1956.

Frank, R.: Parents and the Pediatric Nurse. Am. J. Nursing, 52:76, 1952.

Godbout, R., and Petrick, A.: The Child in the Nurse. Nursing Outlook, 6:460, 1958.

Green, M.: Working out Child-Parent-Nurse Relationships. Nursing World, *127*:10, May, 1953.

Hartrick, P.: Parents and Nurses Work Together. Nursing Outlook, 4:146, 1956.

Ingles, T.: What Is Good Nursing? Am. J. Nursing, *59*:1246, 1959.

Nelson, W. E. (editor): Textbook of Pediatrics. 7th ed. Philadelphia, W. B. Saunders Company, 1959.

Peto, M.: Communicating with Little Children. Am. J. Nursing, 57:602, 1957.

Taylor, R. G.: Some Significant Developments in Maternal and Child Health Nursing. Nursing Outlook, 8:442, 1960.

Webb, C.: Communicating in Pediatrics. Am. J. Nursing, *60*:194, 1960.

# Chapter 4

# The Hospital and the Child

## DIFFERENCES IN THE NURSING CARE OF CHILDREN AND OF ADULTS

THE DIFFERENCES between the nursing care of children and that of adults are based on the anatomic, physiologic and psychologic differences between the immature child and the mature adult. For this reason pediatric nursing must be adapted to the wide range of development from the newborn infant through adolescence. Each unit of this book deals with a progressively older age group. We must consider the basic characteristics of each group and define the general principles of pediatric nursing to meet their needs. We must then consider the diseases most commonly occurring in each age group and the nursing care involved.

### ANATOMIC DIFFERENCES

Anatomic differences between the newborn and the child are obvious. Size is the outstanding difference; it influences the method and equipment used in caring for the child. A more specific anatomic difference between the newborn and the older child is the greater size and weight of the newborn's head when compared with body length and weight. This characteristic, coupled with his immature motor development, makes handling of the little infant quite different from that of the older child. The sutures of the skull in the newborn are not united; the brain is not protected by the skull in the areas of the open fontanels. The head requires gentle washing and careful support so that no undue pressure is brought upon these areas. The little infant's bones are neither as firm nor as brittle as those of the older child. The normal shape of the head and the chest of the infant can be altered by constant pressure from lying in one position. These are but a few of the many examples which illustrate the necessity of adapting basic nursing care to the anatomic development of the child.

Certain diseases are influenced by the interaction of anatomic development with physiologic development. These diseases require specific nursing skills of those who care for the child. An example of such a disease is infection of the middle ear (otitis media), a condition often occurring in young children

**43**

when they have a sore throat because the eustachian tube is both shorter and straighter than that of the older child.

The student will find many other examples of disease related to anatomic development of the child throughout the units of this text.

### PHYSIOLOGIC DIFFERENCES

The differences in the physiologic processes of the newborn infant and of the older child are less obvious than the anatomic differences. But the physiologic characteristics of an age group are more important in the adaptation of nursing care to needs than are the anatomic ones, since they are subject to greater control by medical and nursing procedures.

The little child's physiologic development influences his susceptibility to certain diseases, the symptoms of disease and the probability of lasting harm. The infant or small child requires a greater caloric and fluid intake in proportion to his weight than does the older child, because of his need to support growth and to carry on physical activity and basic metabolic functions. Any pathologic condition which causes loss of fluid—diarrhea or fever, for instance—quickly alters the electrolyte balance.

### PSYCHOLOGIC DIFFERENCES

We shall not stop to consider the psychologic differences between the infant and the older child, since these will be discussed in detail in later units.

### THE GROWTH FACTOR

Growth is not merely a matter of increase in size; it involves a change in both the anatomy and physiology of the body. Important among these developmental changes is resistance to disease.

The infant has a short-lived immunity to certain infectious diseases which he derives from his mother (see p. 96). Immunization against the contagious diseases which he is likely to contract must be given early in infancy,

since many of these diseases may be fatal or bequeath permanent impairment of bodily functions.

In general the differences in the symptoms of a disease in a little baby and in an older child are due to the pathologic state caused by the injurious agents on tissues in different stages of development. It is important in pediatric nursing to learn the cause-effect relation of any pathologic agent to the developmental stage of the child's body, in order to give preventive and curative nursing care and to be prepared for any emergency. For instance, infants and very young children may have convulsions due to the elevation of temperature accompanying the onset of a contagious disease, whereas an older child or adult is likely to have a chill preceding the fever at the onset of an infection.

Mental and emotional reactions to illness differ in various age groups. Both objective signs (those which can be observed) and subjective symptoms (those which cannot be observed and are known only to the person who experiences them) are important in comprehensive nursing. Since the infant and the little child cannot tell how they feel, the nurse is compelled to rely solely on observed signs. She must know both what to expect and the full meaning of her observations.

The older the child, the more successful he is in communicating subjective symptoms to the nurse. Although an infant cannot tell how he feels, and does not localize pain as an older child will do, he may pull at an aching ear, or cry when some part of his body is moved. Such behavior provides an objective sign of a subjective symptom. These signs are important; to learn their meaning is an essential part of pediatric nursing. An older child may use signs of discomfort or pain—whether he feels pain or not—as an attention-getting device. The infant under a year of age does not do this, and behavior indicating pain in a young infant should never be ignored.

Infants and little children are, in general, better patients than adults are

because (1) they live in the present—
easily forgetting the past and not concerned with the future; (2) their attention span is short; and (3) they are
readily interested in other bodily sensations—sights, sounds, a bit of something sweet, the motion of being rocked,
or sucking a finger. This apparent
transience of discomfort often deceives
an inexperienced nurse; she feels that
the child's condition is improving. She
should, of course, endeavor to amuse
the child, but she should not necessarily
regard his response as evidence that
the cause of pain or discomfort has
abated.

Both the infant who cannot understand what is said to him and the older
child who can should be prepared for
treatments and unpleasant procedures,
although they cannot understand the
implications. This preparation in an
infant may be no more than conditioning him to know that an unpleasant
procedure is associated with something
which brings comfort. We cannot explain the purpose or the procedure of
sticking a needle into his arm, but we
can make it appear as one of the unpleasant things which he has learned to
accept as part of a pleasant relation
with other people. We talk to him and
pet him and let him experience this
procedure in a pleasant setting. He
should have learned to trust others
when unpleasant things are done to him
in his routine care (e.g. cleaning his
nose). This trust in others carries over
from routine care to the unfamiliar experiences in the hospital; he cries from
pain, but is not frightened. If his
mother is with him, or a nurse to whom
he is accustomed, he applies this generalized experience with unpleasant
procedures to this particular incident
and is, as we say, a good baby.

A child in the toddler age group or
older should have all procedures which
are to be done to him explained in
terms he can understand. Listening to
the physician's or nurse's heart through
the stethoscope is a type of explanation
he understands. Not all procedures can
be demonstrated in this way, but the
use of such techniques gives the child

a basis for understanding the general
purpose of examinations and treatments. Picture books and dolls have
been used to help a child to understand
what will be done to him before the
examination, treatment or procedure is
undertaken.

The problems and dangers in an environment must be viewed in relation
to the child's development. The infant
and the little child lack experience and
are therefore dependent on adults to
give them the answer to their problems
—problems outside the widening range
of their ability to solve—and to keep
them safe from physical dangers and
emotional harm. To give this help the
adult must have experience in the use
which children are likely to make of
their physical surroundings and social
environment. Precautions to be taken in
the hospital are listed on page 48.

Throughout this book is emphasized
the importance of the problem which
hospitalization presents to a child, and
the ways in which hospital personnel
and the child's parents can help him to
adjust to the situation. There is always
the danger to a child's emotional development caused by long-term hospitalization with separation from parents and siblings. To avoid this, infants
and young children are being treated
whenever possible on an outpatient
basis. Antibiotics can easily be given for
certain acute infections and in order to
limit complications. Outpatient treatment is therefore possible in many
cases for which formerly it was necessary to hospitalize the child. If the child
must be hospitalized, his parents should
be allowed to visit him as often as they
are able and to participate in his nursing care in every way that is practicable
in the private room or unit where the
child is placed.

## DISEASES PECULIAR TO CERTAIN AGE GROUPS

Diseases and other pathologic states
common in children of various age
groups are considered in the following
chapters. Some of these conditions are
acute in one age group and do not ex-

tend into the other periods of life. Other conditions have their origin during one period of life and extend into later life. The various conditions found in children are grouped in this book according to the age level when they most commonly occur.

The student will see that the nursing care of each condition is based on (1) the anatomic, physiologic and psychologic development and the growth factor normal to the age group and on (2) the treatment (preventive or curative) of each disease. This is all the assistance which a textbook can give the student. Adaptation to the needs of the individual child is made at the bedside under the guidance of the instructor.

## THE PEDIATRIC UNIT

### DESIGN OF THE PEDIATRIC DEPARTMENT

The pediatric unit must be built and furnished to meet the needs of children and of their parents. (Parents have needs of their own which are often forgotten.)

Children's needs can be classified under two main headings: protection from danger, e.g. infection, and protection from a psychologically threatening environment. The first refers to the design of the department with isolation facilities and the second to provision of a cheerful, homelike surrounding, with opportunity to be near other children of a like age.

Parents need the same cheerful surroundings the children need. They are rested and relaxed by facilities which conserve their strength and minimize anxiety. Easy chairs should be near the child's bed so that they may hold the child in their arms while they caress him or show him a picture book or toy. If the child is in a private room, his mother should have a bed or cot which is comfortable for a night's rest. Some hospitals have a few rooms for patients and their mothers in the pediatric units, and the parents pay only what they can afford. These rooms are reserved for ill children who need their mothers with them constantly.

A rest room should be provided for the mothers of patients for use when they are not with a child. Thus they are on call when the child wants his mother or when his condition becomes worse. If there is a good parent-nurse-child relation, the mother is a great help to the nurse, for there are some forms of nursing care which the mother can give with more emotional comfort to the child than the nurse can.

### Physical Layout of the Pediatric Unit

The great majority of pediatric departments are designed to care for the needs of children from infancy to ten or twelve years of age. Let us consider the requirements of such a unit.

**Exposure to the Sun.** The unit should have an eastern or a southern exposure. Outside porches and a grassy play space are good for children who must remain in the hospital a long time and should have the benefits of sunlight and fresh air.

**Light, Heat and Ventilation.** All the rooms in the pediatric unit should have adequate window space and sufficient artificial lighting. Indirect lighting from ceiling lights is good. There should be side lights in cubicles for children old enough to read, and all cubicles should have electric outlets suited for any electrical appliance which may be needed in the care of the child. The walls should be light-colored, since dark colors absorb light. Adequate heat must be provided, as well as ventilation without drafts. Air conditioning of rooms or the entire unit is customary in new buildings.

**Segregation from the Rest of the Hospital.** Segregation of the unit from the rest of the hospital is advisable in order that the noise of a child crying or laughing may not disturb adult patients. Soundproof ceilings are an advantage. Segregation of the unit also has the merit of keeping from the children the distressing and perhaps frightening sights and sounds of the adult sections.

**Floor Plan of the Pediatric Area.** In children's hospitals or large pediatric units of general hospitals segregation into various units may be made on the basis of age or type of illness. Possibly there may even be a unit for convalescent or chronically ill children, though such patients really need a separate institution where the buildings and grounds and the plan of administration are adapted to their needs.

In the small pediatric unit all the children may be placed in one cubicled area. Such an arrangement tends to create problems in the individual placement of patients. Yet even in one area children of approximately the same age may be grouped together in units enclosed by glass. Glass is necessary so that all the children may be under constant observation by the nurses, and the children who are in serious condition should be nearest the head nurse's desk. Individual cubicles are advisable, since they make isolation of the patient easier for the nurses and prevent exchange of toys and other small objects between the children. Individual cubicles are generally provided for young children, even if not for the older ones, since the danger of spread of infection is greatest among infants. An arrangement whereby the older children are lodged in rooms or cubicles separated from the infants permits convalescent children to play without too much restraint. Bright-colored curtains may be hung at the cubicle windows to provide privacy when necessary.

The head nurse's desk should be near the center of the pediatric unit so that she may see all the children through the glass of the cubicles at all times. It should also be near the entrance of the pediatric unit so that she may control the number of visitors. Visiting should be restricted to the parents or their substitutes.

The head nurse or her representative should be responsible for the guidance of parents in gifts of toys and food to the children. Toys should not only be safe, but should also be selected in relation to the activity allowed the child; food should be only that permitted by the physician. Food packages should be labeled with the child's name and deposited in the kitchen or other suitable place. If the parents are willing, the food should be shared with other children. Thus they will not be denied a delicacy not brought for them, and food wastage will be avoided when parents bring their child more than he is permitted or able to consume.

*Side Rooms.* Since it is difficult to control activity in side rooms such as playrooms or bathrooms, children should not be permitted there except under supervision.

PLAYROOM. The playroom should be sunny, homelike, colorful and soundproof. The furniture should meet the needs of children of different ages, and the toys should be suited to the interests of the children who will use them. The room should be under adequate supervision at all times. A nursery school teacher or play lady may be responsible for the activities in this room and may also take toys to children who are not permitted out of bed. Some hospitals allow the mother of one of the children to supervise the room, or any mother to take her child there if it is not occupied.

SCHOOLROOM. This room, like the playroom, should be bright and cheerful and adapted to the needs of the children who will use it. Many pediatric units do not have enough children of school age to warrant a schoolroom, or enough space for such a room. Such units may have a teacher who visits each child in his cubicle, but this plan affords no opportunity for group activity. Some hospitals or pediatric units in general hospitals may have a schoolroom large enough to accommodate the beds of children who are not permitted out of bed, thereby permitting the group activity so valuable for hospitalized children.

BATHROOM. The bathroom should be well lighted so that the nurse, while bathing a child, can detect any rash or discharge he may exhibit. Since tubs are difficult to clean properly and may be a source of infection, shower baths should be provided for the older convalescent children. The toilets should be suited to the size of the children using them, and the seats should have a U shape, since this tends to prevent cross-infection among the children should there be a missed case of genitourinary tract infection. (Cross-infection is most likely to occur with little girls who slide on and off a toilet seat which is too high for them.) Small wash bowls should be provided in sufficient number for all children who are ambulatory and able to wash their hands before eating.

A bathroom is not a safe place for little children. They may wet their clothing, and accidents have occurred when a child has turned on a hot water faucet and been burned. Hot water should be thermostatically controlled and so regulated that it will not burn a child.

TREATMENT OR EXAMINING ROOM. This room should be separate from the patient's unit, and every effort should be made to have it attractive. All children should be taken to this room for treatments or examinations, since it is disturbing to other children to hear a distressed child cry. The treatment table should be sufficiently high for convenience in examination and administration of treatments, and for restraint of the child when necessary. The lighting should be adjustable and adequate for any procedure which is to be done.

A KITCHEN or SERVING ROOM is desirable because infants and children are fed at irregular hours and more frequently than adults.

A CLINICAL LABORATORY is advocated for the physician's use.

**Formula Laboratory.** In the past the formula laboratory and its equipment for sterilizing utensils were connected with the pediatric unit and were likely to be under the supervision of the head nurse. Today the laboratory is seldom adjacent to the children's unit and is generally under the direction of the dietary department of the hospital.

In some communities hospitals are able to purchase infant feedings from a commercial milk laboratory which specializes in the preparation of formulas.

### SAFETY MEASURES

Accidents are a major cause of death among infants and small children. Great emphasis should be placed on the prevention of accidents in the hospital, both for the safety of the child while he is there and in order that mothers may have a practical demonstration of how accidents common to little children may be avoided. The following discussion is concerned chiefly with accidents in the hospital, but certain of these accidents also occur in the home.

Many safety measures deal with the construction of the building or unit and are beyond the control of the nurse. Among these are the following:

1. Fireproof, wide stairways.

2. Windows protected by locked screens and window guards and so placed that drafts do not blow upon the children when the windows are opened for ventilation.

3. Gates at the entrance to rooms where small children play, so constructed that a child cannot open them or catch his fingers between the door and its frame.

Other measures for children's safety which are directly under the nurse's control include the following:

1. The catches on the side gates of the crib should be in good condition, and the gates should always be up when the child is in bed. When administering care with the side gate down, the nurse should keep her hand on the infant or little child to prevent his falling, especially if she looks away from the child or reaches for an object on the bedside table.

2. Restraints, if used, should be applied correctly to prevent constriction of any part of the child's body. The greatest danger is that of strangulation through pressure of a jacket restraint which has slipped out of place and encircled a patient's neck.

3. Medicine cabinets should be locked at all times when not in use, and medications should never be left standing on a bedside table.

4. Instruments and solutions should be kept in cabinets or on shelves where children cannot reach them.

5. *Safety pins should be closed* at once when taken from a child's clothing and put out of his reach. An infant

or young child tends to put small objects into his mouth.

6. Toys should have rounded rather than sharp edges. They should never be painted with lead paint and should not have small parts which a child could remove and swallow or aspirate. They should never be left on the floor, because of the danger that a child or a nurse with a child in her arms might trip over them. For the same reason, wet areas on the floors should be dried immediately.

7. Infants and small children should not be allowed to play with tongue depressors or applicators.

8. Electric outlets and fans should be covered when not in use, and the fans should be placed where children cannot reach them.

9. Isolation techniques should be carried out on all children with infectious illnesses. For this to be practicable, adequate facilities must be available for the nurse to wash her hands. She should wash her hands after caring for each child. All other isolation procedures to prevent cross-infection must be rigidly followed. In the children's units of some hospitals ultraviolet rays are used to cut down the number of air-borne organisms. Nurses must be aware of symptoms indicating the onset of infectious disease in both the children and herself. Such symptoms should be promptly reported.

10. Nursing bottles should *never* be propped, *nor should feedings be forced* upon a little child. There is danger of aspiration, which may cause pulmonary disease or even sudden death.

11. In giving medication to an infant or a little child who will not cooperate a second nurse is required to assist in gentle restraint of the child. Oily medications should *never* be given orally to a child who is crying, because of the danger of aspiration (see p. 307).

12. Hot-water bottles must always be tightly stoppered and covered before being placed near a child's body or even in the bed with him. The water temperature should not be over 115° F.

13. The bulb of a thermometer should be checked to be certain that it is not cracked. If the temperature is taken rectally, the nurse must hold the thermometer in place so that it will not be dislodged and so that the child will not injure himself if he rolls over.

## HOSPITALIZATION OF CHILDREN

Admission of a child to the hospital can be considered in connection with the activities involved or from the standpoint of the emotional effect upon the child and his family. We shall consider first the emotional effect, because it is often mistakenly accorded less importance than the physical care given the child. As was pointed out in connection with the nurse-parent-child relation, the nurse's attitude is probably the most important single factor in the emotional atmosphere during the child's admission (Fig. 8).

Hospitalization of children is so common today that we tend to forget its importance as a break in the unity of the family. The feelings of each member of the family must be considered if this break is to result in furthering rather than hindering the emotional and social maturity of all concerned. Although it has been said that the nurse has the major role in helping the child and his parents adjust to the hospital situation, the entire health team (physician, public health nurse, nutritionist and possibly a social worker) is involved in creating the optimum emotional environment on the child's admission.

### EMOTIONAL REACTIONS ON ADMISSION OF A CHILD TO THE HOSPITAL

#### Maternal Reaction

A mother whose child has been admitted to the hospital feels not only that he is separated from her, but also that others are taking her place and, furthermore, giving him necessary care which she, with all her intense love for him, cannot give.

Immediate operation is often necessary to save the life of an infant who is born deformed or deviates from the nor-

**Figure 8.** The nurse must be understanding of the feelings of parents when she admits their children to the hospital. (William H. Rittase.)

mal, or he may be sent home from the newborn nursery with his mother, for deferred admission to the pediatric unit when he has reached the optimal age for correction of the defect. In general the reaction of parents to such a child at birth is that he presents a threat to all their happy expectations centered around the concept of a normal baby. It is natural that when he is readmitted to the hospital, they still feel anger, fear, disappointment and possibly guilt.

The majority of mothers want the understanding, sympathetic support which the nurse can give and thereby gain a realistic view of the difficulties which they and the child must face. Some mothers appear withdrawn, however; these are in greater need of help. To assist them to put into words their deep emotion may be too heavy a responsibility for the nurse to undertake. The psychiatrist or psychiatric social worker should be available to guide both the parents in their trouble and the nurse in her contacts with them in

order that she may learn to take her place in the mental health program.

A mother, particularly with her first child, often feels that his sickness is due to some error that she has committed and is her fault. If he was an unwanted baby, she may consider it a punishment for not having had the normal maternal love for the child during her pregnancy and after his birth.

**Specific Causes of Maternal Anxiety.** In addition to her feelings about the illness itself, a mother may be frightened and excited by the new experience of placing a child in the hospital. Among the many factors which increase her anxiety are the following:

1. Fear of the unknown and of what will happen to the child immediately and in the future. The life of a handicapped child appears the more difficult because mothers have no clear picture of what it will be like.

2. Fear of separation from the child and fear that the nurses may be unloving or that, because they are able to do

so much for him, they will take his love from her.

3. Fear that the child will suffer from his condition.

4. Fear that the condition is infectious and may spread to other members of the family.

5. Fear of unbearable financial obligations incurred through the illness. The social service worker may help in such a case.

6. Fear that society will look upon the illness as a reflection of something wrong with the child's parents.

A mother's anxiety about her child magnifies all other problems. She may enter into long discussions of problems which are extraneous to that of the child's illness. The nurse should accept this as natural and never feel that a mother's dwelling on other difficulties means that she is disinterested in the child.

### The Child's Reaction

Illness or a physical handicap threatens both the physical development of a child and his sense of trust in other people which is important to his emotional development. Sickness causes pain, restraint of movement, long sleepless periods and, in an infant who cannot be fed by mouth, restriction in the fulfillment of his sucking need. When he most needs his mother, he is without her, unless the hospital has provision for her remaining day and night.

Hospitalization is a completely new experience to the infant or young child. When he was taken to the private physician's office or the Child Health Conference, he made friends with doctors and nurses, but he is too young to understand that the hospital personnel are also his friends. Since his mother tends to be anxious, her feeling of fear is communicated to him.

What the hospital means to the individual pediatric patient will depend upon his stage of maturity and upon how accustomed he was to being left with friends of his mother. It appears that even a very young baby becomes accustomed to the ways in which he is cared for. He will soon become adapted to a complete change in the people who care for him and to their new ways of giving care. Although an infant adjusts to a change from his mother to his nurse, he appears to have great difficulty in adjusting to a constantly changing group of nurses or nonprofessional personnel. For this reason it is essential that his care be given by a few nurses all of whom use the same technique and even similar ways of showing affection to him.

Under the case assignment of infants or children to nurses both the child and his parents will develop a personal relation with his nurse. Having unlimited visiting hours during which the mother may care for her young child is ideal. She can use the same procedures and methods of giving care that the nurses use. Under case assignment a child needs only to adjust to one nurse on each of the three shifts of duty, while his mother's presence establishes a continuity of care which is lacking without her. Her presence is particularly necessary if the case assignment method is not used and the child receives units of nursing care from many nurses or subsidiary workers during the twenty-four hours of the day.

### THE NURSE'S ROLE

The role of the nurse in the admission procedure is complementary to that of the mother and the child. To fill her role she must understand that the mother's behavior is the result of the way the child's sickness and hospitalization appear to her. The mother should never be told not to cry or that she is "really fortunate, because the situation could be worse." Such comments cause a mother to repress her feelings and to be ashamed that she spoke so openly. Repression of anxiety or feelings of guilt or inadequacy causes these feelings to increase, while expression of them diminishes their intensity.

In some rare cases the mother may feel ambivalent toward her child, since he is the cause of her anxiety. She may overprotect him either through her loving anxiety for his welfare or to hide even from herself her ambivalent feeling toward him, of which she is ashamed. If she feels inadequate to meet the problems arising from his illness, this attitude is reinforced, but overprotection is likely to be reduced if her anxiety can be relieved and her self-confidence built up.

The nurse should never be critical of a mother's attitude however unreasonable it may appear. Such criticism leads to greater tension and possibly to hostility on the mother's part. In order to be helpful the nurse must understand what the illness means to the mother, who may be misinformed as to the cause, prognosis and necessary treatment.

The following are ways by which the nurse may make the mother feel more secure and calm in the hospital, and the child less restless:

1. The mother should be taken with the child to his bed in the unit or private room. Then she knows where the child is and has a mental picture of his comfortable physical environment. Reducing her anxiety reduces that of the child.

2. The nurse who admits the child should introduce herself and the head nurse to the mother. All names should be clearly pronounced. If the child is old enough, he should be introduced to other children of his own age and to the attending personnel.

3. The mother should be given a friendly welcome and should be seated comfortably. The nurse, even if she has other duties which need her attention, must be unhurried and calm. Her attitude increases the parents' trust in the hospital and medical staff which the nurse, at the time, represents.

4. The admission procedure should be carefully explained, and all questions asked by the parents should be answered clearly, fully and in a way which will not frighten the mother.

The specific routine of admission is as follows:

1. History of Illness. The nurse introduces the mother to the physician who will take the history of the present illness. The child should not be present, for if he is old enough, he will understand and sense his mother's anxiety. Even an infant senses tension and anxiety in his mother.

2. Vital Signs. The nurse takes the vital signs: temperature, pulse, respiration and, if necessary, blood pressure. A temperature reading per rectum should be taken last, since it is likely to make the child cry. Crying influences the respiration and pulse, and an accurate record is not obtained.

3. Weight. The nurse weighs the child on admission (see p. 290).

4. Examination of the Child. The mother should undress the infant or young child and, if possible, assist with the examination. The nurse may have to help in restraint of an infant or young child during examination of the head (eyes, ears, nose and mouth). During this part of the examination the nurse holds the child with his back against her chest. Her right hand, placed on his forehead, steadies his head, and her left arm restrains his arms. With some children it will be necessary to "mummy" (see p. 149) the body and further restrain the child by leaning over his body while placing her hands on either side of his head. Another method of restraint is to place the child upon his back on the examining table. With one hand the nurse grasps the child's hands, which are extended over his head. With the other hand she holds his ankles, keeping one or two fingers between the ankles so that pressure is not brought upon the ankle bones.

The nurse should speak to the child and caress him in order that restraint may not be frightening to either him or his mother.

### Conference with the Head Nurse

The talk should center on the mother's child and not on children in general. To emphasize this the nurse should speak of the child by name rather than use some general term such as "baby" or "little boy." Such an approach in the conference leads up to asking the moth-

THE HOSPITAL AND THE CHILD

er for information about the child which the physicians and nurses need in caring for him. This information should be available to the whole health team. Figure 9 gives a suggested outline for obtaining such information, especially after the period of infancy.

The nurse should tell the mother the hours when she will be allowed to visit the child and should explain why it is advisable for the mother to come as often as possible to see him. If a mother seems reluctant to visit frequently, she may be questioned as to the reason, but should she still be reticent or speak of needing help which the nurse cannot give, arrangements may be made for her to talk with the physician or, with his permission, the social worker.

It should be explained to the mother that during visiting hours she may help in the child's care. There may be little she can do for a critically ill child, but gradually, as she becomes accustomed to his care and his condition improves, she will be able to do more for him, e.g. giving him the "potty," bathing or feeding him or changing his diaper. Helping in his nursing care relieves not only the mother's sense of frustration at not being able to do everything for him, but also her sense of guilt if she feels that his sickness was caused by neglect on her part. At the same time she is learning how to give the care he will require after he has gone home.

If the hospital has written policies about visiting hours and regulations as to food, toys, the wearing of gowns and masks, and so on, this should be fully explained to the mother, who should be given a copy of the rules—if the hospital has printed copies—before she leaves the pediatric area.

The mother should remain, if possible, until the child is comfortable. If she has permission from the hospital for unlimited visiting hours or if the child is in a private room, all facilities for her comfort should be explained to her: the location of the wash room, smoking room, lounge, public telephone, and the place where she may sleep and have her meals. In the majority of hospitals only breakfast is served to the

mother; for her other meals she may go to the cafeteria or snack-bar. To be away from the child for these short periods gives her a needed change of environment.

If the mother intends to remain with the child during treatments, examinations and the taking of specimens, the purpose of these procedures should be explained to her. Although the parents may participate in the child's care, the nurse must be responsible for the total nursing care. With the mother as an assistant she has an opportunity for health teaching which will affect not only the patient, but also the entire family. It is an ideal situation, for the mother learns through observation and discussion rather than through formal teaching, which is only indirectly related to the individual child.

## Nursing Procedures after Admission of a Child

After admission of a child to the hospital the nurse may need to carry out certain additional procedures, including medical aseptic technique, collection of urine specimens, collection of blood specimens and the giving of medications.

**Medical Aseptic Technique.** The *purpose* of medical aseptic technique is to prevent transmission of infection from one child to another or to the personnel who care for him. It is the joint responsibility of the medical and nursing staffs to plan the procedures and techniques and to carry out medical aseptic patient care.

Medical aseptic technique is necessary whenever the patient and his belongings are considered contaminated. Those who care for him are considered to be clean when they enter his unit, but to become contaminated when they touch him or his equipment. If only her hands touch the patient while the nurse gives him brief nursing care, it is not necessary for her to wear a gown. Only her hands will be contaminated, and she will wash them on leaving the cubicle.

*The unit in which the child is isolated*

Pediatric Department
Personal History Sheet

Child's name _____    Date of Birth _____
Child's nickname _____    Religion _____
Date of admission _____ Number of previous hospitalizations _____
Does the child know why he is being hospitalized? _____
Has the child been prepared for this admission? _____
How did he react to the preparation? _____
Does he have any special fears about the hospital?  Needles? _____
        People in white uniforms? _____  Others? _____
Names and ages of child's brothers and sisters - _____
_____
Is the child friendly with unfamiliar adults? _____
Is the child friendly with unfamiliar children? _____
Does the child have a pet? _____ Kind_____ Name _____
Have any changes occurred in the child's environment recently? _____
    Birth of sibling (s)_____  Illness in the home _____
    Death of relative_____  Other_____

Eating Habits

How does the child eat?  Bottle_____ Cup_____ Spoon_____
Eating schedule _____
Who feeds the child?  Adult_____ Child _____
What fluids and solid foods does the child especially enjoy?_____
_____
What fluids and solid foods does the child dislike?_____
_____
Food allergies _____

Sleeping Habits

Usual hour of sleep.  Naptime _____  Bedtime _____
Where does the child usually sleep?  Crib_____ Junior Bed_____ Adult Bed____
Does the child sleep alone? _____ If not, with whom does he sleep?____
Does the child sleep well? _____
Does the child climb out of bed?_____
Does the child have any routines at bedtime? _____ Prayers_____
    Taking a toy to bed_____  Others _____

Toilet Habits

Is the child toilet trained?_____ Bowel movements_____ Urination_____
Terms used for bowel movement_____ Urination_____
What time does the child usually have a daily bowel movement?_____
Does the child wear diapers or panties?_____
Does the child use a toilet chair?_____ Adult toilet?_____
Does the child need assistance with toileting?_____
If the child is taken to the toilet at night, what time is this done?_____

**Figure 9.** *See facing page for legend.*

Personal Care

Does the child need assistance with  Bathing _____
                                      Dressing _____
                                      Combing Hair _____
                                      Brushing teeth _____

Play Habits

With whom does the child like to play?  Alone _____
                                        With other children _____
                                        With adults _____
What are the child's favorite Games _____
                              Toys _____
Did you bring the child's favorite toy to the hospital? _____

School Activities

Does the child attend Nursery school _____
                      Grade school _____
                      Church school _____
Name of school attended _____
Grade in school _____
Name (s) of favorite friend (s) _____
Name of favorite teacher _____

Special interests

Does the child enjoy any particular  Hobbies _____
                                     Radio programs _____
                                     Television programs _____
                                     Books _____

Additional comments which would help make the child's hospital stay as pleasant as possible __
_____
_____
_____

**Figure 9.** The Personal History Sheet may be completed by either the mother, the nurse admitting the child to the hospital or the head nurse. On another sheet the nurse who admits the child should record her observations concerning the mother-child relationship and their initial adjustment to the hospital. Other personnel who care for the child should make additional comments during the course of the hospital stay.

is defined as an area, cubicle, room or part of a unit in which one or more patients having the same infectious disease are given care. The furnishings in an isolation unit should be simple, as few as possible for the comfort of the patient, and easily cleaned. There should be sufficient equipment in the room for the patient's care, but excess articles should not be kept in the same area. The amount of equipment will depend upon the child's age, the type of infection and the number of patients isolated in the unit. All furniture, the sink, walls, floor and equipment are considered contaminated in such an isolation unit. The area where the gown is hung is contaminated, but the inside of the gown is kept clean. A damp cloth or a wet mop is used in cleaning the room to prevent organisms from being dispersed in the air.

*Admission of a patient to an isolation unit* involves a number of procedures. It is customary to send the child's clothing home and give the parents instruction as to its disinfection or sterilization by airing it, washing it thoroughly or boiling whatever can be sterilized in this way.

Each patient should have his own equipment, such as thermometers and bathing equipment, in his unit, and these should not be taken from the room until he is discharged, when they are given terminal disinfection. Toys brought to the hospital with the child should be of the sort that can be easily cleaned; they should be tied to the bed so that they cannot drop to the floor. Care must be taken that the string or tape tying the toys to the crib cannot become twisted around the child's neck.

*Visiting an isolated patient* is permitted because of the importance of preserving parent-child relations. Parents must observe certain precautions, however, for their own safety and that of the child. They should be given instructions about visiting regulations for such patients. It is a good plan to have these instructions printed in order that parents may read them when they are at home and the initial anxiety over the child's hospitalization is passed.

When parents visit, they must wear isolation gowns, to be discarded after use. (In some hospitals these gowns are sent to the laundry with other contaminated linen; in other hospitals they are not only laundered when necessary, but also autoclaved between use.) The parents must be supervised during visiting hours to prevent their breaking the prescribed hospital technique.

*Gown technique* is time-consuming, but is one of the most important factors in medical aseptic technique. Anyone who gives direct care involving close contact with a child must wear a gown over his clothing to protect it from contamination. The gown must be long enough to cover the nurse's uniform; it should open down the back and be ample enough to lap over the other side.

In some hospitals gown technique requires that the gown be discarded after each use, but it is more general practice to have it reused for twenty-four hours unless soiled. If it is to be reused, the inside must be kept clean. The gown must be put on, taken off and hung up in a special way in order that the inside does not become contaminated. If the gown is hung inside the contaminated area, it is hung on a hook with the contaminated side out so that persons or equipment near-by will not contact the gown and contaminate the clean inside surface.

Before anyone puts the gown on he must wash his hands thoroughly. The gown is lifted from the hook by grasping the inside near the shoulder seams. The person putting on the gown inserts one arm into a sleeve while still holding the gown with the other hand. The gown is then supported with the hand that is within the sleeve while the other arm is put into the other sleeve. Both hands are uncontaminated, since only the inside of the sleeves and cuffs has been touched. Next, the top back-strings are tied. Then the back edges of the gown are approximated and rolled together, and the lower strings are tied securely so that the gown will not drop upon the patient as the nurse bends over him.

After the nurse has given the child all the necessary care she removes the gown by first untying the strings at the back of the waist. She then washes her hands. She unties the strings at the back of her neck. Next she slips her right hand under the cuff of the left sleeve and pulls it over her left hand, which, remaining in the sleeve, is used to pull the right cuff of the gown over the hand. The right hand, uncontaminated, is withdrawn from the sleeve and used to grasp the clean neck band and support the gown while she withdraws her left hand from the sleeve. Both hands, still uncontaminated, are used to approximate the sides of the neck band. Holding the gown in her left hand, the nurse with her right hand grasps the outside of the shoulder seams and hangs the gown on the hook. The gown must be hung so that both edges are brought together and the top back strings hang free. The neck band and strings can be adjusted with the clean left hand. Both hands can then be used to complete the adjustment of the gown on the hook. The hands and lower forearms must be thoroughly washed before the nurse leaves the unit or touches her uniform.

*Mask technique* is important since infectious disease is commonly spread through droplet spray from the nose and mouth, which are also the portals through which respiratory infection is most likely to enter the body. The wearing of masks has become a controversial topic, however; some physicians believe them to be of value, but others believe them to be ineffective. If a mask is worn, it should cover both the nose and the mouth to prevent (1) spreading of organisms present in the spray of the nose and throat of the wearer and (2) inhalation of infectious material in the air about a patient suffering from a respiratory infection. A mask should be worn once and then discarded, for it is readily contaminated by the constant passage of air through its meshes, which trap bacteria. A mask should never be dropped loosely around the neck and then be drawn up into position over the nose and mouth.

*Hand-washing technique* varies in different hospitals both as to the soap or cleansing solution used and the precise procedure. The equipment needed is running water, soap, a nail brush and paper towels. Soap containing hexachlorophene is being used in many hospitals. This leaves a film on the skin surface of adsorbed chemical which has a prolonged antiseptic effect. If hexachlorophene soap is used repeatedly, it tends to reduce the normal bacterial flora on the skin surface. It is most effective against gram-positive bacteria. The action of the chemical is reduced when alcohol or water or other soaps which do not contain hexachlorophene are used. The nail brush is kept in a disinfectant near the sink. Paper towels should be available in a suitable container.

The procedure for turning the water on varies with the location of the sink. If it is in the cubicle, the handles of the faucets are usually considered contaminated. If the sink is outside the cubicle, the handles are usually considered clean and must be turned on with paper towels, since the nurse's hands are contaminated. If the water is controlled by a foot pedal, this is always considered contaminated, since it is near the floor. The hands must be soaped and rinsed three times. If they are grossly contaminated, they must be scrubbed with a brush for at least two minutes. The nurse should not give care to isolated patients if she has abrasions on her hands, since she is unable to cleanse them thoroughly. Furthermore, if the patient has an infectious condition which can be contracted through a break in the skin, the nurse might become infected with the organism.

*Concurrent disinfection* is the destruction of pathogenic organisms carried out continuously while the child is isolated. Such articles as dishes, clothing, bedding and equipment for treatment must be disinfected. Any articles brought into the room which are used by or have touched a patient must be disinfected before being used for another patient. Heat sterilization by boiling or autoclaving is used for linens, clothing and eating utensils. Any glass or metal objects which cannot be autoclaved, such as thermometers, must be scrubbed with soap and water and soaked in alcohol or benzalkonium chloride (Zephiran). Certain objects such as mechanical equipment which cannot be cleansed by boiling or washing must be exposed to the air and either sunlight or ultraviolet light to kill the surface organisms. The need for disinfection of excreta, vomitus and sputum depends on the type of organism causing the illness. Specific directions for disinfection are usually outlined by the hospital and are influenced by sewer facilities in the area.

BIRD-SEED CUP

SPICER URINAL

FEMALE T BINDER

A

B

**Figure 10.** Procedures to be used for the collection of a urine specimen from an infant girl. *A*, A bird-seed cup may be held in place by a tightly applied three-cornered diaper. *B*, A bird-seed cup or a Spicer urinal may be held in place with a female T binder.

TEST TUBE

MALE T BINDER

A

B

**Figure 11.** Procedures to be used for the collection of a urine specimen from an infant boy. *A*, A test tube may be held in place with a male T binder. *B*, A test tube may be held in place also by adhesive tape. The ankle or extremity restraint is used to restrain the infant's legs.

*Terminal disinfection* means making the physical environment and the body of the child *clean* so that infection cannot be conveyed to others after he has ceased to be a source of infection. A child released from isolation or discharged from the hospital must be given a complete bath, including washing of his hair. He is then moved to a clean area and dressed in clean clothing. The room can be easily cleaned if the furnishings are simple. Everything, including walls, floor and furniture, must be scrubbed with soap and water. The mattress must be autoclaved or aired. If rugs and window curtains have been used, they too may be autoclaved or exposed to sunlight for some hours. The room should be thoroughly aired for at least a day before another patient is admitted. All articles which cannot be adequately disinfected, such as a child's paper picture book, must be destroyed.

**Collection of Urine Specimens.** Urine specimens are usually requested on admission. Collection of such specimens from older children who can cooperate with either the nurse or the mother is relatively easy, but is more difficult from infants. Procedures have been set up for the collection of single specimens from both sexes. (For the collection of 24-hour specimens, see page 224.) The methods are as follows.

1. Cleanse the genitals with soap and water and rinse them thoroughly. The receptacle is washed with soap and water unless a *clean*

specimen is ordered, in which case the receptacle should be sterilized before using. A sterile specimen is obtained by catheterization (see p. 339).

2. Cover the edges of glass receptacles with adhesive tape to prevent cutting of the genitals.

3. Elevate the head of the bed so that urine will run by gravity into the receptacle.

4. Restrain the child if necessary. A small, inactive infant probably needs no restraint. An older, active infant may be restrained with "mummy restraint" (Fig. 41, p. 149), extremity restraint (p. 224), clove-hitch restraint (p. 168), abdominal restraint (p. 225) or jacket restraint (p. 431), depending on his age.

5. Use as little adhesive tape as possible on the child's skin so as to reduce the irritation caused by its removal. When removing the tape, pull the skin away from the tape, not the tape from the skin. This will lessen the irritation from the process.

6. When a T binder is used, pin the waist band securely. Draw the narrow strips between the legs, under the buttocks, and pin them to the waistband at each side.

7. Encourage the child to take increased fluids.

8. Cleanse the genitals and dry them carefully after removing the receptacle.

*Procedures in Girls.* The Spicer infant urinal (see Fig. 10, *B*) or bird-seed cup (see Fig. 10, *A*) is most commonly used in the collection of a specimen of urine from a girl infant. Either of these glass receptacles can be placed over the urethra after the labia have been spread apart. The receptacle can be held in place by a tightly pinned three-cornered diaper (see Fig. 10, *A*) or by a T binder (see Fig. 10, *B*).

*Procedures in Boys.* 1. A test tube of adequate size is inserted through the hole of a T binder (see Fig. 11, *A*). The tube should fit tightly in the hole so that it does not slip out of place. The test tube is placed over the penis and the T binder secured snugly so that the tube does not slip.

2. The rolled end of a finger cot is placed over the end of a test tube, and a piece of adhesive tape, ½ inch wide, is wrapped around the tube to hold the finger cot in place. The tip is cut from the other end of the finger cot. The finger cot is punctured several times with a pin to allow the air to escape from the tube when the child voids. The test tube is then placed over the penis. A strip of adhesive tape, ½ inch wide, is run under the end of the penis, brought around the penis and crossed over the lower part of the abdomen (see Fig. 11, *B*). This piece of adhesive tape is attached to the finger cot so as to hold it in place. The finger cot must not be long enough to twist and constrict the circulation of the penis.

**Collection of Blood Specimens.** Blood specimens are obtained for various reasons: for determination of the degree of illness, for diagnosis or for evaluation of the therapy used.

The procedure used for adult patients is used for older children whose veins are large enough and who are able to

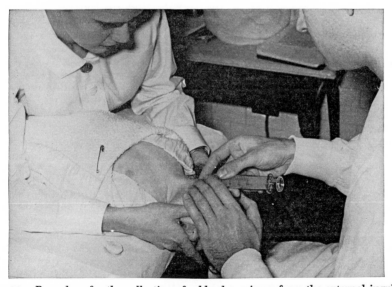

**Figure 12.** Procedure for the collection of a blood specimen from the external jugular vein. The "mummy restraint" (see Fig. 41) is used. The child's head is rotated fully to one side and extended partly over the end of the table to stretch the vein. The nurse places the palm of one hand over the occiput, the fingers of the other hand over the bones of the face. The nurse must avoid making pressure over the child's nose or mouth.

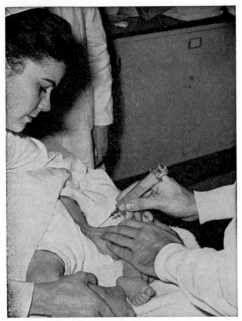

**Figure 13.** Procedure for the collection of a blood specimen from the femoral vein. The "mummy restraint" is used over the upper part of the child's body. The nurse spreads the child's legs apart in a frog position and holds them securely. The infant's genitals are covered with a diaper.

cooperate after an explanation of the procedure has been given them. In infants and young children whose veins are small only the larger veins may be used. Those most commonly used are the femoral or external jugular veins. Since infants and small children cannot understand a verbal explanation, mummy restraint is used, and the procedure is completed as soon as possible.

The nurse's responsibility is to restrain the child's head during jugular puncture (see Fig. 12) or the legs during femoral puncture (see Fig. 13).

After the needle has been removed from the jugular vein firm pressure should be exerted over the vein for three to five minutes while the child is held in a sitting position. After femoral vein puncture firm pressure should be exerted over the vein, also for three to five minutes, in order to prevent leakage of blood into the subcutaneous tissues.

**Medications.** The giving of medica-

tions to a child is a serious responsibility. There is even greater need for accuracy in pouring and giving medications than with adult patients. The dose varies with the size and age of the child, and the nurse has no standard dose which she is accustomed to give as in giving medication to adult patients. Since the dose is relatively small, a slight mistake in the amount of a drug given makes a greater proportional error in terms of the amount ordered than with the adult dose.

Every hospital has its own method of identification for patients. Identification is necessary with all patients, but is more difficult with children. The infant cannot give his name, and a small child is likely to give his nickname or only his first name. The nurse must carefully identify a child before giving him medication. Most hospitals use wrist bands for identifying children, and the child's name is also marked upon his bed. A double check on the child who is out of bed and old enough to tell his name is to ask him his name. (The nurse should never say, "Are you Alice White?" but should ask, "What is your name?") The child's name is checked with that on the medicine card, as is done in giving medication to adult patients.

The nurse should give all medications in a way that helps her to establish a constructive relation with the child. To tell a child that a medicine will taste good when it tastes bad destroys a child's faith in nurses.

Since the possibility of error is greater in the giving of medication to children than to adults, and since a child's reaction to a dose ordered by the physician is less predictable than an adult's reaction, the nurse must be alert to recognize undesirable effects of the medication given the child.

*Drug Dosage.* Since most drugs are put up by drug companies in a convenient form or strength for giving a standard adult dose, children's doses are often computed in terms of fractions of the adult dose on the basis of age or weight. Although the physician prescribes the dosage of medication, the nurse should have a general knowledge of the relation between the customary adult dose and that for children in different age groups from infancy through childhood. The following rules for calculating drug dosages for children are frequently used:

*Clark's Rule*

$$\text{Child's dose} = \frac{\text{Adult dose} \times \text{weight in pounds}}{150 \text{ (weight of average adult)}}$$

*Cowling's Rule*

$$\text{Child's dose} = \frac{\text{Adult dose} \times \text{age next birthday}}{24}$$

*Young's Rule*

$$\text{Child's dose} = \frac{\text{Adult dose} \times \text{age}}{\text{Age plus 12}}$$

Dosages based on the child's weight (Clark's rule) give the most accurate results. Many drugs are calculated entirely on this basis. Although the nurse does not decide the dosage to be given the child, she must be alert to amounts of drugs customarily ordered by the physicians. If an amount ordered seems to her to be excessive, she should call it to the attention of the physician. The nurse should know the expected action of the drug as well as the appropriate dose commonly ordered for a child the size of her patient. She should also be alert to symptoms of overdosage and report such symptoms at once to the physician so that quick action can be taken to counteract the effects of the drug.

*Oral Administration.* Infants will generally accept medication put into their mouths, provided it is in a form which they can readily swallow. A bib should be placed on the infant, and the medication should be given slowly. The nurse should raise the infant to a sitting position or, if this is contraindicated, elevate his head and shoulders. There is then less danger of his choking.

The older child, because he is unhappy in the hospital or has had experience with bad-tasting medicines, may refuse his medication. There is no single technique for winning his cooperation. The child is an individual, and the nurse must study the situation and find the best way to get him to take the medication. Her manner should be positive, firm and kind. When the nurse gives a child a feeling of support, that she understands his dislike of the medication and appreciates cooperation, he is conditioned to take the medication. She must convey in her manner rather than in words that he *must take the medication.* She should never plead or coax. Children will cooperate more readily if they see other children taking their medicine.

It is a good plan to disguise the taste of a drug by putting it in cherry syrup, Karo or honey syrup. Pills should be crushed and the contents of capsules emptied and mixed with syrup for children too young to take bulk medication. In general, medications should not be mixed with milk or food unless specifically ordered by the physician, because the child might develop a serious dislike for that food.

Medication can be given from a medicine glass, the tip of a teaspoon or a rubber-tipped medicine dropper. Fluids may be offered with bright-colored straws through which the child may suck the fluid medication.

The nurse should be careful not to let her own distaste for a drug show in her expression, for the child will quickly adopt this attitude toward his medicine from her.

If a child always struggles when medication is given him and his cooperation cannot be obtained, the nurse should report this to the physician. To struggle may do the child more harm than to go without his medicine. The nurse should never hold the child's nose or force the medication into his mouth, for he may aspirate the medication. Such action shows that the nurse is hostile and not helpful to the child.

If the medication is immediately vomited, the physician should be notified. He may order the dose to be repeated. Unpleasant-tasting drugs should not be given around mealtime, for they may interfere with the child's appetite or nutrition.

The child old enough to take pills should be told to place the pill near the back of his tongue and to drink the fruit juice or milk offered him in order to wash down the pill.

A child who cooperates in taking his medicine should be praised and thereby will know that his nurse appreciates his help.

*Intramuscular Injections.* The giving of the first intramuscular injection is important because on the basis of this experience the child builds up his attitude toward future injections. The procedure is the same as for the adult. The needle should have a sharp point so that it will not cause unnecessary pain.

If the child is old enough to understand, the procedure should be explained to him. He should be allowed to express his fear and resentment of needles. The procedure should be carried out quickly and gently. It is a good plan to have a second nurse assist. She supports or restrains the child, or both, and diverts his attention. Since the injection is painful, the nurse must help him master his feeling about such necessary forms of treatment.

With small children it is customary to use the upper outer quadrant of the buttocks for intramuscular injections. The tissue should be held firmly at the site of the injection. If the child is old enough to have sufficiently large muscles on other parts of the body, the injection site should be varied.

The syringe and the needle are held in a perpendicular position. The nurse must be certain to have the needle in a muscle. She should pull back on the plunger to make certain that the needle is not in a vein.

After the procedure the nurse should show her approval of the infant or child for his cooperation and hold him for a few minutes so that he does not associate only pain with her ministrations. He may then be given some toy to divert his attention from the experience. If he has been uncooperative, the nurse should not show disapproval. He too should be held and comforted and then given a toy.

An older child may be allowed to select the site for injection, subject to the nurse's approval, and cleanse the area for himself.

Verbal explanations can be given the child of school age and the adolescent. They are less fearful, but, like the little child, should be allowed to vent their feelings of dislike or resentment.

*Rectal Administration.* Drugs given by rectum are injected in the same manner as a retention enema. (Paraldehyde may be given rectally.) The medication may be mixed with a little water or a small amount of starch solution. It should be given slowly so that all of it is retained. Some medications to be given rectally are also available in suppository form.

### Summary

The comprehensive nursing care which the nurse will give during hospitalization should meet the physical and emotional needs of the individual child and his family. The child will thereby have minimal anxiety and will learn to trust others than the familiar members of his family. Within the framework of his medical care the nurse will provide for his physical activity, alternating with periods of rest, and in every way reduce frustrations to a minimum. She should help the parents to accept the child's disability, whether temporary or permanent, and, by letting them participate in his care, strengthen their self-confidence in their ability to nurse him when he is discharged.

In order to fulfill her role in the total plan of care for every hospitalized child, the nurse must think through her own feelings about each family. In some hospitals a psychiatrist is available to help her, not only so that she may learn how to handle her own emotional problems, but also so that what she does and says will have an immediate and beneficial influence on the parents' attitudes and on the child's condition. Of all the members of the health team, the nurse, by rejection of a child or his parents, would be the most injurious. If she accepts the child, she will learn, while nursing him, to apply her theoretical knowledge and past experience to his care. Having done this, she is in a position to teach the parents.

The mother of a chronically ill child who has been cared for at home can help the nurse in this adaptation of her general knowledge of pediatric nursing to the care of the particular patient. The mother should be considered a member of the health team, the one who works most closely with the nurses.

### DISCHARGE FROM THE HOSPITAL

The physician or nurse, or psychiatrist if he was attached to the health team, should tell the parents that it is natural for an infant, or even an older child, when he is taken home, to show symptoms of a disturbed relation with his parents. He may be more clinging and seek more affection than before hospitalization, but the reverse may also be true, and he may withdraw from or even reject his mother. He may show his need for comfort by sucking his thumb excessively or reverting to behaviorisms which he had outgrown. His mother must accept this regression as the result of the emotional trauma produced by his separation from her and must help him to regain the normal mother-child relations by her unwavering affection.

Discharge of a child from the pediatric unit to his parents' care requires explicit instructions, especially if his mother has not stayed with him during his hospitalization. Important among these are instructions in the use of any specific article of equipment needed in his care at home, and in the giving of medications; review of the physician's orders; time of the next clinic or physician's appointment; and description of new habits which the child has acquired since his mother last cared for him— e.g. drinking from a cup or eating from a spoon—or new developments in muscular activity. If an infant has learned to roll over, it is important that his mother know it in order to protect him from falling. These new habits change not only the mother's image of her child, but also the way in which she gives him care.

## GUIDES TO FURTHER STUDY

1. What is your understanding of the role of the professional nurse in providing care for a sick child? What should be the nurse's relations with the child and with his parents?

2. Make a survey in your community of the types of agencies which provide care for well and for sick children. List them and their specific functions.

3. Study the *Declaration of the Rights of the Child* (p. 6). To what extent do you believe these "rights" are provided for the children in (a) an urban area and (b) a rural area known to you? How are these provided for in these two areas? What conditions in these areas prevent the achievement of any of these goals?

4. Recall a hospitalization experience during childhood. (This may be your own experience or that of a sibling or friend.) Was this a positive or a negative experience? Give specific memories you have about it and propose ways by which they could have been made more pleasant.

5. Define and differentiate clearly between the following terms: (a) growth and development and (b) eugenics and euthenics.

6. Obtain either your own, a sibling's or a friend's "Baby Book." List the steps of growth and development which have been recorded in it. Summarize the principles of growth and development and apply them to this record.

7. Select a well sibling or a friend's child in any of the following age groups: birth to 1 year, 1 to 3 years, 3 to 6 years, 6 to 12 years or 12 to 18 years. Discuss the growth and development and care of this child with his parents. Define the problems these parents are facing with this child. In class each student will discuss the child she has investigated, highlighting important points about the child's home, type of family, his community, and his physical, emotional, social and mental growth and development, and care.

8. Discuss individually with your own or a friend's grandmother and mother their attitudes about the care of children. State the differences in philosophy or child care practices expressed. What would some of the reasons be for these differences?

9. Immediately after the admission of a child to the hospital, observe the behavior of both the parent and the child. On the basis of specific observations you have made draw conclusions as to the feelings of the parent and the child. What could you as a nurse do to help this parent and child face this situation less anxiously or more positively?

10. What can you observe in the children's area on which you are working that would help a child feel more "at home" in the hospital setting?

11. Evaluate the unit in which you are working as to its safety for the care of children. List your findings and make constructive suggestions for its improvement.

12. List the various kinds of personnel in the pediatric unit who provide some type of care or

guidance for children and/or their parents. Differentiate as clearly as you can between the functions of these persons.

13. Select a patient who is receiving various types of medications. Check the dosages of these drugs according to Clark's rule, Cowling's rule and Young's rule. What would be your professional responsibility if you found a notable discrepancy between the dose ordered and the result of your calculations?

14. Children and adults react differently to disease processes. Explain why this is true and what effect this understanding has or will have on the type of care you give to children.

## REFERENCES

American Academy of Pediatrics: Care of Children in Hospitals. Evanston, Ill., American Academy of Pediatrics, 1960.

Baty, J. M., and Tisza, V. E. B.: The Impact of Illness on the Child and His Family. Child Study, 34:No. 1, 15, 1956.

Benson, M. E.: Handwashing—An Important Part of Medical Asepsis. Am. J. Nursing, 57:1136, 1957.

Blom, G. E.: The Reactions of Hospitalized Children to Illness. Pediatrics, 22:590, 1958.

Erickson, F.: Reactions of Children to Hospital Experience. Nursing Outlook, 6:501, 1958.

Faddis, M. O., and Hayman, J. M.: Textbook of Pharmacology for Nurses. 5th ed. Philadelphia, J. B. Lippincott Company, 1959.

Gofman, H., and others: The Child's Emotional Response to Hospitalization. A.M.A. J. Dis. Child., 93:157, 1957.

Grossman, E. R.: Device for Urine Collections. Pediatrics, 22:778, 1958.

Hart, E. L., and Magee, M. J.: Collecting Urine Specimens. Am. J. Nursing, 57:1323, 1957.

Hemmendinger, M.: Treatment—'Admit Parents at All Times.' Child Study, 34:No. 1, 3, 1956.

Hohle, B. M.: We Admit Parents Too. Am. J. Nursing, 57:865, 1957.

Hunt, A. D.: An Experiment in Teamwork. Child Study, 34:No. 1, 10, 1956.

Idem: Parent Participation in the Hospitalization of Children. A.M.A. J. Dis. Child., 96: 616, 1958.

Hunt, A. D., and Trussell, R. E.: They Let Parents Help in Children's Care. The Modern Hospital, 85:89, September, 1955.

Loeb, D. G.: Problems of Children in Hospitals. Understanding the Child. 24:7, January, 1955.

Moore, B. R.: When Johnny Must Go to the Hospital. Am. J. Nursing, 57:178, 1957.

Musser, R., and Bird, J. G.: Modern Pharmacology and Therapeutics. New York, Macmillan Company, 1958.

Nelson, W. E. (editor): Textbook of Pediatrics. 7th ed. Philadelphia, W. B. Saunders Company, 1959.

O'Connell, E. A., and Brandt, P.: Liberal Visiting Hours for Parents. Am. J. Nursing, 60: 812, 1960.

Report by the Citizens Committee on Children of New York City, Inc.: Liberal Visiting Policies for Children in Hospitals. J. Pediat., 46:710, 1955.

Robertson, J.: Young Children in Hospitals. New York, Basic Books, Inc., 1958.

Terry, F. J., and others: Principles and Techniques of Rehabilitation Nursing. St. Louis, C. V. Mosby Company, 1957.

Work, H. H.: Making Hospitalization Easier for Children. Children, 3:83, 1956.

Wright, H. N., and Montag, M.: A Textbook of Pharmacology and Therapeutics. 7th ed. Philadelphia, W. B. Saunders Company, 1959.

# The Newborn

# Chapter 5

# The Newborn,

# His Family and the Nurse

## ENVIRONMENT AND DEVELOPMENT OF THE FETUS

THE UTERUS of a healthy woman is perfectly adapted to the needs of the fetus. Her body is the medium which adapts conditions outside her to the developmental immaturity of the fetus. Since her heat-regulating mechanism keeps the temperature within the uterus constant, changes in outdoor or room temperature do not affect the fetus. The amniotic fluid which surrounds it in her uterus acts as a sterile insulating medium in which there is no friction.

The fetus, like the infant, needs oxygen and nourishment in order to live and grow. These are supplied through the blood stream of the prospective mother by way of the placenta and umbilical cord. Through the same route the fetus is relieved of the waste products of metabolism.

The fetus is completely dependent upon the mother for all vital functions because the fetal organs have not developed to the extent that extrauterine life is possible. The lungs are not inflated. The circulatory system is adapted only to intrauterine life; little blood flows through the pulmonary artery, since the foramen ovale and the ductus arteriosus are not closed as they are after the birth process. The digestive tract cannot reduce even the simplest foods to the state in which elements can be taken up by the blood stream.

The world we live in reaches the fetus only through the mother's body. If she is healthy and receives good prenatal care, the fetus will thrive. But if she is leading an unhealthy life, its vitality is endangered. Even then, however, the fetus tends to normal development at the expense of the mother, as if its needs take precedence over her bodily requirements. An accident to the woman may involve the fetus. Anything which interferes with the normal transfer of oxygen or nutriment from the

**67**

maternal blood stream to that of the fetus will jeopardize its safety.

# THE NEWBORN

## NEONATAL HAZARDS AND PREPARATION

Birth is associated with the most drastic changes that will ever befall a person. In extrauterine life all functions undergo a radical change. There is a sudden adjustment to be made from a "topsy-turvy aquatic environment" to a so-called sane air existence. After birth the infant must not only continue the vital activities of intrauterine life, but must also initiate other extrauterine processes which were performed for him by his mother. The normal infant is able to do this, provided he receives essential care. If the infant is to survive the crucial neonatal period, three conditions are necessary: that he be in good physical condition, that he experience a safe delivery and that he then receive good care.

### Infant Mortality

Improvement in maternal and infant care has greatly reduced the infant mortality rate in the last fifteen to twenty years, but the decrease has been slower in the neonatal period than in the remaining months of infancy. The highest infant death rate is within the first month of life, and within that month in the first twenty-four hours. The most critical period for the infant is the first hour of life, when the drastic change from intrauterine to extrauterine existence occurs. More than one third of the total deaths occurring in the first year of life are in the first day of life, and more than two thirds in the first four weeks.

The chief cause of death in the newborn period is *prematurity* (see Fig. 5). The causes of premature birth and the characteristics and care of premature infants are of such importance that they are discussed separately in Chapter 8. Other causes of death in the neonatal period are *congenital malforma-tions* which render it impossible for the infant to establish an independent existence, *birth injuries, asphyxia* and *atelectasis.* All these conditions are discussed in succeeding chapters. Here we should take note that the causes of congenital malformations are not clearly understood. The number of those infants who are kept alive and their condition relieved or mitigated by surgery is much higher than it was in the past. Birth injuries are not as common a cause of death as they were even a decade ago. An increasing number of prospective mothers are receiving better prenatal care. Difficult deliveries are anticipated and arrangements made for hospitalization of the mothers. Instrumental and operative deliveries are more judicious. The trained nurse-midwife is replacing the experienced but ignorant midwife of the rural south and has completely replaced her in the slums of the large cities. For these reasons the percentage of infants injured during delivery has been reduced.

**Health and Welfare Measures for Reduction of Infant Mortality.** The environment of a pregnant woman influences her health, which in turn creates a healthful or unhealthful environment for the fetus. Unfortunately not all pregnant women can be provided with a healthful environment, but federal, state and local health and welfare programs have made a great difference in the conditions under which the low-income group lives. Maternal and infant death rates are likely to be much lower in federal-state housing projects than in the surrounding area. Free or "pay-what-you-can" clinics have had a tremendous influence on the welfare of mothers and babies. The infant death rate is falling rapidly in this lower-income group, which often receives more adequate care than the middle-income group. Since newborn infants are prone to suffer infections of the respiratory and intestinal tracts and pyogenic or other skin infections, the death rate among them is influenced more than that of adults by good sanitation in the community, cleanliness in the home, fresh air, sunshine, and avoidance of overcrowding in sleeping and living rooms.

Some pregnant women, because of a lack of self-discipline, are not willing to make the effort to lead wholesome lives. They do not go to a physician early in pregnancy, and when they do, they pay little attention to his advice. To win them over to a different attitude toward their own health and safety

MORTALITY OF INFANTS BEFORE, DURING, AND AFTER BIRTH

UNITED STATES, 1942-58

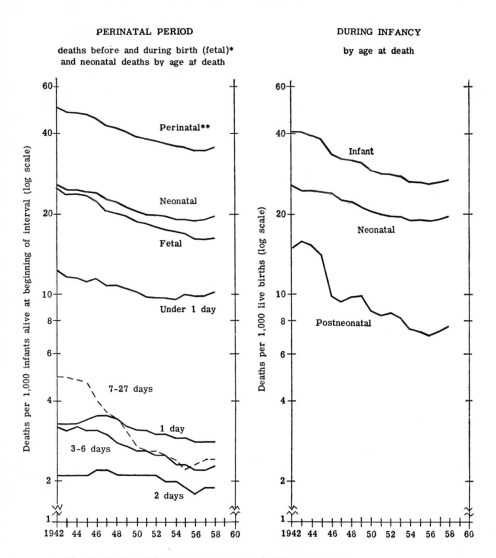

*In pregnancies of 20 or more weeks or duration unreported.

**To the end of the neonatal period.

Figure 14.   Mortality of infants before, during and after birth in the United States, 1942–58. (Department of Health, Education, and Welfare; Social Security Administration, Children's Bureau. Based on data from the National Office of Vital Statistics.)

and to create in them a great desire for the infant is a challenging task for the nurse.

The young student nurse has a special role in working with these mothers. She is likely to have good rapport with the young prospective mother because as a nurse she is intensely interested in pregnancy, knows well the physical processes that are taking place and, by her own attitude toward health and confidence in the medical advice given, influences the patient in a way different from that in which the older nurse, medical social worker or even the physician influences her. The young nurse, working under the direction of her clinical instructor or supervisor, has a special function which has only recently been recognized.

As long as the infant is well his mother can be taught to give him all the care he needs, and she probably gives it better than anyone else because of her innate love for him. There are, of course, some mothers who either do not love their children or are unable to show their love in ways that transmit security to them. The cause for such an unnatural condition is often extremely difficult to determine. The mother may be in need of psychiatric treatment. When the mother cannot give her infant the loving care he needs, some other person must be found to serve as a mother-substitute or to supplement the care she gives.

Although mothers under the direction of their physicians are the best people to care for their well babies, if the baby is not gaining as he should or is ill, the professional services of the nurse are needed. Infants have surprising vitality, but little resistance to disease, particularly disease which interferes with electrolyte balance, such as dehydration because of diarrhea, or massive infection with or without a high fever. Mothers must be taught that they cannot safely wait to see whether the baby will be all right the next morning. He must be seen by a physician, and measures must be taken to prevent the condition from becoming worse.

Clinics, outpatient departments and admitting departments of hospitals, particularly in the low-income areas of large cities, are open twenty-four hours of the day and every day in the week. Immediate availability of the physician and the nurse, and hospitalization if necessary, is extremely important, for the infant lacks the adult's resistance to conditions causing pathologic states. His body is still poorly adapted to meet adverse factors such as infection, injury or improper feeding. All this is doubly true in the premature infant, whose development is even more immature than that of the full-term infant.

Even a healthy infant needs to be kept on a good regimen directed by a physician who examines him at regular intervals. It is often the nurse who welcomes the mother to the physician's office or the Child Health Conference and helps her to understand the physician's suggestions. Nurses in Child Health Conferences and outpatient departments of hospitals observe these well infants brought for routine checkups. They look for signs that the infant is not gaining as he should, has some chronic condition or is in the first stage of an acute disease. They must be particularly skillful in observing symptoms and eliciting information from a mother, since the infant cannot say how he feels.

In the final analysis these great Health and Welfare programs extend care to individual children, through whom the nurse makes her great contribution to the reduction of infant mortality. Whether the student is having her clinical experience in the pediatric unit or in a public health agency, she is working with individual babies. Only by keeping each one healthy and caring for each one when he is sick or in need of operation will infant morbidity and mortality rates be reduced.

### Parental Education

Education for parenthood begins with the general education of the child for responsibilities in family living. More specifically, parental education today begins with the courses which prepare

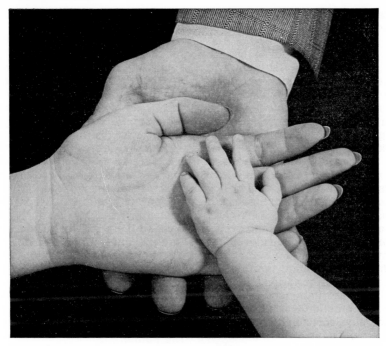

Figure 15.  The child, in addition to physical care, needs the love and affection of his parents.
(H. Armstrong Roberts.)

men and women for family life. Such courses are offered in undergraduate and adult education programs. Lectures or conferences for young wives who are pregnant—their husbands are invited to attend—include discussion of the physical and emotional needs of infants and how these needs can best be met. The emotional needs are considered to be as important as the physical needs, for lack of affection shown in ways a baby can understand has an adverse influence on personality development. Among these needs is that for contact with a soft, warm human body and the slight motion which comes from gentle handling and cuddling in his mother's arms.

## FAMILY RESPONSES TO THE NEWBORN

### The Mother

In caring for the newborn the nurse bases her role on much more than an understanding of his physical attributes. It is her responsibility to help the parents build a happier family life through

Figure 16.  Members of the health team should encourage the close relation between the mother and her newborn child. (William M. Rittase.)

his coming. In order to do this she must understand the mutual dependency of the mother and her infant.

Mother love is supposed to be the strongest emotional tie between two human beings. The influence of the endocrine glands as they function in the pregnant or lactating mother is evident even among the higher animals. They are gentle in handling their young and are likely to be fiercely protective of them. If all her offspring are taken from a mother, she will become restless, may refuse to eat and may evidence her frustration at the blocking of an instinct based on glandular secretion. The human mother has not only this physical basis for her dependency on her infant, but also a love for him which has been developing through the long nine months of gestation. If she is separated from her baby, she is denied relief from an emotional need based in part on her physical condition.

Up to the child's birth there has been a *symbiotic relation* between the mother and the fetus. A symbiotic relation is one of extreme closeness. Before birth the fetus existed as a parasite within his mother. The two—mother and fetus—were necessary to each other. The fetus could not live without her body supplying his needs, and she in turn needed the product of conception to complete the physical changes which pregnancy was producing in her. If the fetus should die, the mother would feel emotionally distraught.

Mothers desire to continue this symbiotic relation after the child's birth, and the nurse should recognize the importance of the tie. Modern obstetrical nursing is planned to keep mother and baby together, his bassinet beside her bed. Mothers are urged to nurse their infants, since breast feeding is the closest approach to a symbiotic relation which can be achieved after the birth of the child. The importance of rooming-in is considered on page 77. Breast feeding is discussed in Chapter 7.

### The Father

The father lacks the glandular basis for feelings of tenderness and gentle-

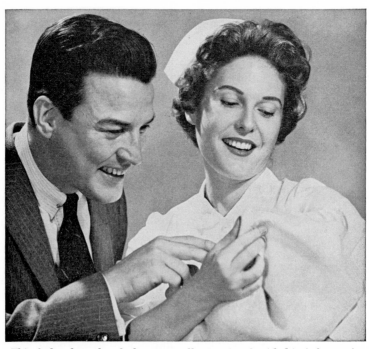

**Figure 17.** This father has already become well acquainted with his infant prior to its discharge from the hospital. (H. Armstrong Roberts.)

ness toward the infant. There is, however, a glandular basis for the attraction of the male and the female for one another. This tends to an acceptance by the male of the offspring she loves. This physical basis for the foundation of the family is socially reinforced, so that the family is the strongest social institution in our society.

The father actually has two responsibilities in the family after the birth of his child. His first responsibility is to his wife. The hormonal changes which are inevitable after childbirth produce in many women a state of depression. The mother needs to feel at this time that she is loved so that she in turn can love her infant. The father, therefore, must not only feel love toward his wife, but must also communicate this feeling to her.

The role of the father is honored in every Christian society. The father, like the mother, has looked forward to having a son or a daughter. Half of the child's heredity is transmitted through him, and the infant is as much a continuation of himself as of his wife. He has also the moral obligation to be a provider. In a family the children need the masculine influence as much as they do the feminine. They need a father's affection as they need a mother's. But because of the newborn's immediate need for his mother, the father's role is likely to appear subsidiary and to be taken as a matter of course, and he may feel left out of this most important event in married life.

The modern father, however, unlike *his* father, is not willing to be left out of all these new activities in the home. He accepts odd chores connected with the baby. He changes diapers, picks his little son up when he cries and cuddles him as successfully as the mother. In this way he reaches the baby's consciousness and lays the basis for affection. As the infant responds, the father becomes increasingly fond of taking an active part in his care. The mother, of course, appreciates this help. So the coming of the baby has strengthened their love for each other through their love for the newborn infant.

## The Siblings

The siblings' reaction to the arrival of a new baby in the family is conditioned by their parents' attitude and the number of other members in the family. Little children are egotistical and are likely to think of a little brother or sister in terms of whether he or she makes life more pleasant or less pleasant for them. If they are allowed to share in the care of the baby and if they feel certain that he is not taking their place in their parents' affection, they are likely to be proud of him and later learn to love him dearly.

## The Grandparents

The grandparents are happy in the coming of the baby. The maternal grandmother is probably most deeply interested in him and can be a real help to the mother. It is seldom a good plan for her to live in her daughter's home, but she makes an excellent baby sitter and, if the mother returns to work outside the home, may assume the entire care of the baby during the day.

### THE NEWBORN'S RESPONSE TO BIRTH

That giving birth to a child is difficult and even dangerous for the mother is common knowledge, but that even an easy normal birth must be a great strain upon the baby is seldom realized. His body sustains the pressure of the uterine contractions and his head the pressure of the resisting cervix. Although good obstetrical care prevents injury to the infant as well as to the mother and makes his passage through the birth canal less exhausting, birth still remains an anxiety-provoking experience. To this is added the necessity to adapt to life as a separate entity, no longer part of the mother. Her body, if healthy, shielded him from the direct influence of cold, heat, trauma and infection. On the other hand, if the mother was unable or unwilling to make of her body a good environment for the child, little could be done to help him until after birth. After birth good hygiene influences the baby not through his mother, but directly. If a mother neglects her infant, he can be legally taken from her and placed in a foster home. The infant of a tuberculous mother, however, should be taken from her at birth and cared for by relatives or placed in a foster home to avoid neonatal infection.

As long as the fetus is nurtured through his mother's body, his health and that of his mother are the concern of the obstetrician and the obstetrical nurse. But the infant's health after birth is the concern of the pediatrician and the pediatric nurse, whether or not he remains with his mother.

### The World as the Infant Experiences It

Since an infant's senses are not acute and discriminating at birth, the world about him must appear to be "one great, blooming, buzzing confusion." Yet the beginning of personality is there; he is not just another baby. How far personality at birth determines that of the older child or adult is not known, but it is certain that environmental factors modify personality early in infancy. The infant has two great drives: to be loved and to love. The physical drives of the infant who is loved are sure to be satisfied, but the unloved infant is likely to be neglected. (Although the need to be loved is evident at birth, the drive to love is not manifested until later.) The infant equates the relief of a need with love. Since hunger is an imperative need, it is natural that his infant love goes to the person who feeds him. Assured of food and cuddling, the infant develops a sense of *trust*. The implication of this is that when the mother holds her baby to her breast while he nurses or when she feeds him from the bottle, she is showing him love in a way that he can sense. The loved, contented baby forms a habit of contentment and does not easily become fretful. Anxiety-arousing stimuli should be kept from the baby, for a habit of anxiety can be as easily aroused as that of contentment.

Some psychologists believe that the infant is capable of fear and anger at birth. If so, these two emotions are difficult to distinguish. Sudden loss of support or a loud noise will produce a reflex startle reaction, and this is said to be evidence of fear. When he is roaring, we infer that he is angry. In either case he is reacting to a stimulus which he does not like and wants to have stopped. He soon learns that crying will bring someone who will make him comfortable. Since it is generally his mother who does this for him, he soon learns to prefer her to other people. This appears to be the basis of his love for his mother. She responds to his flattering preference for her with endearing attention, and so the cycle of mother-baby, baby-mother love is strengthened. Secure in her care for him, he will accept supplementary care from other people, provided it is *like* that which she gives him.

The child who is cared for by a changing group of people fails to form an affectionate attachment to anyone. He is likely to be very self-centered, and this situation, if continued, is one factor in producing the autistic child (see p. 581).

One principle on which child care is based is that the baby needs consistent loving care given by one or two people, a minimal amount of anxiety and a maximum amount of contentment. Only then can the infant learn to adapt to his new environment.

## ROLE OF THE PROFESSIONAL NURSE

### Needs of the Parents

The role of the nurse in caring for the family during the postpartum period must be based not on the needs of the hospital and its staff, but rather on the needs of the parents and their child.

The new family relations which spring from the arrival of the baby are evidenced through all the hours of the day and night, as a new element in the former kinship within the family. The family relations before the first pregnancy were that of one to one, but with the birth of the first child each member

The relations of husband and wife are like this:

Those of a husband, wife and child can be diagrammed like this:

Those of a husband, wife, and 2 children look like this:

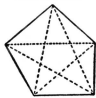

Those of a husband, wife, and 3 children look like this:

Within every family there are 2 variables which submit to precise mathematical determination. One of these is the number of members in the family, i.e., the size of the group; the other is the number of personal relations between its members. If these 2 variables are considered mathematically, what happens with the addition of each new member of the family group may be set forth in the following 2 sets of numbers:

Number of persons. . . . 2, 3, 4, 5, 6, 7, 8
Number of personal relations. . 1, 3, 6, 10, 15, 21, 28

**Figure 18.** Bossard's Law of Family Interaction. (J. H. S. Bossard: The Sociology of Child Development. Rev. Ed. New York, Harper and Brothers.)

is related to two others. Neither parent may now expect the entire love and attention of the other. With the second and succeeding births the change in relations becomes more complex. Figure 18 presents these family relations. Note that the father's place in this diagram is comparable to that of the mother.

The supportive role of the professional nurse in the adjustment of the parents to their new relations to one another and to their child is enacted while giving the mother and her infant physical care. It is this support which gives her role its peculiar significance and makes it more effective than that of the other professional members of the health team. Other team members, of course, give physical help to patients, but it is not characterized by meeting their daily recurrent needs and so is less likely to be helpful in adjustment to a new situation which involves the minute details of family life.

The first mother-father-infant experience is generally set in motion by the nurse, who comes with the baby in her arms. Obviously her role is an important one.

We are apt to concentrate attention on the mother rather than on the father. This is justified, but both parents (particularly if this is their first child) need help in making all the necessary adjustments involved in childbirth and in the care of the newborn infant. The nurse can help them in many ways. She, more than any other member of the hospital staff, makes them feel at home. She is hostess in the hospital and makes the first meeting of the mother and the father, after the birth of their child, emotionally satisfying. The nurse should remember that the mother will be thinking of all that was said and done in this first brief visit until her husband comes again. A satisfying visit promotes tranquil rest; an unsatisfying one, emotional disturbance.

It is true that what the nurse may allow the parents is controlled by hospital policies. If the hospital imposes stringent rules as to visiting hours and viewing the infant, this first meeting of husband and wife may be so emotionally unsatisfying that the mother's physical condition is adversely influenced by her disappointment. In any case, however, the nurse's friendly, cordial manner is helpful.

The nurse should accept the mother's dependency needs and not expect from her all the self-care of which she is physically capable. In the early days of ambulation after delivery it is easy for the nurse to forget the emotional effect of childbirth upon a young mother. If the mother is not emotionally ready for the routine self-care which is customary in the hospital, the nurse should do for her what she feels she cannot do for herself. The mother should never be made to feel that she is failing to live up to the nurse's concept of the modern woman who accepts childbirth as a natural process which incapacitates the mother for only a day or two. (Even the most ardent believer in natural childbirth realizes that not all women are capable of carrying it to completion without emotional trauma. This is true also of early self-care.) Nurses should accept and understand the reactions of each mother and plan her care accordingly. When both the physical and the emotional needs of the mother have been met, the mother feels secure in the hospital and can accept the rest she requires before returning to her duties as homemaker. Because of the close emotional union of mother and child, she will not be content unless she knows that the infant, too, is well cared for and *loved* by the nurses. In such a permissive atmosphere the mother sees the application of what she has learned of child care.

The mother should be encouraged to talk over her recent experience in the delivery room and also any matter which worries her about the infant, her own condition or her home. Past experiences are interpreted in the light of the present. If the nurse makes the mother's stay in the hospital as pleasant as possible, the mother's attitude toward past, present and future pregnancies and deliveries is likely to be optimistic.

### Needs of the Newborn

The needs of the newborn are those of any young animal which nature made helpless and dependent upon its mother, but with this significant difference: he is the recipient of the scientific knowledge which only human beings possess and is himself one of the coming generation who will add to this fund of knowledge.

The nurse's knowledge of what is normal in a newborn baby enables her to know what is abnormal. She should observe and appraise the status of the infant when he is brought to the nursery in order that she may report any abnormalities which the physician may have overlooked or which did not appear until after the examination of the baby was completed. Many potentially dangerous abnormalities of the newborn can be treated before a serious physiologic disturbance results. These require early recognition and diagnosis.

The newborn is likely to be exhausted by the birth process, and gentle handling to conserve his strength is necessary. His personality is being formed by his experiences even during these first few days of life. Gentleness in handling him gives him the feeling of the world as a pleasant place which is necessary to his tranquil rest, enjoyment of feeding and learning to love in his immature way those who care for him. Gentleness in caring for him is an expression of love, and makes physical care—his bath and the changing of his diaper—a pleasure to him. He likes skin-to-skin contact. His heat-regulating system is so poorly developed that he needs external warmth. A soft cuddly blanket wrapped around him gives him the feeling of a closed environment of even temperature such as he experienced in the uterus. He needs frequent changes of position, not merely from lying on one side to the other, but also the many minor changes which occur when he is picked up and cuddled.

Although the healthy newborn is not the fragile little creature that he is sometimes thought to be, he has little resistance to infection of the respiratory or gastrointestinal tract or of the skin, and even less resistance to systemic infection. Fortunately such infections are uncommon.

**Self-Demand Schedule.** Today it is believed that the newborn responds to his bodily needs with sleeping when his body needs sleep and with crying to be fed when his body needs nourishment. He demands sleep and feedings in accordance with his rhythm of bodily functions, a rhythm which is fairly constant from day to day. His schedule should be planned in accordance with his demands and will vary with his physical condition. If he has a fever, he will, of course, want water more frequently, and his sleep will be intermittent. As he matures he will lengthen the interval between feedings and will take more at each feeding. His periods of wakefulness will be longer, and his total time spent in sleep will be less.

The self-demand schedule must be carried out in a stable environment adapted to the infant's immature development. This environment is both physical and social. The physical environment must be hygienic, and the social environment such that he learns to associate a feeling of well-being with the care given him. He should be held lovingly when fed, for feeding is to him an expression of love and conditions him both to want the manifestations of love that accompany the feeding and to love the one who feeds and cuddles him.

After the traumatic experience of birth the newborn needs time to acquire strength before he will begin to gain in weight and vigor. This is a period of adjustment for him in which the self-demand schedule is particularly important. He should be offered the breast or bottle, but never unduly urged. From the time he enters the nursery his comprehensive nursing care includes meeting both his physical and his emotional needs; otherwise he will not reach and maintain his optimum level of well-being and feel secure in the strange environment of the nursery.

### ROOMING-IN

What has been said about the needs of the newborn makes it clear that an environment can be planned which will be suitable for all infants, each of whom requires environmental adaptation to meet his needs. It is extremely difficult to provide this in a nursery where one or two nurses are caring for a large number of infants. Furthermore, babies need affection shown in ways which are peculiar to the mother-child relation and which no nurse can reproduce in the care of a constantly changing group of babies. Rooming-in is a method which provides for the baby, mother and nurse the conditions in which each is most satisfied and can most successfully fulfill his or her role.

Rooming-in is a term applied to the hospital arrangement whereby the mother has her newborn infant by her bedside and takes as much care of him as her condition permits and she desires. It is a family-centered service in the hospital situation. It is an effort to meet parents' requests for more information about the care of the baby, and it gives both the parents and the baby a homelike feeling in the impersonal hospital atmosphere.

The practice of rooming-in gives the young mother with her first child an opportunity to become acquainted with him and accustomed to his care. It relieves her anxiety as to his welfare in the nursery, where she often hears babies crying and is sure that one of them is hers. It permits the baby's father to hold or feed him or change his diaper. This is a different introduction from standing in the hall and looking through a glass window at a room full of infants while a nurse brings *the one* to the nursery side of the window.

The infant who rooms-in receives more individual attention, for his mother can reach over and pat him, change his position, give him water or replace a wet or soiled diaper. Feeding is promoted because when the mother sees her infant hungry, she is motivated to put him to the breast. If the physician approves of the infant's being on a self-demand schedule, the mother can easily feed him whenever he wants to nurse.

In contrast to this individual attention, in the nursery the infant's needs are likely to be met at certain fixed times suited to the average baby's schedule for feeding, sleep and periods of placid rest. The nursery schedule is adjusted to administrative and personnel considerations as well as to the needs of the average infant. Many infants are not average, however. Also, a baby's needs vary from day to day.

We do not know of any scientific study which has proved that rooming-in has a lasting influence on the child's personality, but it appears to be a happy

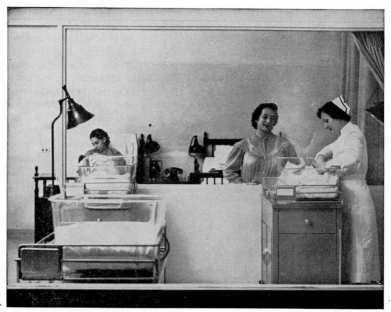

Figure 19.   In this rooming-in unit consisting of 2 double rooms separated by a nursery mothers may participate freely in the care of their babies. They may observe them at all times and still have sufficient privacy for rest and sleep. (Michael Reese Hospital.) (Davis and Sheckler: DeLee's Obstetrics for Nurses, 16th ed.)

experience for both him and his parents. Happiness is a great determinant in the formation of personality, and so rooming-in may conceivably exert a permanently good influence on personality formation.

Some mothers, however, do not want the baby's crib beside their bed. They do not want to feed him on a self-demand schedule, nor do they want to give him care. These are likely to be the mothers of large families who have been overworked up to the time of delivery. They are in need of a complete rest and should not be forced to do more for their infants than give them the breast or, if they are bottle-fed, hold them for a few minutes each day.

There are disadvantages to rooming-in, from the point of view of both the parents and the hospital. We have already noted that some mothers are neither physically nor emotionally able to do their part in the rooming-in care of an infant. The physician may feel that there is danger of infection, although the infectious conditions which the newborn is most likely to contract

are those which are carried from infant to infant by the hospital personnel or through the use of improperly sterilized equipment. The hospital administrator knows that rooming-in requires more well qualified personnel and uses more floor space than does the traditional type of care given to newborns in a central nursery.

For rooming-in to be successful, the staff nurses must have warm, comforting personalities. They must not insist on a rigid plan of nursing care. Rather, they should promote normal relations in the family and help the parents make their own plan for the infant. This they do by sharing with them their own knowledge of child care and giving the parents reassurance in their ability to meet any problems which may arise in the care of the infant.

### Modifications of Traditional Maternity Units

Although rooming-in would seem to be the ideal method by which the needs of both newborns and parents could be met, the practice is still not widely accepted in this country.

If rooming-in is not practical in the maternity area of the hospital, the same objectives may be attained in the traditional maternity unit by the following modifications in arrangement and in assignment of patients to the nursing personnel.

1. *Individual family units* may be assigned to the nurse for study and the making of a plan of care. She can observe the interpersonal relations within "her family" and plan the care of the mother and child with reference to their relation to the father, maternal grandmother or other relatives who are permitted to visit the patient. In this way she can carry out her supporting role with the family as a whole. If attention is focused on only one member, the needs of others are likely to be forgotten, and thereby the nurse may create friction within the family which reacts adversely on her patient. Of course if the hospital policy does not permit nurses who are caring for the mothers in the maternity unit to enter the newborn nursery, this family-centered plan of nursing care cannot be carried out. Nevertheless, the nurse assigned to the care of the mother and the nurse caring for the infant may unite as a team in their study of the family and confer on the needs of the family as a whole.

2. Nurses may be helped by the instructors and supervisors to establish a cooperative learning relationship with the infant's parents whereby (*a*) the parents will realize that the nurse is interested in their baby and in their ability to provide good care for him after his discharge from the hospital, and (*b*) the nurse makes the greatest gain in knowledge and skill from her experience in the nursing care of the infant and his mother.

3. Routines can be made more flexible so that the needs of the individual family may be met through having the nurse use her judgment in the application of hospital regulations. Mothers might be permitted to keep their babies with them for a longer time than is required for feeding. Husbands might be encouraged to talk of their new role of being a father, if this is the first child, or of being the father of an increasingly large family. The nurse will find that successful adjustment to the first baby differs in many ways from that to the second child, and later children.

With the first baby the role of a father is new and at least temporarily appears as the most important of his roles in the many groups to which he belongs. With succeeding children the role of fatherhood is no longer novel and now has the added element of duties and pleasures related to children of different ages and probably sex, and of working with the mother to establish proper sibling relations.

4. Classes of the discussion type may be scheduled for mothers in the maternity unit so that their specific needs can be learned and met. Such classes may be planned by the student nurses under the direction of their instructors.

5. If the mother has had no previous experience in the daily care of a baby, she may be taught to bathe and dress her infant. Even if she is already expert in child care, she may profit by reviewing the hospital technique, and she surely needs to make the acquaintance of her baby in those situations that mean most to him, i.e. in which affection is shown in his direct physical care.

6. Parents may be told of the availability of community resources in case they need assistance after leaving the hospital.

## SHARED LEARNING: NURSE-PARENT EDUCATION

In a narrow interpretation of education, parental education in the hospital is limited to teaching mothers to prepare formulas, to bathe their infants and to give them physical care. In a broader sense it is a continuation of the parental education and prenatal courses which the mother had participated in before the baby came. Such courses give the information needed in making important decisions about the baby, but do not provide ready-made answers to questions about the individual baby in his family setting. It is in the application of what the mothers have already learned that the nurse is most helpful. It is a shared learning experience, for the nurse, like the mother, must apply her knowledge of child care to the individual infant.

If the student nurse has had little experience in caring for infants and if the mother has had several children of her own, it may be that the nurse will learn more from the mother than the mother from her. On the other hand, if the nurse has had considerable experience with children and if this is the mother's first baby, it is the nurse who shares with the mother her greater knowledge, and both learn by applying theory to the infant, who has his own individual wants and for whom a special schedule is to be devised.

The nurse should appreciate the mother's level of understanding and background of experience. This will vary with the mother's socio-economic class and ethnic background and will also depend upon whether this is her first baby and whether she has had experience with the infants of near relatives. The mother may herself be a professional woman working in the area of child care and may be an expert in the daily care of children.

The nurse should know the type of care which will be possible in the home, the equipment available and the level of living which can be maintained. Specific directions should be written down, or if they are given orally, the mother should be asked to repeat what the nurse has said. Instructions should be given slowly over a period of time; a mother cannot absorb all that she is to learn of child care at one time. Knowledge and experience should come gradually. If a mother attended prenatal classes, she has already learned much and will learn more from the physicians and nurses in the hospital. The public health nurse will show her the adaptation of all she has learned to the home care of her baby and its application to the immediate situation.

For the student nurse and the young graduate working with the mother as members of the team caring for the child in the hospital, such teaching is definitely a shared learning experience. The expression *shared learning experience* of mother and nurse is often more truly descriptive of their relations than saying that the nurse teaches the patient.

It is simpler to teach the physical care of children than the psychological care, and this is particularly true of infant care. The tremendous importance of happiness in infancy lies not only in the present, but also in the long-term formation of the child's personality. Today the mother-child relationship is recognized as the normal center of the baby's emotional development and is therefore most important. Other members of the family and the world outside the family are likely to influence the infant through their effect upon his mother.

The love of a mother for her child has been shown throughout this discussion. It is the great incentive to her for learning how best to care for him. Such love is likely to make her somewhat critical of instruction given in a purely professional way. The nurse's manner should be warm and friendly. She should convince each mother that mothers in general are capable of applying the scientific principles of child care.

## RECOGNITION OF MATERNAL DEPENDENCY NEEDS

The mother's physical weakness after delivery of her first-born child is likely to increase her feeling of incompetency in the role of mother to a helpless infant who, when she leaves the hospital, will be completely dependent upon her for his care. This brings us to the problem of meeting her dependency needs so that she feels secure and confident that she will receive the help she has a right to expect from her family and the community. If she worries over the future, her relationship with her baby is influenced by her anxiety and ceases to be the happy fulfillment of her long months of pregnancy. As we have seen, this will influence her ability to nurse the baby at the breast, and her insecurity for the baby and herself on leaving the hospital may be communicated to the infant. He is not likely to be a contented, placid baby.

The mother's dependency needs, both physical and emotional, influence her relations with her baby. She needs her husband's understanding love. She needs to know that he loves the baby not only for itself, but also as the common object of their affection, and that the infant strengthens the emotional bond between them. In contrast, the infant may be made the center of emotional conflicts. The presence of other children may be an emotionally sustaining influence on the one hand, but on the other hand may create many problems caused by their jealousy of the attention given the new arrival.

Probably the crucial factor in the situation is how the mother deals with her dependency needs. In the hospital she may resent being asked to undertake more self-care and more care of the baby than she feels able to undertake. At the other extreme there are mothers who are accustomed to denying the existence of their dependency needs. They find even a few days of enforced hospitalization unpleasant and want to go home too early.

Mothers who feel insecure and fear criticism of their care of the baby insist upon rules to follow or depend upon their own mother's advice in all the little day-to-day problems that arise. The mother who finds dependency humiliating may not ask for the help which she knows she needs in caring for her baby.

Nurses will find that the mother of a first baby is more likely to feel dependent, whether she acknowledges it or not, than is the mother of several healthy children. The baby looks so small and his ways are so different from those of older babies whom she knows that she is afraid he is choking, suffocating or in extreme danger of some sort. Such a mother is apt to feel that his crying is caused by a condition which must be remedied at once. If she is the overdependent type, she will make many demands upon the nurses. If she is accustomed to taking responsibility and denying her dependency needs, she may force herself into the role of the self-reliant, competent mother, but with a suppressed feeling that she is not receiving the help to which she is entitled. Neither extreme leads to a good mother-child relationship. These women need all the help the nurse can give them.

The nurse is close to maternity patients and therefore can have a great influence on them. This closeness, which is of great potential value, is likely to involve the nurse emotionally in her relations with a young mother and, in so doing, hamper her service to her patient. Young nurses who are married or expect to be married soon may develop a feeling of identity with the mother which hinders rather than helps their nursing care. It is important to retain the professional attitude, which need not be cold or aloof, but never becomes too personal.

The reaction of the individual mother to childbirth should be considered and her care arranged accordingly. Sending her home from the hospital within a few days after delivery is necessary, since the bed is needed for another patient. But it is essential that she be given help in the housework and care of the baby. Her own mother or sister or a visiting housekeeper can give her the assistance she needs.

### THE UNLOVING MOTHER

When a mother does not love her baby—as may happen if he is illegitimate—the great stimulus to learn to care for him is absent. Today it is believed that no mother should be urged to keep her illegitimate child against her wishes. It would probably be far better for him and for her if he were placed in an adoptive home where he could be loved and cherished. Such a mother need not be taught the care of the infant.

There are other mothers who are married, however, who did not want to become pregnant and who feel that the baby interferes with their professional or social life. Many such mothers find that they love the baby dearly when he is put in their arms, but others remain indifferent to him and look upon his care as an unwanted chore. In hospitals where it is the routine for mothers to attend the classes, discussion meetings and demonstrations of child care these mothers attend with all the others. They are likely to feel guilty that they do not nurture love for the baby and as a result are overpunctilious in learning all the details of his physical care. Later at home, when the public health nurse sees the mother and child, the baby's fine physical condition under his mother's care may generate in her a sense of achievement and pride in him which may in turn evoke love.

Both the hospital and the public health nurse may stimulate a mother's love for her child by promoting situations in which the baby shows his dependency on his mother and satisfaction in her care of him. This is often true of the unwanted baby whose parents felt that the family was complete without another member.

## TEACHING AIDS AND OTHER INFORMATION*

*Public Affairs Pamphets*
Carson, R.: Having a Baby.
*Ross Laboratories*
Discovering Parenthood.

* Complete addresses are given in the Appendix.

## REFERENCES

Bookmiller, M. M., and Bowen, G. L.: A Textbook of Obstetrics and Obstetric Nursing. 3rd ed. Philadelphia, W. B. Saunders Company, 1958.
Brackett, A. F., and Price, B.: Main Causes of Infant Mortality. Nursing Outlook, 1:355, 1953.
Chenoweth, A. D., and Hunt, E. P.: Current Trends in Infant Mortality. Children, 7:213, 1960.
Corbin, H.: Meeting the Needs of Mothers and Babies. Am. J. Nursing, 57:54, 1957.
Davis, M. E., and Sheckler, C. E.: DeLee's Obstetrics for Nurses. 16th ed. Philadelphia, W. B. Saunders Company, 1957.
Dawson, M. C.: Rooming-in; a Decade's Experience. Child Study, 34:No. 1, 30, 1956.
Donnelly, M. M.: A Four-Step Program for Reducing Perinatal Mortality in the Nursery. Hospitals, 30:56, August 1, 1956.
Donny, E.: Imagination in Maternity Care. Am. J. Nursing, 60:46, 1960.
Fitzpatrick, E., and Eastman, N. J.: Zabriskie's Obstetrics for Nurses. 10th ed. Philadelphia, J. B. Lippincott Company, 1960.
Larsen, E. C.: Terminal Rooming-In. Am. J. Nursing, 56:1442, 1956.
Lesser, M. S., and Keane, V. R.: Nurse-Patient Relationships in a Hospital Maternity Service. St. Louis, C. V. Mosby Company, 1956.
McFarland, M. B., and Reinhard, J. B.: The Development of Motherliness. Children, 6:48, 1959.
Smith, C. S.: Demand Feeding in the Newborn Nursery. Nursing Outlook, 6:514, 1958.
Stitt, P. G., Babbott, J. G., and Salber, E. J.: Teamwork in Helping Families to Launch a Life. Children, 6:53, 1959.
Stott, K. B.: 'Rooming-in' Is Not a Passing Fad. Hospitals, 29:80, May, 1955.
Van Blarcom, C. C., and Ziegel, E.: Obstetrical Nursing. 4th ed. New York, Macmillan Company, 1957.
Wiedenbach, E.: Family-Centered Maternity Nursing. New York, G. P. Putnam's Sons, 1958.
Wrieden, J. E.: A New Baby Is 'One of the Family' in This Hospital. Hospitals, 32:47, February 16, 1958.

# Chapter 6

# Examination and

# Characteristics of the Newborn

IN ORDER for the nurse to care for the newborn adequately, she must understand his physical attributes and functional disturbances. Anatomically, physiologically and psychologically the baby differs from adults and even from older children. His characteristics are those of his age group. Every baby is an individual and should never be regarded as a typical infant, one unit of a group in which all are alike. But the averages and the range of normality should be remembered so that each baby may receive medical care if he deviates too far from the so-called normal. It is impossible to study the infant except as a living whole; it is essential to understand his anatomy in order to understand his physiologic activity, which in turn is strongly influenced by his emotional state.

## PHYSIOLOGIC RESILIENCE

Nature provides the fetus and the newborn with a certain physiologic re-silience. The normal neonate is relatively indifferent to a wide range of body temperature from as low as 97° to as high as 100° F.; in premature infants the body temperature may even drop to 94°. By indifference is meant that the newborn does not seem uncomfortable or show the concomitant signs of low or high temperature which would appear in the adult. The infant has an unstable heat-regulating system, and his body temperature is influenced by the environmental temperature. If the room is cold, so is his body; if he is covered with too many blankets, his body temperature rises. Regulate the temperature about him, and his returns to normal. A casual observer may feel that a change in temperature has done the infant no harm and that the condition can be ignored. Often this is true, and no bad results follow a drop in or elevation of temperature.

The infant is also indifferent to abnormal levels of substances carried in the blood. The levels usually found in predictable concentration in the blood of normal children are less standardized in the neonate and can be expected to be even more unpredictable in premature infants.

Although the blood glucose level may be low, the usual hypoglycemic reaction of the adult is not seen. The infant shows some departure of the blood hydrogen ion content and carbon dioxide tension from the adult level. There is also an increase in the range of their normal values. The infant can survive without breathing for a relatively longer time than the adult, but here too there are definite limits to his tolerance for lack of oxygen.

This physiologic resilience of the newborn has many obvious advantages, and because of it many infants have survived who otherwise would have died. Yet it has one great disadvantage: it conceals or minimizes physical signs of diagnostic value. For instance, infection of the newborn may not be accompanied by fever as it is in older children or adults. In other cases an infant who is moderately dehydrated may have respirations which seem to be barely perceptibly increased, yet he may have a blood pH of 7.2 or even lower without having acidotic Kussmaul respirations. Also, infants do not conform to a pattern in their reactions to drugs; this fact makes it essential that the nurse observe infants carefully for untoward reactions.

All in all, this passive resistance of the infant is an ally. But there are limits to his resistance which cannot safely be overstepped. This is particularly true of the premature infant, who shows few defense mechanisms against those unfavorable circumstances which in the end do him harm.

The first few days of life are normally a time when the infant is in a state of negative balance. Examples of this are postnatal weight loss, loss of body fluids, and decreases in hemoglobin, calories, nitrogen, sodium chloride and inherited antibodies. There is danger of feeding him too much and too early in an attempt to make up for these losses.

Although many deaths occur on the first day of extrauterine life, this is not due to wasting of resources. Negative balance is normal, and only harm results from attempting to force it to positive.

## LENGTH AND WEIGHT

The newborn, in order to be measured, must be placed flat on his back and extended as much as possible. A scale is necessary for weighing him; it should be accurate and one in which he can lie comfortably without danger of falling.

The length of the average newborn male is 20 inches, or 50 cm.; of the female 19.6 inches, or 49 cm. The normal range for both sexes is from 19 to 21½ inches, or 47.5 to 53.75 cm.

The weight of the normal newborn, like the length, tends to vary. About two thirds of all full-term infants weigh between 2700 and 3850 gm., or between 6 and 8½ pounds. Many infants, of course, weigh more or less than this. The average girl weighs approximately 7 pounds, the average boy approximately 7½ pounds.

During the first few days after birth the infant tends to lose about 6 to 10 ounces, or 5 to 10 per cent of his birth weight. Factors contributing to this initial weight loss are the withdrawal of hormones originally obtained from the mother's body, the withholding of water and the loss of feces and urine.

At birth Negro infants tend to be smaller than white ones. A first-born child is likely to be smaller than his later siblings. Finally, the size of the parents has a bearing on the weight of the newborn: smaller parents tend to produce smaller infants.

## TEMPERATURE, PULSE, RESPIRATION AND BLOOD PRESSURE

The temperature of the newborn, though unstable, is normally about 98.6° F., and the pulse rate is rapid, around 120 to 150 per minute, as are the respirations, which vary from 35 to 50 per minute. The blood pressure is low.

The temperature, pulse and respiration of the newborn vary in an unpredictable way with changes in the surrounding temperature and with relatively slight stimuli. He appears to have a passive resistance or resilience, within a wide range of bodily responses, to such stimuli; yet when these limits of tolerance are exceeded, because he lacks the adult's reserve vitality, he may suddenly appear ill. This need for constant observation is an essential of infant nursing care. The nurse must learn from experience to recognize the significance of his response to sensations which he cannot let her know about in words or actions—e.g. pushing off the covers if he is too hot, shivering if too cold, or putting his hand to "the place that hurts" as an older child might do.

## Temperature

The infant's temperature at birth is slightly higher than his mother's, since the uterus lies deeply insulated within her body. It drops immediately after birth in adjustment to the temperature of the delivery room and then rises to normal within about eight hours. His hands and feet are colder than the rest of his body, since his circulation is poor. This lack of stability, due to underdevelopment of his heat-regulating system, requires that external heat be applied. He is generally wrapped in warm blankets in the delivery room. The nurse who puts him in his crib in the nursery or his mother's room will have to remember that too much heat for too long will send his temperature far above normal.

## Pulse

The infant's pulse is irregular, owing to immaturity of the cardiac regulatory center in the medulla. Extreme irregularity results from any one of many physical or emotional stimuli. When the infant is startled or cries, his pulse rate not only increases, but also becomes more irregular. Irregularity of rhythm of the pulse may follow that of the respiration.

## Respiration

Respiration in the newborn is irregular in depth, rate and rhythm. Like the pulse rate, it is readily altered by internal or external stimuli. Normally respirations are gentle and quiet. They can be observed most easily by watching abdominal movement, since respiration in the newborn is carried on largely by the diaphragm and abdominal muscles. Dyspnea or cyanosis may occur suddenly in an infant who is breathing normally. These signs may be the first indication of the presence of a congenital anomaly or other condition from which an infant may suddenly expire if he does not receive adequate care. The nurse should notify the physician if respiration drops below 35 or exceeds 50 per minute when the infant is at rest or if dyspnea or cyanosis occurs.

## Blood Pressure

The blood pressure is characteristically low. It is difficult to determine accurately and may vary with the size of the cuff used. When using a cuff 1 inch in width, the average blood pressure at birth is 80/46.

## THE SKIN

The skin of the newborn is dark pink, soft, covered with lanugo and overlain with vernix caseosa. There is slight desquamation. Good elasticity or *turgor* is one evidence that an infant is in good condition.

*Lanugo* is a slight downy distribution of fine hair over the body. It is most evident on the shoulders, back, extremities, forehead and temples. Since lanugo begins to appear on the fetus by about the sixteenth week of gestation and to disappear after the thirty-second week, it is often an evidence of immaturity when present. The premature infant has a heavier showing than the full-term infant. Lanugo tends to disappear during the first weeks of life.

*Vernix caseosa* is a cheeselike, greasy, yellowish-white substance, sometimes likened to cream cheese or cold cream, which covers the newborn's skin. It consists of secretions from sebaceous glands and epithelial cells. Its distribution over the body is variable, being heavier in the folds of the skin and between the labia. It dries or fades spontaneously and is rubbed off as well on the infant's clothing.

*Tissue turgor* refers to the sensation of fullness derived from the presence of hydrated subcutaneous tissue. Elasticity of the skin is demonstrated when a fold of skin is grasped between the thumb and forefinger. When released, the skin promptly springs back to form the smooth, soft surface of the infant's body.

Observation may reveal the following additional normal findings. *Desquamation* or peeling of the skin occurs during the first two to four weeks of life. Because of its natural delicacy, denuded areas may occur where the skin has been rubbed off the nose, knees and elbows because of pressure and erosion on the sheets. The skin of the buttocks needs special care so that it does not become chafed. A wet or soiled diaper should of course be changed at once.

Transient *rashes* may occur. *Milia* is a condition in which tiny white papillae occur, particularly on the nose and chin, owing to obstruction of the sebaceous glands. These blemishes disappear in a week or two. *Physiologic jaundice* becomes definite between the third and seventh days. It is likely to appear gradually on the second or third day and is seen in the majority of infants. (See also page 89.)

There may be one or more of a number of types of marks upon the infant's body. Some are temporary, caused by the trauma of birth; others are due to immaturity, even in the infant born at term; still others are permanent birthmarks. Among the temporary marks are *hemangiomas*, or pink spots, on the upper eyelids, between the eyebrows, and on the nose, upper lip or back of

the neck. The mother may be reassured that they will disappear spontaneously. If forceps were used during delivery, temporary marks may be left upon the part of the body or head where the blades exerted pressure. In a breech delivery there may be edema and extravasation of blood into the tissues of the buttocks and genitals due to trauma to the presenting parts. In fact, there may be bruising of tissues on almost any part of the infant's body as he progresses through the birth canal.

Another type of mark which may be present is the so-called *Mongolian spot*. These spots, which are slate colored, usually occur on the buttocks or lower portion of the back of infants whose parents are Negro, Oriental or from the Mediterranean area. They fade during the preschool years without treatment.

By two weeks of age the infant should have the typical rosy, soft, dewy skin which we associate with babies. The sweat glands, which do not function during the neonatal period, become active by the end of the second week.

## THE HEAD

The head is proportionately large, averaging 34 to 35 cm., or 13.6 to 14 inches, in circumference. The normal limits of head size are 33 to 37 cm., or 13.2 to 14.8 inches. The head is one fourth the total length of the infant. In the adult the length of the head is one eighth of the total height (see Fig. 3b). The infant's cranium is large and the face relatively small when compared with the adult cranium and face. The jaws are relatively small, and the chin is receding. The circumference of the head equals or exceeds that of the chest or abdomen.

The fontanels are openings at the points of union of the skull bones. The anterior fontanel is diamond-shaped and located at the juncture of the two parietal and two frontal bones. It is 2 to 3 cm. or 0.8 to 1.2 inches in width and 3 to 4 cm. or 1.2 to 1.6 inches in length (see Fig. 20). The posterior fontanel is triangular and located between

Figure 20.   The size of the fontanels varies considerably from infant to infant. They are palpated to ascertain their tension. (Courtesy of Pfizer Laboratories, Brooklyn, New York.)

the occipital and parietal bones. It is much smaller than the anterior fontanel and may be nearly closed. The fontanels bulge when the infant cries or strains or if there is increased pressure within the skull. Increased intracranial pressure may be due to a number of causes, among them hydrocephalus (see p. 218). The anterior fontanel normally closes by the time the infant is twelve to eighteen months old, and the posterior fontanel by the end of the second month.

The bones of the cranium are held together by membranes at the suture lines. During delivery, pressure may mold the head into asymmetrical proportions. In general the head assumes its normal shape by the time the infant is a week old.

*Caput succedaneum* is represented by swelling or edema of the presenting portion of the scalp and may be localized or fairly extensive. It usually disappears by the third day.

*Cephalhematoma* is an accumulation

Figure 21.   Caput succedaneum. Extensive soft tissue swelling of the scalp is evident.

of blood between the periosteum and a flat skull bone. The collection of blood does not cross a suture line. The mass may be described as soft, irreducible and fluctuating. It does not increase on

A                                    B

Figure 22.    Cephalhematoma. *A*, The collection of blood lies between the periosteum and the
skull bone. *B*, Cephalhematoma of the right parietal bone.

crying. A cephalhematoma may not be evident during the first few days of life because of the presence of a large caput succedaneum. Aspiration of this sanguineous collection should not be done because of the danger of infection and because the condition usually clears within a few weeks. While a cephalhematoma is in process of absorption a firm ring can sometimes be palpated around the edge. This ring may simulate a skull defect, but is of no significance (see Fig. 22).

### Face

The infant's face is expressionless. The receding mandible quivers at the slightest stimulation, especially if the infant is startled or whimpers. The ears are flabby until the cartilage calcifies. The eyes, before they acquire their permanent color, are an indeterminate blue or slate gray. Their movements are not coordinated, and both eyes momentarily may turn inward or outward. The lids are shut or only partly opened. There are no tears until the infant is a few months old. The neck is short and creased. These creases, particularly in a fat infant, are deep and likely to become sore unless carefully cleaned.

### THE CHEST

The chest is bell-shaped and at birth is approximately the same circumference as the abdomen and less than the head. For this reason it appears small. By the time the child is two years old the size of the chest exceeds that of the head, and he begins to take on more nearly adult proportions.

The thorax is almost circular. The anterior and lateral diameters are the same because of the pressure of the arms against the chest wall in utero. In breathing the infant does not use the thoracic cage as does the older child or adult; he uses the diaphragm and abdominal muscles to exhale and inhale.

The breasts of infants of either sex may be swollen because of hormone activity originating from the mother, and pale milky fluid ("witch's milk") can be expressed. The condition disappears in two to four weeks without treatment, but as long as it lasts the breasts are tender and should be touched only when necessary and then very gently.

The *thymus* is usually proportionately large in the newborn and triples its weight by the time the child is five years old; it then remains approximately the same size until he is about ten years old, when it begins to decrease. A large thymus in the past was thought to be the cause of respiratory difficulty or of sudden death by asphyxia, but this has been disproved. Usually some other factor is accountable for cyanosis or apnea.

## RESPIRATORY SYSTEM

The mechanism of respiration is established before birth, but at birth it undergoes profound changes. Prerespiratory movements begin in the fourth month of gestation. In fact, the amniotic fluid may move in and out of the lungs as a result of these tidal movements. Oxygen is, of course, obtained through the placental circulation. The hypoxia resulting from severance of the cord assists in initiating breathing through stimulation of the respiratory center by the accumulation of carbon dioxide. The process of birth and the environmental change also stimulate the respiratory center. The first breath, usually taken within thirty seconds after birth, helps to expand the collapsed lungs, though full expansion does not occur for several days.

## CIRCULATORY SYSTEM

At birth sudden changes occur in the circulatory system. The circulatory pattern must change from fetal dependency on the placenta to include the expanding lungs. The functional structures (i.e. foramen ovale and ductus arteriosus) of intrauterine life must be obliterated. The circulation of the pulmonary system is perfected, and a short time after birth oxygenated blood flows through the infant's body in the same manner as that of the adult. The foramen ovale (see Fig. 70) closes by the third month. The ductus arteriosus is occluded when the infant is from several weeks to four months old. Approximately 2 per cent of newborns have transitory, insignificant heart murmurs caused by blood leaking through openings not yet closed. These disappear within a few weeks.

The *vascular system* and *heart* are large in the newborn in comparison with their size in adult life. The blood volume of the newborn is about 10 to 12 per cent of his body weight. This percentage is influenced by the amount of blood he received from the placenta before the cord was clamped off.

### Blood

The infant's blood contains a relatively high number of red blood cells and a high hemoglobin level at birth. These characteristics are essential to provide adequate oxygenation in utero and during the first few postnatal days before the lungs expand fully. Oxygenation improves during the first two weeks of life to the extent that a high red cell count and hemoglobin level are no longer necessary, and hemolysis occurs.

### Physiologic Jaundice (Icterus Neonatorum)

All infants have an excessive amount of bilirubin in the blood at birth. During the first week there is a further breakdown of hemoglobin, thereby increasing the blood bilirubin level. At this time the immature liver cannot excrete bilirubin in sufficient quantities. The result is a jaundice of the skin and sclerae. This occurs in approximately 55 to 70 per cent of all newborns, from 36 hours to 3 days after birth. It increases for a few days and usually disappears by the fourteenth day. The urine may become dark and the infant appears sluggish, even showing anorexia. Continuing jaundice indicates a pathologic condition such as an obstruction of the bile ducts, syphilis or erythroblastosis fetalis.

### Physiologic Hypoprothrombinemia

During the first few days of life the prothrombin level decreases in all infants. Thus the blood-clotting time is prolonged. This condition is most acute between the second and fifth postnatal days. It can be prevented to a great extent by giving vitamin K to the mother during labor or to the infant after birth. Recovery usually occurs between seven and ten days of age.

## GASTROINTESTINAL SYSTEM

### Sucking Pads, Mouth and Jaw

The sucking pads are deposits of fatty tissue in the cheeks which persist even when the infant is extremely malnourished. They disappear when sucking is no longer the infant's only way of taking food.

The infant has a receding chin, which trembles when he is startled. His tongue is relatively large and protrudes when the mouth is open. The young infant cannot move food from his lips to the pharynx. Later, when food is given, it must be placed at the back of his tongue so that he can swallow it. At two or three months of age salivation occurs. Since the infant has not yet learned to swallow facilely, he may drool.

### Esophagus, Stomach and Intestines

The cardiac sphincter is not as well developed as the pyloric sphincter. For this reason the infant should be "bubbled" several times while being fed so that air which he has swallowed may be eructed. (A little milk may come up with the air.) If the air were to remain in the stomach, there would be danger of vomiting or, if it passed into the intestine, of colic.

Occasionally the action of the pyloric valve may not be normal, and regurgitation (the vomiting of food immediately after it has been taken) may be so constant that an infant fails to gain in weight. This pathologic condition will be taken up in Chapter 13.

It is difficult to measure the size of the infant's stomach. The contents are emptied almost immediately into the duodenum. When we look at the infant and the amount of milk he is taking, it is evident that the fluid is leaving the stomach before the feeding is completed. It is likely that at birth the stomach holds from one to 2 ounces, at 2 weeks 3 ounces, at 5 months 7 ounces and at 10 months 10 ounces.

The entire digestible formula should be out of the infant's stomach in two and a half to three hours. Digestion is slowed by food high in protein or fat.

Although the fetus has no need of the intestinal tract in order to obtain nourishment, the tract functions as an outlet for amniotic fluid as early as the fifth month of intrauterine life. The normal gastrointestinal tract assumes its function readily after birth. *Meconium*, the first fecal material, is a sticky, odorless material, greenish black to brownish green, which is passed from eight to twenty-four hours after birth.

The nature of the *stools* changes daily in the first week. They are called transitional stools. From the third to the fifth day they are loose, contain mucus and are greenish yellow. After the fifth day the nature of the stools depends on the feeding. The stools of the breast-fed infant are yellow and pasty and have a rather pleasant, sourish odor. The breast-fed infant will normally have from two to four stools a day. The stools of an infant fed on a formula of modified cow's milk are light yellow and hard and have a distinctly unpleasant odor. One or two stools a day are normal. Later, when the infant is receiving a soft diet, the stools are brown or colored from the type of food given him.

### Abdomen

The umbilical stump begins to shrink and become discolored soon after birth and within a few days turns black (see p. 99). It sloughs off between the sixth and tenth days, but leaves a granulating area which heals in another week. Extreme care must be taken that this lesion does not become infected, since the blood vessels of the cord and their extension into the abdomen afford a potential portal of entry for organisms until the umbilical wound is completely healed. If a belly band is used to hold an umbilical dressing in place, it should be clean and not so tight as to interfere with the free exercise of the abdominal muscles, especially necessary in respiratory activity.

## ANOGENITAL AREA

The infant's buttocks are plump, firm and pink. In the anal region there should be no redness or fissures.

### Genitals

**Male Genitals.** The size of the penis and the scrotum varies. The prepuce or foreskin of the penis may adhere to the glans, and if it cannot be loosened by the physician, circumcision may be necessary. The testes have usually descended into the scrotum by the eighth month of intrauterine life, but in some cases they remain in the abdomen or the inguinal canal. This condition is commonly known as undescended testes or cryptorchidism (see p. 633).

**Female Genitals.** The female genitals may be slightly swollen, owing to hormone activity originating from the mother. The labia majora are undeveloped, and the exposed labia minora appear large. The vagina exudes a mucous discharge which may occasionally be blood-tinged during the first week. This is also caused by hormones transmitted from mother to infant. The condition should disappear by the second or third week.

### Urine

The infant has urine in the bladder at birth and may void immediately or after several hours. In a small percentage of newborns, however, urination may be delayed until the second day. The urine is dilute because of the immaturity of the kidneys and their lack of ability to concentrate. Loss of a large amount of water may result in a temporary hemoconcentration. A pink stain may be found on the diaper which is usually due to deposition of uric acid crystals.

## EXTREMITIES

The legs are small, short and bowed or curve outward as the infant lies with his legs abducted and flexed, so that the soles of the feet nearly touch each other. The feet appear to be flat, owing to the presence of the plantar fat pad (a pad of fat in the longitudinal arch of the foot). The arms, like the legs, are relatively short, and the position of the neonate is often that of the tonic neck reflex (see p. 93). The hands are plump, the fingers relatively short, and the nails are smooth, soft and long enough to extend over the finger tips.

The bones of the newborn are soft because they are composed chiefly of cartilage in which there is only a small amount of calcium. The skeleton is flexible and the joints are elastic to ensure a safe passage through the birth canal.

## MUSCLES

The muscular contour in the healthy, plump infant is smooth, and his muscles, in spite of their lack of strength and his inability to control them, feel hard and slightly resistant to pressure. The nurse should note whether the infant offers a normal resistance to passive movement of his extremities. If he does not, such lack may indicate that he is suffering from cerebral injury, narcosis or even shock. If an infant feels limp in the hands of the nurse, the condition should never be mistaken for a mere characteristic of his immaturity.

The movements of the newborn are random and uncoordinated; he wriggles and stretches. When the nurse picks him up, she must support his back and head, for he lacks the muscular strength to hold even his head steady and would slump if placed in a sitting position.

## NERVOUS SYSTEM

The nervous system of the newborn is strikingly immature. His bodily functions and responses to stimuli from outside his body are carried on chiefly by the midbrain and reflexes of the spinal cord. The cerebral influence characteristic of even the preschool child is lacking. The immaturity of his nervous system in control of bodily functions is evidenced by such manifestations as inadequacy of the heat-regulating system and irregularity of both pulse and respiration.

As soon as the nerve fibers become myelinated and make the necessary connections with one another, control from the higher cerebral centers begins, and increasingly more complex and purposeful behavior is possible. One can observe the neurologic development from week to week as it proceeds caudally from above.

### Reflexes

Certain reflexes are absolutely essential to the infant's life, and many are protective. Among these latter are the *winking reflex,* which is aroused when something comes near the eyes or when the infant is subjected to a bright light, and the *reflexes of coughing and sneezing,* which clear the respiratory tract. The *yawn reflex* is in a sense protective, since thereby the infant draws in an added supply of oxygen.

A number of reflex actions are involved in feeding. The *rooting reflex* causes the infant to turn his head toward anything which touches his cheek and is his way of reaching for food. It helps the infant to locate the nipple with his mouth when the breast touches his cheek. The *sucking reflex* provokes sucking movements when anything touches the lips. It is difficult in an artificially fed infant to keep the bottle nipple from touching the area around the mouth before he gets it into his mouth. This reflex is normally present at birth and is accompanied by the *swallowing reflex.* The *gagging reflex* comes into play when he has taken more into his mouth than he can successfully swallow. He can also cough if a little of the fluid is "swallowed the wrong way" and enters the trachea.

The infant is not skillful in coordinating all these reflexes and requires help from the mother or nurse. He may have trouble getting the nipple into his mouth, and when he does succeed, the nipple may be under rather than on the tongue. These reflexes essential to successful nursing are absent or underdeveloped in the premature infant, but their absence in the full-term infant would indicate narcosis, brain injury or mental retardation. If the sucking reflex is not stimulated, it ceases to exist.

The *grasp reflex* is present in both hands and feet. An infant will grasp any object put into his hands, hold on briefly and then drop it. At birth he may be able to hold on so securely to an adult's forefinger inserted into his fists that he may be lifted from the crib to a standing position (the "Darwinian reflex"). This grasping action in its reflex form fades. As the infant matures it becomes conscious and purposeful and obviously is one which brings him pleasure—shaking his rattle, for instance. Although he cannot literally grasp with his feet, his toes react to stimulation with an attempt to get hold of the object which touches the sole of the foot or the toes (see Fig. 23).

The neonate can take a few prancing steps when supported in a standing position. This appears to be purely a reflex movement and soon disappears. Not until he is trying to stand and walk does he again make any attempt to move his legs as in prancing, though he gets great fun from kicking as he lies on his back.

The newborn has one great unlearned reaction to strong stimuli: the *startle reflex* pattern. At birth or soon after this reflex is aroused by a sudden loud noise or loss of support. The reaction is a generalized, aimless muscular activity. The startle or *Moro reflex* demonstrates an awareness of equilibrium in the newborn and is seen during the first month or two of life. This reflex can best be elicited when the infant is quiet and without the restraint of clothing. A sudden stimulus such as jarring the table or bassinet will cause the infant to draw up his legs with the soles of the feet turned toward each other and the under surface of the toes almost touching. The arms assume the embrace position. These movements, followed by a rather fixed and rigid position, normally are symmetrical. The Moro reflex is a normal reaction; in its absence the possibility of brain damage must be considered (see Fig. 23).

The *tonic neck reflex* is a postural reflex in which the infant, when lying on his back, turns his head to one side and extends the arm and the leg on the side to which the head is turned at right angles from his body; he flexes the other leg and the arm. He may make a fist with both hands. This position has been aptly called the infant's fencing position; it occurs in fetal life by about twenty to twenty-eight weeks of gestation and in the newborn and infant up to about the eighteenth or twentieth week (see Fig. 23).

Successful use of the reflex mechanism is evidence of the normal functioning of the nervous system. If a reflex is impaired or absent, it is possible that the central nervous system has sustained injury. Although it may not be possible to correct the condition, the care of the infant can and must be adapted to his disability. For instance, if he cannot suck, he must be fed by gavage. Certain reflexes present in the newborn disappear as he matures, and the cerebrum exercises greater control over the nervous system. This brings about changes in behavior to which the care given him by the mother or nurse must be adapted.

**The Conditioned Reflex.** This is the only way by which the infant learns, and it is largely limited to carrying over the satisfaction from feeding to the concomitants of the process. He sees the nurse's or mother's face, although it is blurred for him, and learns to like those who feed him because of

Figure 23.   Reflexes and motor development of the newborn infant. *A*, Grasp reflex. *B*, Startle reflex (Moro reflex). *C*, Tonic neck reflex. *D*, Lifts head slightly from the bed.

their association with the relief of his hunger and the general comfort of being fed.

## Motor Activity

The movements of the newborn are rapid, varied and diffuse. Any specific movements he makes are simple reflex actions or those which are prompted by a reflex action, such as swallowing prompted by the sucking reflex. Although he begins soon after birth to learn about his little world through the conditioned reflex, practically all his behavior is still due to reflex response to stimuli. His whole body is likely to be involved in his activity, and his responses appear to be aroused by some generalized state such as hunger, pain or discomfort from lying too long in one position. He does not localize the feeling of pain or hunger, and he has a wide indifference to changes in temperature.

When the infant feels that something is wrong, he reacts with his whole body and may try out reflex movements which he associates with relief. For instance, although he does not yet connect the breast or the bottle with relief from hunger, he makes sucking movements with his lips and will try to suck anything which comes in contact with them. Specific responses to specific stimuli are an outgrowth of this generalized activity; the useless movements are dropped, and the useful movements which bring him a reward are perfected through practice. This is not due primarily to practice, however, but rather to maturation of his nervous system, muscles, bones and, in fact, his entire body. Maturation does not proceed at the same rate in all the systems of the body, but the general pattern makes possible the typical behavior of infants at certain ages. Naturally they must be given opportunity to try out and practice new responses, or their behavior will be atypical.

At birth the infant can raise his head slightly when lying on his stomach, but not when on his back. If he is pulled to a sitting position, his head falls back and his spine is curved in a bow from shoulders to hips, like that of an old person unable to sit or stand upright. At an early age the infant can make crawling movements when on his abdomen and a little later push himself up in his crib by kicking movements.

## EMOTIONAL RESPONSES

The signs of emotion in the newborn are extremely difficult to interpret. Probably all that can be said is that two emotional states are evident: in one he lies peacefully, and in the other he appears in discomfort—his face is twisted, and he cries. To this could be added his emotional response to the startle stimulus.

Since vocalization shows his emotion and, increasingly as he grows older, will express *the emotion* he wishes to convey to mother or nurse, we will consider vocalization under emotional responses.

## Vocalization

The newborn vocalizes solely by crying, and this he does in response to any form of discomfort or pain. He is an egocentric little person entirely dependent upon adult care and unable to make his wants known in any other way. His birth cry is the beginning of vocalization and serves two purposes: to supply the blood with sufficient oxygen and to inflate the unexpanded lungs.

If the cry is weak and not sustained, an abnormal condition must be suspected. It should be a lusty cry even with only the stimulation of the birth incident. No one knows whether the birth cry has any connection with discomfort or is a pure reflex evoked by his physiologic needs.

Soon it is evident that crying is used to express discomfort. If crying brings the infant relief and pleasant sensations from the care given him by mother or nurse, he soon learns through the conditioning of this reflex to cry for attention. Even within the first twenty-four hours the cry varies in pitch, intensity and continuity, so that it has meaning to those who are accustomed to caring for infants.

The stimulation to cry comes from the immediate environment or from his own body. He may be hungry, in pain or in need of exercise such as comes from being picked up and moved about. Infants often cry for unknown reasons, and the cause of their discomfort cannot be ascertained. Assuming that an infant is neither hungry nor wet, if he stops crying when cuddled, we can infer that this is what he needed, and after being quieted he may be put back in his crib. But the infant who continues to cry while he is being held and petted is probably in distress and should be watched carefully for other symptoms of illness.

Hunger is said to be the most common cause of crying, and this is an argument for putting the infant on a self-demand feeding schedule (see p. 135).

The infant's cry is made almost exclusively from vowels produced in the front of the mouth. Soon he makes other sounds which are as important as crying as a forerunner of speech. These sounds are explosive—coos, grunts and gurgles. They probably have no meaning other than that they occur only when he appears contented. But the next stage of vocalization—that of repetition of syllables, as in "ma ma" —is built upon his practice in phonation.

## SPECIAL SENSES

An infant shows by his general discomfort that he can feel pressure and temperature change and pain.

### Touch

The sense of touch is the most highly developed of the special senses and is most acute on the lips, tongue, ears and forehead. Failure to grasp the nipple is therefore one indication of brain damage.

### Sight

The eyes are blue or gray at birth, changing to the permanent color in from three to six months.

It is difficult to know what an infant sees. His eyes are only half open, and the lids are swollen. There may be a purulent discharge from the use of silver nitrate (see p. 99). The pupils react to light, and bright lights appear to be unpleasant to the infant.

### Hearing

The newborn is deaf until his first cry. He normally makes some response to sound from the third to the seventh day, and there is evidence that he hears ordinary sounds before the tenth day. By the fourth week he is likely to react to the voice of his mother or nurse more frequently than to a loud noise.

### Taste

The infant's sense of taste is more highly developed than that of sight or hearing. He accepts sweet fluids and resists fluids with an acid, sour or bitter taste.

### Smell

The only evidence of the sense of smell is that many infants appear to smell breast milk and reach for the nipple. There is a wide difference among infants in their apparent ability to smell.

### Skin Sensations

Sensations of touch, pressure, temperature and pain are present soon after birth, and at the end of ten days the infant reacts violently to cutaneous irritation.

### Organic Sensations

The infant appears to be highly sensitive to organic stimulation, since hunger and thirst are the most common causes of his crying. The newborn and the very young infant are not likely to have pain from gas in the intestines, but the infant of a few weeks appears to suffer intensely if his feeding produces colic.

## SLEEP

In the newborn, sleep can hardly be distinguished from tranquil rest. The neonate sleeps from fifteen to twenty hours out of the twenty-four hours of the day. Short waking periods occur every two hours, but are fewer and shorter during the night, probably because there are fewer external stimuli to arouse him. He is awakened by internal discomfort such as hunger or pain. Hunger is by far the most common cause of an infant's waking before his physiologic need for sleep has been satisfied. As he grows older the length of unbroken periods of sleep and also of wakefulness increases.

## IMMUNITY

Antibodies for certain infectious diseases pass through the placenta from mother to infant. Among these antibodies are those of smallpox, mumps, diphtheria and measles if the mother is immune to these diseases. This passive immunity of the infant lasts from a few weeks to several months. Little immunity is passed on for chickenpox or pertussis, and young infants may contract these diseases. It is not feasible to immunize very young infants, since they are not sufficiently mature to form antibodies successfully, as can the infant who is several months old.

If an infant does contract a con-

tagious disease, it is likely to be more severe and to be followed by more complications than in an older child.

## REFERENCES

Adams, M. M.: Appraisal of the Newborn Infant. Am. J. Nursing, 55:1336, 1955.
Berrien, C. D.: Evaluating the Newborn. Nursing Outlook, 9:93, 1961.
Bookmiller, M. M., and Bowen, G. L.: A Textbook of Obstetrics and Obstetric Nursing. 3rd ed. Philadelphia, W. B. Saunders Company, 1958.
Davis, M. E., and Sheckler, C. E.: DeLee's Obstetrics for Nurses. 16th ed. Philadelphia, W. B. Saunders Company, 1957.
Fitzpatrick, E., and Eastman, N. J.: Zabriskie's Obstetrics for Nurses. 10th ed. Philadelphia, J. B. Lippincott Company, 1960.
Grulee, C. G., and Sanford, H. N.: The Newborn; in Brennemann, J.: Practice of Pediatrics, Hagerstown, Md., W. F. Prior Co., 1959, Vol. 1, Chap. 42.
Hurlock, E. B.: Child Development. 3rd ed. New York, McGraw-Hill Book Company, Inc., 1956.
Koop, C. E.: Emergency Surgery of the Newborn. Clinical Symposia. Ciba Pharmaceutical Products, Inc., Summit, New Jersey, 11:35, 1959.
Nelson, W. E. (editor): Textbook of Pediatrics. 7th ed. Philadelphia, W. B. Saunders Company, 1959.
Peto, M.: The Normal Newborn Infant. Am. J. Nursing, 52:1353, 1952.
Richmond, J. B., and others: A Hearing Test for Newborn Infants. Pediatrics, 11:634, 1953.
Silver, H. K., Kempe, C. H., and Bruyn, H. B.: Handbook of Pediatrics. 3rd ed. Los Altos, California, Lange Medical Publications, 1959.
Smith, C. A., and Cook, C. D.: Special Problems of the Newborn, Pediatrics, 15:348, 1955.
Smith, C. A.: The Newborn Patient. Pediatrics, 16:254, 1955.
Idem: The Physiology of the Newborn Infant. 3rd ed. Illinois, Charles C Thomas, 1959.
Van Blarcom, C. C., and Ziegel, E.: Obstetrical Nursing. 4th ed. New York, Macmillan Company, 1957.

# Chapter 7

# Care of the Newborn

THE FAMILY-CENTERED care which the nurse provides for parents and their newborn infants should be based on her understanding of the physical status of the newborn and the emotional reactions of the infant and of his parents to the process of childbirth. In the preceding chapter the physical and physiologic characteristics of the normal newborn were given. This chapter is concerned with his care immediately after delivery, in the nursery, and after discharge from the hospital. Immediate care of the newborn includes gentleness and prevention of infection, establishing and maintaining respiration, care of the umbilical cord, care of the eyes, identification of the infant, establishing and maintaining his temperature, putting him to the breast and maintaining a record of observations on his condition.

While the newborn remains in the hospital daily care must be provided for him. This is an intermediate step between the care given directly after birth and his care at home. Since many infant deaths occur in the first few days of life, his physical care and the observations made and charted by the nurse are fully as important as those in the first few hours of life.

## CARE IN THE DELIVERY ROOM

In the delivery room the infant is inspected for any gross anomalies such as spina bifida, cleft lip and cleft palate, imperforate anus, hydrocephalus, birthmarks, or for evidence of shock or birth trauma. Many anomalies are not immediately evident on inspection, however, and these are the concern of the physician and the nurse in the nursery.

The nurse has several responsibilities in the care of the infant immediately after his birth.

### ESTABLISHMENT AND MAINTENANCE OF RESPIRATION

The infant's respirations must be established and maintained. For this it is necessary that he cry lustily. Full expansion of the lungs provides oxygen for the blood, which until birth was supplied through the placental circula-

**97**

**Figure 24.** Position in which the infant should be held after delivery. If the infant's first breath occurs in the head-up position, respiratory obstruction follows. Note the identification band on the wrist. (From Resuscitation of the Newborn Infant. American Academy of Pediatrics, Inc.)

tion. Removal of this source of oxygen stimulates respiratory movements within the infant's body, movements which took place in a superficial manner even during intrauterine life. Any infant who does not breathe within thirty seconds after birth is in danger of asphyxia. The need for close observation of the infant and for having everything in readiness for his resuscitation is evident.

Some infants need further stimulation than that provided normally through separation from the mother. Failure to cry may be due to several causes, a common one being obstruction of his air passages with mucus. In order to clear these passages the infant may be held by his feet with the head down and the neck curved backward. In this position the mucus drains out by gravity. Drainage of mucus may also be facilitated by stroking the neck in the direction of the mouth. This is known as milking the trachea. Respirations may be further stimulated by gently rubbing the infant's back or spanking his buttocks or the soles of his feet. The mucus may be gently wiped from his mouth with the nurse's gloved finger.

If these measures fail, it may be necessary to remove mucus by suction. A soft rubber catheter, no. 14 or 16 French, attached to a De Lee mucus

**Figure 25.** Aspiration of the newborn. *A*, De Lee glass trap and rubber catheter may be used for aspiration. Movement of the nurse's finger is the silent method of indicating the heart rate of a newborn. *B*, Method of suctioning the pharynx of a newborn. (From Resuscitation of the Newborn Infant. American Academy of Pediatrics, Inc.)

trap may be used to reach farther down into the throat through the mouth. A no. 8 to 10 French catheter is used for suctioning through the nostrils. When the catheter is in position, suction is made on the mouthpiece of the mucus trap. It is important that mucus be removed before the infant draws his first breath in order to prevent him from aspirating the mucus. When as much mucus as possible has been removed, the infant should be placed in the head-down position to induce further drainage unless this is contraindicated.

If the infant does not cry after such resuscitative measures, the physician will clamp the cord, and more drastic means of stimulating the infant to breathe will be used.

## CARE OF THE UMBILICAL CORD

Two clamps are used to compress the cord. They are placed about 2 inches from the abdomen. If possible, this is not done until the cord has stopped pulsating, for the infant will then receive approximately 100 ml. of blood from the placenta, which will provide him with a store of iron and other desirable blood constituents. He will need this iron during the first few months of life when the iron content of his diet tends to be below his needs. But if the mother has been deeply anesthetized, he may evidence signs of depression from passage of the anesthetic or analgesic agent across the placental barrier.

After the cord has been clamped a ligature is tied in a square knot about 1 inch from the abdominal wall. After removal of the clamp the cord should be turned back on itself and tied a second time with the same ligature. Instead of a ligature a clamp which crushes the vessels may be placed on the cord and removed after several hours, or another type of clamp may be used which may be left on the cord until it drops off. Some institutions favor the use of a special type of broad rubber band.

There is a difference of opinion as to whether an antiseptic solution and a dressing should be applied to the cord. The custom of the hospital or the physician's order should be followed. If a dressing is applied, an abdominal band must be used, kept clean and changed whenever it is soiled. Extreme care must be taken that the cord does not become contaminated. The cord is connected with the great blood vessels of the abdomen through which infection could be carried, with septicemia a likely result.

## CARE OF THE EYES

If the mother has gonorrhea, the infant's eyes may be inoculated with the organism during delivery. If the eyes are not adequately treated at once, ophthalmia neonatorum is likely to develop (see p. 162). A prophylactic treatment against ophthalmia neonatorum is required by legal statute in every state. A germicide must be instilled into the eyes of the newborn shortly after delivery. Silver nitrate, 1 per cent solution, has been used for many years. Penicillin, which is a gonococcide, has been used more recently.

If silver nitrate is used, it may be dropped between the eyelids at any time after the head has been delivered until the third stage of labor is completed. The eyelids should be cleansed carefully with a sterile cotton ball moistened with sterile water; wiping should proceed from the nose outward. The lower lid should be pulled down, and 2 drops of a 1 per cent solution of silver nitrate should be instilled into the conjunctival sac. After a minute or two the eyes should be irrigated with warm physiologic salt solution; this washes out the excess silver nitrate and forms a precipitate with the remainder. In about 50 per cent of infants a chemical irritation may result from the silver nitrate. Although within a few hours a profuse discharge may appear in the eyes, there is no permanent ill effect from the treatment and the chemical conjunctivitis.

Penicillin may be administered as a topical application in the form of penicillin ophthalmic ointment or may be given intramuscularly.

### STABILIZATION OF TEMPERATURE

The temperature of the newborn usually drops immediately after birth, but returns to normal in about eight hours. The temperature in the delivery room is lower than that in utero, and this accounts for the drop in the infant's temperature after delivery. To raise his body temperature to normal, he should be wrapped in a warm sterile cotton flannel blanket immediately after birth.

### IDENTIFICATION OF THE INFANT

All infants must be identified in some manner before they are removed from the delivery room. Several methods are in use, the most common among them being an adhesive label bearing identification information applied to the infant's back, a name bracelet or necklace placed on the wrist or about the neck, identification tapes marked with identification numbers for both the infant and the mother placed about their wrists (see Fig. 24), and foot or palm prints of the infant taken while he is still on the delivery table. This last is the most "mistake-proof," but must be used in conjunction with a form of identification which can be used in caring for the infant. The name necklace or bracelet is popular.

### BAPTISM

If there is danger of death of the newborn, the majority of Christian parents wish to have their child baptized immediately. This may, of course, take place in the delivery room, but is more likely to be the responsibility of the nurse in the nursery. If the parents are Roman Catholics, a priest should be called if it appears that the infant will live until he arrives. If death is imminent and a priest is not present, the nurse may perform the baptism by pouring water on the infant's forehead while saying, "I baptize you in the name of the Father and of the Son and of the Holy Spirit." The Roman Catholic Church teaches that every fetus and embryo should also be baptized if possible. Conditional baptism can be carried out if it is not certain whether the subject is capable of receiving baptism, by saying, "If you are capable of receiving baptism, I baptize you in the name of the Father and of the Son and of the Holy Spirit."

If the parents are Protestant and wish to have their child baptized, a minister of their faith should be called. In case of emergency the physician or the nurse can baptize the child by placing water with the palm of the hand on the child's forehead and saying, "I baptize thee ( *or* you ) in the name of the Father and of the Son and of the Holy Ghost." Although it is not essential to repeat the Lord's Prayer or the Apostles' Creed, or both, it is well to do so.

### PUTTING TO THE BREAST

Some physicians believe that the infant should be put to the breast as soon after delivery as the condition of the mother and of her infant permits. They believe that this early suckling assists in involution of the uterus, stimulates lactation and also provides emotional satisfaction for both mother and child. Other physicians believe that nursing should be postponed until four to twenty-four hours after birth. This would allow time for the infant's throat to be cleared of mucus and for the infant to sleep after the exertion of birth and of being handled by physicians and nurses in the necessary care after birth. This interval also permits the mother to rest before giving her infant the breast. This first feeding is difficult, for he must learn to take hold of the nipple and to suck.

### ESSENTIALS OF NURSING CARE

Nursing care is begun in the delivery room immediately after birth and is continued in the nursery or the mother's room if the infant rooms-in with her.

The great need for *gentleness* in caring for the newborn has already been stressed. He has undergone a difficult if not exhausting experience and is now initiating bodily functions for himself which his mother's body performed for him while he was in utero. He has been accustomed to his "marine bath," and even the softest fabric is irritating. Being moved about independently is a novel experience after the confinement of the uterus.

*Avoidance of infection* is imperative. The only source of infection in utero was through the mother's blood stream, but now there are many portals of infection. In general his nursing care is that of strict aseptic nursing. Clothing and the linen and blankets for his crib, the gown which the nurse wears, and all equipment used in his care should be surgically clean if not sterile. His bedside equipment is, of course, for his personal use only. The nurse who cares for him should never be on duty if she has a cold, sore throat, loose stools or any type of septic skin infection.

## CARE IN THE NURSERY

The newborn, wrapped in a warm receiving blanket, is transferred to the nursery in either a warm crib or the nurse's arms. He is then dressed in a diaper, shirt and gown, and is loosely wrapped in a blanket and placed in a warm crib. If the father has not seen him previously, the infant is shown to him at this time.

### GENERAL NURSING PROCEDURES

Only when the nurse is fully aware of the physical attributes, the physiologic activities and the common functional disorders of the newborn can she appraise the infant put under her care in the nursery. (See Chapter 6 for characteristics of the normal newborn.)

It was mentioned previously that the first day of life is a most hazardous period for the infant, and the mortality rate is highest during these hours. The nurse must therefore observe the infant closely. On his admission or soon after

she should appraise his physical status. This appraisal can be accurate only when she knows what is normal and what is abnormal in the newborn. (There is a wide range of individual differences among normal infants.) This knowledge cannot be learned solely in class or from books; it comes only with experience in the care of the newborn. For this reason the student should be particularly careful to query her instructor or supervisor whenever she is in doubt about the significance of variations in an infant's physical state and behavior.

The two factors of gentleness in handling and prevention of infection, which were considered in carrying out all procedures in the delivery room, are equally essential in the care of the neonate in the nursery or his mother's room. Rapid or rough movements in handling tend to produce fear and provoke crying. Infection which might be of little consequence in an older child may cause the death of a newborn.

In order for a nurse to apply her knowledge of what is normal to a particular infant, she should know something of his history. As has been shown, hereditary traits differ in races, subracial groups and families. Some infants by inheritance are short and plump, and others long and slender. Coloring also is an inherited trait.

The nurse should read the physician's notes on the mother's prenatal record and labor chart, for a difficult delivery may have brought pressure on the infant's soft bones and caused a temporary abnormality. The length and weight of the infant are charted. The circumference of the head, chest and abdomen should be noted. The infant's position when lying still, his activity and facial grimaces need not be charted if they are normal, but any unusual circumstance should be reported. The infant is seldom quiet for any length of time; he stretches and makes grimaces apparently in his sleep. Many an inexperienced nurse has mistaken the normal tonic neck reflex (see p. 93) for an abnormal position. Nevertheless it is better to err and report what is normal than to fail to report an unusual condition. When the infant is lying on his back and begins to cry, the nurse should note whether his head is held in the midline and both sides of the face are mobile or whether there appears to be a partial paralysis of one side of the face. Absence of symmetry and contour is an evidence of some abnormality.

Even infants need freedom of movement. When an infant is awake and crying, there is movement of the entire body, and restraint arouses resistance. The startle or Moro reflex (see p. 92) demonstrates symmetry or its lack in the movement of the arms and legs.

The nurse should note the color of the skin. In an infant of the Caucasian race it should be red or dark pink, in the Negro a reddish black, and in the Mongolian the color of a tea rose. The skin is covered with a light coat of downy hair (lanugo). A substance called vernix caseosa, somewhat of the consistency of thick, sticky cold cream, is smeared over the body of the newborn. The skin and subcutaneous tissue should be firm and resistant when the nurse takes up a fold of skin and tissue between her thumb and forefinger. The skin should be elastic; i.e. when she removes the pressure of her finger and thumb, the skin instantly springs back to its normal smooth state (see p. 86). There may be slight nevi of the skin, but these, unless they are extensive, are of little significance. Birthmarks are not uncommon and should, of course, be charted. There may be marks from the forceps used in an instrumental delivery. Mongolian spots (see p. 86) are often seen in Negro infants and in those of the Mediterranean subraces.

### Preliminary Examination

The nurse should look for obvious malformations and then systematically examine the infant's entire body, beginning with the head.

1. She should observe the skull and palpate for cephalhematoma and caput succedaneum. She should turn the head gently from side to side to ascertain

**Figure 26.** The infant is observed for obvious malformations before the detailed examination begins. (Courtesy of Pfizer Laboratories, Brooklyn, New York.)

whether there is rigidity. The sternocleidomastoid muscles may have been injured during delivery. The eyes should be tested to determine whether the pupil reaction to light is normal. To test his hearing a bell may be gently rung (held a little distance from his ear). If he hears it, he will respond with generalized activity of his whole body.

2. The infant's chest is relatively small in comparison with the abdomen. The breasts may be slightly swollen, and so-called witch's milk may be present in infants of either sex. The respirations are rapid and shallow. The normal cry is lusty, frequent and often apparently without cause. If the infant does not cry, he should be stimulated to do so at approximately hourly intervals in order to force expansion of his lungs by the concomitant deep respirations.

3. The abdomen is relatively large in relation to the torso, but it should not be distended. The umbilical cord must be examined for any trace of bleeding, which should be reported to the physician at once. Close observation should

be continued for at least the first twenty-four hours after birth. If bleeding occurs, the cord should be clamped or retied immediately, and the infant's condition reported at once. After the first day there is less danger of bleeding, but signs of infection may appear and should be reported.

4. The genitals should be closely examined. In the female infant there may be evidence of a mucoid discharge. A slight reddish discharge has no significance, since it is due to maternal stimulation. The genitals are much larger in some infants than in others; the size should be noted, though it seldom exceeds normal limits. In the male infant the testes may possibly not have descended into the scrotum. Sometimes the foreskin can be retracted easily and the glans can be cleansed, but in many infants the foreskin adheres to the glans. Force should never be used in an attempt to retract the foreskin; the application of force is not only painful for the infant, but also may make it difficult to replace the foreskin after retraction, since manipulation induces edema.

5. The infant's back is normally straight and flat. The lumbar and sacral curves develop later when the infant sits up and begins to stand.

6. Many of the common anomalies of infancy are noted in the extremities (e.g. clubfoot or syndactyly, the latter a union of the fingers or toes). Although these do not interfere with vital functions as do anomalies of the heart, bladder or other internal organs, they are a cause of great anxiety to the parents. The physician should tell the mother of the infant's condition and what can be done to correct any anomalies. The nurse should note whether the arms are of equal length and roundness. She may do this by holding the

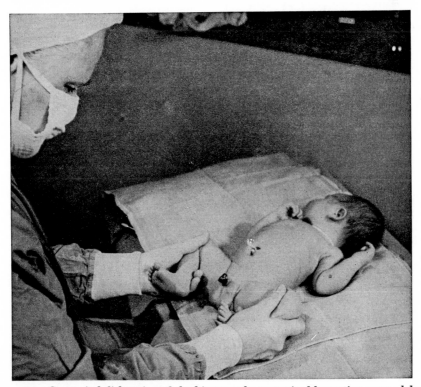

**Figure 27.** Congenital dislocation of the hips may be recognized by testing gross abduction of the thighs and observing for protrusion of the femoral heads. (Courtesy of Pfizer Laboratories, Brooklyn, New York.)

infant's arms extended and close to his side. The newborn's hands are clenched in little fists. The nurse should separate the fingers and examine them. The normal grasping reflex is so strong that if the nurse puts her forefingers into the infant's fists, he can be raised from the crib.

The infant normally holds his legs flexed and somewhat bowed. With the infant on his abdomen, the nurse should grasp his ankles and straighten the legs, noting whether they are the same length and whether the gluteal and knee folds are symmetrical. Next she should turn the infant on his back, move the legs and note whether there is limitation of movement (see Fig. 27). If the nurse holds the infant with her hands around his chest and his feet touching the examining table or crib, he will attempt prancing movements with his legs. This is called the *dancing reflex.*

After examining the infant's head, body and extremities the nurse should observe his movements. When prone, the infant can raise his head for a moment, but cannot hold it steady, and it soon falls, to rest on one cheek. When placed on his back, the infant cannot raise his head.

Finally the nurse should note whether all normal reflexes are present, especially the rooting, sucking, Moro and grasping reflexes.

Some physicians like to have the nurse complete the appraisal of the newborn with three additional tests; designed to uncover anomalies which prevent normal physiologic processes, in contrast with those deformities which have no influence on the general condition of the newborn, such as a clubfoot. These anomalies, not obvious on general inspection, are of such importance that their early discovery and correction may mean the saving of the infant's life. Such anomalies include imperforate anus, omphalocele and esophageal atresia.

**Imperforate Anus.** In order to test for the presence of this condition, in the absence of a meconium stool, the nurse need only insert into the infant's rectum

Figure 28. Digital examination ascertains whether there is rectal atresia. (Courtesy of Pfizer Laboratories, Brooklyn, New York.)

a thermometer, a gloved finger (since the infant's rectum is very small, it is well to use the index or little finger) or a soft rubber catheter.

**Omphalocele.** The nurse should examine the point of juncture of the umbilical cord with the abdomen to make certain that a loop of intestine is not protruding into the base of the cord.

**Esophageal Atresia.** In order to test for the presence of an esophageal atresia, a soft rubber catheter may be passed through the esophagus into the stomach. Any obstruction should be reported immediately, for the infant will be unable to take nourishment. Repair should be made before his condition is weakened by lack of nourishment or before pneumonia develops, owing to aspiration of formula.

These simple tests are not dangerous to the newborn and may safely be performed by the student nurse under the direction and supervision of the physician or her instructor (Koop, *op. cit.,* p. 37). The nurse does not, of course, make a diagnosis of a medical condition, but through intelligent observation and description of her findings she is able to inform the physician of conditions which require his consideration.

The nurse's responsibility in the appraisal of the newborn is in part determined by the policy of the agency which employs her. It may be that she is responsible for appraisal not only when the infant is brought to the nursery, but also when he is discharged. If so, she should understand the normal maturation which takes place in the infant during the first few days of life. She cannot use the same standards of normality for a three-day-old infant that she used during his first hour of extrauterine life.

The role of the professional nurse is being enlarged to include many functions which formerly belonged exclusively to the physician. This is made necessary by (1) the extreme shortage of medical personnel as compared with the increasing demand and (2) the greater competency of the modern professional nurse in assisting the physician by accurate, intelligent observation. Whatever the policy of the hospital, the nurse can best fulfill her responsibility for the infant's complete nursing care by frequent observation of his condition. This is necessary not only for the infant's safety, but also for improvement of her own ability to make discriminating judgments between normal and abnormal states.

### Continuous Observation

General observation of an infant must be made at frequent intervals during the day and night for evidence of malfunction in vital bodily functions, including respiratory distress.

*Respiratory distress* is shown by the rate and nature of an infant's respirations, his cry, color and general behavior. If the infant appears to be choking, mucus may be found in the nose or mouth. The air passages may be cleared immediately by placing the infant with his head lower than his body and stroking his neck in the direction of his mouth. If these procedures do not give relief and the physician cannot be reached, the nurse should use an aspirator and provide oxygen if she considers that it is necessary. To meet such an emergency, equipment for aspiration and oxygen administration should always be kept in the area where newborns are cared for.

**Position of the Infant.** Because of the possibility of respiratory distress during the first 24 hours of life, the foot of the crib or the mattress should be elevated at a 15- to 20-degree angle. The infant should be placed on his side in this head-down position. He should be rotated to the other side every two or three hours.

The infant's bones are soft and molded by pressure. This fact gives us another reason for changing his position frequently, since lying constantly upon one side will cause the bones of the skull to be flattened. The shape of the chest is also influenced by the position in which he lies, but seldom to the extent of deformity such as occurs in the skull. Since infants like to face the light and it is essential that they do not lie always upon the same side, the infant's head will be alternately at the "top" or "foot" of the crib. (In the majority of cribs both ends are alike, and there is no "top" or "foot," so that this arrangement makes no difference to his comfort or the appearance of the nursery.)

After the infant has learned to roll over he may show a preference for lying on one side. This is less likely to be so unless his mother has conditioned him to one position, or some skeletal deformity makes that position more comfortable than any other, or he is placed so that he must lie upon that side in order to face the light. If deformity has occurred, he should be placed in the crib so that, in facing the light, he lies in a corrective position. This position can be alternated with the supine position or the prone position.

The newborn should become accustomed to sleeping on his abdomen, but since there is danger of suffocation, he should be placed on his abdomen only when it is possible to watch him closely.

The position in which the infant is held should be determined with reference to his level of maturation, par-

**Figure 29.** Isolette Incubator. *A,* The Isolette features an easy-to-clean conditioning chamber, optimal humidity and oxygen control, and unequalled isolation through the use of the exclusive Micro-Filter or the outside air adaptor. The infant can be weighed in the incubator by using the scale seen on the top. A "background" air temperature of about 86° F. is maintained by the standard Isolette temperature control. *B,* By means of the Infant Servo-Controller mechanism, supplementary temperature control is provided and the infant's temperature is automatically maintained at a predetermined optimum. This supplementary temperature is provided by infra-red lamps mounted in reflectors on the top of the Isolette hood. (Courtesy of Air-Shields, Inc., Hatboro, Pennsylvania.)

ticularly that of his neuromuscular system, which together provide for muscular control. Even a normal infant cannot hold his head up without support until he is six weeks old. To hold an infant upright in her arms, the nurse should support his head and shoulders with one hand and his buttocks with the other. Her hold upon him should be firm and steady so that he has no fear of loss of support. (Some child psychologists hold that such fear is one of the few fundamental fears of infancy.) An infant enjoys being held, and holding him gives the nurse an opportunity to help him develop a sense of trust in those who care for him.

**Temperature.** Proper temperature and humidity control must be maintained in the nursery or, if the infant is rooming-in, the mother's room. Room temperature and humidity are important in respiratory considerations, and this is particularly true with the newborn infant. During the day the temperature should range from 68 to 76° F., and the humidity from 45 to 55 per cent. The infant's heat-regulating centers are poorly developed, and he reacts quickly to any divergence in temperature of his environment. The air in the room should be fresh, but there must be no drafts. Fresh air usually has sufficient moisture to prevent drying of the mucous membranes of the nose and throat.

The body temperature of the newborn upon admission to the nursery may be subnormal (see p. 85). He should be dressed in dry clothes and external heat applied, if necessary, until his temperature is normal. Hot-water bottles placed outside the crib covers may be used to provide an accessory heat source. Electric pads should not be used, for there is always danger of overheating or of shock from faulty connections.

Since heat perception is poorly developed in the newborn, three precautions in the use of hot-water bottles must be remembered: (1) the temperature of the water must not be over 115° F. (2) The bag must be covered with flannel or a towel and should be checked for leakage before it is used. (3) The bag must not be placed upon the infant's chest or abdomen, where its weight might interfere with respiratory movements. Ordinarily three hot-water bottles are used, one under the legs and one on either side of the body. These provide heat for the extremities, where the circulation is poor, without overheating the chest. Hot-water bottles cool quickly and need to be refilled frequently. If three are used, they may be filled in rotation.

An incubator is the most satisfactory method of applying external heat. The incubator maintains a controlled, uniform temperature. The heat regulator of the incubator should be set at 80° F. (26.7° C.). The infant's temperature must be checked frequently in order that the regulator of the incubator may be adjusted to meet his needs. An infant's temperature responds readily to external heat, and his temperature should be taken every hour until his body heat is established at normal. The average newborn may then be removed from the incubator to his crib, but those who weigh less than average or those who are debilitated from a difficult delivery may need confinement in the incubator for a longer time.

The amount of clothing and covering which an infant needs depends upon the temperature of the room. In general the nursery is kept at a higher temperature than the mother's room, and so the infant who rooms-in will need extra covering. Mothers tend to dress their babies too warmly because they

use as their guide the temperature of the infant's hands and feet. Both the hands and the feet are cooler than the rest of the infant's body, since the blood circulates less freely in the extremities. Mothers will learn from the nurse that a more accurate way of determining whether an infant is warm or cool is observing the color of his face. If it is flushed, the infant is too warm; if pale or bluish, he is too cool. The mother may feel the arms and legs of the infant, rather than the hands and feet, to check on her observation of the color of his face. She will then have an adequate basis for determining the amount of clothing and covering he needs.

Infants cannot adjust their body temperature to the rapid changes in environmental temperature which may occur when they are carried from the nursery through the hall to the mother's room. For this reason they are wrapped in blankets when taken to their mothers. The blanket may be adjusted, wrapped closely about or thrown open, as need be.

After the temperature of the newborn

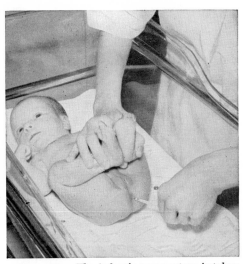

Figure 30. The infant's temperature is taken twice a day, rectally. If the infant has a fever, the temperature should be taken every 4 hours. When taking the temperature, the nurse should place her index finger between the infant's ankles and should hold the thermometer securely in place. (Davis and Sheckler: DeLee's Obstetrics for Nurses. 16th ed.)

*A*

*B*

**Figure 31.**   Weighing the infant. *A*, The infant is lifted carefully from his crib onto the scoop basket of the scale, which is covered by sterile impervious paper. *B*, The daily weight is a good index of the general well-being of the infant as well as the adequacy of the diet. (Davis and Sheckler: DeLee's Obstetrics for Nurses. 16th ed.)

has become stabilized it is taken every four hours during the first day and after that twice a day. The temperature may be taken by either the axillary or the rectal method. Each infant should have his own thermometer so as to reduce the possibility of cross-infection in the nursery. If temperatures are routinely taken by rectum, care must be exercised to prevent injury to the rectal mucosa. The thermometer bulb should be examined carefully for imperfections. The infant's legs should be grasped firmly with the nurse's index finger between the ankle bones. The rectal thermometer should be well lubricated and inserted for at least one minute. Some physicians prefer that the infant's temperature be taken by the axillary method. If this is done, the thermometer must be held firmly in the axilla, with the infant's arm pressed against his side, for five minutes or until the mercury stops rising.

**Weight.** The infant is weighed at birth and each following day at approximately the same time, usually when he is given his morning care. Newborns are usually weighed completely naked in a warm nursery. A fresh sheet of paper or a diaper should be balanced on the scale before he is placed upon it.

If the infant is immature or not in good health or the nursery is not sufficiently warm, he may be weighed dressed and wrapped in his blanket. Then, when he is undressed for morning care, these articles are weighed and their weight subtracted from the combined weight of the infant, his clothes and his blanket.

Certain types of incubators contain all necessary equipment, including scales. An infant can then be cared for and weighed without removing him to a cooler atmosphere.

The infant's weight is compared each day with that of the day before. If he loses more than the usual physiologic weight loss during the first few days or if, after a week, he shows little or no gain in weight, the physician's attention should be called to the weight chart.

### SPECIFIC NURSING CARE

The care of the newborn has varied through the years and in different hospitals to such an extent that a review of all the methods which have been used would result in confusion in the mind of the student.

In the past the face was cleansed with water and the body with sweet oil or liquid petrolatum (liquid petrolatum is less likely than sweet oil to be a culture medium for bacteria). When the umbilical cord had healed, the infant was bathed with soap and water. Today no

cleansing of the body is given, for the vernix caseosa is believed to have a beneficial effect upon the tender skin. The vernix is dissipated in a few days.

The technique given here is based on principles which are now generally accepted.

### Care of the Skin

The majority of pediatricians today accept the theory that the less the skin is handled and abraded by even gentle friction, the better is its condition. Even under this regimen skin irritation may occur in some infants. Today neither soap nor oil is used in the cleansing of the infant immediately after delivery.

The following method is in accordance with modern concepts of child care.

1. Soon after birth the blood on the face and scalp is washed away with a very soft cloth or cotton balls and water.

2. No attempt is made to remove the vernix caseosa, which adheres to the skin and has a protective value. It has been likened to vanishing cream in its softening effect upon the infant's peeling skin.

3. The infant should not be exposed, since he would become chilled. While the nurse is wiping off the amniotic fluid and blood he should be covered with his blanket. The nurse exposes only that part of his body which she is wiping at the moment. In this way his entire body is not uncovered at any time. He is then dressed in a diaper and shirt and loosely wrapped in a fresh blanket.

4. During the first day the vernix caseosa rubs into the skin or comes off on the infant's clothing. On the second day any remnant adhering to the skin in the creases of the body may be wiped off with a soft cloth or cotton balls.

**Daily Morning Care.** The following technique for bathing the infant is typical of the procedure in many hospitals.

1. His condition is observed at bath time, since he is naked. In bathing him, special attention is given to the condition of the skin, eyes, nose, ears, mouth, umbilicus and genitals. The bath is a time when the infant is free of restraint from diaper or clothing, and his spontaneous movements may be observed better then than at any other time. Any unusual condition or abnormal movements should be reported.

2. The infant may be washed with a

soft cloth or absorbent cotton and clear water. No soap or oil should be used. A soft dry cloth should be used to dry his face and body and, if cotton was used, to prevent wisps of cotton from clinging to the skin or body orifices.

3. Wherever two areas of skin lie in close contact with each other, chafing is likely to occur. Such sites are the creases of the neck and, if the infant is fat or the weather warm, the creases behind the ears, on the inner surfaces of the thighs, the axillae and the groin. These areas may need to be cleansed several times a day if they are soiled or sticky with secretions.

4. It is normal for the outer layer of skin to peel off, either in minute grainy particles or in fairly large flakes. These areas may be bathed with clear water and dried and have oil applied to them. Cracks in the skin may appear around the wrists and ankles and should be cleansed and oiled. It is often difficult for a mother to believe that these lesions are normal and of no significance. Fortunately they improve readily under proper treatment.

5. Care of the buttocks and genitals is extremely important. The area should be washed with warm water, and in the male infant, special attention should be given to the areas of skin contact about the scrotum and the penis. In some institutions a bland soap is used if it is difficult to remove the stool with clear water. There is a difference of opinion as to whether oil should be used on the buttocks. Some physicians believe that its use increases the danger of infection, while others order it to be applied routinely.

6. Talcum powder is contraindicated and is seldom, if ever, used in the nursery. Some mothers, however, believe that it prevents chafing. Its use, then, with the infant who rooms-in with his mother depends upon her insistence on its value and the policy of the hospital. The harm it may cause to the skin is slight. There is some danger that the mother may shake the can too vigorously and that some of the fine powder particles may drift where the infant can inhale it. Even the better powders on the market may be irritating to the infant's delicate respiratory tract. Powder accumulated in the folds of skin may become saturated with body secretions. If powder is used with oil, it forms a paste which is likely to retain urine, feces or bodily secretions and prove irritating. Zinc stearate powders should never be used because of their intensely irritating effect upon the respiratory tract. Powders made for use with infants do not contain zinc stearate, but the ordinary commercial powders may.

7. Other items included in the daily morning care are taking the infant's temperature, weighing him, changing the covering on the umbilical cord (see p. 113), changing the sheets and pads of his bed, and cutting his fingernails and toenails if they extend beyond the ends of the fingers and toes. The nails should be cut square, the corners slightly rounded, so that the infant cannot scratch himself.

**Skin Irritations.** In spite of good care, skin irritations are prone to develop in some infants.

Probably the most common skin irritation seen after the newborn period is *miliaria* (prickly heat). It is caused by a superficial bacterial action after excessive sweating during hot weather or fever. The signs are small erythematous papules and vesicles which cause itching. The treatment is cleanliness, washing with warm water and a mild soap, rinsing with clear water and drying thoroughly. Soothing lotions may be used, of which calamine lotion is the most common. It dries the skin as powder does and stays on the irritated area without caking. Talcum powder is sometimes used, but should be used with care to avoid inhalation. In general, miliaria is a sign that the infant has been too warmly dressed. Even in hot weather it is not likely to occur in areas freely exposed to the air.

*Intertrigo* or chafing is most often seen in infants with very sensitive skins. It occurs where two surfaces of skin are in contact—behind the ears, in the creases in the neck, axillae and groin and, in the male, under the scrotum—

and is particularly likely to occur where there is moisture from sweat, urine, feces or milk which has dripped into a fold of skin. The condition is also caused by friction, although this is seldom the case in the newborn, whose clothing is soft and whose physical activity is limited.

The manifestations of intertrigo are raw, red, moist areas in the skin folds. The lesions do not itch, and they do not heal by forming a crust or scab. Instead, the area becomes dry and gradually assumes its normal texture and appearance. Prevention lies in cleanliness, particularly in the folds of the skin, and in keeping the skin dry and free from contact with organisms which would cause the area to become infected. The nurse is not likely to see intertrigo in an infant born in the hospital, but rather in those brought into the hospital by mothers delivered at home and sent to the hospital after a few days because of some complication which required hospital care. In such a case the hospital policy might permit a breast-fed infant to be isolated on the obstetrical area, where it could be taken to its mother for feedings. But it is

much more likely that the infant would be placed on the pediatric unit and given a formula or his mother's milk, expressed manually or by a breast pump.

There may be *abrasions* on the heels, knees, toes and elbows from rubbing against the crib linens. These seldom occur in the healthy, well cared for newborn, but are frequently seen in a neglected, undernourished infant who lies crying and engages in aimless crawling or kicking movements. Such an infant may be brought to the hospital for some illness. The irritated areas should be bandaged lightly and kept scrupulously clean.

*Diaper rash* is caused by irritation from urine and stool. It is seldom seen in the breast-fed infant, but is common in the infant on a formula. If the stool is irritating and the diaper is not changed immediately, the buttocks may become red, and then shiny and raw. The lesions smart when the infant urinates and are a frequent cause of crying among infants who are not receiving sufficient care. The treatment consists in exposure of the area to warmth and air by placing a diaper under the infant

**Figure 32.** Ammoniacal dermatitis or diaper rash. (Courtesy of Dr. Ralph V. Platou and the American Academy of Pediatrics.)

and laying him on his abdomen with his shirt folded up above the buttocks. The diaper should be changed, of course, whenever it is soiled.

If possible, the area should be exposed to the sunlight, but if this cannot be done, the buttocks may be exposed to the warmth of an electric light bulb (25 to 40 watts) placed in a goosenecked lamp. The lamp stands by the crib, and the neck is bent so that the bulb is perhaps 12 to 16 inches from the infant's body. Ointment should not be put upon the infant's skin at the same time the light is used. If the area is raw, the bulb should be farther from the buttocks, for excessive heat will be painful and may cause injury. Great care should be taken that the lamp is secure and the bed clothing in no danger of touching the bulb.

When exposure to the sunlight or the use of a lamp is not practicable or is insufficient therapy, a soothing ointment such as zinc oxide, A and D ointment or methylbenzethonium chloride (Diaparene) will aid the healing process. Diaparene contains a germicide inimical to harmful bacteria which decompose urine in the diaper area and cause irritation.

Diapers which have been improperly washed and rinsed may cause a rash and certainly aggravate the condition, whatever its cause.

If diapers are to be washed at home, they should be soaked in cold water, then washed with a mild soap, rinsed thoroughly and, if possible, dried in the sun. One crushed tablet of Diaparene in 2 quarts of water makes an excellent antiseptic terminal rinse for 6 diapers. This should be poured over the diapers after they have been washed and rinsed. They should soak for a few minutes and then be dried. Commercial laundries do excellent work, and many hospitals as well as private families are using their services.

Cleanliness is the major factor in the prevention of diaper rash in the well infant. Plastic pants are seldom put on infants, but, when used, may predispose to diaper rash because the diaper is likely not to be changed often enough.

### Care of the Eyes, Nose, Ears and Mouth

Care should be given only as necessary to the infant's eyes. Any secretions that have accumulated in the corners should be washed out with a soft wash cloth and clear water, stroking from the inner canthus outward. The eyes should not be irrigated even if there is a discharge unless the physician orders irrigation. If irrigation is prescribed, physiologic salt solution should be used. Boric acid should not be used. Since boric acid solutions are both odorless and colorless, they may be mistaken for water. Boric acid is harmful when taken internally.

Because any severe discharge from the eyes may be evidence of a serious infection, the physician will probably order warm saline irrigations and isolation precautions and send smears of the discharge to the laboratory for culture. He may prescribe antibiotic drugs or ointment to counteract the infection.

The infant's nose and ears may be cleansed externally by using a twisted cotton cone moistened in water. All excess water should be squeezed out since it annoys the infant if it drips upon his face. Oil should never be used because of the danger of aspiration with resulting harm to the infant's respiratory tract. No attempt should be made to cleanse the nose or ears internally. Toothpicks or wooden applicator sticks covered with cotton should not be used because of the danger of injury from deep penetration if the infant moves unexpectedly. There is also the risk that the cotton may become loose and lodge in the nose or ear; it will then be necessary for the physician to remove the cotton with instruments.

The mouth should not be cleansed except by offering sterile water between feedings. There is danger of injuring the tissues and thus predisposing to infection.

### Care of the Genitals

**The Vulva.** The vulva should be cleansed gently with a bland soap and warm water. Some of the vernix caseosa may be removed each day at bath time and when the buttocks are cleansed after passage of a stool. Mothers should be especially instructed to cleanse the vulva from the urethra toward the anus, using a different section of the wash cloth with each stroke. With this method there is less likelihood that the urethra will become contaminated with fecal organisms, thereby minimizing the possibility of cystitis due to infection traveling up the urethra to the bladder.

**The Penis.** In cleansing the penis, the foreskin should be retracted, when possible, each day if the infant has not been circumcised. Irritation will result if smegma, a malodorous cheeselike substance, and bacteria are not removed from beneath the foreskin. The cleansing process should be done very gently, and the foreskin should be retracted only as far as it will go without pressure. The foreskin must be returned to its normal position immediately afterward to prevent painful paraphimosis due to constriction and edema.

If the foreskin is adherent to the glans during the neonatal period, the physician may postpone retraction. Nevertheless the mother should be taught the procedure so that later, in cleansing the penis, she will be familiar with the technique.

*Phimosis.* In this condition the foreskin is so tightly hooded over the tip of the glans that it impedes the discharge of urine and predisposes to irritation. The treatment is by circumcision —surgical removal of the foreskin. The operation is performed to prevent infection, to facilitate the discharge of urine and to make the area easier to clean. A written order for the operation must be obtained. The operation is generally done on the sixth to the eighth day of life, at which time the infant has recovered from physiologic hypoprothrombinemia and the bleeding and coagulation times are usually within normal limits. (The religious rite of circumcision, comparable to baptism in the Christian faith, is one of the fundamental tenets of the Jewish law and must be performed on the eighth day after birth unless the infant's condition necessitates postponement.)

Although circumcision is a minor operation, the infant needs care after it. The nurse must watch for bleeding. A soothing ointment may be applied to the raw area after the diaper has been changed (some physicians prefer that no diaper be used). Such care should continue until the area is healed.

### Care of the Umbilical Cord

During the first twenty-four hours after the infant's admission to the nursery the cord must be observed closely for bleeding. Sometimes the cord contains an excessive amount of Wharton's jelly. When this shrinks, as part of the normal process, a ligature or clamp which was tight becomes loosened, and there is danger of hemorrhage. Normally a clot forms at the end of the cord stump and may prevent bleeding even if the ligature or clamp is loose. But if the clot is dislodged through manipulation, bleeding will occur. To prevent further loss of blood the nurse should apply a sterile hemostatic forceps as far from the abdominal wall as possible. The physician or nurse can then apply another clamp or ligature to the cord, closer to the abdominal wall.

The umbilical area provides a portal of entry through which infection can be carried to the infant's blood stream. It is important, therefore, that asepsis be maintained until the cord drops off and the navel is healed. The cord may heal in one of two ways: by dry or moist gangrene. Dry healing is preferred because a dry area is a poor medium for the growth of bacteria. Normally, the umbilical wound is completely healed in a week.

The umbilical area should be cleansed each day with 60 to 70 per cent alcohol, which has a drying effect and promotes antisepsis. If a cord dressing is used, it should be changed promptly when soiled. If infection develops around the umbilicus, as shown by redness in the area, malodor, or moisture or discharge from the cord, the physician should be notified at once. Treatment of such infection usually consists in frequent applications of an alcohol dressing and an antibiotic applied locally or given systemically, or both. Opinions vary as to the use of a cord dressing. Some physicians believe that it is necessary to protect the area from infection, but others believe that a soiled dressing increases the danger of infection.

### Inanition or Dehydration Fever

Between the second and fourth days of life the infant may have fever as a result of his low fluid intake with normal fluid loss. His temperature may rise to 102° to 104° F. (38.9° to 40° C.). His skin becomes dry, urine output is decreased, and his face and body show that he has undergone a sudden loss in weight, a loss confirmed when he is weighed. Treatment consists in increasing the amount of fluid taken, giving water between milk feedings, or in administration of parenteral fluids.

### PREVENTION OF INFECTION

The newborn has little resistance to disease. For this reason all nurses caring for the newborn must understand the importance of aseptic technique. Probably the fundamental rule to be followed by parents and hospital personnel is that they wash their hands thoroughly before handling the infant. In the nursery this is done on entering the room. Antiseptic detergents are better for this purpose than toilet soap, and the hands should be washed under running water. No rings or wrist watch should be worn, since either may be the site of lodgment of bacteria. Even nail polish is forbidden, for it too may be a source of transmission of infection. It is possible for an infant to be orally infected with organisms from his own stool. For this reason the nurse should wash her hands thoroughly after changing his diaper and before feeding him.

In some nurseries all personnel routinely wear masks. Their value is questionable, however. If they are not changed frequently or if they become soiled when adjusted, they are a source of contamination rather than of protection to the infant.

No one who has symptoms of a respiratory, intestinal or skin infection should enter the nursery or rooms where infants are with their mothers; such persons absolutely should have no contact, direct or indirect, with the infants. If the mother acquires an infection, her infant should not be taken to her; if he rooms-in, he should be isolated from her. If she has been in contact with the infant, he should be isolated not only from her, but also from the other infants in the nursery so that he may not be a source of transmission if he has contracted his mother's disease.

Infection is far more likely to be carried by direct contact with an infected person than by indirect contact through contaminated equipment. Nevertheless contaminated equipment is definitely a source of infection. Each infant should have his own personal articles for his bath and other care. These may be kept in his stand or in a drawer underneath the bassinet and taken with him to his mother's room if he is to room-in with her.

An infant in the nursery who shows signs of infection should be isolated at once. The other infants must be closely observed for symptoms of the specific infection which he has contracted. Symptoms of the most common infections are refusal of feedings, frequent loose stools, elevation of temperature, drainage from the umbilicus, and discharges from the eyes or nose. Respiratory infections are first evidenced by a running nose and a rise in temperature. Skin lesions are easily observed when the infant is undressed for morning care or when the diaper is changed.

### RECORDS AND BIRTH REGISTRATION

The nurse caring for an infant in the nursery is responsible for all notations on his permanent record. When the infant rooms-in, the mother tells the nurse of the care she has given her infant and her observations on his condition and behavior. This the nurse charts.

In addition to the permanent records, some nurseries have *daily record sheets* which are not permanent records. These are composite tally sheets used for the total nursery population. The auxiliary personnel as well as the nurses record on these sheets the care they have given the infants and their observations, such as morning care, feedings, stool passages and urination. The nurse copies from these temporary daily sheets the notations about each infant onto his individual chart. In some instances she summarizes the information, e.g. the number of stools during the day and the total amount of feeding taken. Important notations commonly included in the nurse's notes on individual permanent records include the following:

The infant's name, day of life, birth weight and daily weight

Observations on his condition: his cry, respirations, temperature, the condition of the cord, mouth, eyes, skin, frequency and nature of stools and urine

The time of feedings and the amount taken and retained; frequency and volume of regurgitation

Medication and treatments given

Execution of all physician's orders, such as administration of oxygen, irrigations, and the like.

The physician, midwife, nurse or attendant who delivers the infant is responsible for the birth registration with the local registrar. The information necessary for the birth certificate includes the child's name, date and place of birth, names of each of the parents, and other data of local option. This information should be accurate and easily read, since it is filed permanently with the state Bureau of Vital Statistics. Some form of notification of the registration is sent to the parents, who should keep it as proof that the infant's birth has been registered. Proof of birth registration may be important in later life to determine whether a child is of school age, whether a youth is of legal age for employment or voting, or whether a person is old enough for social security benefits, and so on.

## FEEDING THE NEWBORN INFANT

The nurse should be able to recognize the signs of hunger in the helpless newborn. The infant becomes restless, cries, moves his head in search of food (the rooting reflex) and makes sucking movements which, bringing no relief, are likely to end in crying.

The infant may be hungry immediately after birth or may show no signs of needing food for the first or even the second day. Usually he goes to sleep for several hours after being fed, wakening when he again needs food or is uncomfortable from any cause. The most common causes of crying in a healthy infant are hunger and discomfort from a soiled diaper.

If an infant is on a self-demand feeding schedule, it is particularly necessary for the nurse to recognize signs of hunger in order to satisfy his demand for food, rather than use the bottle to pacify him whenever he cries.

### BREAST FEEDING

Breast feeding is not as important a consideration in infant morbidity and mortality rates as it was some years ago. Probably the psychological and emotional factors are more important than the physical factors in breast feeding today, since satisfactory artificial feedings can now be easily obtained.

The typical breast-fed infant is contented, and active in a happy, playful way. At six weeks his smile is easily provoked. He will normally have two to four stools a day; these are spongy, bright yellow, almost orange, and with a characteristic odor which is not at all unpleasant. After his initial weight loss he should gain from 6 to 8 ounces a week.

If he is underfed, he is likely to be constipated. He may have colic, may vomit, may be irritable and may alternate crying with sucking his fingers. Vomiting and colic are also characteristic of the overfed infant. In general, however, the breast-fed infant shows a steady gain in weight and is less prone

**Figure 33.** The typical breast-fed infant is contented and happy.

to intestinal upsets than is the infant on an artificial feeding plan.

**Advantages to the Mother.** The mother as well as the infant benefits from breast feeding. The infant's sucking at the breast promotes involution of the uterus after parturition. Many mothers find great emotional satisfaction in feeding the infant at the breast, for it is the culmination of the symbiotic unity which existed during the infant's intrauterine life. The fact that breast feeding saves time and trouble appeals to some women. Breast milk is less of a strain on the family budget than buying fresh or even evaporated milk.

**Objections to Breast Feeding.** For some women the advantages of breast feeding may be outweighed by other factors. The mother may feel that it ruins the firm contour of her breasts and so makes her look older than her age. Breast feeding may be too great a strain upon her vitality and thus may lead to a state of exhaustion which interferes with the supply of milk. If the mother works outside the home or has many social engagements, it may be impossi- ble for her to be at home promptly at feeding time, provoking infant distress and discomfort from engorged breasts.

The subject of infant feeding should be an integral part of the parental edu- cation course. Although the mother and the father have talked over the whole problem before the child is delivered, the actual decision on breast feeding comes after the infant's birth. The nurse is likely to be the one who interprets the physician's recommendation to the par- ents. A sickly infant is more in need of breast feeding than is a healthy one. But the mother's condition may make it inadvisable for her to nurse her infant. The mother's attitude toward breast feeding cannot be ignored; she is the one most vitally concerned. The physi- cian and the parents must consider what is best in their individual case.

If the mother has worked and her salary is needed for the family to con- tinue to live on the accustomed level of expenditure, the all-round implica- tions of giving up her position to breast- feed the infant must be considered. Then, too, many professional women find their work so satisfying that they are reluctant to stay at home.

Nursing an infant every three or four hours interferes not only with work, but also with recreation outside the home. This is obviously more of a problem for the society woman than for the young middle-class mother whose friends have babies and whose recreation consists in visiting among their contemporaries and comparing their mutual experiences of motherhood.

Unless the mother wants to remain at home to breast-feed her infant, she is not likely to be successful, for her milk supply depends not only on her diet, but also on her emotional state. Although the nurse should never advise parents on the question of breast feeding, she should be sure that they understand the physician's recommendation and help them to clarify their thinking before a final decision is made. In order to do this the nurse herself must have some knowledge of the value and the process of both breast feeding and bottle feeding.

**Maternal Personality and Breast Feeding.** Studies have shown that there is a difference between women who want to nurse their infants and those who do not. The desire to breast-feed their infants is commonly found among women who obtain satisfaction in fulfilling the feminine role. They do not feel that childbirth is an ordeal to be feared and consider that wives may lead domestic lives as rewarding as their working husbands'. Wanting to breast-feed an infant appears to be closely related to motherly attitudes. Women of this type are likely to be successful with breast feeding and to be rewarded by the health and vitality of their offspring. Voluntary breast feeding increases their feeling of competency in child care. They are less likely to worry about the child than the mother who has reluctantly consented to breast-feed her infant and who lives in fear that her milk supply will not be sufficient to meet the infant's nutritional needs.

**Advantages to the Infant.** There are many reasons why physicians hold breast feeding to be superior to even an adequate formula properly prepared and given with loving care. The most important arguments for breast feeding from the point of view of the infant's health are as follows:

Breast milk is more easily digested than is cow's milk and is designed by nature to satisfy the needs of the human infant just as cow's milk meets the needs of the calf.

Breast milk is available at all times. This fact is important if the infant is to be on a self-demand schedule. Breast feeding can be used to comfort an infant, although this should not be done to excess.

Breast-fed infants have greater immunity to certain childhood diseases. Certain antibacterial and antiviral substances may be transmitted in the milk which increase the infant's resistance to infectious diseases. The extent of this protection in the infant has not been proved.

Breast-fed infants are less likely to have gastrointestinal disorders and food allergies in infancy.

Breast-fed infants are less likely to suffer from colds and severe respiratory infections.

Breast-fed infants are less likely to acquire infections in homes where cleanliness is difficult to attain. This is because breast milk is sterile, and the mother's nipples are easily cleaned.

Breast-fed infants enjoy the watchfulness and close contact with their mothers' bodies and can take as much or as little milk as they desire. They can regulate the rapidity of the intake and can never be forced to take more than they want.

Breast-fed infants are less prone to anemia or vitamin deficiency.

In spite of all the advantages of breast feeding, physicians and nurses should not stress its value to the extent that a mother feels guilty if she is unsuccessful in her attempts to breast-feed her baby or if for any reason she is definitely opposed to breast feeding.

**Factors in the Supply of Breast Milk.** The majority of women who have been delivered of a healthy full-term infant and are themselves in good health are capable of breast-feeding their infants.

*Physical factors* in the supply of breast milk include (*a*) an ample diet with a sufficient supply of calcium from milk and other sources. Cigarettes or an occasional cocktail have not proved harmful to the infant.

(*b*) The stimulus of the infant's sucking. If the infant does not fully empty the breasts, the remaining milk should be manually expressed (see p. 120).

(*c*) The nursing mother should avoid fatigue. She should have from eight to ten hours of sleep at night and a nap during the day. It must be remembered that her rest is broken by the infant's night feeding.

(*d*) The mother requires an ample supply of vitamins, especially vitamin D, for her needs and also for the baby, since he receives vitamins through her milk.

(*e*) Her fluid intake should be adequate for her needs, and should supply 16 to 32 ounces of milk for the infant.

(*f*) She needs normal exercise. Housework, if it is not too exhausting, is excellent, but she should also have exercise out of doors every day.

(*g*) The amount of milk-producing tissue in the breasts affects the supply. Large breasts may contain a great deal of fat or supporting tissue and an inadequate amount of glandular secreting tissue.

(*h*) The amount of chemical stimulation by the lactogenic hormones cannot be controlled by any known means, but since the hormones are related to pregnancy, they are in general sufficient in amount.

*Psychologic factors* in the supply of breast milk are extremely important. The mother needs to feel an easy competency in her capacity to supply the feedings day and night and in amounts sufficient to satisfy the infant. She needs to feel secure, happy and relaxed in her family life. Naturally she will become emotionally disturbed at times and the quantity of her milk will be decreased, but the quality remains unchanged; when she has regained her

**Table 1. Comparison of Human Milk with Whole Cow's Milk**

|  | Human Milk (Per Cent) | Whole Cow's Milk (Per Cent) |
|---|---|---|
| Water | 87.0–88.0 | 83.0–88.0 |
| Protein | 1.0–1.5 | 3.2–4.1 |
| Lactalbumin | 0.7–0.8 | 0.5 |
| Casein | 0.4–0.5 | 3.0 |
| Sugar (lactose) | 6.5–7.5 | 4.5–5.0 |
| Fat | 3.5–4.0 (More olein and less of the volatile fatty acids) | 3.5–5.2 |
| Minerals | 0.15–0.25 | 0.7–0.75 |
| Calcium | 0.034–0.045 | 0.122–0.179 |
| Iron | 0.0001 | 0.00004 |
| Vitamins (per 100 cc.) |  |  |
| A | 60–500 I.U. | 80–220 I.U.* |
| D | 0.4–10.0 I.U. | 0.3–4.4 I.U. |
| C | 1.2–10.8 mg. | 0.9–1.4 mg.* |
| Reaction | Alkaline or amphoteric | Acid or amphoteric |
| Bacteria | None | Present |
| Digestion |  | Less rapidly |
| Emptying of stomach |  | Less rapidly |
| Curd | Soft, flocculent | Hard, large |
| Calories per fluidounce | 20 | 20 |

Adapted from W. E. Nelson: Textbook of Pediatrics. 7th ed.
* Values are for pasteurized milk.

composure, her breasts will again be full. She should be told that the emotional strain of coming home from the hospital and undertaking the entire care of the infant may produce a state of tension which will diminish the flow of milk, but that the condition is only temporary.

**Secretion and Composition of Breast Milk.** The secretions of the mammary glands are under the influence of a lactogenic hormone derived from the pituitary gland and are stimulated through the influence of pregnancy.

*Colostrum* is secreted during the first two to four days after delivery. It is yellow, and thin or watery in consistency. It has more protein and minerals and less fat and carbohydrate than breast milk. It is easily digested and has a mild laxative action.

Mature milk appears two to four days after delivery. By the end of the first month the breast milk is constant in composition and remains so. The amount increases as the infant's need for food increases. By the end of the first week 6 to 10 ounces (180 to 300 cc.) a day is the normal amount of milk for a healthy mother to produce; by the end of the first month, 20 ounces (600 cc.), and later, 30 ounces (900 cc.) a day.

Breast milk is slightly bluish and has a relatively high sugar content. The presence of antibodies has not been proved, but they are thought to be present. In the infant's stomach breast milk forms a soft, flocculent curd. If the mother is taking an adequate diet, the vitamin content of her milk is sufficient, or nearly so, for the infant. Mothers should be told that drugs which they take may be eliminated in the breast milk; for instance, if a mother takes opiates, alcohol, nicotine, belladonna or penicillin, a small amount of the drug will be present in the milk.

Table 1 shows the relative composition of breast milk and cow's milk. Breast milk has more carbohydrate and less protein than cow's milk, has approximately the same amount of fat and is of equal caloric value.

## Technique of Breast Feeding

The mother should be told that the supply of breast milk will be well established by the third or fourth day and only in exceptional cases as late as the fourteenth day. During the latent period before an adequate supply of milk is available, the infant loses weight. This is a normal phenomenon and should not cause the mother anxiety. Glucose water may be given to supply the required amount of fluid.

The general procedure is to put the infant to the breast immediately after birth or from four to twelve hours after delivery. Those physicians who advise waiting give as their reasons that the infant and his mother should be given time to rest after the birth process and that time should be allowed for the mucus to be cleared from the infant's throat before he attempts to suck and swallow milk. The length of time spent in nursing at the breast and the number of feedings are increased after the first day or two.

Healthy, supple nipples are important in making the feeding time comfortable for the mother. Erect nipples favor ease of sucking. The skin should be cleansed carefully and thoroughly dried. This will keep the tiny nipple openings from becoming clogged. If the skin is dry and sensitive, the physician may order an ointment to be applied. If the nipples are flat, an ointment should be applied with a gentle, rolling motion of the fingers from the outer rim of the nipple to the tip.

The mother's clothing should not be too tight over the breasts. If a little milk tends to exude from the nipples, she should be careful to keep the area and her clothing clean and dry.

The mother should wash her hands thoroughly with soap and water and should cleanse the nipples before the infant is put to the breast. She should be in a comfortable position, sitting or lying on her side. Her head should be slightly elevated. In presenting the nipple to the infant and while he is sucking she should support the breast tissue away from his nostrils so that he may breathe easily. After feeding it is important that the nipples be washed.

If the nipples are cracked and painful to the mother, they may be lubricated with petrolatum jelly, or a protective nipple shield may be used to minimize the trauma of nursing.

The room should be quiet while the infant nurses, and the mother should not be disturbed in any way. Although the infant obtains 85 to 90 per cent of his feeding in the first 5 to 8 minutes of vigorous sucking, he should be allowed to nurse from 10 to 20 minutes. He enjoys this, and the added milk he gets is to his advantage. Since sucking stimulates the secretion of milk, he should nurse from both breasts at each feeding. It is important that the infant grasp the whole nipple within his mouth; otherwise he cannot achieve adequate suction and may gulp air, since the tip of the nipple is so small that he does not close his lips closely around it.

If the mother's milk is not sufficient to meet the infant's needs, supplementary feedings of modified cow's milk may be given. It is customary to weigh the infant before and after his feedings if there is doubt about the quantity of breast milk. This, however, is likely to make the mother tense and fearful that she cannot supply his needs. Her anxiety reacts on the physical process of milk production and tends to decrease the supply.

It is not as necessary to bubble the breast-fed infant as it is the bottle-fed one. Yet the infant who nurses eagerly at a breast from which the copious flow of milk is more than he can swallow readily may need to be bubbled several times during the feeding. In bubbling the infant, he should be held over the shoulder or seated erect in his mother's lap and gently patted or stroked on the back (see Fig. 37). Thereby the air he has swallowed will rise to the top of his stomach and be eructated. It may be advisable with some infants to do this several times during a feeding and with all infants after the feeding, before laying them in the crib. If the infant's stomach is too full, he may spit up a little milk with each eructation or even after he has been put back in the crib. He may also hiccup. In that case he should be given a little warm water and comforted until the hiccups cease.

Sterile water may be offered between feedings, but it is not necessary for the infant to take it. He should not be urged, for water may interfere with his capacity to finish his next feeding. Giving water is an excellent way to accustom the infant to the rubber nipple so that he will nurse from the bottle in case breast feedings for some reason must be suddenly discontinued. It likewise prepares him to take orange juice in water when the physician orders it.

Infants like to cling to the breast after they have ceased to suck. To remove the infant if he does not voluntarily release the nipple, gentle pressure may be made on his cheeks, or the mother may insert her finger into his mouth. These methods allow air to enter his mouth; suction is then lessened, and he cannot maintain his hold on the nipple. This method is not painful to the mother, nor does it irritate the soft skin covering the nipple.

Rigid feeding schedules are not advisable for the infant. No child should be raised on a clocked schedule. An infant may become hungry before or after the set time for his feeding. If he is allowed to set his own pace, he will eventually work out a fairly regular demand schedule, and the process is accomplished with little frustration on his or his mother's part.

**Manual Expression of Milk.** The technique of emptying the breasts when the infant has not done so is as follows:

Grasp the breast with the thumb above and the index finger below the outer edge of the areola. Press the thumb toward the fingers at the base of the nipple with firm, deep pressure. Support the breast with the other fingers. Use a forward stripping movement. Repeat this about thirty times a minute until the breasts are empty; the process usually takes from ten to fifteen minutes. If the milk is to be used for the infant (for instance, if the mother will be away at the next feeding period), it can be kept in a sterile container under refrigeration.

A hand breast pump or an electric pump may be used instead of manual expression, and many mothers find the electric pump superior to the other two methods. It is fairly expensive, however, and seldom used in the home.

**Wet Nursing and Breast Milk Stations.** Milk from wet nurses is rarely used, for the wet nurse cannot be housed in the apartments or small homes which are customary today. Neither are wet nurses commonly housed in the large modern hospitals as they formerly were to furnish a steady supply of breast milk for premature infants or for infants who could not tolerate modified cow's milk, or for research in feeding problems. If wet nurses are used, they should have serologic tests and roentgenograms to assure the absence of syphilis and tuberculosis. In hospital practice the infant is never put to the wet nurse's breast. Her milk is expressed, usually by the electric breast pump, and given to the infant by bottle, medicine dropper or gavage.

Breast milk stations are found in a few of the large cities, but the milk is expensive, and constant supervision of the mother is required to prevent its dilution with cow's milk or water. It is best to have the mother come to the milk station and express the milk with the electric breast pump. Unless she lives close by it is impractical for her to come to the station three or four times a day, yet if she fails to come, the supply of breast milk for the day runs short.

Since such mothers cannot be as closely supervised as the wet nurse who lives in the hospital, there is need of constant testing for disease. (A rough gauge of the wet nurse's health is, of course, the condition of her own infant, but more precise testing is needed.) In the past immigrant mothers or Negroes from the rural South were willing to undertake the responsibility of providing breast milk for the station for profit. Today breast milk is difficult to obtain.

Breast milk may be pasteurized and kept in sterile containers under refrigeration. It can be frozen and shipped to distant points where it may be thawed and prepared for use as directed by the physician.

## Contraindications to Breast Feeding

The great contraindication to nursing is *serious illness of the mother*. If she has tuberculosis, her condition may be aggravated by lactation, and her infant would be in grave danger of contracting the disease through intimate contact of nursing. A mother may lack the vitality to nurse her infant, owing to some serious complication which developed during pregnancy. For instance, she may be anemic after excessive loss of blood. She may have a chronic disease which is not infectious, but which prevents her undergoing the strain of lactation. Examples of such a condition are cancer, heart disease or impairment of the kidneys. Her labor and delivery may have been complicated by an intercurrent illness or emergency operation which requires prolonged convalescence.

If her condition permits breast feeding, in the presence of intercurrent infection, her milk may be expressed, boiled and given to the infant. In this way the milk supply will be maintained until she is able to give the infant her breast.

The milk from a *mother addicted to drugs*—e.g. morphine, heroin or codeine—will contain small amounts of the drug. The amount the infant receives may not be enough to hurt him, but it may prove habituating. Penicillin may be passed to an infant through breast milk and produce allergic sensitization.

*Menstruation* is not a contraindication to breast feeding unless the mother's nutrition is disturbed. *Pregnancy* is a contraindication to breast feeding only because of the strain upon the mother.

*Mothers working* outside the home often find it difficult if not impossible to return home at feeding times. Likewise the rigors of employment and lactation impose too great a strain upon their health.

*Insanity* is not in itself a contraindication to nursing, although grave danger is involved when a small infant is entrusted to a mentally disturbed patient. Since her milk is normal in amount and certainly in composition, it may be expressed and given to her child if the procedure does not disturb or aggravate the mother and if there is a probability that her condition will improve to the extent that the infant may safely be put to the breast at some future time.

*Local lesions* such as cracked nipples, tumors or breast abscess may contraindicate breast feeding. The milk may be manually expressed to relieve the mother's discomfort from engorgement and to maintain breast function so that she can nurse her infant if the local condition is cured. If the milk is not contaminated, it can be given to the infant.

Some mothers have so-called *inverted nipples;* i.e. the nipples do not stand out so that the infant can grasp them with his mouth. A breast shield will help the infant to attain suction and secure the milk, or the milk may be extracted with a breast pump and prepared as a bottle feeding. If a shield is used, a small amount of colostrum or milk may be expressed into it before it is applied, or it may be partially filled with sterile water.

The *infant's condition* may contraindicate breast feeding. He may be too weak to suck, or sucking may exhaust his strength. The premature infant may not only be too weak to suck, but also may lack the necessary reflexes. The infant with a cleft palate or harelip is unable to suck, as is the infant with facial nerve paralysis. For such infants the breast milk may be manually expressed and given by medicine dropper.

Erythroblastosis fetalis is not a contraindication to breast feeding, since Rh antibodies in the mother's milk are inactivated in the infant's intestinal tract.

## ARTIFICIAL FEEDING

Today artificial feeding is based on scientific principles of nutrition and sterilization. When adequate artificial feedings cannot be provided, the morbidity and mortality rates among the artificially fed infants are far higher than those among breast-fed infants.

The following conditions may adversely affect the success of artificial feeding: contaminated cow's milk; a formula not suited to the infant's needs, either in composition or quantity; lack of cleanliness in preparation of the formula and improper refrigeration of the 24-hour supply of feedings; haphazard and irregular feeding; and feeding entrusted to strangers, with implications of lack of interest and affection.

The importance of this last cause is seldom realized and is rather difficult to analyze. An infant becomes accustomed to one person's ways and responds with restlessness on being fed in an unaccustomed way. Some students of the matter believe that the mother responds more quickly to the infant's needs in regulating the flow of milk by tipping the bottle, bubbling him when he needs to expel air, and in general makes the procedure a more personal service adapted to her infant's needs.

The modern station wagon has made it easy to take the infant and all his equipment wherever the mother goes. He can be left in the station wagon for a few minutes while she shops. The new type of stroller with provision for carrying the baby-bag and groceries is also extremely convenient, and many stores in the suburbs of large cities have rest rooms where mothers can not only change the infant's diaper, but also feed him in comfort.

There are many factors in the mother-child relationship, but in general for the breast-fed infant the relationship is closer, warmer and more demonstrative of affection. The artificially fed infant, then, may not be likely to feel as contented and secure as the breast-fed infant.

The stools of the artificially fed infant are firmer and fewer than those of the breast-fed infant. The color varies somewhat with the type of carbohydrate used in the formula; with cane sugar the stools are yellowish, with a strong, unpleasant odor. The number of stools depends upon the frequency of feedings, the amount taken and the type of food. The typical infant has one to three stools in twenty-four hours.

Cow's milk in the infant's stomach forms large, tough curds which can be rendered more digestible by pasteurization, boiling, homogenization, evaporation or the addition of an acid or alkali. In these processes the curd tension is favorably altered.

### Requirements for Artificial Feeding

**Low Bacterial Count of Milk.** The fundamental requirement of a satisfactory artificial feeding mixture is that the milk, when taken from the cow, have a low bacterial count. Tuberculosis and undulant fever (brucellosis) can be acquired through milk from infected cows. Dairy herds are screened with the tuberculin test for tuberculosis and the Bang test for brucellosis.

The second requirement is that all milk handlers be free from diseases which are transmitted through milk, e.g. scarlet fever, streptococcal sore throat, typhoid fever, diphtheria and tuberculosis.

A third requisite is cleanliness in the care of the cows and in the milking process. In most cities there is strict inspection of the handling of commercial milk from the dairy to the retail store where it is sold to the consumer. The bacterial count and the fat content must conform to certain standards. The milk must be free from preservatives or any injurious substance. It must be pasteurized. Even this clean, pasteurized milk should be pasteurized again or boiled for use in an infant's formula.

**Economy and Availability of Milk.** In the homes of the low-income group it is necessary that an artificial feeding be inexpensive. This is one reason for the extensive use of sterile evaporated milk. It can be bought in small quantities, and if refrigeration is not available, a small tin can be opened for each feeding. What is not used for the infant can be used by the older children or by adults in their coffee.

**Ease of Digestion of Milk.** The average infant under six months of age cannot tolerate undiluted cow's milk. For this reason the milk is diluted with boiled water. For some infants it may be necessary to reduce the large, tough curd formed in the stomach to a softer, finer curd which they can more readily digest. Sometimes lactic acid or lime water is added for this purpose.

**Nutritional Requirements of Formula for Metabolism and Growth.** An *adequate fluid intake* should be 2 to 3 ounces per pound of the expected body weight of the infant, allowance being made for loss of water in urine and stools, by evaporation from the skin and in expired air. The general rule is that a child of one year should take 1000 cc. a day, and an additional 100 cc. should be added for each year of life; e.g. a child of 2 years should take 1100 cc. of fluid per day.

The *protein requirement* is 1.5 to 2 gm. per pound of body weight. One ounce of cow's milk provides 1 gm. of protein. An adequate amount of protein is necessary for growth and for repair of tissue.

The *carbohydrate requirement* in the typical formula for the infant under five months is supplied in the form of Karo or cane sugar. One to 1½ ounces (30 to 45 gm.) is added to the formula. The addition of sugar brings the carbohydrate content of the formula to approximately that of breast milk. For other forms of carbohydrate suitable for use in infant formulas see page 125.

The *caloric requirement* for the infant under 3 months is approximately 50 calories per pound, and over 4 months approximately 45 calories per pound. In contrast, the average adult requirement is 20 calories per pound of body weight.

The *basal metabolic needs* remain low during the neonatal period. Basal heat production rises rapidly, however, during the first year of life. The caloric requirements for basal metabolic needs are proportionately higher in infancy than at any other time of life. During the neonatal period about 80 calories per kilogram of body weight per day are needed to satisfy the infant's nutritional requirements. This amount must be increased rapidly because, although basal metabolic needs do not change, the caloric requirements for growth and energy are much greater in the older infant. Soon a caloric intake of 100 to 130 calories per kilogram (45 to 60 calories per pound) of body weight is needed; this requirement remains constant until the age of 4 months. Caloric needs vary with the infant's activity, his general well-being and his weight gain.

The *fat content* of the formula is not of great importance in the modification of cow's milk and is seldom mentioned in the calculation. Many of the proprietary milks, however, substitute varying proportions of olive, coconut, palm or peanut oil for the butter fat.

*Vitamins* are usually lacking or in insufficient amount in the artificial feeding. Vitamin A, a fat-soluble vitamin, is needed for growth and for resistance to disease or infection. It, in conjunction with vitamin D, which prevents rickets (see p. 345), is derived from cod liver oil or some form of concentrate. The infant needs approximately 400 International units of vitamin D each day. Vitamin B complex is needed for optimum health. Vitamin C prevents scurvy (see p. 349). The infant needs 25 to 50 mg. a day. Since vitamin C is easily destroyed in pasteurization of the milk, it must be provided from some other source. Breast-fed infants usually receive a sufficient amount in the mother's milk, though this depends upon her diet. Vitamin C may be supplied by giving the infant 2 ounces of orange juice daily or ascorbic acid, 25 to 50 mg. a day.

In summary, the infant up to 6 months of age needs approximately 130 to 190 cc. of fluid per kilogram (2 to 3 ounces per pound) of body weight per day. The total caloric, protein and fluid needs for the twenty-four hours of the day determine the composition of the formula. The number of feedings decreases as the infant grows older. At one month he will probably be taking five or six feedings. The amount given at each feeding increases as the intervals between feedings lengthen and the infant requires a greater total fluid intake.

## Types of Milk and Ingredients for Artificial Feeding

The caloric value of whole cow's milk is 20 calories per ounce.

**Certified Milk.**   This is the purest form of raw milk. It contains less than 10,000 bacteria per cubic centimeter and no pathogens, even before pasteurization. It is produced under special hygienic conditions; i.e. manure piles must not be near the barn, and the area should be sprayed liberally with DDT. All milk containers must be sterilized before use. The personnel who handle the milk must be inspected for evidence of disease which might be transmitted through milk. (Throat cultures are taken, and other tests are made.)

**Pasteurized Milk.**   In pasteurization raw milk is heated to 145° F. for 30 minutes. It is then cooled rapidly. In the great majority of cities pasteurization of commercial milk is required by law. Pasteurization kills pathogenic organisms, but does not sterilize the milk; it renders harmless *Bacillus typhosus,* tuberculosis bacilli, organisms causing diphtheria and those in the paratyphoid group, and hemolytic streptococci. Pasteurization destroys vitamin C, which is a heat-labile vitamin, and makes the curd in the infant's stomach smaller and softer. Pasteurized milk should be boiled for infant feeding purposes.

Pasteurized milk is graded A and B. Both are suitable for infant use.

**Vitamin D-Reinforced Milk.**   This is whole cow's milk to which has been added vitamin D, the sunshine vitamin which prevents rickets. Milk from cows at pasture contains more vitamin D than that of cows which do not graze on fresh grass. The vitamin D content of milk may be increased by feeding the vitamin to the cow. In practice it is more satisfactory to add the vitamin directly to the milk. This is done in most large commercial dairies and in the production of evaporated milk. The procedure ensures the desired content of vitamin D in all the milk offered for sale.

**Homogenized Milk.**   In homogenized milk the fat globules are broken down and distributed in a state of colloidal suspension throughout the milk. The curd is rendered softer and thus more digestible, and the flavor of the milk is improved. Digestion is thereby aided, since a larger surface area is offered by the smaller fat moieties for interaction with intestinal enzymes (lipase).

**Evaporated Milk.** This is whole milk from which 60 per cent of the water has been removed. The caloric value is 44 calories (usually considered 40 calories) per ounce. There are 2 gm. of protein per ounce. It is sterile, relatively inexpensive, available in all grocery shops, and can be stored in the home without refrigeration if the can is unopened. Evaporated milk is usually both irradiated and homogenized. It has a fine curd because of the homogenization process and because the casein has been altered in the evaporation process. To use as whole milk it is only necessary to dilute it with an equal quantity of water.

**Condensed Milk.** This is evaporated whole milk to which has been added 45 per cent of sugar. The caloric value is approximately 100 calories per ounce. It should not be used for infant feedings since the sugar content is far too high. An infant fed on condensed milk is likely to be pale and fat, have flabby muscles and be subject to diarrhea due to fermentation of the excessive carbohydrate content of his feeding.

**Dried Milk.** In dried milk the water from whole or skimmed milk has been completely evaporated.

*Modified dried milk* contains various amounts of fat. It is valuable in the formulas of infants who cannot tolerate the amount of fat present in whole milk. Dried milk produces a fine curd, and any dilution desired can be easily made from the dry powder. It is packed in airtight cans and will keep for months without spoiling; for this reason it is useful in traveling with a baby and under conditions when fresh or evaporated milk is not available. In the drying process vitamin C is destroyed. One ounce by weight or 3½ packed level tablespoonfuls of dried milk mixed with seven ounces of water gives a mixture having the composition of liquid milk. For infant feeding the powdered milk is mixed with enough cool water to make a paste; to this the desired amount of water is added gradually while the mixture is stirred to prevent the formation of lumps.

**Carbohydrates.** Carbohydrates are added to the formula to increase its caloric value and improve the flavor, and for their laxative effect. They contain, on the average, 120 calories per ounce. In order to dissolve the carbohydrate it is mixed with a warm fluid.

All types of carbohydrates must be broken down into monosaccharides in the intestinal tract before they can be utilized by the body. The carbohydrates commonly used in infant feedings include the following:

   a. Dextrose or glucose. This is easily digested
   b. Sucrose or cane sugar, the cheapest and most convenient form for use in the infant's formula, but with the disadvantage of being too sweet
   c. Lactose or milk sugar. Milk sugar is not sweet to the taste, is similar to the carbohydrate in breast milk and has a laxative value
   d. Dextri-Maltose, a relatively expensive form, but easily digested. This proprietary product consists of a mixture of maltose and dextrins. These are simplified by digestive processes prior to absorption
   e. Karo (corn) syrup, a cheap and easily digested carbohydrate. It should be kept in the refrigerator and carefully covered, since it is a good liquid culture medium for bacteria
   f. Starch, a polysaccharide. It is difficult for the infant to digest unless it is thoroughly cooked (cooking breaks down the starch molecules).

**Proprietary Infant Milk Products.** These are made by commercial firms and have evaporated milk or dried milk as the basis. In some the fat has been removed or replaced, and in others still different modifications of the original milk have been made. A few proprietary milks are said to closely resemble breast milk in composition. These preparations are relatively expensive, but have the advantages of convenience, sterility and compactness. The law requires the ingredients to be listed on the container. Usually only boiled water is added to the preparation in order to prepare the formula.

### Preparation of the Formula

The basic principles in the preparation of the infant's formula relate to cleanliness and accuracy. The formula must be clean and preferably sterile, since it can be a source of infection to the infant. In the milk laboratory of the hospital, personnel should wear gowns and caps, and many hospitals require that they also wear masks. The formula room should not be in the line of traffic of hospital personnel or visitors, nor near the area housing patients. In the home the formula is prepared in the kitchen. The mother should wear a clean wash dress or large coverall apron.

All equipment must be sterile. The formula should be kept in individual bottles, nippled, capped and clearly labelled. The bottles must be kept under efficient refrigeration until ready for use. When the infant is discharged, the mother is sometimes given a 24-hour supply of his formula in a sterile jar.

**Equipment.** All equipment and ingredients should be ready before preparation of the formula is begun. The ingredients are milk, sterile water and some form of carbohydrate. Figure 34 shows the equipment needed, besides bottles, nipples and bottle caps.

*Bottles.* Enough 8-ounce feeding bottles should be provided for the entire 24 hours' feedings, and at least one extra bottle to replace any that might be broken. Wide-mouthed bottles are commonly used since they are more easily and thoroughly cleaned with a brush and the nipple more nearly approaches the rotund form of the mother's nipple. Many hospitals and mothers are still using the small-necked bottles, however.

*Nipples.* The newborn requires a firm nipple. A nipple which has become flabby from use and repeated sterilization makes sucking difficult for the infant. The aperture in the nipple should be a cross cut, i.e. two 4-mm. incisions in the shape of a cross. Some nipples on the market have this cross cut, but others have the traditional three small holes dispersed in the shape of a triangle. The holes may be enlarged to suit the needs of the individual infant. Factors determining the size of the holes are the infant's ability to suck (the immature and feeble infant may become exhausted if he has to pull vigorously in order to obtain the milk through tiny holes) and the consistency of the formula.

To enlarge the holes in the nipple, the blunt end of a darning needle is inserted into a cork. The point of the needle is held in a flame until red hot and is then used to puncture the nipple. Since the point is red hot, the rubber melts to form a round aperture. It is better to make three small holes in the shape of a triangle than to make a single hole. The nipple is then placed in cold water to harden the rubber. The flow should be tested before the nipple is used. Milk should drip slowly from the nipple when the bottle is tipped upside down at the rate of one drop per second.

*Bottle Caps.* Since the nipple must be sterile when it enters the infant's mouth, airtight sterile bottle caps are used. These may be made of glass or plastic and are cone-shaped, covering the nipple. They are used if the nipples are put on the bottles when the formula is made. If the sterile nipple is to be put on the bottle just before being given to the infant, a close-fitting rubber or plastic cap may be used to cover the bottle top.

*Preparation of Formula.* Figure 34 shows the steps in the preparation of a formula using the aseptic method.

In the hospital each bottle is labeled clearly and accurately with the infant's name. The formula in the individual feeding bottles should be kept in the refrigerator until feeding time.

*Terminal Heating.* Terminal heating is now used in many hospitals and homes for all formulas which can tolerate the degree of heat necessary for this form of sterilization. This process produces a bacteriologically safe formula and eliminates one source of infection; it saves time and causes less work; it destroys bacteria, but does not cause nutritive damage or physical change to the formula.

The formula is prepared with clean but not sterile technique and poured into thoroughly clean bottles. Nipples are put on the bottles, and caps are placed over the nipples.

## FORMULA EQUIPMENT NEEDED

Teakettle or pan

Bottles, nipples, rubber bottle caps
(*or waxed paper, see step 14*)

Measuring cup (*8 oz.*)

Measuring tablespoon

Pitcher or quart jar

Covered kettle or large pan
(*for boiling equipment*)

Long-handled spoon
(*for stirring formula*)

Table knife

Funnel

Can opener

Tongs

Small pan (*to boil nipples and rubber bottle caps*)

Bottle brush

Small jar with screw type lid
(*for storing nipples*)

**1.** Wash all equipment in hot, soapy water and rinse in hot, clear water.

**2.** Use the bottle brush to scrub the bottles and funnel. Rinse in hot clear water.

**3.** Scrub the nipples and rubber caps with the bottle brush in hot, soapy water. Rinse in hot, clear water. Squeeze water through nipple holes during washing and rinsing.

**4.** Place equipment, including bottles, in sterilizer or kettle and pour in 2 inches of water. Cover with lid and boil for 5 minutes.

**5.** Place nipples and rubber caps in small pan and cover with water. Boil for 3 minutes.

**6.** Store nipples in the small jar that was sterilized with the other equipment. Screw on sterile lid and keep jar covered.

**7.** Boil water in teakettle or large pan for 5 minutes and measure the required amount in the sterilized measuring cup.

**Figure 34.** Preparation of the infant's formula by the aseptic method. *Continued on following pages.*

**8.** Pour into the sterilized pitcher or quart jar.

**9.** Measure the required amount of syrup or sugar in the measuring tablespoon. If syrup is used, pour it from the bottle or can into the spoon. If dry sugar is used, level off measuring tablespoon with table knife. Add syrup or sugar to water in pitcher. Stir until dissolved.

**10.** Scrub top of the can of evaporated milk with soapsuds and rinse with scalding water.

**11.** Measure the required amount of milk in measuring cup. Open fresh can daily.

**12.** Pour milk into water sugar mixture and stir with long-handled spoon.

**13.** Use the funnel to pour the formula into the bottles. Drinking water previously boiled may be poured into one or two bottles and given between feedings. (The following instructions apply to the drinking water as well as the formula.)

**14.** Cover bottles with rubber caps, or with the special caps that come with some bottles, or with waxed paper held in place with rubber bands or string. Any one of the 3 ways shown may be used.

**Figure 34** (*Continued*).

**15.** Cool the formula rapidly by placing the bottles in a pan of cold water for 10 minutes. The water should come up to the level of the milk in the bottles.

**16.** Place the bottles in refrigerator until needed.

**17.** When it is time to feed the baby, take one bottle from the refrigerator and remove cap. Use sterile tongs to take one nipple from the jar. Replace cover.

**18.** Place nipple on bottle.

**19.** If screw-cap bottles are used, lift nipple and disk from bottle. Use disk to push shoulder of nipple through cap.

**20.** Remove disk and screw the cap on bottle. Flow may be regulated by tightening or loosening.

**21.** Warm bottle in pan of hot water, not boiling.

**22.** Before giving the formula to the baby, test the temperature by shaking a few drops on the inside of your wrist. It should feel warm, but not hot.

Figure 34 (*Concluded*).    (Courtesy of Pet Milk Company, St. Louis 1, Missouri.)

In the hospital the bottles are placed in racks and autoclaved for 10 minutes at a temperature of 246° F. and 15 pounds' pressure.

For the home a sterilizer may be bought and the technique adapted to its use. The formula should be sterilized for 25 minutes at 212° F. The lid of the sterilizer should not be removed until it is cool enough to handle with the bare hand. This is a rough gauge of the time required for the nipples to cool slowly. (Under rapid cooling the holes in the nipples tend to become clogged by a thin coagulum which tends to form at the surface. Remove the bottles and place them in the refrigerator at a temperature of 40 to 45° F. (4.4 to 7.2° C.) until they are to be used.

Figure 35 shows the steps in formula preparation by the terminal heating method.

**Calculation of Formula.** The following example may clarify the general statements made about an infant's daily nutritional need and fluid intake.

An infant one month of age weighing 8 pounds requires the following:

Fluid: 2 to 3 ounces per pound of body weight
  Total fluid per day: 16 to 24 ounces
Whole cow's milk: 1½ to 2 ounces per pound of body weight
  Total amount of milk: 12 to 16 ounces, *or*
Evaporated milk: 1 ounce per pound of body weight
  Total amount of milk: 8 ounces
Water: A total of 24 ounces of fluid is required for the formula. Sufficient water is added to the milk to bring the amount of the mixture up to the required 24 ounces: e.g. 16 ounces with evaporated milk, 8 to 12 ounces with whole fresh cow's milk
Calories: 50 calories per pound of body weight
  Total caloric requirement: 400 calories per day
Sugar: $\frac{1}{10}$ ounce per pound per day
Volume per feeding: The infant's age in months plus 2 or 3; in this instance, 3 to 4 ounces of formula per feeding
Number of feedings: Total volume of feedings per day (24 ounces) given in 4-ounce feedings results in 6 feedings per day; given in 3-ounce feedings results in 8 feedings per day. During the first 6 months up to 7 ounces may be given at a feeding. More than 8 ounces is rarely given at a feeding
Schedule: 6 feedings (every 4 hours) of 4 ounces each, or 8 feedings (every 3 hours) of 3 ounces each.

An infant, regardless of his age, is seldom given more than 1 quart of whole milk or one can (13 fluid ounces) of evaporated milk during a 24-hour period.

## Technique of Bottle Feeding

The nurse or mother should wash her hands thoroughly with soap and water. The bottle should be placed in a pan of water at a temperature of 120° F. for 10 minutes or in an electric thermostat-controlled warmer. For acid milks (see p. 328) the water temperature should be 110° and the time 5 minutes. Check the name of the infant and that on the bottle before giving the infant his feeding. A mistake in the formula may be as dangerous as a mistake in the giving of medication. To test the temperature and the rate of flow of milk, the nurse lets a few drops fall on the inner side of her wrist. She takes a bib and a diaper to the infant's crib and places the bottle on the bedside stand. She changes his diaper and places the soiled one in the pedal-controlled can, if there is one, or on a piece of newspaper or paper towel at the foot of the crib.

After washing her hands again the nurse picks up the infant, wrapped in a blanket if the room is chilly, and sits down in a rocking chair, holding the infant in her lap with his head supported on her left arm. If for any reason the infant cannot be held in the lap, the nurse should sit beside the crib, elevate the infant's head and hold his bottle. The mother may hold the infant in her arms to feed him while she rests in bed during the postpartum period.

*A bottle should never be propped on a pad,* for an infant is apt to lose his hold on the nipple and be unable to get it in his mouth again; there is also danger that the flow of milk will be too rapid and that the infant might choke. The bottle should be slanted so that the nipple is always filled with fluid; otherwise the infant will suck in air. He may need to be bubbled frequently, and always at the close of the feeding, usually in ten to twenty minutes. After this he should be placed on his right side or prone in his crib. In either of these positions the formula can most easily drain through the pylorus into the intestinal tract.

Any milk left in the bottle should be

## FORMULA EQUIPMENT NEEDED

Pitcher or quart jar

Bottles and nipples

Nipple covers (*see step 10*)
   Brown paper cut 7 inches
   square may be used.

Measuring cup (*8 ozs.*)

Measuring tablespoon

Can opener

Long-handled spoon
   (*for stirring formula*)

Funnel

Bottle brush

Table knife

Sterilizer (*see pictures, step 11*)

**1.** Wash all utensils to be used. Use the bottle brush to scrub the bottles, nipples and nipple covers in hot, soapy water. Soap or a good detergent may be used. Rinse well in hot, clear water, and let drain—do not wipe. Squeeze water through nipple holes during washing and rinsing.

**2.** Measure the required amount of hot water from the tap. (Water does not need to be boiled.)

**3.** Pour into a pitcher or quart jar.

**4.** Measure the required amount of syrup or sugar in the measuring tablespoon. If syrup is used, pour it from the bottle or can into the spoon. If dry sugar is used, level off measuring tablespoon with back of table knife. Add syrup or sugar to water in pitcher. Stir until dissolved.

**5.** Scrub the top of the can with soap suds and rinse in hot water from the tap. Open can by punching two holes in top. Open fresh can daily.

**Figure 35.** Preparation of the infant's formula by the terminal heating method. *Continued on following pages.*

**6.** Measure the required amount of milk in measuring cup.

**7.** Pour milk into water-sugar mixture and stir with long-handled spoon.

**8.** Use the funnel and pour the formula into the bottles. (Drinking water for the baby may be sterilized in a bottle at the same time you are sterilizing the formula.)

**9.** Put the nipples on the bottles.

**10.** Place the nipple covers over the nipples. Three different ways are shown. (*CAUTION—be sure covers are not pressed or screwed down to form a tight seal. They should be loose enough to allow steam to circulate.*) If nipples are covered with brown paper, fasten with string or rubber bands.

**11.** Three different types of sterilizers. Any one of them or a deep cooking utensil with lid may be used.

**a.** Tall sterilizer (9 inches high including lid) with rack for bottles.

**b.** Standard height sterilizer (7 or 8 in. high) showing screw cap type bottles with nipples inverted. Can be used only with this type bottle.

**c.** Pail with wire mesh or washcloth in bottom. Handle of pail must be removed and handle fasteners bent down so that a lid will fit evenly.

**12.** Place rack, wire mesh or washcloth in bottom of sterilizer. Stand the bottles of formula on it, and then pour in two inches of water.

Figure 35 (*Continued*).

**13.** Cover the sterilizer with lid and place on stove. Turn on heat.

**14.** When water starts to boil, write down the time. *BOIL 25 MINUTES BY THE CLOCK.* After water has boiled "*25 minutes*" set sterilizer off the burner.

**15.** *CAUTION*—DO NOT REMOVE LID FROM STERILIZER. DO NOT EVEN LIFT THE LID until sterilizer has cooled enough to allow you to hold your hands against the sides. Then remove bottles and press or screw the nipple covers down firmly over nipples.

**16.** Place covered bottles in refrigerator until needed.

**17.** When it is time to feed the baby, warm the bottle in a pan of hot water (not boiling).

**18.** If screw-cap bottles are used, lift nipple and disk from bottle. Use disk to push shoulder of nipple through cap.

**19.** Remove disk and screw the cap on bottle. Flow may be regulated by tightening or loosening.

**20.** Before giving the formula to the baby, test the temperature by shaking a few drops on the inside of your wrist. It should feel warm but not hot.

**Figure 35** (*Concluded*). (Courtesy of Pet Milk Company, St. Louis 1, Missouri.)

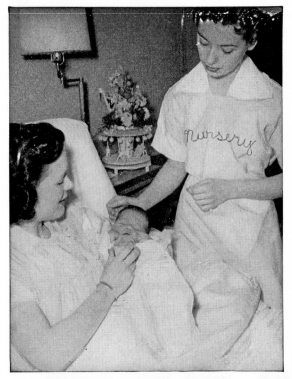

**Figure 36.** Mother learns the art of feeding her baby. (Davis and Sheckler: DeLee's Obstetrics for Nurses. 16th ed.)

**Figure 37.** Bubbling the baby. *A*, The newborn can be bubbled most satisfactorily in the sitting position while gently leaning over the nurse's arm. This procedure is less likely to contaminate the newborn than if he is held over the shoulder. (Davis and Sheckler: DeLee's Obstetrics for Nurses. 16th ed.) *B*, The infant can also be bubbled by holding him firmly against the shoulder, supporting his back and head. His back may be patted or rubbed gently in order to help him relax.

discarded. The bottle and the nipple are rinsed in cold water. If the infant is in isolation, all equipment should be boiled before being returned to the milk laboratory. The nurse should return to the infant after a few minutes to see whether he has regurgitated or vomited part of his feeding.

The feeding should be charted: the time when given, the amount taken and whether any was regurgitated or vomited. Words which may aid the nurse in charting are eructate, bubble, ruminate, regurgitate and vomit. Eructate means to belch. Bubble has almost the same meaning, but implies that air is expelled while the nurse is holding the infant upright or is patting or rubbing him on the back. Rumination means voluntary or habitual regurgitation of formula into the mouth after it has been swallowed. Such milk may be swallowed again or spit out. An infant who spits out milk may lose a considerable amount of his feeding. Regurgitate means to express—"spill over" as it were—a small amount of formula. Vomit means to bring up an appreciable amount of the feeding. If the infant is sick, vomiting may be projectile.

### SELF-DEMAND FEEDING

Infants are best satisfied when they are placed on a self-demand or self-regulating schedule. The infant nurses when he wants food. Then he sleeps until the contractions of an empty stomach waken him. He cries, but when the warm formula is given him, the muscular contractions cease and he experiences a pleasant sensation of fullness. If he is fed whenever he is hungry, he will develop a good appetite. Whether he is breast-fed or bottle-fed, he will establish his own rhythm of feeding. This self-demand schedule is more easily managed in the breast-fed infant, for whom the milk is always ready, than in the bottle-fed infant.

### CARE AT HOME

The hospital gives essentially the same care to the newborn whether his mother is a private, semiprivate or ward patient. When he is taken home, his environment is extremely different. An infant in the low-income group is likely to receive as much loving care as one in the high-income group, but he may be handled by many neighbors, a number of whom may be young children who will be awkward in their handling of him. This is in decided contrast to the more concentrated love and attention which the infant in the middle or upper class receives from a few relatives and friends who are "allowed" to hold him. This difference is an important one.

The physical environment of the home of those in the low-income group is likely to be unhygienic, owing to poor neighborhood sanitation, to overcrowding and to parental attitudes toward health. Poorer parents are likely to accept sickness and a high infant mortality rate as inevitable, for they are accustomed to sickness and death among the infants and little children in the neighborhood. Adjustment between the care an infant should have and what his parents can and will give him is one of the problems with which social workers and public health nurses in clinics, dispensaries and hospitals are constantly faced. It is essential that all these infants be under the supervision of a pediatrician and a public health nurse. This advice should be stressed in the prenatal course and stressed again by the hospital nurses caring for the mother and her infant on the obstetrical and pediatric units.

### Shelter

Here we can consider only an ideal home in a good neighborhood. In her experience in public health nursing the student will see many homes in poor neighborhoods and will be aware of the adaptations in child care which must be made under such conditions.

It is important that the sewer and water systems be adequate and the house well built, with adequate equipment for comfort and safety. The infant should have a room of his own. The floor covering and walls should be easy to keep clean; light colors are preferable. The heating and ventilation should be adequate. For the young infant the temperature during the day should be 70° to 75° F., and at night 55° to 60°; for the older child the temperature should be 68° to 70° during the day and 50° at night. There should be no drafts; ventilation can be secured by any of the modern devices for maintaining fresh air or indirectly from another room. The humidity should be 55 per cent. In winter any device providing for evaporation of water will raise the humidity; a receptacle full of water may be placed on the radiator, or one of the patented devices which fit the radiator may be used.

### Room Furnishings

The furnishings should be simple, durable and easily cleaned. Paint containing lead is no longer used on household equipment, but paint in old homes or on old cribs may be a source of lead poisoning if the infant bites the painted surface or puts broken bits of paint-covered plaster from the wall in his mouth.

The infant should have a bed of his own. It is a needless expense to buy a bassinet which is soon outgrown. A better plan is to buy a crib suitable for a child of four or five years. This will give the infant room to roll and creep in as he becomes able to move about and will keep him happy when he wakes and his mother does not come at once. The bars of the crib should be close together and the side gates high enough to prevent his climbing over. The latch should be out of his reach.

The mattress should be firm, but not hard. The cover should be of thin rubber or other waterproof material and large enough to tuck in at the sides and ends. One type of mattress cover is made to cover both sides of the mattress and fastens with a zipper or snaps. A quilted pad large enough to cover the entire mattress is needed, as well as sheets long enough and wide enough to tuck 12 inches under the mattress at the sides, foot and top. The blankets should be of cotton or wool or a mixture of both. A sleeping bag is good if the infant tends to kick off the covers and the room cannot be kept sufficiently warm. He should not have a pillow until he is old enough to be propped up against it in a corner of his crib. A little infant is no more comfortable with a pillow placed under his head than without it; he may turn on his abdomen with the danger of suffocating as his face presses against the pillow.

Scales are expensive and not necessary for a thriving, full-term infant. To weigh an infant every day or even every few days is likely to worry the mother, for she expects a steady, even gain and is disturbed if he loses an ounce or two. There should be a small chest of drawers for the infant's clothing and personal equipment. As a preschool child he can use the chest and can be taught to put away his own things. There should be chairs for adults, one of them a low rocking chair. When the infant is old enough to sit up, he should have a small chair of his own, low enough for his feet to touch the floor, or the supporting foot rest if it is a high chair. The modern high chair can be lowered so that the infant is on a level with a small table. If the infant is to be left alone, it is safer to have the lower chair. There should also be a shelf for toys, and a playpen raised off the floor.

The infant needs his own bathtub or bathinette. The modern plastic tubs are light, durable and smooth for the infant's skin. An enamel tub is likely to chip, and the sharp edges left may scratch the infant's skin. He will need a diaper pail, preferably of the pedal-controlled type, with a closely fitting cover, and later on a toilet seat or training chair. There should be a gate at the door of the nursery, or at the top of the stairs if the family live in a two-story house.

### Bathing

The infant is bathed once a day and may be sponged off several times a day during warm weather. The temperature of the room should be 75 to 80° F. Either a bathinette or tub is used. The infant over two months enjoys a bath in the family tub, but the mother may find that stooping tires her. If a tub is used, a bath towel is placed over the bottom. This feels soft and warm to the infant, prevents sliding and adds to the pleasure of the bath. The temperature of the water should be 100 to 105° for the newborn or little infant; for the normal healthy infant it can soon be reduced to 95°. The mother tests the temperature with her elbow or a bath thermometer. Soft towels and a wash cloth are needed.

There should be a bath tray containing the following articles:

Jar of cotton swabs or cotton balls
Dish for soap (soap should be white and unscented)
Bottle or jar of baby oil or lotion
Pin holder
Hair brush and comb
Orange wood stick
Paper bag for waste
Powder (if the mother wants to use it)

The mother should be taught that there is no one set procedure to be followed in bathing the infant, but that certain principles must be remembered.

The scalp should be washed frequently. Mothers caring for their first babies may be fearful of washing over the "soft spot" or anterior fontanel. *Cradle cap,* a greasy crust or scale formation on the scalp, often occurs. Treatment of this seborrheic condition is by application of oil or a bland ointment with repeated scalp shampoos until the crust is removed.

The care of the eyes, nose and ears requires special attention to prevent injury. The creases of the body must be carefully cleansed and wiped thoroughly. The genitals and the buttocks are bathed after each stool and, if the infant has a tendency to be chafed, after urinating.

The mother should be given complete directions on the care of the umbilicus before the infant is discharged from the hospital. She should be told, if she does not already know, that there may be a slight bloody discharge from the navel and that the umbilicus will heal in a few days after separation of the cord. She should not give the infant a tub bath until the area is completely healed. Before the infant is discharged the mother may give a return demonstration to the nurse to ensure that she (the mother) will not be anxious about her ability to care for the infant when she is home.

If an abdominal band is used to hold the cord dressing in place, it must be applied firmly and frequently readjusted when it becomes loose. Abdominal bands may be purchased, or can be made at home from strips of stockinet, muslin or flannel. They should be 4 to 5 inches wide and 18 to 20 inches long. They need not be used after the umbilicus has healed. Many physicians do not favor such covering and prefer that the umbilical stump and navel remain totally exposed.

### Clothing

Infants today wear very little clothing. Houses are comfortably warm in winter, and the less the infant wears in summer, the more comfortable he is. Children outgrow their clothing rapidly, so that it is best to buy only enough for several days' wear and to wash their clothes frequently. All articles of infants' clothing should be (a) soft and nonirritating, (b) simple in design, (c) comfortable, (d) loose for activity, (e) washable, (f) suitable for the weather, (g) easy to put on, (h) absorbent, (i) safe—e.g. no ties around the neck which, if caught in any way, might choke the infant and in any case are uncomfortable, and (j) tailored with safe fastenings to avoid the danger of loose or awkward buttons.

In general, shirts for infants are of cotton knitted material.

Diapers are made of gauze, knitted cotton, bird's eye or cotton flannel. They should be either square—27 by 27 inches—or oblong—18 by 36 inches.

To dress the infant, if the shirt is of the slip-over type, it should be gathered in the hands so that it is easily pulled over the infant's head. The double-breasted type of shirt which ties is more

**Figure 38.** The simplest way to dress the infant is to put the entire hand through the sleeve, grasp the infant's hand and pull it through gently. (Davis and Sheckler: DeLee's Obstetrics for Nurses. 16th ed.)

popular, for it is easier to put on, gives double warmth across the chest and does not tear easily. To put the infant's arm through the sleeve, the nurse or mother should put her fingers through the end of the sleeve and put the infant's hand through the armhole. She can then take his fingers in hers and gently pull his hand through the sleeve. The diaper is put on like a pair of pants and pinned at either side to the shirt. The shirt is less likely to tear if it is turned up and the diaper is pinned through the two thicknesses. Turning it up also keeps it clean and dry when the infant voids or has a stool. The diaper should also be pinned securely around the leg openings. For laundering the diapers, see page 112.

Stockings or socks as a rule are used only if the infant's feet are cold and should be large enough to allow the infant to move his toes without being cramped. If long stockings are used, they are pinned to the diaper, above the knee on the outside of the leg. They are likely to become wet whenever the

infant voids. Socks are pretty, but tend to come off when the infant kicks and rubs his legs together.

Bibs are used when the infant is fed. The young infant needs no other clothes, but as he grows older he should be provided with nightgowns, overalls or dresses, sun suits and outdoor clothes for all weather.

### Elimination

The nature of the stool of a well infant depends on his diet. The breast-fed infant has several stools a day which are soft and rather spongy and may contain a little mucus. They are not likely to chafe the infant. Their odor is rather aromatic and not unpleasant. The stools of the infant fed on cow's milk and cane sugar are yellow and more solid than those of the breast-fed infant and have an unpleasant odor. One or two stools a day is normal.

### Sleep

The newborn infant sleeps or appears to be sleeping practically all the time he is not feeding. His sleep is light, and there are frequent spontaneous movements of the face and body. He stretches and puckers up his face. When he is only a few weeks old, his sleeping periods are longer and more quiet, but he is also awake and alert for longer periods. This trend continues as he grows out of early babyhood.

### Weight

Mothers should learn, while in the hospital, how to weigh their infants if they have or intend to have scales at home. Safety factors should be emphasized. The mother should keep one hand over the infant at all times when she is weighing him. She should place the head end of the scale near, but not touching, the wall so that he may not slide out that end. She should hold her hand close enough to his body to prevent his sliding down and over the other end of the scale.

In the home weekly weighings are sufficient. If they are attempted daily, mothers tend to worry about minor fluctuations. Scales are not absolutely necessary, for the infant can be weighed when taken for his check-up to the physician's office or the Child Health Conference. The average infant will gain between 7 and 8 ounces (210 and 240 gm.) each week. Some infants, however, gain within a range of 5 to 12 ounces (150 to 360 gm.) a week. If the gain is more or less than this, the mother should notify the physician.

### Temperature

Although mothers should be taught how to take the infant's temperature, this should not be considered part of the daily care. The temperature should be taken only when the mother believes that it is not normal.

### Feeding

The feeding of the infant should be considered part of the routine activities of daily living in which all the members of the family are engaged. If everyone in the home is to be subordinated to the infant, he is likely to become a disturbing factor in the family. This consciously or unconsciously creates a feeling that he is privileged and influences the emotional relations of parents and siblings toward him and indirectly toward each other. All plans for his care, from the first day in the hospital on, should be made with reference to what is best for him in the family situation. Feeding is so essential that the way an infant is fed (see Fig. 36) and bubbled (see Fig. 37) conditions him to feeling that this world is a friendly place to live in or a place of unpleasant sensations in which he is anxious all the time. It is easy to recognize an unhappy infant: he is a whining child with a puckered forehead who is always sucking whatever he can get hold of and put into his mouth.

Feeding time should be a pleasant time for both the infant and the family. The infant learns to like the one who feeds and cuddles him. The average infant at six weeks of age will return his mother's smile when she picks him up and smiles at him. In time he is conditioned to smile because smiling always brings more cuddling and expressions of love from his mother. He is a little egotist, and his own comfort is all he cares about. But in time he learns to like a smiling mother and wants to have her smile. This is his way of wanting to please her, and it lays the foundation for willingness to do what she wants (obedience), so essential to the willing acceptance of discipline, which in turn leads to self-discipline.

While the mother is in the hospital the nurse should give her (1) a recipe for the formula, (2) a set of instructions, and (3) a demonstration of formula preparation. The mother may be taught either the aseptic technique or the terminal heating method, or both. Teaching may be supplemented by the use of booklets from milk companies; these illustrate the steps by which formulas can be prepared by either method (see Figs. 34, 35).

### Follow-up Care

If the mother has a private physician, she will put her baby under his care after she and the baby have been discharged from the hospital. But the mother who is a clinic patient will come to the postnatal clinic for the further care she needs. The infant is routinely referred by either the social service department of the hospital or the head nurse (or supervisor) of the obstetrical unit to the public health Child Health Conference in the district in which he lives. The public health agency will be notified of his discharge from the hospital, and a public health nurse will visit in the home to instruct the mother in the adaptation of all she has learned to the home situation. She will check on the equipment for the infant's care and demonstrate his bath and the making of his formula. If further guidance or help is needed, she may refer the mother to The Family Service Society or equivalent agency.

After discharge the infant should be under continuing medical care. He should be seen by the physicians in the outpatient department of the hospital, by the family physician or by those in the community-sponsored Child Health Conference in which the public health nurses work.

## TEACHING AIDS AND OTHER INFORMATION*

*American Academy of Pediatrics*
Resuscitation of the Newborn Infant, 1958.
Suggestions for Control of Staphylococcal Infections in Newborn Nurseries, 1958.

*H. J. Heinz Company*
Nutritional Data. 3rd ed. 1959.

*U.S. Department of Health, Education, and Welfare*
Aseptic Nursing Techniques, 1960.
Breast Feeding, 1947.
Infant Care, 1955.
The Confidential Nature of Birth Records.
Your Well Baby, 1949.

## REFERENCES

Adams, M. M.: Appraisal of the Newborn Infant. Am. J. Nursing, 55:1336, 1955.
American Academy of Pediatrics Committee on Fetus and Newborn: Standards and Recommendations for Hospital Care of Newborn Infants, Full Term and Premature. Evanston, Ill., American Academy of Pediatrics, 1957.
Bookmiller, M. M., and Bowen, G. L.: A Textbook of Obstetrics and Obstetric Nursing. 3rd ed. Philadelphia, W. B. Saunders Company, 1958.
Canice, Sister M.: Circumcision of the Newborn. Am. J. Nursing, 60:1431, 1960.
Committee on Medicolegal Problems: Review of Status of State Laws Requiring Use of a Prophylactic in the Eyes of Newborn Infants. J.A.M.A., 169:1950, 1959.
Cooper, L. F., Barber, E. M., Mitchell, H. S., and Rynbergen, H. J.: Nutrition in Health and Disease. 13th ed. Philadelphia, J. B. Lippincott Company, 1958.
Davis, M. E., and Sheckler, C. E.: DeLee's Obstetrics for Nurses. 16th ed. Philadelphia, W. B. Saunders Company, 1957.
Fitzpatrick, E., and Eastman, N. J.: Zabriskie's Obstetrics for Nurses. 10th ed. Philadelphia, J. B. Lippincott Company, 1960.
Grayson, R., and Cranch, G. S.: Care of the Foreskin. Am. J. Nursing, 56:75, 1956.
* Complete addresses are given in the appendix.

György, P.: Trends and Advances in Infant Nutrition. Nursing Outlook, 6:516, 1958.
Kirkes, L.: Hints on Helping Mothers. Am. J. Nursing, 59:1740, 1959.
Koop, C. E.: Emergency Surgery of the Newborn. Clinical Symposia. Ciba Pharmaceutical Products, Inc., Summit, New Jersey, 11:35, 1959.
Krause, M. V.: Food, Nutrition and Diet Therapy. 2nd ed. Philadelphia, W. B. Saunders Company, 1957.
Larsen, E. C.: Terminal Rooming-In. Am. J. Nursing, 56:1442, 1956.
McClure, M. H.: When She Chooses Breast Feeding. Am. J. Nursing, 57:1002, 1957.
Mellin, G. W., and Kent, M. P.: Ophthalmia Neonatorum: Is Prophylaxis Necessary? Pediatrics, 22:1006, 1958.
Miller, H. C., and Conklin, E. V.: Clinical Evaluation of Respiratory Insufficiency in Newborn Infants. Pediatrics, 16:427, 1955.
Nelson, W. E. (editor): Textbook of Pediatrics. 7th ed. Philadelphia, W. B. Saunders Company, 1959.
Newton, N.: Maternal Emotions. New York, Harper and Brothers, 1955.
Ormsby, H. L.: Prophylaxis of Ophthalmia Neonatorum. Am. J. Nursing, 57:1174, 1957.
Parmelee, A. H.: Management of the Newborn. 2nd ed. Chicago, Year Book Publishers, Inc., 1959.
Riker, A. P.: Successful Breast Feeding. Am. J. Nursing, 60:1443, 1960.
Senn, M. J. E.: Fads and Facts as the Bases for Child-Care Practices. Children, 4:43, 1957.
Silver, H. K., Kempe, C. H., and Bruyn, H. B.: Handbook of Pediatrics. 3rd ed. Los Altos, California, Lange Medical Publications, 1959.
Smith, C. S.: Demand Feeding in the Newborn Nursery. Nursing Outlook, 6:514, 1958.
Spock, B.: Baby and Child Care. New York, Duell, Sloan & Pearce, Inc., 1957.
Spock, B., and Lowenberg, M. E.: Feeding Your Baby and Child. New York, Duell, Sloan & Pearce, Inc., 1955.
Stott, K. B.: 'Rooming-In' Is Not a Passing Fad. Hospitals, 29:80, May, 1955.
Van Blarcom, C. C., and Ziegel, E.: Obstetrical Nursing. 4th ed. New York, Macmillan Company, 1957.
Volinsky, T. J.: Care of the Newborn. Nursing World, 131:24, July, 1957.
Wiedenbach, E.: Family-Centered Maternity Nursing. New York, G. P. Putnam's Sons, 1958.
Wishik, S., Watson, N. D., and Bullock, A.: Breast, Bottle or Both for Your Baby? Parents Magazine, 31:36, September, 1956.

# Chapter 8

# The Premature Infant

THE CARE of the infant born prematurely illustrates remarkably well the continuity of care from that of the fetus through care of the mother to the infant's care after delivery, since in this instance care after birth is based on the needs of an infant so immature that he is adapted only to life in utero.

Approximately 10 per cent of all live births are premature. The standard of prematurity should be the number of days of gestation, but this standard correlates with the weight, length and activity of the newborn. Prematures are therefore often defined in terms of weight, length and behavior. *Prematurity* may be defined as the termination of pregnancy in the period from approximately the twenty-eighth to the end of the thirty-seventh week of gestation. Because weight is often indicative of an infant's prematurity and physiologic immaturity, a premature infant is now considered to be one who weighs 2500 gm. (5 pounds 8 ounces) or less at birth. The length of such an infant from crown to heel is likely to be close to 18.5 inches (47 cm.). His behavior shows his immaturity: he lacks the normal reflexes and general ability to carry on the vital functions which the normal full-term infant has.

### Incidence and Causes of Prematurity

In a large number of cases the cause of prematurity is not known, partly because the incidence is highest among the low socio-economic groups. Prospective mothers in such groups are least likely to have adequate prenatal care, which includes observation and recording of a woman's condition throughout pregnancy. Many of these women are first seen by an obstetrician when they are in labor.

Multiple births are a frequent cause of prematurity; few triplets are carried to term. Toxemia of pregnancy is an important cause, particularly among women who are not under observation of a clinic obstetrician or their own physician. Antepartum hemorrhage is likely to occur in two important complications of pregnancy: premature separation of the placenta and placenta praevia. Both conditions may contribute to premature birth of the infant. Pre-

**141**

**Figure 39.** The infant on the left was 28 days old when the picture was taken and weighed 585 gm. It was born at 25 or 26 weeks' gestation and weighed 780 gm. at birth. It survived and is normal. For comparison the infant on the right is a normal full-term infant who weighed 3150 gm. (Davis and Sheckler: DeLee's Obstetrics for Nurses. 16th ed.)

mature rupture of the membranes invariably causes premature birth.

Among maternal diseases related to premature delivery are (1) those of noninfectious origin—e.g. cardiac disease, diabetes mellitus and severe sensitization to the Rh blood factor—and (2) those of infectious origin, whether acute or chronic. Chronic maternal malnutrition may also cause premature birth of the infant.

Fetal abnormalities or injury to the mother or fetus, or both, may make it impossible for the infant to be carried to term. Overwork and inadequate diet are important factors in the high incidence of premature births in the low socio-economic groups. They are seldom the immediate cause of a premature delivery, but predispose to poor health, if not chronic or acute illness, which interferes with carrying the fetus to term.

### Prevention of Prematurity

The great preventive measure to reduce the number of premature births is adequate prenatal care for all prospective mothers, including both medical care and a healthy environment. Maternal and child health programs—federal, state and local—have provided good obstetrical care for thousands of women who otherwise would have lacked even a minimum of medical supervision during the prenatal period. It will be impossible, however, to provide an adequate environment for many of those mothers until the slums of large cities are wiped out and the level of living of the lowest economic group is raised. Maternal care is provided to protect the infant as well as the mother, since *the longer the fetus can be retained in utero, the better are its chances for survival.*

### CHARACTERISTICS OF PREMATURE INFANTS

#### Physical Characteristics

The premature infant that we see in the incubator is at the same stage of development as the fetus of the same gestational age. The age of viability is commonly said to be seven months. Many premature infants, then, will resemble the fetus of seven months' gestation. The premature infant is adapted to life in utero. His immaturity is evident as we look at him. He is small and limp. His skin is thin, wrinkled and red; there is an excess of lanugo and little or no vernix caseosa. His head is relatively large with prominent eyes, soft ears and receding chin. The thorax is less firm than that of the full-term infant. The abdomen protrudes, and the genitals are small. The extremities are thin, the muscles small. The fingernails and toenails are abnormally soft and short. The subcutaneous tissue is deficient, so that he has a wizened appearance. (Extremely small prematures may have a plump appearance due to edema. This is lost, however, in a few days.) Engorgement of the breasts, normal in the full-term infant, is absent in the premature, since it is due to hormones from the mother which are passed to the fetus in the late months of gestation. The normal sucking, swallowing and gag reflexes are absent in very immature infants.

## Physiologic Handicaps

The nursing care of the premature infant, so far as it differs from that of the normal infant, is based on the physiologic handicaps of immaturity: (1) poor control of body temperature, (2) difficult respiration, (3) inability to handle infections adequately, (4) tendency to hemorrhage and anemia, (5) tendency for rickets to develop, (6) disturbances of nutrition, and (7) impairment of renal function.

**Poor Control of Body Temperature.** What was said of the normal newborn's de-pendency on the temperature of his environment to maintain a normal body temperature (p. 85) is even more important in planning the care of the premature infant. His nervous system is poorly developed, and the heat-regulating center in the brain is immature. The skin surface of the premature is great in proportion to his weight. He lacks the insulation of the subcutaneous fat layer, which is developed in the last month of gestation. His muscular development being poor, he is inactive. The metabolic rate is low. If the environment is too warm, he becomes overheated, since his sweating mechanism is underdeveloped. Yet internal conditions which would cause a fever in a normal infant may be present in the premature without an elevation of temperture (this often happens in the dehydrated premature or one with an infectious condition).

**Difficult Respiration.** Respirations are difficult and irregular in the premature infant. Since his lungs are immature, there is incomplete development of the alveoli and weakness of the thoracic cage and of the respiratory muscles. Gaseous exchange is retarded by the immature alveolar membrane. Then, too, if mucus lodges in his throat or if a few drops of feeding enter the trachea, his gag and cough reflexes are too weak to clear the airway.

*Cyanosis.* The premature's tendency to cyanosis is evidence of inadequate

**Figure 40.** A premature infant delivered after 25 weeks of intrauterine life. It weighed only 710 gm.; its length was 34 cm. Few infants of this age and weight survive. (Davis and Sheckler: DeLee's Obstetrics for Nurses. 16th ed.)

oxygenation of his arterial blood. This may be due to increased intracranial pressure from birth trauma, obstruction of the respiratory tract, poor development of the respiratory muscles or some interference with the normal expansion of the lungs. There may be interference with the action of the diaphragm from abdominal distention.

*Apnea.* Apnea is a condition of suspended respiration. It may result from excessive analgesics or anesthetics given the mother during labor. Expert care during delivery decreases the danger of birth trauma with resulting cyanosis. General immaturity of the nervous system and the respiratory tract is a cause of apnea which is inherent in the premature infant's condition and cannot be controlled by the obstetrician, although modern methods of resuscitation keep many such infants alive who formerly would have died at birth.

**Inability to Handle Infections Adequately.** The premature infant is very susceptible to infection, and his ability to handle infection of any sort is poor. He is listless and hardly responds to stimulation. His body has little ability to produce the necessary immune responses, and he does not react to infection with fever or an elevation of the white blood cell count. He lacks immune substances from his mother, which are transmitted to the fetus during the last months of gestation.

The immature infant has more avenues for access of infection than does the normal infant. His skin and mucous membranes are not as protective as the more mature skin and membranes of the full-term infant.

**Tendency to Hemorrhage and Anemia.** The blood vessels of the premature infant are incompletely developed and therefore more fragile, the supporting tissue lacks normal elasticity, and the plasma is hypoprothrombinemic. He lacks the normal supply of vitamin K. Anemia results from hemorrhage as with the normal infant, but the premature suffers more from loss of blood than does the normal infant because he lacks iron and other essential hematogenous factors which the fetus receives

during the last months of gestation. His body growth is rapid and therefore requires a greater blood supply. He still has an increased proportion of fetal hemoglobin. His red blood cells are easily destroyed, and even a slight loss of blood is of great consequence to him.

**Tendency for Rickets to Develop.** The premature infant lacks the calcium, phosphorus and usually the vitamin D normally stored in the body of the full-term infant. Yet his potentially rapid rate of growth requires an ample supply of these minerals, and vitamin D is needed for their utilization. He also lacks the ability to absorb fat-soluble vitamins given in his feedings. The result of these adverse factors is that the premature is more likely to acquire rickets than is the normal infant.

**Disturbances of Nutrition.** Good nutrition requires an adequate intake of the essential nutritional requirements. The premature infant, because of his weak sucking and swallowing reflexes, is often unable to take a sufficient amount of feeding to meet his needs. It may be necessary to feed him by gavage or medicine dropper. Frequently he does not retain the entire feeding. The value of what he takes and retains is reduced through his faulty absorption of fat-soluble vitamins and certain minerals. The low acidity of his gastric secretions interferes with the normal digestive processes. He is prone to disturbances of nutrition, since his digestive system is unable to handle even undiluted breast milk.

**Impairment of Renal Function.** The incomplete development of the kidneys of the premature causes difficulty in concentration of urine, and a proportionately large amount of fluid is lost.

## CARE AND TREATMENT OF THE PREMATURE INFANT

Differences in the nursing care of the premature infant from that of the full-term infant are based on the anatomic and physiologic characteristics of prematurity in contrast to those of the infant of nine months' gestation. The needs of the premature cannot be met in the same way, for he is not fully adapted to extrauterine life.

## CARE IMMEDIATELY AFTER BIRTH

The nursing care of the premature immediately after birth is based on his peculiar needs and includes the following.

**Warmth.** The infant is placed in a warm incubator provided with the necessary facilities for increasing environmental oxygen and humidity.

**Initiation of Respirations.** The airways should be cleared. To accomplish this the mucus may be removed from the nose and throat by gentle suction. A mucus trap may be used with a no. 8 to 10 French rubber catheter. The infant is placed in a level position or with his head down and his body and feet slightly raised. This position increases the natural drainage of secretions.

If the infant has hypoxia, he may be given artificial respiration with a mechanical device providing measured positive pressure. If no mechanical device is available, *gentle* mouth-to-mouth insufflation by blowing "puffs" of air through several layers of gauze may be used. Air enriched with oxygen may be given to the infant if an oxygen tube is placed in the operator's mouth. Other more vigorous measures may cause the infant to gasp once or twice, but are not helpful in establishing respiration.

**Oxygen Administration.** Oxygen should be in readiness if respirations are not established in the first few seconds of life, and later if the infant shows signs of cyanosis. Immediately after birth he may be placed in an atmosphere having an oxygen content of 30 to 40 per cent. To stimulate respiration once it has been established, oxygen, 95 per cent, and carbon dioxide, 5 per cent, may be used for short periods only.

**Medications.** The nurse should know the drugs commonly used in treating conditions usual in premature infants, and such drugs should be in readiness in case of emergency. Epinephrine is given intramuscularly as a cardiovascular stimulant, and caffeine and sodium benzoate is given intramuscularly for respiratory stimulation. To reduce the tendency to bleeding, Menadione (vitamin K) may be given intramuscularly in the lateral aspect of the thigh. Excessive doses are to be avoided, since the drug may cause increased bilirubinemia. Nalorphine hydrochloride (Nalline) should be given intravenously into the umbilical cord to counteract the respiratory depression due to morphine, codeine or other opiates given the mother before delivery and transmitted to the infant via the placenta.

## CARE IN THE NURSERY

**Environment.** In general, the premature nursery is close to the nursery for normal infants and is under the direction of the obstetrical supervisor. No nurses may enter the premature nursery except those assigned to it. There is usually an isolation nursery for prematures brought to the hospital from other hospitals or from the home. This nursery may be operated in connection with either the obstetrical or the pediatric unit. The trend is to consider the nursing of premature infants as a pediatric departmental responsibility and to assign students to their care during the experience in pediatric nursing.

The infant should be taken from the delivery room to the nursery in a heated carrier. The nursery should be isolated from all other units to ensure protection from infection. It should be air conditioned, although this may not be possible in old buildings. The humidity of the nursery should not be below 55 or above 65 per cent, the temperature not below 77° or above 90° F. Each infant should have his own incubator or crib.

Good nursing care is essential to the preservation of the premature, and the survival rate is highest where nursing care is adequate in both quantity and quality. Such care must be constant. Any omission lessens the infant's chance for survival. Nurses caring for premature infants must know the principles on which care of the premature is based and must be skilled in its adaptation to the needs of the individual infant. They must be able to judge his needs at any time and be devoted to providing the best possible care. In no other area of pediatric nursing is the ability to observe and accurately record all symptoms of greater importance. Manual skill is also required. Procedures must be carried out with extreme gentleness and precision. The underdeveloped condition of premature infants makes them liable to injury from the slightest error in medication or treatment.

An adequate physical environment is necessary, but more important is the nursing personnel. The nursing care of the premature is a special area of nursing, and only nurses experienced in such care should be placed in charge at any time during the day or night. Student nurses cannot acquire the knowledge and skill to give adequate care during the short time they are assigned to the care of the premature, and the head nurse or instructor should be available at all times to assist them.

### Maintenance of Body Temperature

The premature infant is unable to maintain a stable body temperature. Even minor deviations from the optimum environmental temperature cause a corresponding change in his body temperature. In caring for the premature the danger of his being cold is always stressed. A warm nursery and the use of incubators (see Figs. 29, 45) make it possible to provide the required environmental heat to maintain each infant's body temperature at 96 to 98° F. (35.5 to 36.5° C.). Ideally, the infant's body temperature should be 98°, but stability of temperature is more important than maintenance at exactly 98° F. Overheating is as bad for the infant as being cold. The ideal temperature and humidity of the nursery prevent loss of water through the skin and excessive loss through breathing.

Incubators are indicated for infants of 3 pounds or less. If for any reason a premature is placed in the general nursery, the incubator will probably be used until he weighs well over 3 pounds, and even longer if he cannot maintain his temperature, has difficulty in breathing or becomes cyanotic. One great advantage of the incubator is that it can be regulated to meet the needs of the individual infant. In general, the temperature in the incubator should not be over 90° F. (32.2° C.); it may be raised or lowered, according to whether the infant requires more or less heat.

If an incubator is not available, other methods of applying heat must be provided. The most commonly used is the hot-water bottle. The temperature of the water should be 115° F. The rubber bag must be covered with a cotton flannel square fastened with safety pins or a bag with a draw string to hold the cover in place. The bottle must never be placed next the infant, but rather outside his blankets. It is well to use three hot-water bags and refill them in rotation. In this way a more even heat is maintained about the infant. One may be placed on either side of him and one under his legs.

If no other method of keeping the crib warm is available, hot bricks may be used. They are, of course, hard and unyielding, even when well covered and placed outside the blankets. Extreme care must be exercised to avoid overheating the bricks, which must be covered with several layers of soft cotton flannel.

Since the objective of applying external heat is to maintain the infant's temperature within a normal range, it is necessary to take his body temperature in order to determine the amount of external heat required. It may be necessary to take the temperature every hour until it is stabilized. The temperature should be taken when the infant is first brought to the nursery. This is done rectally, thereby simultaneously detecting the presence of anal occlusion if the condition is present (see p. 104). After this initial trial the temperature is routinely taken by the axillary method as often as ordered.

**Preparation and Use of Incubators.** Types of incubators include, among others, the Armstrong, the Isolette and the heated crib. Each varies from the others in some detail of operation, and the nurse must study the operating instructions of each; these are provided by the manufacturer.

In the selection of an incubator the points on which it is to be evaluated are (1) easy maintenance of heat and humidity, (2) ease in administration of oxygen, (3) transparent top for easy visibility, and (4) safety alarms to indicate overheating or lack of circulating air.

The incubator should be prepared before the infant arrives. The regulator is set at approximately 90° F. Thereafter it is adjusted so that the infant's temperature is maintained between 96 and 98° F. The water chamber is filled so that the humidity can be increased if necessary. For the newborn premature infant the bed is adjusted as ordered so that his head is level with his body or slightly lower than his body. The oxygen flow is adjusted and tested every five minutes for concentration, to determine whether it is what the physician ordered. After the concentration has been stabilized it should be rechecked every four hours and the results recorded on the patient's chart. Prematures should be kept in 30 to 40 per cent oxygen only as long as they have symptoms of respiratory distress or cyanosis.

### Maintenance of Respirations

The respirations of the premature may be rapid, shallow and irregular. The abdominal muscles are used, and there may be some periods of apnea. Gentle suction may be needed to clear the respiratory tract of mucus and other fluid. Stomach lavage may be ordered if the secretions are excessive.

A vaporizer should be used to produce the high humidity necessary for premature infants or those born by cesarean section. This is adjusted to produce a humidity within the incubator of 55 per cent or higher. If the respiratory difficulty is relieved, the vaporizer may be discontinued after twen-

ty-four to thirty-six hours. Routine nebulized water is not necessary and may predispose to skin infections and sepsis. High humidity may be obtained in the home through the use of steam kettles, inhalators, or wet towels placed over a radiator. The towels are kept wet by immersing one end in a pan of water.

Oxygen 95 per cent and carbon dioxide 5 per cent may be necessary for 30 to 120 seconds every half-hour to one hour for at least 12 hours to stimulate respirations. It is always necessary to clear the pharynx before giving oxygen and carbon dioxide so that the infant does not aspirate the secretions when he inspires.

The infant should be on his side in the incubator in order to get the maximum amount of air into his lungs. If he is inactive, as he probably will be, his position should be changed every one to three hours. If artificial respiration is necessary, it should be given very gently (for the technique, see p. 145).

When the oxygen concentration in the incubator is above 40 per cent, there is danger of retrolental fibroplasia developing (see p. 153). Several methods may be used to limit the concentration of oxygen to the percentage ordered by the physician. The oxygen flow can be adjusted until analysis shows that the desired concentration has been established. A mixture of 40 per cent oxygen and 60 per cent nitrogen can be used in the incubator; by this means the infant cannot receive more than 40 per cent oxygen, and there will be no danger of inducing retrolental fibroplasia. An oxygen-diluting meter can be used to regulate the concentration of oxygen. This device mixes the air of the room with pure oxygen and can be set to produce any concentration ordered by the physician. It is not, however, a substitute for oxygen analysis (see p. 154), but keeps the range of concentration within limits.

**Charting Oxygen Intake.** Each infant's chart should contain a separate oxygen record, which should include (1) the physician's written order for oxygen and its method of administration, (2) the duration of administration, (3) the oxygen concentration, and (4) the infant's response to the concentration and to its duration. The extent of time during which the infant received oxygen must be determined accurately (all interruption in therapy required when caring for the infant must be noted). The oxygen concentration should be analyzed at four-hour intervals, or more frequently if necessary, and charted. The infant's response, including changes in his color, respirations, pulse, and degree of activity, should be carefully observed and accurately charted.

Today the danger of giving more oxygen than the infant requires is so well understood that the nurse has a greater responsibility than formerly, when excessive oxygenation was not considered dangerous. The ability to judge an infant's need for oxygen is acquired only by long experience. The student should observe the infants closely and understand the reason for giving oxygen of a particular concentration in each case.

### Nutrition

The problem of nutrition in the premature infant is complicated by his difficulty in sucking and even in swallowing. Often these reflexes are absent, and he makes no response to stimulation of his lips by a nipple or medicine dropper; feeding placed in his mouth either runs out or causes him to choke. If he is able to take the feeding or is fed by gavage, the small capacity of his stomach often results in distention and vomiting, which may cause respiratory embarrassment. The gastric acidity is low, and the capacity for absorption of fat is not that of the normal full-term infant. His entire digestive enzyme system is incompletely developed, and he may be unable to handle satisfactorily any type of feeding, even breast milk.

The problem is accentuated by his need for a nutritional intake higher than that of the normal infant, whose weight at birth allows for the initial loss which normally occurs until feeding is established. The premature needs 60 to 80 calories and 3 to 4 gm. of protein per pound of body weight, plus an adequate carbohydrate and liquid intake. Since his ability to absorb fat is poor, skimmed milk rather than whole milk is generally used as the basis for his formula.

Because of the edema present at birth, the premature infant is seldom given a feeding or water by mouth during the first eighteen to twenty-four hours. The initial feeding may be as little as 2 to 4 cc. and may consist solely of a 5 per cent sugar solution. Feedings are slowly increased, and both fat and protein are added to the carbohydrate given in the first few days.

There is no set standard for his feeding; it must be adapted to his individual needs. In general he does not tolerate cow's milk unless the fat and protein content has been altered. If possible, he should be given breast milk, though it may be necessary to dilute the milk with water. The mother may be able to provide breast milk. If so, it should be expressed manually and given to the infant. The supply is thereby maintained, and the infant may be put to the breast when he is able to suck and swallow adequately.

Mention has been made of breast milk stations where human milk can be bought (see p. 121). Such milk is expensive, however, and it may be difficult to secure a steady supply. Often mothers on the obstetrical unit who have an overabundance of milk will donate the excess to the premature infants in the nursery.

The formula for the premature should be high in protein, low in fat and of average carbohydrate content. Proprietary milks which resemble breast milk in composition are often used.

**Methods of Feeding.** The method of feeding is extremely important, since there is danger that the infant may aspirate a little of the milk and also since no formula is of advantage to the infant unless it is taken and retained. The infant takes so little milk at a feeding that it is generally ordered in cubic centimeters rather than ounces.

Figure 41.   Mummy restraint. *A,* One corner of a small blanket is folded over. The infant is placed on the blanket with his neck at the edge of the fold. *B,* One side of the blanket is pulled *firmly* over one shoulder. *C,* The remainder of that side of the blanket is tucked under the opposite side of the infant's body. *D,* The procedure is repeated with the other side of the blanket. The blanket should be pinned in place. (Note: When applying a mummy restraint, be certain that the extremities are not forced into an uncomfortable position.)

Figure 42.   Alternate method of applying a mummy restraint so that the infant's chest is exposed. *A,* Pull the blanket firmly over both arms and tuck it under the infant's back. *B,* Wrap the legs in the remainder of blanket on both sides of the body and pin it in place.

Tongue

Stom.

**Figure 43.** The catheter tip is just within the stomach. (Davis and Sheckler: DeLee's Obstetrics for Nurses. 16th ed.)

The feedings are given slowly in small amounts and at frequent intervals. The infant is bubbled frequently. He should never be forced to take the feeding. Underfeeding is less harmful to him than overfeeding.

A fixed schedule or an occasional missed feeding may be indicated for weak infants or those whose condition is complicated by vomiting, convulsions, cyanosis or hemorrhage. For an older premature who is gaining weight a flexible schedule is advantageous.

*Gavage.* The infant who is unable to suck or swallow or who becomes fatigued with the effort of nursing or is apt to become cyanotic after feeding by bottle or medicine dropper should be fed by gavage. An indwelling catheter may be used for the small infant who cannot suck or swallow. If necessary, mummy restraint may be used.

*Mummy restraint* is used with infants and young children during treatments and examinations involving the head and neck. The equipment needed is a square sheet or an infant blanket, depending upon the size of the child, and two safety pins. For the method of application, see Figure 41. Figure 42 gives an alternate method of application. If the nurse talks to the infant while she gently applies the restraint, it will not in any way disturb him. The young child

will need to be reassured, for the procedure is more or less frightening, particularly if he knows that it is likely to be followed by an unpleasant or painful experience.

For gavage feeding the following equipment is needed: (1) a plastic catheter, no. 5 to 8 French, with a rounded end, sterilized with Zephiran solution (benzalkonium chloride), (2) the barrel of a glass syringe (sterile), (3) medicine glasses (sterile), (4) sterile water, (5) the warmed formula.

The method of *gavage feeding with an indwelling catheter* (generally inserted by the physician) is as follows:

1. Measure the distance from the bridge of the nose to the lower end of the sternum and place a mark on the catheter.
2. Lubricate the tube with water. Do not use oil, because of the danger of aspiration with subsequent lipoid pneumonia.
3. Insert the catheter through a nostril until the mark is reached.
4. Check for placement of the catheter in the stomach by placing the free end under sterile water in one of the three medicine glasses. If many bubbles rise and then cease, the catheter is in the stomach and the infant is relieved of air which might cause him to vomit during or after the feeding. If, however, bubbles rise periodically, they are caused by air expelled with each respiration, an indication that the catheter is in the trachea. The infant is then likely to choke and become cyanotic. The tube should be withdrawn at once and reinserted.

Another method of testing to determine the

location of the catheter in larger infants and children is by gently aspirating a small amount of stomach contents. This may not be possible in a premature who receives extremely small amounts at each feeding. Only slight suction should be used because of the danger of traumatizing tissue at the end of the catheter.

5. When it is certain that the tube is in the stomach, it is taped to the infant's cheek.

6. The barrel of the syringe is connected to the catheter by means of a no. 20 needle which acts as an adaptor.

7. The syringe is held 6 to 8 inches above the level of the bed and the milk poured very slowly into the syringe barrel. No air should precede the milk, and no pressure is used. The milk flows into the infant's stomach by gravity.

8. After the feeding a small amount of sterile water is poured into the syringe to wash out the milk and prevent clogging of the catheter. In a very small infant the amount of sterile water to be used may be ordered by the physician, since overdistention of the infant's stomach may result in vomiting.

9. When the syringe is empty, the catheter may or may not be occluded, depending on the physician's order. Some physicians believe that the tube should be left open, but elevated above the infant's body. If vomiting occurs, the tube acts as a safety valve so that the possibility of aspiration of vomitus is minimized. If the catheter is to be changed, it must be compressed while being withdrawn. This prevents milk from dripping into the pharynx and causing the infant to gag or aspirate it.

10. Place the infant on his right side with a blanket rolled behind him for support.

11. The catheter should be changed at least every four days.

*Gavage feeding without an indwelling catheter* differs in several respects from the foregoing procedure. A soft rubber catheter, 8 to 10 French, is used. This is passed through the mouth toward the back of the throat. Its location must be tested carefully. The catheter is held in place with the hand near the infant's mouth. The catheter is withdrawn after the feeding and during withdrawal is compressed firmly for the reason given above. Before withdrawal it is a good plan to run sterile water through the catheter at once to clear it of milk and to avoid drippings which might be aspirated.

*Feeding with a Medicine Dropper.* This method of feeding is used for small prematures who have a good swallowing reflex, but cannot suck with sufficient strength to draw the milk through the nipple or cannot swallow rhythmically as they suck. The tip of the medi-

cine dropper is protected with a bit of rubber tubing pulled well over the end of the glass dropper. The soft rubber tubing is less irritating than glass to the delicate mucous membranes of the mouth, and also less dangerous should the tip break. The feeding is given a few drops at a time, with time allowed for the infant to swallow before the bulb is again compressed. If the infant becomes exhausted by this method, he should be fed by gavage until he is stronger.

*Bottle Feeding.* Bottle feeding is used with more mature prematures or those with an unusually strong sucking reflex (and adequate ability in swallowing) for their stage of development. There are special nipples on the market for small prematures. If these are not available, a regular nipple which is soft but not flabby may be used. The holes in the nipple should not be so small that the exertion of sucking tires the infant, nor too large, for he might not be able to swallow the milk which fills his mouth as he sucks and as a result might gag or aspirate it. Furthermore, the infant who drains the milk too easily is deprived of the natural satisfaction which sucking brings. The bottle should be held during the entire feeding. Infants large and strong enough to be fed from a bottle also need the closeness and cuddling a mother gives when feeding her child.

## Medications

Here are considered only those medications necessary for growth and health.

The premature infant's vitamin requirements are greater than those of the full-term infant, since his antenatal storage of vitamins is incomplete, his growth rate is greater, and the milk given him is both small in amount and has been boiled (if he is not breast fed), thereby reducing the vitamin C content. His defective fat absorption reduces the utilization of such fat-soluble vitamins as he receives in his formula. In general he requires 50 mg. a day of vitamin C (this is started as soon as he receives a formula) and 1000 units a day of vitamin D, which is given him within two weeks after birth.

Iron must be added to his intake by about 2 months of age, but may be given earlier if his hemoglobin level is under 8 gm. or if he has lost blood. In general, iron is not well utilized until the second or third month of life.

### Prevention of Infection

The premature infant has little resistance to the strains of extrauterine life. He lacks the vitality to resist pathogenic organisms or to localize infection, and he also lacks immune substances which are transmitted placentally to the full-term infant.

**Gastrointestinal Infections.** Infections of the gastrointestinal tract are common in premature infants and are most likely to be caused by contaminated nipples, bottles or other appliances used in feeding.

**Skin Infections.** Infections can find entrance through slight trauma to the skin. Some skin infections are transmitted by contact, however. Infections of this sort are likely to be transmitted from infant to infant if equipment is shared in common or if the nurses fail to wash their hands thoroughly after care of each infant. Skin infections may also be contracted from linen which has not been sterilized before use.

**Respiratory Infections.** Organisms that cause respiratory infections are likely to be carried to an infant by the personnel who care for him. As has been noted, the staff caring for prematures should wear gowns and caps. In some hospitals masks are also required, but in other hospitals are considered unnecessary. Organisms causing respiratory infections may be carried by the air from infant to infant. For these reasons each infant should be in strict isolation, and any infant showing signs of a respiratory infection should be removed from the nursery.

In the majority of hospitals air-borne organisms are prevented from drifting into the premature nursery, when the door is opened, by an antechamber between the main hall and the nursery.

All equipment used for the infants and for their examination should be kept in the nursery, and traffic within the nursery should be kept at a minimum.

Supplies such as linens, blankets and cotton should be sterile when brought into the nursery and as far as possible sterile when used in the care of the infants. The outer wrapping of all such equipment should be removed before being brought to the nursery, in an area set aside for the purpose.

Nurses caring for a premature infant who exhibits evidence of infection must not care for the other, well prematures in the nursery.

**General Suggestions for Prevention of Infection.** There should be no dry dusting or sweeping in the nursery. A damp mopping should be done daily with hot water and a cleansing powder. The daily dusting should be done with a damp cloth.

Minimal handling of the infant lessens the danger of infection and conserves his strength. The premature sleeps practically all the time. Nursing care should be planned around the feeding time. This not only minimizes the danger of infection, but also does not interfere with his rest more than is necessary and tends to keep the concentration of oxygen at the prescribed level in the incubator.

## DISEASES OF THE PREMATURE INFANT

The ability to observe and describe symptoms so that the physician has an accurate and reliable account of an infant's symptoms and behavior is one of the chief distinguishing characteristics of the professional nurse. Important among the observations which a nurse should make of the premature infants under her care are (1) nature of the cry, respirations, color, activity, condition of the skin and umbilicus, and bladder and bowel function; (2) stability of body temperature under slight variations of external environmental conditions; (3) response to feedings in relation to the method used, the swallowing and sucking reflexes, and the amount taken and retained; (4) symptoms of unfavorable response to the environment; (5) symptoms of illness, knowledge of which is necessary to the physician's diagnosis and treatment, especially of serious conditions likely to occur in the premature. Such conditions are considered here in some detail.

### Retrolental Fibroplasia

**History.** The condition was diagnosed and the cause discovered within the last twenty years. The condition is peculiar to infants under 1500 gm. in weight and of gestational age of 6 to 7 months.

**Incidence.** Retrolental fibroplasia is the chief cause of neonatal blindness and has replaced ophthalmia neonatorum as the most common cause of blindness in children. It occurs in the smaller, less mature infants more frequently than in the larger and more fully developed prematures. The condition involves both eyes and may produce complete or almost complete blindness. The effects are not immediately apparent, but can be detected by the physician when the infant is several weeks or months of age.

**Etiology.** The cause of this condition is oxygen poisoning, the oxygen acting upon the primitive vasculature of the infant's eyes. A high concentration of oxygen causes spasm of the retinal vessels; this leads to exudation of blood and serum through the walls of these vessels.

**Pathology.** The retinal veins dilate and become tortuous. There is hemorrhage with exudate into the retina, and finally areas of separation of the retina from the inner surface of the eye occur. Some of these changes may regress, but in other instances they continue until the retina detaches and floats forward in the eye. Eventually the retina may become atrophic, a completely detached and useless fibrotic mass (see Fig. 44). Some light perception may be present, but the child has no useful vision. Glaucoma may occur in the late stage of the disease, and corneal opacities may result.

**Diagnosis.** Routine ophthalmoscopic examinations of the eyes of premature infants should be made so that the condition may be detected early. Such examinations should be begun in the nursery.

**Prevention.** Oxygen therapy should be given only when an infant is in immediate need of oxygen, and then only in the lowest concentration which will satisfy his need. The concentration should never exceed 40 per cent unless it is needed as a lifesaving measure. Even in this situation oxgen should be discontinued as soon as possible. Physicians today order oxygen by concentration rather than by rate of flow. The nurse must check the oxygen concentration in the incubator and adjust the flow so that it does not exceed 40 per cent

A          B

**Figure 44.** Retrolental fibroplasia. *A,* Photograph of eyes of an infant to show the complete white opacification of the tissues behind the pupil. This is the end-stage of retrolental fibroplasia. *B,* Sagittal section of an eye removed from this child. One sees the entire retina detached and pulled forward toward the lens and a band of scar tissue encircling the posterior aspect of the lens. The whole disorganized mass makes up the retrolental eschar. (From the collection of Dr. Arnall Patz, Baltimore.) (Schaffer: Diseases of the Newborn.)

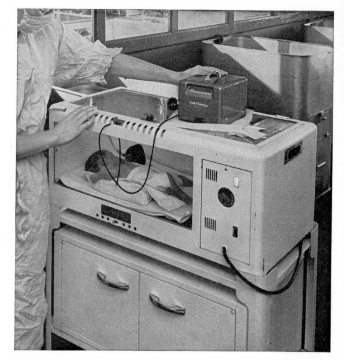

Figure 45. Oxygen analyzer. The regulation of oxygen flow does not guarantee that the atmosphere inside the incubator is in accordance with the prescribed atmosphere. The only certain method for determining actual oxygen concentration is to make periodic checks using an oxygen analyzer. (Beckman Scientific and Process Instruments Division, 2500 Fullerton Road, Fullerton, California.)

concentration unless ordered. This requires that an accurate oxygen analyzer be part of the standard equipment of every nursery (see Fig. 45). Frequent analysis of oxygen concentration is necessary even if oxygen-limiting devices are used on the incubator.

If the infant's condition is such that he should have a higher oxygen concentration, the exact concentration should be ordered by the physician and not given on the judgment of the nurse, except in dire emergency (the pediatric staff may be asked for routine orders to cover such emergencies). Oxygen therapy should be discontinued as soon as there is no further need for it.

There is no obvious contraindication to the use of oxygen therapy in infants over 5 pounds, but such infants seldom need oxygen, since their respiratory and circulatory systems are more completely developed.

### Pulmonary Hyaline Membrane

**Incidence.** This condition is found in about 50 per cent of premature infants who die within a few days after birth. It seldom occurs in full-term infants, but may develop in infants whose mothers have diabetes or in infants delivered by cesarean section.

**Pathology.** A membrane is deposited along the walls of the bronchioles, the alveoli and the alveolar ducts.

**Etiology.** The membrane has been thought to be due to inhalation of amniotic fluid, or it may be formed from extravasated blood or edema fluid.

**Course.** The infant's respirations are normal for the first two or three hours after birth. Then dyspnea develops. There is retraction of the ribs and lower portion of the sternum. The infant becomes cyanotic, and his rapid, grunting respirations give evidence of his difficulty in breathing. Although death may occur, improvement may come about rapidly if the infant survives for several days.

**Prevention and Treatment.** *Prevention* involves many of the factors already mentioned in the delivery and care of the newborn. Cesarean section should be avoided if possible. Mucus and amniotic fluid should be aspirated from the respiratory tract and the gastric contents from the stomach. If the infant shows signs of difficult breathing, the oxygen content in his environment should be increased and the humidity raised. Secondary infections are prevented by the use of antibiotics. If an infant has respiratory distress, he should be given nothing by mouth because of the danger of aspiration.

**Nursing Care.** The nursing care is that of the premature or normal newborn, but with added precautions against aspiration of feeding and with closer observation for a change in condition. The obstetrical nurse rather than the pediatric nurse aids in prevention by good prenatal care and immediate care after birth of the infant while he is still in the delivery room.

## Vomiting

The most common cause of vomiting is overfeeding or too rapid feeding, or both. The great preventive, therefore, is reduction of the intake and slow feeding. If the infant's condition permits of his being held for his feeding, he may be bubbled several times during the feeding and before he is put back in his incubator. Abdominal distention not only causes vomiting, but also hinders respiration because of elevation of the diaphragm. Congenital malformation of the esophagus hampers the swallowing of milk, and that taken into the mouth is ejected. Increased intracranial pressure is a serious cause of vomiting, which may be projectile.

The nurse should chart not only the amount, color and nature of the feeding vomited, but also the conditions under which it occurred. This will aid the physician in his diagnosis and may also indicate defective feeding technique on the part of the nurse which she will be anxious to correct.

## Diarrhea

A premature infant normally has more stools a day than does a full-term infant; it is normal for the premature

to have four or five stools a day. Increased frequency or loose stools are serious in the premature, since he needs all the nutriment of his feeding for metabolism and growth; also he cannot easily tolerate excessive fluid loss. Because of the low tolerance of his gastrointestinal tract for fat, the fat content of his feeding may be the cause of the diarrhea, or overfeeding may be responsible.

Diarrhea in infancy may occur with either an enteral or parenteral infection. The physician should be notified at once and the infant placed on strict isolation so that the infection—if that is the cause of the diarrhea—is not transmitted to other infants in the nursery. Vomiting often accompanies a diarrhea and should be carefully observed and charted, since these observations will help the physician in making his diagnosis and planning therapy.

## Dehydration

Dehydration is more important in infancy than in childhood and even more serious in the premature than in the normal infant. In the premature, dehydration is often caused by excessive warmth of the environment, which is likely to be accompanied by relatively low humidity. This condition is easily corrected in the hospital, but in the home or a rural hospital which is not equipped with modern incubators, hot, dry weather is likely to cause dehydration in the premature infant, and means must be found to place him in an environment of suitable temperature and humidity.

Dehydration is certain to follow an inadequate fluid intake. We have already noted that diarrhea and vomiting cause dehydration.

## Jaundice

Jaundice in the premature, as in the full-term infant, may be physiologic, i.e. due to bilirubinemia in the early postnatal period. Physiologic jaundice is of no great importance, but jaundice which persists or becomes excessive is indicative of some serious condition, such as erythroblastosis fetalis, congenital anomaly or obstruction of the bile ducts, congenital toxoplasmosis or septicemia. The nursing care is that of the condition causing the jaundice.

*Pallor*

Pallor accompanies shock and hemorrhage in the premature as in the full-term infant. It is often seen in infants who fail to breathe at birth and may be a symptom of intracranial injury.

*Convulsions*

One reason why premature infants should be under constant observation is the danger of convulsions. The accompanying anoxia and stress are threatening to his welfare. The nurse must be there to render care. A description of the convulsion may assist the physician to arrive at a diagnosis and correct the cause if correction is possible. A convulsion may be a symptom of intracranial hemorrhage or of a congenital cerebral defect, or may be the result of prolonged anoxia. It may be caused by hypoglycemia or hypocalcemia or an overwhelming bacteremia.

## PROGNOSIS IN PREMATURITY

The premature's chances of survival are much less than those of the full-term infant. Twelve to 20 per cent of prematurely born infants die. About half of all deaths in the first month of life occur in infants classified as prematures. The smaller the infant, the less are his chances of survival. About half of the deaths in the premature group occur on the first day of life.

**Causes of Death.** Immaturity itself is the fundamental cause of the high death rate among premature infants. Only a small number of those who weigh less than 1000 gm. survive. Respiratory failure, from whatever cause, is responsible for many deaths. Birth injury such as intracranial hemorrhage with resulting damage to brain tissue may cause immediate death. Congenital

malformations may make vital physiologic functions impossible. Infection, as already noted, is far more likely to be fatal to the premature than to the full-term infant, since the premature can neither combat the infection nor withstand its systemic effects.

**Factors Favoring Survival.** Favorable prognostic signs in the premature are a birth weight of more than 1500 gm., good muscle tone and normal respiratory activity. If the infant is not cyanotic and exhibits an active response to stimulation, his immediate condition is likely to be good. When the gag and swallowing reflexes are present, he will be able to take his feedings with less danger of aspirating fluid. The importance of stabilization of body temperature has been shown. This is less of a problem in the modern hospital than in the home, where makeshift methods must be used to maintain the stable environmental heat necessary to his well-being. Absence of other serious conditions is additionally hopeful.

## PARENTAL PROBLEMS DUE TO PREMATURITY

Mothers of premature infants often worry for fear that the infant will not develop into a normal child, and that he will be mentally retarded, frail and small. This is not wholly so, and the nurse may tell the mother that studies of children born prematurely show that by and large they develop more rapidly than infants born at term, and that if age were dated from the time of conception rather than from birth, prematures are frequently on a par with infants born at term. Any lag in development of the premature in comparison with term infants tends to decrease with age and at the end of several years to become indistinguishable.

All this does not imply that the months of intrauterine life which the premature lost, and spent in the premature nursery, have had no influence on his development. No one can tell what the optimum development would have been had he been born at term. Nevertheless prematurity does not necessarily handicap a child throughout later life.

In his early infancy the premature may appear backward in motor control, less so in sensory acuity, but still not up to the level of the normal infant. Prematurity does not influence intelligence, but emotional and social behavior are likely to be less mature than in children who were born at term. This is largely due to the overprotective attitude of his parents in infancy and to later pressure upon him to catch up with other children of his age. He is confused by the change of attitude and finds it difficult to adjust to the new demands made upon him.

The parents of a premature infant are likely to show their anxiety for him in oversolicitude. They may doubt their ability to give him the care he needs. They may feel that they dare not let themselves love him too much since they fear to lose him. Their love for him may be mixed with longing for the healthy infant they had planned for and expected.

The nurse can do a great deal toward helping the parents to adopt a more normal attitude. Before the infant goes home they should have an opportunity to become familiar with his daily care and the way in which he responds to that care. For instance, the mother should bathe and dress the infant. She should give him his feedings, and his response to her care should be explained by the nurse. The mother should be encouraged to show him affection in ways which give him pleasure. She will have to be more gentle and unhurried in her movements than with the infant born at term. She will have to understand that his response will appear to be that of a retarded infant when his age is calculated from the day of his birth, but may be advanced when age is calculated from the date of conception. If the mother is a clinic patient whose infant will be followed up by a public health nurse and will attend the Child Health Conference, she should meet the nurse who will visit her home and should be made familiar with the help which will be given her.

The public health nurse should visit the home before the infant's discharge to evaluate the setting and to make suggestions as to how conditions may be improved for the infant's welfare. She should make suggestions as to his physical environment, including the equipment needed in his care, and should evaluate the mother's feelings about the infant. The public health nurse should also visit the family after the infant's discharge from the hospital in order to give necessary guidance and assistance.

Mothers in the middle class have probably read a great deal about premature infants and may have studied their characteristics and their care in college classes on child development. These mothers understand the theory of premature care, but need help in putting it into practice. Since they are not likely to be clinic patients and therefore do not receive the routine help of a public health nurse, they are in even greater need of an opportunity to care for the infant while he is still in the hospital.

Some premature infants tend to develop undesirable behavior patterns. They may be overdependent and are likely to be negativistic. This may be due in some cases to resistance to overprotection, or to a sudden change on the parents' part from overprotection to pressing the child to catch up with his age group. Among the traits which may develop in prematures are thumb-sucking, speech defects and general emotional instability. Their emotional and social lag is demonstrated in delay in learning toilet habits. Mothers should be told that such problems are common in prematurely born children and that they should blame neither the child nor themselves. A mother, while helping her child to lead a normal life, must remember that prematurity is a handicap which is outgrown gradually.

The premature infant looks so frail and helpless that many mothers concentrate on his physical care and forget his emotional needs. Like an infant born at term, during the first year of life he should learn to trust those about him. This requires that he feel secure in their love. He learns to trust others not only through being well cared for, but also through all the expressions of affection so familiar to mothers of full-term, healthy infants. So-called maternal love takes the form in some mothers of anxiety about the infant. These are the overprotective mothers who do not let the infant develop at his own rate, but hold him back for fear that he will in some way be harmed by activity. Infants do not feel love which is expressed in terms of anxiety; they miss the happy, playful ways of mothers with normal infants.

Probably helping the mother to feel secure in her ability to care for the premature is the most important factor in forming good mother-child relations. If such a relation exists, a mother is not afraid to correct the child. (An infant of one year should understand what is meant by "No, no.") She should let the child experience the minimal frustrations that occur in daily life and develop early independence, as would an infant born at term.

### TEACHING AIDS AND OTHER INFORMATION*

*National Society for the Prevention of Blindness*
  Prevent Retrolental Fibroplasia in Premature Infants with Oxygen Control.
*U.S. Department of Health, Education, and Welfare*
  Your Premature Baby, 1954.

### REFERENCES

American Academy of Pediatrics Committee on Fetus and Newborn: Standards and Recommendations for Hospital Care of Newborn Infants, Full Term and Premature. Evanston, Ill., American Academy of Pediatrics, 1957.
Association for the Aid of Crippled Children, Proceedings of the First Scientific Conference: Prematurity, Congenital Malformation, and Birth Injury. New York, Association for the Aid of Crippled Children, 1953.
Bookmiller, M. M., and Bowen, G. L.: A Textbook of Obstetrics and Obstetric Nursing. 3rd ed. Philadelphia, W. B. Saunders Company, 1958.

* Complete addresses are given in the Appendix.

Cole, W. C. C., Sr.: Oxygen and the Premature Infant. Hospitals, 31:33, May 1, 1957.
Crosse, V. M.: The Premature Baby. 4th ed. Boston, Little, Brown and Co., 1957.
Davis, M. E., and Sheckler, C. E.: DeLee's Obstetrics for Nurses. 16th ed. Philadelphia, W. B. Saunders Company, 1957.
Drorbaugh, J. E., and Fogg, M. F.: Respiratory Distress in the Newborn Infant. Am. J. Nursing, 56:1559, 1956.
Eggli, O. W.: Follow up Care of the Premature Baby. Am. J. Nursing, 58:231, 1958.
Fitzpatrick, E., and Eastman, N. J.: Zabriskie's Obstetrics for Nurses. 10th ed. Philadelphia, J. B. Lippincott Company, 1960.
Geddes, A. K.: Premature Babies: Their Nursing Care and Management. Philadelphia, W. B. Saunders Company, 1960.
Kagan, B. M.: The Premature Infant; in Brennemann, J.: Practice of Pediatrics. Hagerstown, Md., W. F. Prior Co., Inc., 1959, Vol. I, Chap. 43.
Letourneau, C. U.: Preventing Retrolental Fibroplasia — A Continuing Responsibility. Hospital Management, Part I, 86:47, August, 1958; Part II, 86:46, Sept., 1958.
Lundeen, E. C., and Kunstadter, R. H.: Care of the Premature Infant. Philadelphia, J. B. Lippincott Company, 1958.
Lynch, M. J. G., and others: Hyaline Membrane Disease. J. Pediat., 48:602, 1956.
National Society for the Prevention of Blindness: Retrolental Fibroplasia Still a Problem. Nursing Outlook, 8:549, 1960.
Nelson, W. E. (editor): Textbook of Pediatrics. 7th ed. Philadelphia, W. B. Saunders Company, 1959.
Newman, D. S., and Sutherland, J. M.: Diagnosing Hyaline Membrane Disease. Am. J. Nursing, 61:72, Jan. 1961.
Ott, E. W., and Lubchenco, L. O.: The Premature Infant's Reaction to Illness. Am. J. Nursing, 57:1431, 1957.
Owens, C.: Parents' Response to Premature Birth. Am. J. Nursing, 60:1113, 1960.
Patz, A.: The Role of Oxygen in Retrolental Fibroplasia. Pediatrics, 19:504, 1957.
Prugh, D. G.: Emotional Problems of the Premature Infant's Parents. Nursing Outlook, 1:461, 1953.
Schaffer, A. J.: Diseases of the Newborn. Philadelphia, W. B. Saunders Company, 1960.
Silver, H. K., Kempe, C. H., and Bruyn, H. B.: Handbook of Pediatrics. 3rd ed. Los Altos, California, Lange Medical Publications, 1959.
Silverman, W. A.: Care of the Premature Infant. Pediatrics, 21:857, 1958.
Idem: Dunham's Premature Infants. 3rd ed. New York, Harper and Brothers, 1961.
Smith, C. A., and Cook, C. D.: Special Problems of the Newborn. Pediatrics, 15:348, 1955.
Unsworth, A. C., and Parkinson, J. E.: Oxygen Administration to Premature Infants. Hospitals, 32:56, June 16, 1958.
Van Blarcom, C. C., and Ziegel, E.: Obstetrical Nursing. 4th ed. New York, Macmillan Company, 1957.

# Chapter 9

# Congenital

# Diseases and Birth Injuries

IN THE preceding chapters it has been noted that hereditary diseases, of which there are few, and a tendency to certain diseases are fixed at the time of conception. In contrast, congenital disease is acquired while the infant is in utero. Congenital disease, then, is subject to preventive medicine, as is disease in the newborn infant and in the child. Prenatal care of the prospective mother is not only for her sake, but also for the health of the fetus.

Congenital disease, however, is only one of the problems related to the condition of the mother. The infant's general well-being depends upon her ability to provide for him the essentials for normal development. If her diet has been insufficient or her general hygiene poor, the infant as well as she suffers. If she is injured, he also may be injured.

This relation of the welfare of the fetus to that of the mother usually means that what is beneficial for her is also good for him, but this is not always so. Drugs, x-ray treatments or the use of radium necessary in treatment of the mother may have an adverse effect upon the development of the fetus.

Prevention of disease in the newborn has been a problem for the obstetrician rather than the pediatrician, and the obstetrical rather than the pediatric nurse. But as the two areas of medicine and of nursing are being brought close together in present-day maternal and child health programs, the dichotomy of the infant's care before and after delivery is no longer found. Congenital disease, deformity and prematurity are studied from their inception to their full implications in the welfare of the infant and the child.

## CONGENITAL DISEASES

### HEMOLYTIC DISEASE OF THE NEWBORN (ERYTHROBLASTOSIS FETALIS)

Hemolytic disease of the newborn includes a number of hemolytic processes occurring in the fetus and in the newborn. The two most important hemolytic diseases are (1) that due to iso-immunization to the Rh factor and (2) that due to iso-immunization to A or B substances.

**Etiology.** Hemolytic disease is due to the development of an isohemagglutinin in the maternal serum. Antibodies traverse the placenta and produce agglutination of the infant's red blood cells.

### Hemolytic Disease Due to Rh Incompatibility

This condition occurs when the mother is Rh negative and the father—and therefore the fetus also—Rh positive. About 15 per cent of the white population are Rh negative and 85 per cent positive. Very few Asian or Negro women are Rh negative.

Erythroblastosis fetalis does not always occur in the infant born of an Rh-incompatible mating, because of the vagaries of maternal sensitization, paternal heterozygosity and small families. The first child is less apt to be affected than are later ones. The reason for this is that the mother who produces antibodies easily will begin to do so in response to the stimulus of the first fetus. The titer is further stimulated by succeeding pregnancies. Subsequent infants are therefore more likely to be affected than was the first child, as the titer accumulates.

**Etiology.** In an Rh-negative mother the alien Rh-positive red blood cells of the fetus crossing the placental barrier induce the formation of anti-Rh antibodies. This may also result if the mother has had a transfusion or an injection of Rh-positive blood cells. These anti-Rh agglutinins are carried in turn from the mother's blood across the placenta into the blood stream of the fetus and destroy the fetal erythrocytes by their specific reaction with the Rh-positive cells.

**Clinical Manifestations.** The vernix caseosa is often yellowish; in some cases there may be severe edema (*hydrops fetalis*). Jaundice appears on the first day, and there is progressive anemia due to the severe hemolysis. Enlargement of the liver and spleen is common. In severe cases the central nervous system may be affected, as evidenced by opisthotonos, spasticity, abnormal Moro reflex, inactivity, and anorexia present from the third to the fifth day after birth. Under such circumstances kernicterus (jaundice of the basal ganglia) may be present.

**Laboratory Findings.** The mother's blood is found to be Rh negative and the infant's Rh positive. The Coombs test on the infant is positive. His blood picture shows anemia with an increased number of nucleated red blood cells. The indirect serum bilirubin is increased. The anti-Rh titer of the mother's blood is elevated.

**Course.** In severe hemolytic disease the infant may be born dead or may die within the first few days of life. On the other hand, with prompt therapy complete recovery is the rule.

*Kernicterus* sometimes follows severe hemolytic disease of the newborn. The symptoms may appear within the first week of life or months later. The more important symptoms are absence of the Moro reflex, opisthotonos, spasticity, lethargy, convulsions and defective sucking activity. It is believed that such sequelae can be avoided through the use of exchange transfusions when the serum bilirubin threatens to rise above a critical level of 20 mg. per 100 ml. If the infant survives, there may be central nervous system damage.

**Prevention.** Prevention begins in the prenatal period. All pregnant women should have their blood typed. Any woman who is Rh negative should have her antibody titer ascertained after the thirty-sixth week. Thus in the event of a rising titer a tentative diagnosis can be made even before the birth of the child. If the newborn infant is Rh positive, if the Coombs test is positive, and if the infant exhibits a rapidly rising bilirubin level, treatment is indicated.

**Treatment.** The infant should receive an exchange transfusion with fresh Rh-negative blood which is compatible with the mother's serum by the indirect Coombs test. This should be done as soon as possible after delivery and repeated later if necessary.

*Exchange Transfusion.* A polyethylene catheter through which blood is to be given is inserted into the umbilical or other large vein. Small amounts (approximately 10 to 20 ml. at a time) of the newborn's blood are withdrawn and equal amounts of Rh-negative blood injected. This process is continued until most of the newborn's blood has been replaced; i.e., approximately 500 ml. of blood are generally used in this procedure. Antibiotics are given after transfusion to prevent infection. Repeated small transfusions may be necessary later.

**Nursing Care.** Skillful nursing is needed. An incubator to maintain the infant's temperature should be in readiness, as well as oxygen in case he becomes cyanotic. Preparation for exchange transfusion should be made when it is known that the birth of a possible erythroblastotic infant is expected or as soon as possible after it has been proved that the infant is erythroblastotic. His condition must be closely watched during and after treatment, and special attention must be paid to respirations, pulse, temperature and evidence of increasing lethargy. At all times the nurse should watch for and report to the physician the following symptoms: increasing jaundice, pigmentation of urine, edema, cyanosis, convulsions, and changes in any of the vital signs. She should change the lethargic infant's position frequently to prevent atelectasis and infection. If kernicterus is present, however, the infant should be handled as little as possible, since movement is likely to result in increased spasms. Because the infant is weak and may have difficulty sucking, a soft nipple with a large hole should be given him or he should be fed with a medicine dropper. These infants may be breast fed, since it is doubtful whether agglutinins in the breast milk would affect their circulating erythrocytes to a great extent.

### Hemolytic Disease Due to ABO Incompatibility

**Etiology.** The etiologic process is the same as in Rh incompatibility. Clinical manifestations of hemolytic disease are more commonly due to ABO incompatibility than to Rh incompatibility. In ABO incompatibility the difficulty is caused by the presence of the blood group A or B factors instead of the Rh substance.

Hemolytic disease due to A or B incompatibility is not usually anticipated unless there is a history of this problem among previous children in the family.

**Course.** A or B iso-immune disease of the newborn is usually mild and may even pass unnoticed. It should be treated, however, if signs are well developed.

**Clinical Manifestations.** Mild jaundice appears during the first thirty-six hours of life. On physical examination the physician may find enlargement of both the liver and the spleen. Central nervous system complications are rare. There is little or no edema.

**Treatment.** The majority of cases need no treatment, but an exchange transfusion may be needed if the infant's serum bilirubin level approaches 20 mg. per 100 ml. Treatment is aimed at the prevention of kernicterus.

**Nursing Care.** The nursing care is like that of erythroblastosis fetalis and needs no further comment.

### OTHER DISEASES

### Hemorrhagic Disease of the Newborn

**Etiology.** This disease is due to a deficiency of prothrombin resulting from either immaturity of the liver or a deficiency of vitamin K. Vitamin K, which is ordinarily elaborated by bacterial action within the intestinal tract during later life, is lacking in the sterile newborn. It is essential to the formation of prothrombin by the liver.

**Clinical Manifestations.** There is bleeding from the skin, retina, conjunctiva, mucous membranes, umbilical wound or viscera. The infant may have tar-colored stools, owing to blood in the fecal matter, or hematemesis (vomiting of bright red blood). Such bleeding may occur with or without trauma and is most likely to appear between the second and fifth days of life, when the available prothrombin is at the lowest level (see Physiologic Hypoprothrombinemia, p. 89).

**Laboratory Findings.** The prothrombin time is prolonged; the coagulation time may be normal or prolonged.

**Treatment.** Vitamin K is given intramuscularly once or repeated as necessary. The effect is much slower, however, than if the vitamin is given intravenously. A transfusion of fresh, matched whole blood may be given. If the bleeding is from accessible bleeding areas, pressure dressings may be applied with topical application of anticoagulants (thrombin or fibrin foam).

**Prevention.** The mother may be given synthetic water-soluble vitamin K intravenously or intramuscularly 4 to 12 hours before delivery, or she may take it daily by mouth for several days before the beginning of labor is expected. This will help to correct maternal hypoprothrombinemia due to poor diet and thus may help to raise the prothrombin level of the infant at the time of birth. Direct administration of vitamin K to the full-term infant is more effective than administration to the mother before delivery. Vitamin K may be given intramuscularly to the infant immediately after birth or orally if there is any bleeding. Large doses of vitamin K have recently been found to be conducive to the development of hyperbilirubinemia in the newborn.

**Nursing Care.** The nursing care is that of the normal or premature newborn, with special care in handling to avoid the slightest danger of trauma and resulting bleeding. The nurse must observe these infants even more carefully than others for evidence of bleeding from the umbilical wound or gastrointestinal tract, as shown by tar-colored blood in the stool or bright red blood in the vomitus.

### Ophthalmia Neonatorum (Gonorrheal Conjunctivitis)

**Etiology.** The causative organism, *Neisseria gonorrheae* (a gram-negative, coffee bean-shaped diplococcus), is found in a smear or culture taken from the purulent exudate from the eye. This pus contains organisms both intracellularly and extracellularly.

The newborn acquires the infection during the birth process by direct contact with infected material in the vagina of the mother. The condition is to be reported to the Board of Health as a contagious disease.

**Clinical Manifestations.** The onset of the disease is usually within two or three days after birth, but symptoms may appear earlier. There is redness and swelling of the lids and a profuse, purulent discharge.

**Complications.** The common complication is corneal ulceration with resulting opacity and partial or complete loss of vision. The extent of the handicap depends on the duration and severity of the untreated condition.

**Treatment.** Penicillin is the preferred drug and is administered parenterally and locally. The infant is kept in strict isolation. Symptomatic therapy consists in removing the discharge thoroughly with irrigations, usually of physiologic saline solution.

**Prognosis.** Excellent results are obtained by the use of penicillin. Ophthalmia neonatorum was formerly the greatest cause of blindness in infancy, but today the incidence is slight.

**Nursing Care.** The nursing care is based on the physician's plan of treatment and on the need for strict isolation technique. It is difficult to instill drops into the eyes of a newborn infant at the time of delivery. The nurse must be absolutely sure that the drops are instilled within the eyelids. The medication may cause a slight irritation and redness of the eyes and the lids for a few days.

The nursing care of an infant with fully developed ophthalmia neonatorum requires strict isolation technique. The infant's arms must be restrained so that he does not rub his eyes. If only one eye is affected, a shield is placed over the other one to protect it from infection. The mainstay of treatment is penicillin. The purulent discharge is removed by frequent irrigations. When irrigations are done, the infant should be restrained in mummy fashion (see p. 149), and a second nurse should steady his head. As in all eye irrigations, the fluid should be warmed to body temperature, and the flow should be directed from the inner canthus outward. The nurse must be extremely careful that no drop of the return flow splashes into her own eyes as she leans over the infant.

**Prevention.** The great prophylactic measure is to keep the mother free of infection. This, of course, is one objective in the prenatal care of pregnant women. If the mother does not come under the care of a physician until the time of delivery, however (this is often unfortunately the case with unmarried mothers or those in the low-income group), instillation of silver nitrate or penicillin safeguards the infant. State laws require prophylactic treatment of all infants at birth even though there is no reason to believe that a particular newborn is infected (see p. 99).

### Thrush (Oral Moniliasis)

**Etiology and Mode of Transmission.** The causative agent of this infection is *Candida (Monilia) albicans*. The organism is normally present in the vagina of the mother, and is a saprophyte in the mouth of older children and adults. Thrush is a fungus infection; the spores grow on the delicate tissue of the buccal mucosa, producing mycelia. The infant may also become infected from improperly sterilized nipples or the uncleansed breast of his mother.

**Clinical Manifestations.** The mouth of the infant who has thrush contains white patches which resemble milk curds. They are different from milk curds, however, in that they are difficult to remove from the mucous membrane and, when removed, leave a bleeding area. These pearly-white, elevated lesions, which occur on the tongue margin, inside the lips and cheeks and on the hard palate, are painless. If the infection is localized in the mouth, the systemic symptoms tend to be mild, although the infant has anorexia. Esophagogastritis or pneumonitis may develop, however, as a result of invasion by the infective organism.

**Treatment and Prognosis.** Nystatin is effective in the *treatment* of these lesions and may be applied locally with a soft swab. (It will not hurt the infant to swallow whatever is left in his mouth.) Aqueous gentian violet, 1 per cent solution, or 1:1000 aqueous solution of benzalkonium chloride (Zephiran) may be used. These latter drugs are only moderately effective.

The *prognosis* in general is very good, recovery taking place in three or four days.

**Nursing Care.** Preventive nursing is

**Figure 46.** Thrush. *A*, Candida in scrapings of thrush. *B*, Characteristic lesions of thrush. (Pillsbury, Shelley and Kligman: Dermatology.)

based on absolute cleanliness of all articles which enter the infant's mouth: the mother's nipples, or the rubber nipples used in artificial feeding. Applicators used in the infant's mouth should be sterile. An older infant's toys and pacifiers must be clean.

To prevent the spread of thrush, the infant should have his own feeding equipment, which should be sterilized before being returned to the milk laboratory. It may be difficult to coax an infant to take enough nourishment. If the nipple irritates his mouth, a medicine dropper may be used.

If the physician orders the infant's mouth to be swabbed with gentian violet, the mother should be warned of the purple discoloration of the infant's mouth, since the dye produces a startling effect.

### Congenital Syphilis (Lues)

**Etiology and Description.** The causative agent of syphilis is a spirochete, *Treponema pallidum.* Here we will consider congenital syphilis and childhood syphilis.

*Congenital syphilis* has declined in incidence in recent years, owing to the universal serologic testing of pregnant women and to the follow-up treatment if the disease is present. The mode of transmission to the fetus is by direct inoculation into the blood stream through the placenta during the latter half of pregnancy. Thus the disease is beyond the primary stage when the infant is born.

**Clinical Manifestations.** Although a variety of other conditions have symptoms similar to those of syphilis, a typical combination of symptoms points to the diagnosis of syphilis. The symptoms may be divided into two groups: those which appear early and those which appear later in the course of the disease.

*Early Symptoms.* The more severe the infection, the earlier will the symptoms be apparent; in general they appear before the sixth week. Characteristic symptoms are as follows: (1) a persistent rhinitis, which has been given the name of "snuffles." This is a

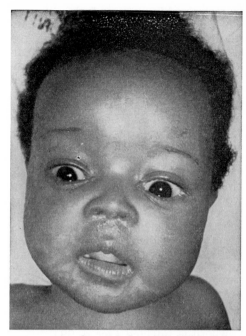

Figure 47. Congenital syphilis. This infant has "snuffles." (Courtesy of Dr. Ralph V. Platou and the American Academy of Pediatrics.)

profuse mucopurulent nasal discharge, which may be blood-tinged and is irritating to the upper lip. The lip may become excoriated from the discharge. (2) There is a rash, heaviest over the back, buttocks and backs of the thighs, and involving the palms and soles. (3) In some cases there may be bleeding ulcerations and moist lesions of the mucous membranes of the mouth, lips, anus and genitals. (4) The infant is anemic. (5) There may be osteochondritis or periostitis, or both, of the bones. (6) Pseudoparalysis or pathologic fractures may be present. (7) The liver and the spleen are enlarged. (8) There may be chorioretinitis with later atrophy of the optic nerve.

*Later Symptoms.* Later clinical manifestations of syphilis are as follows: (1) destruction of the bones of the nose, so-called saddle nose, in which the nose dips slightly beyond the bridge and rises again toward the tip; (2) a periostitis of the tibiae in which these bones develop a sharp forward curve, a condition called saber shins. (3) The deciduous teeth are normal, but the central incisors of the permanent teeth are peg-shaped with a characteristic V-shaped notch, so-called Hutchinson's teeth (see Fig. 49). (4) The lesions of early syphilis around the mouth and nose become linear fissures which form radiating scars on healing (rhagades). (5) Interstitial keratitis may develop when the child is six to twelve years old. Photophobia, lacrimation, general discomfort and impairment of vision are symptoms of this condition. (6) Neuro-

**Figure 48.** Maculopapular eruption of congenital syphilis. (Katharine Dodd in Nelson's Textbook of Pediatrics. 7th ed.)

**Figure 49.** Hutchinson's teeth in congenital syphilis in a boy 10 years of age. (Katharine Dodd in Nelson's Textbook of Pediatrics. 7th ed.)

syphilis, manifestations of which may appear at any time from one to ten years of age. The symptoms are hemiplegia, spastic paralysis and mental retardation. The child is slow in talking and is irritable and restless.

**Diagnosis.** The diagnosis is confirmed by serologic tests. A Wassermann reaction may be determined at any time, or blood may be obtained from the cord at delivery. Blood tests, however, are less accurate in providing proof of the presence of syphilis in the newborn than later in life. When the infant is six months of age, positive serologic test results are more indicative of a syphilitic infection. A second test should be done, however, before the diagnosis is confirmed even at this age if no other manifestations of the disease are evident. Scrapings from the mucous lesions or a specimen of the nasal discharge may show *Treponema pallidum* (darkfield examination is done on the scrapings).

**Prognosis.** Prompt treatment of early congenital syphilis will usually result in a cure and in normal growth and development. Although late congenital syphilis may be cured, the pathologic changes will remain for life.

**Prevention.** A serologic test is required in most parts of the United States before marriage or during pregnancy. This is probably the greatest preventive measure exercised against congenital syphilis. Case finding in adults is furthered by the requirement of physical examinations in many types of work and in the armed services. The almost universal custom of prenatal care during pregnancy has increased the opportunity for early treatment of syphilis if a woman is found to have the disease. Cure may then be effected before the infant is born. Even later treatment may prevent syphilis in the infant or mitigate his condition.

**Treatment.** For early syphilis penicillin is usually given for 15 days with a total dose of not less than 50,000 units per pound of body weight. Penicillin is always given by injection. If the patient is sensitive to penicillin, chlortetracycline may be given. Follow-up serologic tests should be done every three months for at least a year. Both the infant's and the mother's condition should be followed up.

**Nursing Care.** Basic to the nursing care is the danger of transmission of the disease. Although the organism dies rapidly on exposure, it may be transmitted by direct or indirect contact. The organisms are found in the skin lesions and the nasal discharge of the host and invade the body of another through a break in the mucous membranes or skin. In many hospitals nurses caring for syphilitic infants are required to wear rubber gloves and a gown. During the infectious period no pins should be used in the infant's clothing because of the possibility of the nurse sticking herself with a contaminated pin. Diapers should be tied in place temporarily. After a few days of treatment the infant is probably no longer infectious.

Feeding is made difficult by the presence of snuffles. The nose should be cleaned of discharge before the bottle or breast is offered the infant. The upper lip should be kept clean and cold cream should be applied to prevent excoriation from the irritating nasal discharge. Careful handling of the infant is necessary, for bone lesions cause him pain on movement. If the nurse is caring for an older child who shows signs of photophobia due to interstitial keratitis, she should darken the room for his comfort; if he is old enough, he may wear dark glasses.

Public health nurses are stressing the need of prenatal care, including serologic examinations, treatment if necessary and follow-up study on infants on whom treatment has been started.

## Toxoplasmosis

**Incidence, Etiology and Transmission.** This is an uncommon disease of the central nervous system. The causative organism is the *Toxoplasma gondii,* which is considered to be a protozoon. The severe infantile form occurs when the fetus acquires the infection in utero. The fetus may be prematurely born, stillborn or born at term. The disease may also be acquired after birth.

**Clinical Manifestations, Prognosis and Treatment.** Evidence of chorioretinitis (inflammation of the choroid and of the retina) may be detected in the eyegrounds. Cerebral calcifications may be present. Hydrocephalus (see p. 218) or microcephalia (see p. 227) may occur. Psychomotor retardation and convulsions are also symptoms. During the acute stage symptoms of encephalitis may appear. The organism may be isolated from cerebrospinal fluid or from other tissues of the body.

In the infantile form the *prognosis* is poor. Although active congenital toxoplasmosis may cause death in days or weeks, the illness may regress, leaving one or more of the various types of disabilities mentioned above.

The use of pyrimethamine (Daraprim), which is a folic acid antagonist, and sulfadiazine as a combined *treatment* shows promising results. When these drugs are used, frequent leukocyte counts must be made, since both may produce leukopenia.

**Nursing Care.** The nursing care is based on the relief of symptoms, and the child is made as comfortable as possible. The nurse should keep in mind both the symptoms and the complications which may occur so that she may give an accurate account to the physician.

## BIRTH INJURIES

This is an inclusive term embracing both avoidable and unavoidable trauma at birth and also permanent damage occurring soon after birth.

### Intracranial Hemorrhage

**Etiology, Incidence and Diagnosis.** Trauma to the cranium is especially apt to occur when the infant's head is large in proportion to the size of the mother's pelvic outlet, when labor is prolonged and during a breech presentation or a precipitate delivery. It may also be seen in newborns with hemorrhagic disease. The two common types of hemorrhage are *subdural* and *subarachnoid.* Hemorrhage may extend into the ventricles or the brain substance itself.

Intracranial hemorrhage is the most common and severe type of birth injury. It occurs more frequently in premature infants than in full-term infants.

*Diagnosis* is based on a history of difficult delivery and an increase in cerebrospinal fluid pressure. The presence of a few blood cells in the cerebrospinal fluid is not of particular diagnostic value, because a minute amount of bleeding into the cerebrospinal fluid may normally be present in the newborn.

**Clinical Manifestations, Treatment, Prevention and Prognosis.** Intracranial hemorrhage may be evident at birth or may be diagnosed later in an infant apparently normal at birth. The nurse may observe somnolence or limpness in the infant, or irritability and restlessness. Opisthotonos may be present, the Moro reflex absent, muscular twitchings and convulsions may occur, and the cry may be high-pitched and shrill. The cardiac and respiratory functions may be abnormal with resulting pallor and cyanosis. His temperature may be even less stable than that of the normal newborn. The fontanels may bulge if the increase in intracranial pressure is great. Paralysis may appear in a few days.

The results of *treatment* may be quite satisfactory. The infant needs warmth and rest and may be placed in an incubator. His head should be elevated. Hemorrhage may be controlled by the administration of vitamins C and K. The control of increased intracranial pressure can be achieved by mechanical means. The physician may order a sedative such as phenobarbital to control the convulsions. Prophylactic antibiotics are given. If a subdural hematoma is present, it is generally treated as described on page 382.

As with many other birth injuries, better obstetrical care is the best *preventive.*

In the majority of cases the *prognosis* is good, and the child may completely recover. Other infants may show mental retardation or a tendency to convulsions or may be handicapped by cerebral palsy. Those who do not survive usually die within the first three days after delivery.

**Nursing Care.** These infants are generally placed in incubators. Since the sucking and swallowing reflexes are weak or absent, the infant must be fed with great care. If he vomits after feedings, he should be placed on his abdomen or on his right side with a rolled blanket at his back, unless the physician has ordered that this is not to be done. In this position drainage from the stomach to the duodenum is favored, and vomiting may be decreased. The infant must be observed for increased intracranial pressure and for convulsions (see p. 379).

Medications such as sedatives, vitamins or prophylactic antibiotics may be designated to be given orally or by injection. The nurse may assist the physician with treatments such as spinal punctures or aspiration of a subdural hemorrhage.

### PERIPHERAL NERVE INJURIES

### Brachial Plexus Palsy (Erb-Duchenne Paralysis)

**Etiology and Clinical Manifestations.** Brachial plexus palsy is a paralysis of the upper arm. The cause is trauma involving the fifth and sixth cervical spinal nerves or their trunks. The injury results from pulling the infant's shoulder away from the head during delivery. The arm on the affected side is adducted, extended and internally rotated with pronation of the forearm. The hands and fingers are not affected. The arm cannot voluntarily be abducted from the shoulder or externally rotated, and the forearm cannot be supinated. The Moro reflex is absent on the affected side, and there may be sensory loss on the lateral portion of the arm.

**Treatment.** The arm should be immobilized in a position of maximal relaxation, i.e. abducted and rotated externally with the elbow flexed. Later an airplane splint may be used to keep

*A*                                    *B*

**Figure 50.** Brachial plexus palsy of the left arm. *A*, The arm at rest. *B*, Asymmetric response to Moro reflex. (R. J. McKay, Jr., and C. A. Smith in Nelson's Textbook of Pediatrics. 7th ed.)

**Figure 51.** Clove hitch restraint. *A*, In the middle of a strip of gauze make a figure-of-eight. Place one loop over the other. *B*, Place the restraint over the wadding wrapped around the wrist (or ankles). Pull the gauze restraint securely, but not tightly enough to cut off the circulation. The response of this infant, namely crying, is the typical response to restraint. When the clove hitch restraint is used on an infant having brachial plexus palsy, the affected arm should be elevated and the ends of the gauze tied to the head of the crib.

the arm in this position. To prevent contraction deformity, the physiotherapist may manipulate and massage the arm gently. In persistent cases neuroplasty may be necessary.

**Nursing Care.** The arm is to be immobilized as the physician may order. In general a clove hitch restraint is used. The equipment needed for this is (1) a strip of gauze bandage 2 inches wide and 1½ yards long, and (2) cotton wadding covered with gauze, cut to 2 inches wide and long enough to encircle the infant's wrist.

To apply the restraint, spread the gauze strip out on the bed with one end toward the nearer side of the bed. In the middle of the strip make a figure of eight, as shown in Figure 51. Place the gauze wadding around the infant's wrist. Place circles of restraint around the padding on the wrist. Pull the ends of the bandage to the desired tightness. Tie the ends of the gauze to the bedsprings at the head of the bed so that the arm is elevated to the proper angle. Care must be exercised to prevent cutting off the circulation and yet have the bandage tight enough not to slip over the infant's hand.

The fingers and hand should be observed for coldness or discoloration and the skin under the restraint for signs of irritation. These infants need even more petting and affectionate caresses than the normal infant.

**Prognosis.** The prognosis usually cannot be determined for several months. If the paralysis is due to edema and hemorrhage around nerve fibers with no laceration, the prognosis is good. If laceration of the nerve has occurred, operation must usually be considered.

### Facial Nerve Paralysis

**Etiology, Clinical Manifestations and Prognosis.** Facial nerve paralysis results from pressure over the facial nerve in

**Figure 52.** Left facial nerve paralysis following delivery by forceps. (Davis and Sheckler: DeLee's Obstetrics for Nurses. 16th ed.)

front of the ear. This pressure may have occurred in utero during labor or may have been due to the use of forceps during delivery. The paralysis is generally unilateral. When the infant cries, movement is observed on only one side of his face. The mouth is drawn to that side. The eye on the affected side is partially open. If the nerve is only injured by pressure, recovery can be expected in a few weeks; if the nerve is torn, however, neuroplasty may be required.

**Nursing Care.** The nurse must be very patient when feeding the infant, since sucking may be difficult for him. The physician will order care of the exposed eye. If a shield is applied, it may be necessary to restrain the infant's arms so that he does not pull it off. He can be held and cuddled like a normal infant.

### INJURIES TO BONES

**Etiology and Types of Fractures.** Although the newborn's bones bend easily on pressure, as when traction is applied during delivery, a fracture may occur. Fractures occur mainly in the skull, clavicle or long bones.

*Fractures of the skull* are of two types: (*a*) linear fractures, which are the more common type, do not produce symptoms and require no treatment; (*b*) depressed fractures appear as a dent in the infant's head. Treatment is by early operation, which prevents injury to the cortex due to prolonged pressure.

*Fracture of the clavicle* is the most common type of fracture of the newborn. It may occur when delivery of the shoulder is difficult. The infant fails to raise his arm on the affected side, and the Moro reflex is possible only with elevation of the unaffected arm. The infant may be able to raise his arm, however, if the fracture is of the greenstick type, which is common in infants and little children. The prognosis in either type of fracture is excellent. Treatment is by immobilization of the arm and the shoulder on the affected side.

*Fractures of the long bones* of the

arms or legs, unless of the green-stick type, prevent the infant from moving the limb. The treatment of a fracture of the humerus is strapping the arm to the chest and later placing it in an airplane splint or shell cast. For a fracture of the femur the leg is placed in Buck's extension (see p. 460). Splints are used for immobilizing other bones of the extremities. Excessive callus formation is likely to accompany rapid healing.

**Nursing Care.** Nursing care of these infants includes maintenance of good body alignment, splint or cast care (see p. 237) and prevention of pressure areas. Care has to be adapted to the position in which they must lie or the part of the body which is immobilized. Demonstrations of affection for the infant must also be adapted to his condition. The infant in traction cannot be fed at the breast, but his mother's milk may be expressed and given him. In this way the supply of breast milk will be maintained. Whether the infant in traction should go home as soon as other infants do is for the physician to decide, but the infant is likely to have a longer hospital stay than is customary.

### INJURY TO THE STERNOCLEIDOMASTOID MUSCLE

**Etiology, Pathology and Treatment.** About two weeks after birth, or even earlier, a small firm mass may be noted in the midportion of the sternocleidomastoid muscle. This may be caused by a small hematoma resulting from injury or may be a fibromatous malformation in the muscle itself. The injury generally, but not always, results in torticollis (wryneck), a condition in which the head inclines to one side (see Fig. 53). The majority of these tumors resolve under treatment before the infant is one year old.

*Treatment* lies in gently extending the neck so that the face is in the opposite direction. The mother can be taught to turn the infant's head to the normal position and flex the neck toward the unaffected side. This may be done as often as twenty-five times twice

**Figure 53.** Congenital torticollis (wryneck). (From G. A. Caldwell and H. D. Morris, in Christopher's Minor Surgery. 8th ed., edited by Ochsner and DeBakey.)

or three times a day. If the condition is present when the child is two years old, operation may be required.

**Nursing Care.** Nursing care must be adapted to the limitation of movement of the infant. The nurse should talk to the infant, and she should cuddle him before and after the exercise.

### TEACHING AIDS AND OTHER INFORMATION*

*Public Affairs Pamphlets*
  Gould, J.: Will My Baby Be Born Normal?
*U.S. Department of Health, Education and Welfare*
  Blood and the Rh Factor, 1960.

### REFERENCES

Allen, F. H., and Diamond, L. K.: Erythroblastosis Fetalis. Boston, Little, Brown and Co., 1958.
Bookmiller, M. M., and Bowen, G. L.: A Textbook of Obstetrics and Obstetric Nursing. 3rd ed. Philadelphia, W. B. Saunders Company, 1958.
Burchall, D. P.: Caring for the Infant with Thrush. Am. J. Nursing, 61:55, Jan., 1961.
Feldman, H. A.: Toxoplasmosis. Am. J. Nursing, 56:1270, 1956.
Idem: Toxoplasmosis. Pediatrics, 22:559, 1958.

* Complete addresses are given in the Appendix.

Fitzpatrick, E., and Eastman, N. J.: Zabriskie's Obstetrics for Nurses. 10th ed. Philadelphia, J. B. Lippincott Company, 1960.

Harvie, F. H.: Pediatric Methods and Standards. 3rd ed. Philadelphia, Lea & Febiger, 1958.

Ingraham, F. D., and Matson, D. D.: Neurosurgery of Infancy and Childhood. Springfield, Ill., Charles C Thomas, 1954.

Kiesewetter, W. B., Nelson, P. K., Palladino, V. S., and Koop, C. E.: Neonatal Torticollis. J.A.M.A., 157:1281, 1955.

Kozinn, P. J., and Taschdjian, C. L.: Candidiasis. Am. J. Nursing, 61:52, Jan., 1961.

Larsen, L. J.: Congenital Torticollis. Am. J. Nursing, 57:610, 1957.

Larson, C. B., and Gould, M.: Calderwood's Orthopedic Nursing. 4th ed. St. Louis, C. V. Mosby Company, 1957.

Lindsay, M. E.: Nursing the Child with Torticollis. Am. J. Nursing, 57:612, 1957.

Nelson, W. E. (editor): Textbook of Pediatrics. 7th ed. Philadelphia, W. B. Saunders Company, 1959.

Ochsner, A., and DeBakey, M. E. (editors): Christopher's Minor Surgery. 8th ed. Philadelphia, W. B. Saunders Company, 1959.

Paterson, D., and McCreary, J. F.: Pediatrics. Philadelphia, J. B. Lippincott Company, 1956.

Pillsbury, D. M., Shelley, W. B., and Kligman, A. M.: Dermatology. Philadelphia, W. B. Saunders Company, 1956.

Reed, S. C.: Counseling in Medical Genetics. Philadelphia, W. B. Saunders Company, 1955.

Schaffer, A. J.: Diseases of the Newborn. Philadelphia, W. B. Saunders Company, 1960.

Scheinfeld, A.: The Human Heredity Handbook. Philadelphia, J. B. Lippincott Company, 1956.

Silver, H. K., Kempe, C. H., and Bruyn, H. B.: Handbook of Pediatrics. 3rd ed. Los Altos, California, Lange Medical Publications, 1959.

West, J. S.: Congenital Malformations and Birth Injuries: A Handbook on Nursing. New York, Association for the Aid of Crippled Children, 1954.

# Chapter 10

# Conditions of the

# Newborn Requiring

# Immediate or Short-Term Care

CONGENITAL diseases and birth injuries were discussed in the preceding chapter. There are several other conditions of the newborn which it is equally important for the nurse to understand in order that she may adapt her nursing care of the infant to the physician's plan of treatment. These conditions may be divided into two groups: those which require immediate or short-term care and those which require long-term care. The former are discussed in this chapter, and the latter in the next chapter.

Conditions requiring immediate care are divided into three groups: (1) congenital anomalies, (2) respiratory conditions, and (3) infections.

## CONGENITAL ANOMALIES

Congenital deformities are extremely important in the life of a child, since

many of them, in our present state of medical and surgical knowledge, permanently disable him. The influence of abnormalities upon the child's personality cannot be disregarded; many of them limit his social life and activities of daily living.

**Parents' Reaction to an Imperfect Infant.** Parental education should include the possibility of giving birth to an imperfect infant. In a class with other prospective parents, husbands and wives together can consider this possibility objectively. If their first knowledge on the subject comes when their child is born with a congenital anomaly, it is difficult for them to maintain an objective point of view. Men and women of marriageable age should know that prevention of anomalies in children begins with conception, i.e. impregnation of the ovum by a spermatozoon, neither of which carries genes causing hereditary abnormality. Once the ovum has been impregnated, medical care is no longer centered on the unfortunate combination of disease- or abnormality-bearing genes which might have been avoided, but rather with the developing fetus.

The objective of treatment and nursing is to give the fetus as good an intrauterine environment as possible. This means keeping the mother healthy in body and emotionally contented. Because nursing care influences the infant through its effect on the mother, the subject is generally considered under obstetrical nursing. But the integration of obstetrical and pediatric nursing in maternal and child health programs stresses the union of the health of both the mother and the fetus. This is a truism, of course, but pediatric nurses often forget the part which the obstetrical nurse plays in child health.

If the mother can be helped to see that an abnormal condition in her infant is not her fault, nor that of her husband, and that the physician is not to blame, she is more likely to accept the condition realistically and adjust to the infant's needs in the activities of daily life. She is also more likely to welcome and follow professional advice. The nurse, from her knowledge and experience, can explain to the mother all that can be done for the child. Because the nurse is actually caring for the infant and may have him in her arms while they talk about him, she is likely to have greater rapport with the mother than any other of the professional team in the hospital. The emotional makeup of the family of the newborn has a great deal to do with the way the family accepts the child and his abnormal condition. When surgical correction is possible, the parents face the problem of the danger to the infant. When surgical correction is essential to maintain life, the parents face the possibility of immediate death of the infant.

**Definition and Incidence.** *Congenital anomalies* are structural anomalies present at birth. They may be obvious on examination of the newborn, or they may be defects of histologic structure.

One of the reasons why more deaths occur in the first month of life than during the remaining months of the first year of life is that many congenital abnormalities are compatible with intrauterine life, but not with extrauterine life. Approximately 15 per cent of deaths in the neonatal period are caused by such gross malformations.

**Etiology.** The major organ systems of the body are formed from the initial to the final stage in the first twelve weeks of fetal development. Little has been scientifically proved about the causes of fetal malformation. Certain causes are known, however, and their incidence has been lowered. It has been proved that maternal rubella in the first trimester of pregnancy may result in deformity of the fetus. Some congenital anomalies are transmitted from parents to children and follow the Mendelian Law of inheritance of unit characteristics.

The mother's nutritional state is important, since the fetus requires adequate nutrition. Without it, either death in utero or deformity may result. Experience with infants born in concentration camps during World War II and in areas where the level of living is down to little more than the maintenance level has shown the deleterious influence of poor maternal nutrition upon the fetus. Nevertheless the fetus tends to be nourished at the expense of the mother's body. It is possible that an abnormal chemical environment may cause deformity of the embryo. This might be the case in the diabetic mother or one who is in the late childbearing period.

In summary, we may say that the great majority of congenital deformities are the result of the interaction between genetic and environmental factors, and that often more than one anomaly may occur in the same fetus. There may be abnormal development of any part of the body or of any organ.

**Treatment.** The application of medical knowledge to the prevention of congenital malformations has not changed the incidence to any great extent, and the problem remains one of the most important in the field of preventive medicine. Nevertheless better prenatal care of the mother, and therefore of the fetus, has resulted in fewer fetal deaths due to this cause. When the influence of this upon the incidence of anomalies among the newborn is considered, it is probable that considerable progress has been made. The frequency of abnormalities which require operation has increased the importance of surgery for the newborn. This is a specialty which requires surgical competency and an extensive knowledge of the ways in which the newborn reacts to operation and to both preoperative and postoperative care. The surgeon requires a team of experts accustomed to working with him; of these, the nurse is probably one of the most important.

**Emergency Surgery and the Newborn.** The normal newborn is an excellent surgical risk during the first forty-eight hours of his life, but the mortality rate rises rapidly when the infant is more than seventy-two hours old. After this period there are several factors which make operation more dangerous. The most important of these factors are (1) changes in the fluid and electrolyte balance, (2) the normal breakdown of the red blood cells, and (3) the lessening of the infant's physiologic reserve, i.e. all the elements necessary for carrying on the vital functions which he received through the placenta from the mother while still in utero.

There are many problems in surgery of the newborn which make it a specialty for surgeons and nurses alike. The newborn infant does not show gradually increasing signs of loss of blood as do older children and adults. Because of the elasticity of his blood vessels, the infant may show no danger signs until he suddenly goes into shock. Then he is pulseless, and the blood pressure is low and the skin mottled. Because of this characteristic response of the newborn undergoing operation, hemorrhage must be anticipated and blood given before his condition is serious. It is difficult to give the correct amount of blood when he is in shock, since too much fluid given then may cause pulmonary edema.

*Preparation for Anesthesia.* Adequate preoperative medication will prevent secretions from accumulating in the respiratory tract, and emptying the stomach of the gastric contents will prevent vomiting with the danger of aspiration of vomitus. An environment with a high oxygen content is required so that the infant's intake may be sufficient without his becoming exhausted by his efforts to have a sufficient intake.

To be successful, surgery of the newborn requires early diagnosis, minimal preparation and an expert team, including an anesthesiologist who is experienced in working with infants, and nurses who are thoroughly accustomed to nursing the newborn who undergoes operation.

Preoperative preparation gives diminishing returns if it is prolonged.

*Nursing care of the newborn after operation* depends upon his condition and upon the operation which was performed. A few general comments can be made. Infants have a remarkable resilience; on the other hand, they lack the physiologic reserve which older children and adults have. If all goes well, an infant's recovery is rapid, but if complications arise, a state of emergency exists which may develop with little warning. All in all, this type of nursing requires both skill and knowledge of signs and symptoms of trouble arising from the operation which the infant has undergone. It is an exceedingly important area of pediatric nursing. The details of nursing care of infants having various conditions will be discussed when the conditions are described.

## SPECIFIC CONDITIONS WHICH MAY REQUIRE SURGICAL CORRECTION

### Congenital Laryngeal Stridor

When the newborn infant has noisy respiration—a crowing sound on inspiration—he has a condition which may be due to a number of factors. The physician will determine the etiology of the stridor, and the treatment is based upon his findings. No therapy may be required, or immediate treatment may be necessary if the child is to survive. The nursing care will be based upon the plan of treatment outlined by the physician.

**Etiology.** Laryngeal stridor lasting after the first few days of life is due to some abnormal condition in or around the larynx. The most common cause is flabbiness of the epiglottis and the supraglottic aperture. Other causes include epiglottal redundancy, relaxation of the laryngeal wall, absence of the rings of the trachea, deformity of the vocal cords, or a web which partially occludes the larynx. In the older infant or child stridor may be caused by laryngeal infection (see p. 437), tetany (p. 347) or a foreign body in the larynx (p. 306).

**Clinical Manifestations, Diagnosis and Treatment.** The main diagnostic symptom is the noisy breathing, often a crowing sound on inspiration. This is most noticeable when the infant cries and is present at birth or shortly thereafter. This symptom may be accompanied by mild or severe intercostal and supraclavicular retractions. The infant may become cyanotic and dyspneic. The difficulty in the newborn is due to some abnormality in or around the larynx which may be located by laryngoscopy (see Fig. 54).

*Treatment* is based on correction of the underlying cause. For mild stridor there is no specific therapy, but for severe stridor operation may be necessary. If the infant appears unable to take in sufficient oxygen on inspiration, an emergency tracheotomy (see p. 441) may be done. Such an operation may be only a step toward further corrective surgery. For deformity of the larynx laryngoplasty may be necessary.

**Course and Prognosis.** If the condition is uncorrected, constant retractions of the thorax may cause deformity, since

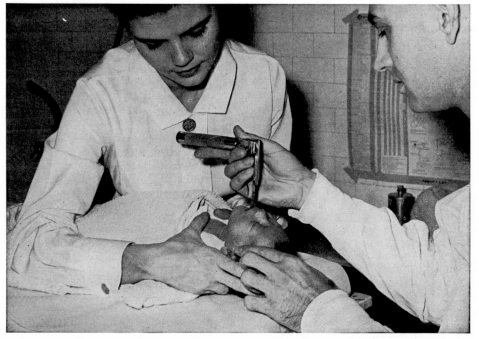

**Figure 54.** Laryngoscopic examination. A mummy restraint is applied, and a small blanket roll is placed under the infant's neck. Note the position of the nurse's hands in holding the infant's head.

the bones readily bend under pressure. If the infant has difficulty in nursing, he may not take sufficient nourishment, and malnutrition may result. Naturally a respiratory infection increases the difficulty and may cause a mild chronic condition to become severe.

The mild, simple form of congenital laryngeal stridor usually subsides by the time the infant is six to eighteen months old. The child does not become cyanotic, and he shows no other symptoms than his noisy breathing. But the *prognosis* in congenital stridor due to some malformation of the larynx will depend upon the etiology.

**Nursing Care.** Feeding may be a problem, since any interference in breathing makes sucking difficult. The infant will have to be fed slowly, stopping frequently for him to breathe unimpeded by nursing. The respiratory process is more imperative than his desire for food, and so he will stop to breathe without the hindrance of sucking. This does not mean that his hunger is satisfied. The nurse should wait a few moments and then offer him the nipple again. If he appears to have difficulty in swallowing the milk which is in his mouth, the nurse should remove the nipple from his mouth at once. A small nipple probably will give the best results. The size of the hole in the nipple should be carefully chosen to give the rate of flow which the infant finds easiest to handle. All infants, of course, should be held when fed and never left with the bottle propped on a pad, but with these infants it is imperative that they be held in the correct position and the bottle supported at the proper angle.

The mother should have ample opportunity to become accustomed to the infant's noisy breathing before she leaves the hospital; otherwise she has no standard by which to judge whether his condition becomes worse. The difficulty in breathing is likely to increase if a respiratory infection develops or if the infant aspirates a little of his feeding or in some other way undergoes an added strain on his already inadequate breathing. The mother should give the infant his bottle with the nurse

beside her to show her the proper technique. The nurse should call her attention to the infant's reaction to too rapid feeding or failure to withdraw the nipple from his mouth if he appears unable to take the milk. If he is a breast-fed infant, the mother will have had ample opportunity to learn the technique of feeding him before she takes him home.

Since a respiratory infection increases the infant's breathing problem, it is important that he be kept from every source of respiratory infection. He should be kept warm, dry, and away from drafts at all times. Raising the humidity in his environment is helpful.

### Choanal Atresia

Choanal atresia is a congenital obstruction of the posterior nares at the entrance to the nasopharynx. The condition may be unilateral or bilateral. The obstruction is usually caused by a membrane, but in rare cases by a bony growth.

**Clinical Manifestations, Diagnosis and Treatment.** The *symptoms* of bilateral obstruction are mouth-breathing and, since the infant cannot suck and breathe at the same time, difficulty in taking his feedings. There may be dyspnea because he cannot obtain enough oxygen when breathing through his mouth. If the obstruction is unilateral, the infant may do well unless infection occurs and persists on the side of the obstruction.

The *diagnosis* is confirmed by passing a sound, probe or soft rubber catheter up the nostril until it meets the obstruction.

Bilateral atresia should be relieved as early as possible, since it is one cause of asphyxia of the newborn. By using a nasoscope the physician is able to pierce the obstruction if it is membranous. A bony obstruction requires extensive operation. Unilateral choanal atresia need not be corrected until the infant is in optimum condition.

**Nursing Care.** There is little in the nursing care of these infants which is specifically directed toward the relief of their condition. The nostrils should be kept clean. Feeding the infant is difficult, since he has trouble in breathing and sucking at the same time, and since there is danger of aspiration of the formula. The precautions and techniques are similar to those outlined in the nursing care of the infant with congenital laryngeal stridor.

## CONDITIONS INCOMPATIBLE WITH LIFE, BUT AMENABLE TO SURGICAL CORRECTION

There are several congenital anomalies of the gastrointestinal tract which, though incompatible with life, may be corrected by surgical treatment. These anomalies are imperforate anus, atresia of the esophagus, omphalocele, diaphragmatic hernia and intestinal obstruction. These lesions are many times associated with other congenital anomalies and are frequent in premature infants. Early diagnosis and treatment are essential in saving life. Operation immediately after birth is indicated when the infant has a diaphragmatic hernia or a large omphalocele.

The difficulties of surgery of the gastrointestinal tract in the newborn increase hour by hour. The infant swallows air, and the gastrointestinal tract becomes distended. He becomes progressively more exhausted because of his increased respiratory rate and is less able to withstand operation.

Three procedures were outlined under Preliminary Examination of the newborn (p. 104) which nurses may carry out, with permission of the hospital administration, to determine the presence of anomalies which require immediate treatment. The nurse should report her findings to the physician, who would then check the symptoms and determine the treatment to be given.

In addition, the nurse should observe an infant closely for four important signs which indicate the possibility of a lesion incompatible with life. These signs are cyanosis, vomiting, absence of stools and abdominal distention.

*Cyanosis* is indicative of many conditions. Those we are concerned with here are diaphragmatic hernia and atresia of the esophagus. *Vomiting* of bile-stained material is a sign of intestinal obstruction. An infant with a diaphragmatic hernia may have repetitive vomiting. In atresia of the esophagus there is immediate vomiting of the undigested formula. *Absence of stools* is the characteristic sign of any form of intestinal obstruction, as is *abdominal distention*. Although these four signs may be seen in the normal newborn, they should be reported promptly to the physician in order to lead to early diagnosis and treatment of conditions incompatible with life, but amenable to surgical correction.

### Imperforate Anus

**Incidence and Etiology.** This is the most common congenital anomaly of the newborn which is incompatible with life. In the eighth week of embryonic life the membrane which separates the rectum from the anus normally is absorbed, and thus a continuous canal is formed whose outlet is the anus. If this membrane is not absorbed and union does not take place, an imperforate anus results. A fistula between the rectum and the vagina, perineum or fourchet in the female, or the urinary tract, scrotum or perineum in the male, is likely to be formed when the infant has an imperforate anus.

**Diagnosis.** The initial diagnosis is made when (1) no anal opening is found on cursory examination of the infant in the delivery room; (2) the nurse is unable to insert the thermometer when taking the infant's temperature on his admission to the nursery; (3) there is no meconium stool; and (4) later abdominal distention occurs. In the presence of these signs the distance between the closed end of the rectum and the anal dimple is ascertained by x-ray examination. The infant cries, and the air which he swallows goes only to the closed end of the rectum. In order to force air down through the bowel, the infant is held upside down or on his side with his knees pushed against the abdomen. An opaque object is placed at the anal

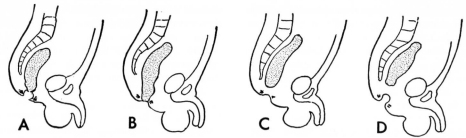

**Figure 55.** Diagrammatic illustration of 4 types of congenital anorectal malformation. (From P. Hanley and M. O. Hines, in Christopher's Minor Surgery. 8th ed., edited by Ochsner and DeBakey.)

**Figure 56.** Schematic representation of imperforate anus, type III (Fig. 55, *C*), with associated fistula in the female. *A*, Low rectovaginal. *B*, High rectovaginal. *C*, Rectoperineal. (From P. Hanley and M. O. Hines, in Christopher's Minor Surgery. 8th ed., edited by Ochner and DeBakey.)

**Figure 57.** Diagrammatic representation of imperforate anus, type III (Fig. 55, *C*), with associated fistula in the male. *A*, Rectovesical. *B*, Rectourethral. *C*, Rectoperineal. (From P. Hanley and M. O. Hines, in Christopher's Minor Surgery. 8th ed., edited by Ochsner and DeBakey.)

dimple, and the roentgenogram thus shows the distance of the rectum from the anus.

The obstruction in a male infant must be relieved at once, for the stool cannot be passed, but an emergency is not so likely in a female, since a fistula probably exists into the vagina, perineum or fourchet. The outlet of the fistula is easily found on inspection. The urine should be watched for flecks of meconium.

**Treatment.** The surgical procedure depends upon the type of anomaly. The anal defect may be such that the opening is covered by a thin membrane through which meconium can be seen. In this case the physician is able to perforate the membrane with a blunt instrument, and no further treatment is required. If the distance between the anal dimple and the blind end of the colon is not more than 1.5 cm., correction is made through the perineum, but if the distance is greater than 1.5 cm., a colostomy is performed while awaiting definitive operation, or the colon is brought down through the anal dimple by an abdominal-perineal procedure. If the anus is normal, but the closed end of the rectum ends in a blind pouch a few centimeters from the sphincter, the condition, called atresia of the rectum, must be surgically corrected as would any other colonic obstruction.

**Nursing Care.** We have noted before that one of the most important characteristics of the professional nurse which set her off from the nonprofessional is her ability for intelligent interpretation of meaningful observations. The detection of imperforate anus is a case in point. In her appraisal of the newborn in the nursery the nurse should observe the infant for the indications of imperforate anus: that the rectal thermometer meets with an obstruction, that there is meconium stain in the urine, but that no passage of meconium such as is normal in the newborn has occurred.

After the diagnosis of occlusion has been made the physician may order gastric suction. If operation is to be done, there may be no specific preoperative preparation. Postoperatively, if the operation has involved only the anal area, that site should be kept dry and clean. If a colostomy has been made, the skin around the wound must be kept clean. The infant's skin is more readily irritated than that of the older child or adult, and cleanliness is very important.

**Figure 58.** Photograph of imperforate anus, type III (Fig. 55, *C*). (From P. Hanley and M. O. Hines, in Christopher's Minor Surgery. 8th ed., edited by Ochsner and DeBakey.)

Aluminum paste or zinc oxide ointment is used to protect the skin. The adhesive straps with ties which hold the colostomy dressing in place should be adjusted so that they remain clean and so that the dressing may be easily changed.

## Atresia of the Esophagus

**Incidence, Pathology, Clinical Manifestations and Diagnosis.** Among the obstructive anomalies of the gastrointestinal tract in the newborn, this condition ranks second (imperforate anus holding first place). The esophagus, instead of being an open tube from the throat to the stomach, is closed at some point. A fistula is common between the trachea and the esophagus. In approximately 80 per cent of these newborns the esophageal atresia is proximal and the tracheo-esophageal fistula is distal.

At birth the infant has excessive mucus in the nasopharynx and therefore is cyanotic. When the mucus is withdrawn by aspiration and oxygen is given, the difficulty in breathing subsides and the infant acquires the normal pink of the newborn. But as the secretions in the nasopharynx accumulate, he again becomes cyanotic. When he is fed, the first mouthful goes down, but since the fluid can go no farther than the atretic area, the second is immediately expelled through the nose as well as the mouth. The infant chokes, sneezes, coughs and shows his discomfort by generalized movement. He is likely to aspirate some of the feeding, and pneumonia results. If he has a distal tracheo-esophageal fistula, the stomach contents may be vomited into the tracheobronchial tree.

In some hospitals the nurse, in making her appraisal of the newborn brought to the nursery, passes a soft no. 8 rubber catheter through the infant's nose into the esophagus; in other hospitals it is customary for the physician to do this. Atresia blocks passage of the catheter. An x-ray film taken with the catheter in this position shows the tip of the catheter coiled back upon itself in a dilated esophageal pouch. No radiopaque substance should be instilled into the esophagus because of the dan-

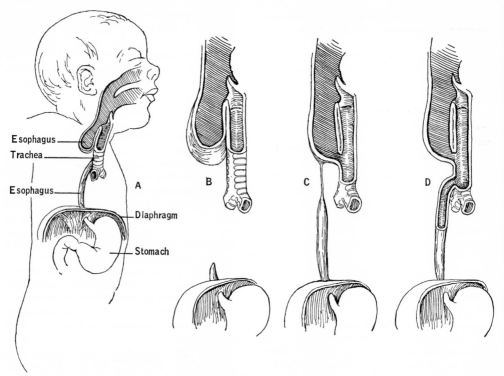

Esophagus
Trachea
Esophagus
A
B
C
D
Diaphragm
Stomach

**Figure 59.** Atresia of the esophagus. *A,* Most common form. The upper esophagus ends in a blind pouch. The lower esophagus communicates with the trachea. *B,* The upper esophagus ends in a blind pouch. The lower segment does not communicate with the trachea. *C,* The upper esophagus ends in the trachea. A cordlike connection with the lower esophagus may or may not be present. *D,* Both upper and lower portions of the esophagus connect with the trachea.

ger of the infant's aspirating it. If the infant has a tracheo-esophageal fistula, the roentgenogram will show air in the gastrointestinal tract.

**Treatment.** Immediate operation is necessary. Depending upon the type of atresia, the following operations are performed: (*a*) an end-to-end anastomosis of the upper and lower segments of the esophagus is done and the fistula ligated. (*b*) If there is no lower portion of the esophagus or if the distance between the lower and upper esophageal pouches is too great for anastomosis, a cervical esophagostomy is done and the fistula closed. A gastrostomy is then made, and the infant is fed through a tube inserted into the stomach. After three to six months a second operation is performed in which either the right or transverse portion of the colon is brought into the chest to join the upper normal portion of the esophagus with the stomach. If a stricture occurs at the site of the anastomosis, it can be dilated later. The chance of survival depends upon the age, weight and general condition of the infant and upon whether other anomalies are present.

**Nursing Care.** It is advisable to place the infant in an incubator where he can easily be kept warm and is protected from infection. He should also be in an environment of high humidity, since this will tend to liquefy the thick mucous secretions which accumulate in the trachea. The nurse should observe the infant's respirations constantly to determine the need for aspiration of secretions. The physician will perform tracheal aspirations if necessary, but the nurse may do nasopharyngeal aspirations. Tracheotomy may be necessary if respiratory difficulty persists (see p. 441).

The use of antibiotics will depend on the type of organism cultured from the blind end of the esophagus. As in other conditions involving the gastrointestinal tract, blood or plasma is given as necessary, and fluids are administered parenterally. There should be a minimum of salt content in these fluids so that the tissues do not become edematous. Depending on the infant's condition, feedings may be given by mouth, or through a tube into the esophagus or through a gastrostomy, if that operation has been performed, for two to three days after operation. Feeding by mouth should be done as soon as it is safe to do so, for fluid passing through the esophagus lessens the danger of a stricture which will require dilatation.

In some cases operation is done in two stages. If in the first stage the opening into the esophagus has been made through the neck, the exposed portion must be protected and kept clean with saline solution. The skin around the opening must be kept dry and clean. The infant's position should be changed frequently to prevent respiratory infection. If a gastrostomy has been done, feedings are begun several hours after operation. The feeding may be given by slow drip (by gravity) from an infusion bottle or by gastrostomy tube, according to the following procedure.

*Gastrostomy Feeding and Care.* The equipment for feeding includes a tray on which is the warm formula, a sterile funnel or Asepto syringe and a sterile nipple filled with sterile cotton.

Attach the funnel or syringe to the gastrostomy tube and fill with the formula before the clamp is removed. This will prevent air from being forced into the stomach. The funnel or syringe is then elevated to allow the fluid to run slowly into the stomach. Force should never be used. Since up to this time the stomach has not received food, distention by introducing air or feeding too rapidly must be avoided. When the formula is passing through the lower outlet of the funnel or syringe, the clamp should be applied to prevent air from entering the stomach.

Some physicians prefer that for infants under one year the gastrostomy tube remain open at all times, but elevated above the infant's body. If vomiting then occurs, the tube provides a safety valve.

The infant fed through a gastrostomy tube must be given the opportunity to satisfy his need for sucking. He is given the sterile nipple filled with sterile cotton to suck on while the milk is running into the stomach through the gastrostomy tube. Sucking on the nipple provides him with a normal pleasure, and he relaxes while being fed. This facilitates the flow of milk. When the feeding is finished, the infant should be held quietly in the nurse's arms while she sings, rocks or plays with him. He should not be bubbled.

The psychological needs of these infants must be met, for they are in the hospital for a relatively long time and might easily become typical hospitalized children—those who are emotionally starved, although physically well cared for.

The care of the skin around the gastrostomy is exceedingly important. This area must be kept clean and protected with aluminum paste or zinc oxide ointment. To prevent displacing the tube when the dressings are changed, the inner side of the adhesive strap which holds the dressing in place should be covered with a second strip of tape so that the part of the tape which extends over the dressing will not stick to it. The adhesive straps can then be tied together over the dressing.

### Omphalocele

**Incidence and Diagnosis.** An omphalocele is a herniation of abdominal viscera at the point where the umbilical cord connects with the abdomen. The defect occurs from the sixth to the tenth week of intrauterine life. The sac which covers the hernia is composed of transparent avascular membrane.

The *diagnosis* is made by inspection. Although the condition is easily seen, the omphalocele is sometimes so small that it appears to be part of the normal umbilical cord.

**Clinical Manifestations, Treatment and Prognosis.** On examination of the large omphalocele the mass of abdominal

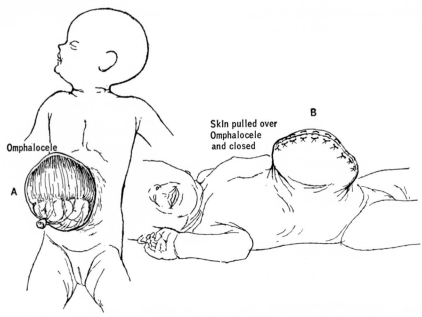

Omphalocele

B

Skin pulled over
Omphalocele
and closed

A

**Figure 60.**    Omphalocele. *A,* An omphalocele is a herniation of the abdominal viscera at the
umbilicus. *B,* The skin is closed over the omphalocele.

viscera seems to be larger than the size of the abdominal cavity into which the viscera must be placed.

The *treatment* must be immediate operation—replacement of the viscera into the abdomen and closure of the abdominal wall—before the bowel is expanded by swallowed air and before the sac dries or is contaminated by bacteria. Even if it is protected by a sterile dressing, the sac may become infected by air-borne bacteria. The operation may be done in one or two stages. Owing to the difficulties we have just noted, plus the fact that the condition is often only one of several anomalies, the mortality rate is relatively high even with expert care.

### Diaphragmatic Hernia

**Incidence, Pathology, Clinical Manifestations and Diagnosis.**    Although this condition is reported today more frequently than it was in the past, this may be due not to an increase in the number of infants who are born with the anomaly, but rather to earlier and more accurate diagnosis.

A diaphragmatic hernia is more common on the left side. The lesion ranges from a slight to an extensive protrusion of the abdominal viscera through an opening in the diaphragm into the thoracic cavity.

The *symptoms* form a characteristic clinical picture, and the diagnosis can often be made in the delivery room if the lesion is extensive. On the other hand, in less severe states no symptoms may appear until later. The symptoms are (1) severe respiratory difficulty, often with resulting cyanosis; (2) a relatively large chest; (3) failure of the side of the chest which is under pressure from the viscera to expand at the same moment as does the unaffected side; and (4) a relatively small abdomen. When the herniated bowel fills with gas, all these symptoms increase in severity.

The *diagnosis* is made by physical examination and confirmed by roentgenograms of the chest. These show air from the intestinal tract in that part of the bowel which has protruded into the hernia and is pressing against the organs of the chest.

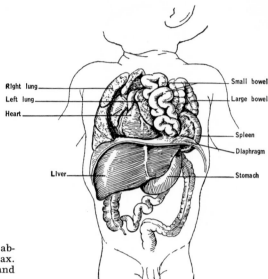

Right lung

Left lung

Heart

Liver

Small bowel

Large bowel

Spleen

Diaphragm

Stomach

**Figure 61.** Diaphragmatic hernia. The abdominal viscera have herniated into the thorax. The thoracic viscera have been displaced and compressed.

**Treatment, Prognosis and Nursing Care.** Immediate operation is indicated. Gastric suction is used to remove secretions and swallowed air from the stomach and the intestinal tract. The operation consists in replacing the abdominal viscera in the abdominal cavity and in repair of the diaphragmatic defect. The lung on the affected side will then fill with air, and normal breathing will occur. If operation is not done immediately, the *prognosis* is very poor: the infant will probably die within the first month of life.

Postoperative *nursing care* is extremely important. Gastric suction is used to prevent abdominal distention immediately after operation. Transfusions of plasma or whole blood are given when necessary, and intravenously administered fluids are given until the infant can take fluids by mouth without abdominal distention. Feedings may be given by gavage on the second or third postoperative day. When fed by gavage, the infant is not so likely to swallow air as he is when sucking.

### Intestinal Obstruction

**Etiology.** Intestinal obstruction in the newborn may result from a number of conditions—congenital atresia or stenosis of the intestine, malformation of the colon with volvulus of the midgut, internal hernias, peritoneal bands or meconium ileus.

*Congenital Atresia or Stenosis of the Intestine.* This condition is due to an arrest in development during the second and third months of intrauterine life. Stenosis (a narrowed lumen) may occur when the intestine develops from a solid structure into a hollow tube. In the course of normal development the diameter of this tube is sufficient throughout its length for the intestines to perform their physiologic functions, but in stenosis at one point only a minute passage is open. In atresia (no lumen) the intestinal tube is completely occluded at one or more points. The intestine may be divided into separate segments connected, in some cases, with fibrous bands.

*Malrotation of the Colon with Volvulus.* During the tenth week of embryonic development the emerging ileocecal structure normally rotates so that the cecum lies in the lower right quadrant of the abdomen and is fixed there by the mesentery. If this process does not occur, the colon may remain in the right upper quadrant. Here an abnormal membrane may obstruct the duodenum. This obstructing band is one of the most significant findings in mal-rotation. A more serious complication is volvulus of the midgut, which happens because of lack of mesenteric attachment. The freely mobile loops of small intestine twist on themselves, and obstruction results.

*Internal Hernias and Obstruction Caused by Peritoneal Bands.* Internal hernias are caused by a loop of bowel slipping out of the normal position and becoming caught in a defective area of the mesentery or becoming compressed between bands of the peritoneum. In either case intestinal obstruction occurs.

*Meconium Ileus.* This condition may occur in infants born with mucovisci-dosis or cystic fibrosis of the pancreas (see p. 352). The infant lacks the enzymes normally supplied by the pancreas and discharged into the intestinal tract. While the infant is still in utero this deficiency causes the meconium to be more sticky than is normal. It is of a putty-like consistency which causes it to adhere to the mucosa of the intestinal wall, and obstruction results. Fortunately, less than 10 per cent of newborns suffering from cystic fibrosis have meconium ileus.

**Clinical Manifestations.** The three main symptoms of intestinal obstruction are (1) absence of stools. If the infant has no stool within four hours after birth, examination for the presence of meconium may be made by inserting a gloved finger into the anus. If no indication of meconium is found, a colonic irrigation with not more than 10 ml. of physiologic saline solution may be ordered. (2) Vomitus stained with bile is diagnostic of intestinal obstruction, though obstruction may produce nonbile-stained vomitus as well. (3) Abdominal distention is a symptom of intestinal obstruction, though it may be physiologic in a normal child until meconium is passed. All infants have these symptoms to a degree, but the presence of two of these manifestations should suggest investigation.

The higher the obstruction, the earlier do the symptoms appear, and the earlier can the diagnosis be made and treatment instituted. For this reason the lowest mortality rate is among infants with high obstruction.

**Diagnosis.** The decisive factor in the diagnosis is the roentgenogram, which shows the presence or absence of an obstruction.

**Treatment.** The treatment is surgical. The majority of operations performed upon the newborn are for intestinal obstruction. The mortality rate is relatively high, but lowest among those cases in which the diagnosis is made early and relief is obtained before the infant's condition has degenerated.

**Nursing Care.** It is the nurse who is most likely to observe the main symptoms of intestinal obstruction in the newborn infant brought to the nursery. She observes more readily whatever has meaning for her. That is why the pathology and etiology of this condition have been given in somewhat extensive detail.

## RESPIRATORY CONDITIONS

Respiratory distress in the newborn may be due to a number of causes, but for a better understanding of the nursing problems of these infants we shall consider two main groups of pathologic conditions which seriously interfere with normal respiration. (1) Failure of the respiratory center of the central nervous system may be due to anoxia, intracranial hemorrhage, anomaly, trauma or narcosis. (2) The second group includes peripheral respiratory difficulty (alveolar exchange of oxygen and carbon dioxide) due to atelectasis, hyaline membrane syndrome, pneumonia or aspiration pneumonia. Conditions not discussed in this chapter are treated elsewhere (see Index).

### Anoxia of the Newborn

**Types, Incidence and Etiology.** Anoxia of the newborn is a condition in which his organs, especially the brain, receive much less oxygen than they need for optimum functioning. Anoxia is not a clinical entity in itself. Some of its causes are known, but others have not yet been identified. Anoxia is an important cause of perinatal death or lasting damage to the tissue of the central nervous system. Cerebral palsy may result or mental retardation be evident later in life.

*Fetal anoxia* may be due to any cause which limits the oxygen supplied by way of the maternal and fetal circulations from reaching the brain of the fetus. Causes include systemic conditions of the mother such as poor oxygenation of the blood due to cardiac failure or low blood pressure. Anoxia may also be caused by conditions of the uterus and the placenta which impede the maternal-fetal circulation or by physical obstruction to adequate circulation due to a knot or kink in the umbilical cord.

*Postnatal anoxia* may be due to any cause which limits the supply of oxygen or renders the cells unable to use the oxygen available. This is the case, for example, if an overdose of barbiturates has been given. During severe shock, oxygen is not sent to the cells in adequate amounts. Even obstruction of the air passages by mucus may drastically diminish the supply of oxygen reaching the brain. Lasting causes of anoxia include severe anemia due to hemorrhage or hemolytic disease, poorly oxygenated blood due to a cyanotic type of congenital heart disease, or inadequate pulmonary ventilation due to malformation of the lungs.

**Clinical Manifestations.**  It is extremely important that the nurse know the signs of both fetal anoxia and anoxia in the newborn. Fetal anoxia is evidenced by an increase in activity of the fetus followed by diminished activity. The fetal heart beat slows and weakens. When fetal anoxia is present, the infant is delivered immediately in order to save his life.

Symptoms of anoxia in the newborn include (1) signs of yellow, meconium-stained amniotic fluid and yellowish vernix caseosa, (2) pallor or cyanosis (even duskiness of the skin), (3) lack of muscle tone, and (4) variable heart beat.

**Treatment.**  The treatment depends

upon the stage of the anoxia and the cause of the condition. Mechanical techniques include mouth-to-mouth insufflation, administration of oxygen by moderate pressure (20 to 30 cm. of water for less than 0.2 second) or through an intratracheal catheter, and the use of "seesaw" respirators. Artificial respiration is of no value unless some expansion of the lungs has taken place. Nalorphine hydrochloride (Nalline) may be given intravenously to reverse respiratory depression due to narcotics given to the mother.

The method of *artificial respiration* for infants and small children advocated by the American Red Cross is as follows:

Clear the child's mouth of any foreign matter.

Place the child on his back, and use the middle finger of each hand to lift the lower jaw from beneath and behind so that it juts out. Hold the jaw in that position with one hand. Place your mouth over the child's mouth and nose, making a reasonably leak-proof seal, and breathe into the child smoothly and steadily until you observe the chest rise. As you start this action, move your free hand to the child's abdomen, between the navel and the ribs. Apply continuous moderate pressure to the abdomen to prevent the stomach from filling with air. When the lungs are inflated, remove your lips from the child's mouth and nose and allow the lungs to empty. Repeat this cycle, keeping one hand beneath the jaw and the other hand pressing on the stomach at all times. The rate should be about 20 cycles per minute. After every 20 cycles rest long enough to take a deep breath.

Carbon dioxide should not be given before spontaneous respiration occurs. Stimulants frequently used include caffeine and sodium benzoate given intramuscularly. After the immediate emergency 5 per cent carbon dioxide and 95 per cent oxygen may be given for ½ minute to 2 minutes every half-hour to 2 hours in order to stimulate deeper respirations.

Infants with respiratory distress should be wrapped in a warm blanket or placed in an incubator. Aspiration to remove mucus from the throat is a routine procedure.

**Nursing care** is the same as that of atelectasis (see p. 187).

**Prevention.**  Preventive measures ap-

**Figure 62.** Mouth-to-mouth insufflation. *A,* Air is breathed into the infant's lungs. *B,* The lungs are allowed to empty. The stethoscope is placed over the abdomen in order to determine whether air is being forced into the stomach.

plying to the management of labor include reduction of analgesia and anesthesia and administration of oxygen during the second stage of labor. Preventive measures applying to the care of the infant include maintenance of an open airway, administration of oxygen as needed, provision of skin stimulation and keeping the infant warm.

### Atelectasis

The lungs are collapsed in fetal life, and the fetus receives oxygen through the maternal circulation. After birth, with the infant's first breath, the lungs normally expand to a variable degree. It may be days or weeks before full expansion takes place.

Atelectasis—collapse or imperfect expansion of lung tissue which carries air—is found in greater or less degree in almost all infants dying soon after delivery. The condition may be either primary or secondary. In *primary* atelectasis the alveoli fail to expand initially. This is common in premature infants and in full-term infants who have suffered brain injury. In *secondary* atelectasis the alveoli collapse after they have once been expanded by air; this may occur when the infant has pulmonary disease.

**Clinical Manifestations.** The symptoms are irregular, rapid, shallow respirations accompanied by a respiratory grunt and flaring of the nostrils. The skin is mottled. Cyanosis may be persistent or in-

termittent; it decreases if the infant cries or is given oxygen. There are intercostal and suprasternal retractions. Fine rales may be heard. On auscultation of the chest poor respiratory exchange is evident. X-ray films reveal increased density in small and large areas which may be present throughout both lungs.

**Treatment.** By bronchoscopy the physician determines whether any obstruction is present and removes it if possible. Oxygen may be given so that the open areas of the lungs will have the benefit of a sufficient supply. The environmental humidity is raised in order that secretions may be liquefied and that the infant may be able to cough up the material. The physician may order 5 per cent carbon dioxide and 95 per cent oxygen to be given in order to stimulate respirations. Caffeine and sodium benzoate may be given intramuscularly. The infant's skin may be stimulated in order to induce crying. His position should be changed every hour or two to provide opportunity for collapsed areas to expand. Antibiotics are given for persistent atelectasis in order to prevent secondary infections. The fundamental treatment is directed toward the underlying condition.

**Course, Prognosis and Prevention.** The *course* of the condition is difficult to predict. Even with early diagnosis and treatment the *prognosis* is poor and death not infrequent. *Prevention* of atelectasis in the infant includes prenatal care of the mother. Premature labor or a difficult delivery in which intracranial hemorrhage occurs is the cause in many cases. Fetal or neonatal anoxia is evidently a predisposing factor, as are pneumonia and hyaline membrane disease.

**Nursing Care.** The nurse should keep in mind the infants under her care who are likely to have atelectasis. Such infants are those who were born prematurely or by cesarean section, those whose mothers had problems during pregnancy, and those who have had intracranial injury or are sick from pneumonia or other respiratory conditions. The nurse must observe these infants closely to detect the first symptoms of distress and also to give an accurate description of their condition to the physician. These infants should be kept warm, preferably in incubators where oxygen can easily be given and the humidity raised. It may be necessary to aspirate the upper respiratory tract if the infant's nose and throat appear to be clogged with mucus. The physician may also order aspiration of the gastric contents in order to prevent aspiration of vomitus should vomiting occur. The infant must be fed with great care, and the physician may order that he be gavaged. All possible measures to prevent abdominal distention must be taken; the infant must be fed slowly and the hole in the nipple be suited to his needs.

The nursing care should be planned so that the infant is disturbed as little as possible; there is more than the usual need for gentle handling. Every precaution should be taken to prevent infection, since even a simple respiratory infection may prove fatal.

*Pneumonia*

**Incidence and Pathology.** Pneumonia is responsible for approximately 10 per cent of neonatal deaths. The disease may accompany an infection which is not of the respiratory tract. Pneumonia in the newborn and the older infant is usually bronchopneumonic rather than lobar.

**Etiology.** In the newborn, pneumonia may be due to bacteria or viruses. The causes of pneumonia of the newborn are connected with the birth process as well as with contact with infection after birth. During delivery, infection may come from aspiration of infected amniotic fluid or vaginal secretions. Infection may be carried to the respiratory tract by way of the blood stream. After birth the infectious organism is most commonly acquired through contact with the mother or with a nurse who has a cold. Although slight respiratory infections in the newborn do not always result in pneumonia, the danger is so great that no one with even a simple cold should care for him. Skin infections caused by a staphylococcus are also a cause of pneumonia in the newborn, whose resistance to any type of infection is low. Organisms which may cause pneumonia in the infant are not the same as those responsible for the disease in older children and adults. The chief causative agents in pneumonia occurring within the first few weeks of life are coliform organisms, enterococci, Klebsiella, Pseudomonas, Proteus, Salmonella and Staphylococcus.

**Clinical Manifestations.** The first sign of pneumonia in the newborn is rapid respiration, which may reach 80 per minute, more than the nurse can count with accuracy. Respiratory distress is evident in flaring of the nostrils. The infant appears listless, is pale or cyanotic, and has an abnormal temperature—higher or lower than normal. He is likely to refuse his feedings and suffers from abdominal distention.

**Treatment.** In general the plan of treatment includes chemotherapeutic agents against the common organisms causing pneumonia in infancy (usually coliform or staphylococcal organisms). Large doses of penicillin and streptomycin are frequently ordered, but chloramphenicol is probably given most often, since it is effective against the majority of strains of coliforms and staphylococci. If the exact etiologic organism can be isolated through laboratory tests, treatment can be made more specific. Gamma globulin is commonly given intramuscularly to increase the infant's resistance to the infection. Oxygen is routinely used to relieve the respiratory distress.

### Aspiration Pneumonia

The first *symptom* of aspiration pneumonia is generally an attack of coughing or, since the cough reflex of the newborn is imperfect, of choking. The usual symptoms of pneumonia are likely to follow within a short time. *Prevention* lies in careful feeding of infants and is therefore the responsibility of the mother and the nurse.

One advantage of breast feeding is that aspiration is not too likely. The newborn has not learned the technique of correlating sucking and swallowing. If the flow of milk is too rapid for him to swallow, he can pull away from the breast more readily than from a bottle held in a nurse's hand. The size of the hole in the nipple is important, and the nurse should be sensitive to the infant's need to swallow what he has in his mouth before more flows in.

If the infant chokes on the feeding and is in immediate danger, the emergency measure is to suspend him by his feet. This permits aspirated milk to drain from the lungs. (For artificial respiration see page 185.) After feeding, the infant should not be placed on his back, but on his right side or abdomen so that if he vomits, the material will drain from the mouth.

Treatments which by their nature disturb the infant emotionally or physiologically, e.g. punctures of the jugular or femoral veins, should be done two hours or more after feedings. Before operation on the newborn the physician will probably order (unless it is a routine procedure in the hospital) aspiration of the stomach contents to prevent aspiration when the anesthetic is given.

### INFECTIONS

Certain congenital infections are discussed in the preceding chapter. This chapter is concerned with infections acquired postnatally.

**Organisms Causing Infection after Birth.** Any pathogenic bacteria or virus may cause infection in the newborn. Many which do not cause disease in older children and adults may cause serious disease in the newborn. The chief organisms affecting the newborn are coliform organisms and *Staphylococcus aureus;* others include enterococci, Klebsiella, Pseudomonas, Salmonella and Proteus.

**Types of Infections.** The most common types of infection occurring in the nursery are septicemia, pneumonia and skin and umbilical infections. Diarrhea is still a common infection, although its incidence has been reduced in this country.

**Clinical Manifestations and Treatment of Infection.** It is extremely difficult for the nurse to recognize infection in the newborn, since his reactions to it may be so general that infection is not suspected. This is one reason why the nurse should report anything abnormal in an infant's condition even though it appears trivial and might easily be caused by some transient indisposition. The pediatrician makes his diagnosis by appraising the significance of every factor in the total clinical picture. Nonspecific symptoms are those which accompany many types of congenital diseases.

Signs that something is radically wrong with an infant include cyanosis, convulsions, listlessness, anorexia, vomiting, jaundice and diarrhea. Fever may or may not be an indication of infection, since it may be the result of keeping the infant too warm or the weather being so hot that no cool place can be found for him. Absence of fever has little diagnostic significance, since the newborn may not react to even a massive infection with an elevation of temperature. The difficulties in making a diagnosis of infection are even greater in the premature than in the normal newborn. Laboratory studies and x-ray examination may be necessary.

If a specific infecting organism is

found, *treatment* is mainly by administration of the appropriate chemotherapeutic agent; if a specific organism is unknown, an agent effective against a number of organisms is given.

### Infections Caused by Escherichia Coli

*Escherichia coli* is the most common cause of serious infection of the newborn and is capable of producing a number of pathologic conditions, among them septicemia, pneumonia, meningitis and diarrhea. The drugs especially useful against this organism are chloramphenicol, tetracycline and streptomycin. Neomycin is commonly used for intestinal infections.

### Infections Caused by Staphylococcus Aureus

**Etiology, Onset, Types, and Modes of Entry.** *Staphylococcus aureus* is a gram-positive organism which under the microscope appears in clumps. It is second only to *Escherichia coli* as a cause of infection in the newborn. Unfortunately the incidence of this type of infection in newborn nurseries is increasing. Many strains of the organism appear to be resistant to the majority of known chemotherapeutic agents.

The initial infection with *Staphylococcus aureus* usually occurs while the infant is in the hospital, but may appear weeks or months later. This is one of the many reasons why all infants should be under the care of a private physician or be visited by a public health nurse and taken regularly to a Child Health Conference or clinic. An infection of this type acquired while the infant is in the nursery is likely to spread to other infants even though the customary isolation technique has been followed.

If the infant is breast-fed, the mother may acquire mastitis due to infection of the nipple from the organisms in his mouth. An infant may also infect other members of the family if he is discharged before the infection has been recognized and treated.

The primary infection with *Staphylo-coccus aureus* is commonly but not always of the skin. Pneumonia, septicemia or enteritis may represent either a primary or secondary infection with *Staphylococcus aureus*. Osteomyelitis or meningitis may be a complication of septicemia. The umbilical wound may become infected, or a leaking meningocele, a break in the skin or a circumcision wound may all be the site of a primary infection.

*Sources of Infection in the Nursery.* Pathogens may be brought into the nursery by the nurses caring for the infants or by the other personnel. The mother also is a possible source of infection to her child. Infection is readily spread from one infected infant to others.

**Treatment and Prevention.** Systemic *therapy* requires the giving of an antibiotic effective against the specific organism infecting the infant. The drugs given include Staphcillin, chloramphenicol, and novobiocin. Skin lesions in general are treated by bathing the infant with a soap or a detergent containing hexachlorophene. Bacitracin ointment may be applied to the skin lesions, but in some cases it may be necessary to drain the lesions surgically.

*Prevention* is as important as treatment. No one with a skin infection should enter the nursery or the rooms occupied by the mothers. A mother who becomes infected should be isolated, and her child, if there is any reason to believe that his contact with her may have caused him to become infected, should be isolated from other infants in the nursery.

Every infant in the nursery should have his individual equipment, and all personnel caring for the infants should use soap or a detergent containing hexachlorophene when washing their hands to lessen the risk of carrying infection to the infants upon the skin of the hands. Personnel should be aware also that the anterior nares are the main reservoir in carriers of *Staphylococcus aureus*. (See page 114 for the advisability of wearing masks when caring for infants.) Infants may be bathed with soap or a detergent containing hexachlorophene to lessen the chance of skin infection, and the umbilical cord stump may be routinely painted daily with bactericidal dyes. The nursery must not be overcrowded, for then it is almost impossible to maintain isolation technique.

If an epidemic starts, certain measures are routine. New cases are isolated. Rigid isolation technique is enforced. Another nursery should be opened for newborns delivered after the epidemic started and therefore not exposed to the infection in the contaminated nursery. Contaminated equipment should be thoroughly scrubbed with soap and water and sterilized if possible. The floor and walls should be cleaned and aired, curtains and furnishings washed. Nose and throat cultures should be taken of all nurses and other personnel who have cared for the infants in the infected nursery. It is imperative that each nursery have its own staff of nurses. As a preventive measure, chloramphenicol or erythromycin may be given to each infant in the clean nursery from his admission until discharge.

If these drastic measures are carried out for three weeks, the epidemic will probably come to an end. Such an epidemic is one of the most serious which may occur in a nursery for newborns.

### SPECIFIC TYPES OF INFECTIONS

#### Impetigo of the Newborn

**Etiology, Incidence and Transmission** The causative organism may be staphylococci or streptococci. These organisms invade the superficial layers of the skin. The condition occurs more readily in the newborn than in older children and adults because their resistance is lower. Impetigo may be carried from one infant to another in the nursery.

**Clinical Manifestations, Treatment, Prognosis and Nursing Care.** The first symptomatic lesions are erythematous papules. Then superficial vesicles containing fluid appear. The covering of these vesicles is loose and wrinkled. The fluid soon becomes purulent, and an area of

**Figure 63.** Impetigo neonatorum. (R. J. McKay, Jr., and C. A. Smith in Nelson's Textbook of Pediatrics. 7th ed.)

erythema develops around each vesicle. The pustule ruptures, and crusts may develop, although this is more common in older children than in the newborn. The lesions usually occur on moist surfaces or body creases, and last from one to two weeks. Constitutional symptoms are rare.

*Treatment* consists in removing the epidermis with alcohol sponges and exposing the denuded areas to dry heat. Bacitracin or neomycin ointment may be applied locally. Systemic antibiotic therapy may be necessary.

Impetigo of the newborn was formerly a dangerous infection which led to sepsis and pemphigus, but today, with antibiotic treatment, the *prognosis* is good. Superficial lesions heal without scarring, although more extensive and deeper lesions may leave scars. Strict isolation technique should prevent the occurrence of impetigo in the nursery. If impetigo occurs, however, the nurse carries out the treatment ordered by the physician, which will probably be similar to that outlined here.

#### Furunculosis

**Etiology, Incidence, Pathology and Clinical Manifestations.** Staphylococci are, in general, the pathogenic organisms which cause furunculosis. Although the condition may occur at any time during childhood, it is most frequent and most dangerous in malnourished newborn infants. Furuncles are most likely to occur on the head, but may appear on the back or the back of the extremities.

Furunculosis is an infection of the sebaceous glands or hair follicles. The furuncle soon develops into a red, pointed or rounded lump. In a few days it softens, and a core is formed. When a number of such lesions are present, the condition is called *furunculosis*. The infant seldom shows systemic symptoms. In extreme cases, however, anorexia and toxemia may occur.

**Treatment.** Local applications may be made of 10 or 20 per cent ichthammol ointment or other mild antiseptic ointment. The infant should be bathed daily, using pHisoHex or a similar antiseptic to prevent spread of the infection. Antibiotic therapy depends upon the specific organism causing the condition. In severe cases staphylococcal toxoid is given or an autogenous vaccine is made. Hot compresses may be ordered to further maturation of the furuncle and, after it has opened spontaneously or been incised, to further drainage.

The diet should be low in carbohydrate and high in vitamin content. The caloric content should be sufficient to meet the infant's nutritional needs. A sufficient fluid intake is necessary, and the electrolyte balance must be maintained.

**Nursing Care.** Good hygiene and general nursing care are the best preventives of furunculosis. Aseptic nursing technique in the nursery is important. Particularly in hot weather the infant's position should be changed so that all surfaces of the skin are exposed in rotation to the air.

If furunculosis develops in an infant in the nursery, he should be removed and isolated elsewhere. With the first sign of the lesion the area should be cleansed with care. If the lesion is on the scalp, the area around the furuncle should be shaved. The nurse will carry out the physician's orders for treatment, which will probably be along the lines just indicated. The infant must not be allowed to rub the area; arm restraints (see Fig. 69) should be applied if necessary. The nurse should be careful that she herself does not become infected; the slightest scratch or abrasion on her hand may easily be a point of entrance for the organism.

### Epidemic Diarrhea

**Etiology, Incidence and Transmission.** No single organism has been identified which is invariably the cause of epidemic diarrhea, though severe epidemics have been caused by virulent strains of colon bacilli. Diarrhea is a highly contagious disease easily carried from one infant to another even if aseptic technique customary in newborn nurseries is maintained. If an infant acquires the condition, he should be taken from the nursery and isolated elsewhere.

An infant may contract the disease through a contaminated formula or from the hands of his mother or nurse who themselves carry the organism, but are without clinical symptoms, since they have the adult's resistance to the infection. The importance of this source of infection is seldom realized. Yet we know that it is impossible to sterilize human hands completely, and even careful washing may not eliminate the risk of carrying the pathogenic organism to the infant.

**Clinical Manifestations, Treatment and Course.** The main *symptom* is frequent watery stools, which are likely to be expelled with considerable force. The infant has abdominal distention; he may refuse his feedings or, if he takes them, vomit. As a rule there is elevation of the temperature. The weight loss is largely due to loss of fluid, which may be extremely rapid. Loss of fluids results in electrolyte imbalance and dehydration. Acidosis may result.

The *treatment* is similar to that given infants with diarrhea (see p. 314). The newborn infant with diarrhea, even if it is not proved to be infectious, should be isolated immediately and preferably cared for by nurses who do not handle the other infants. The obstetric unit should be closed unless all new cases can be cared for in other quarters by nurses who have not been in contact with the infants suffering from this infectious condition. If the cause of the infection is the enteropathic strain of the colon bacillus, neomycin may be ordered and given orally. Fluids and electrolytes are given parenterally to supplement or replace the oral intake.

The disease must be reported to the health authorities because of its infectious nature. The *course* is severe, and the neonatal mortality rate may be as high as 25 to 50 per cent of affected infants.

**Nursing Care.** Nursing care is both preventive and supportive. Rules and regulations safeguarding infants from all sources of infection are an administrative responsibility, but conscientious application of these regulations in the direct care of infants is the function of the nurse. It is she who will see the first loose stool and note the presence of mucus in it, observe the infant's refusal of part or all of his feeding—probably vomiting what he has taken—and note his rise in temperature. The pathologic organism must be isolated in the laboratory examination of a stool specimen before the diagnosis of infectious diarrhea is made, but as soon as infection is suspected, measures to protect the other infants in the nursery must be taken at once. In the majority of hospitals the nurse has a standing order to place an infected infant in isolation even before the physician has made his diagnosis and given her written orders to do so.

The probable treatment which the physician will order has been outlined. All but the parenteral administration of fluids is carried out by the nurse. There are few infants having medical conditions who require such constant attention as those suffering from epidemic diarrhea.

Prevention of excoriated buttocks is an immediate problem in the nursing care. The diaper must be changed frequently. If the room is warm enough, it is advisable not to diaper the infant, but rather to place a pad made of folded diapers under his buttocks and legs and leave him uncovered. If the temperature of the room requires application of heat, a cradle with an electric light bulb in the top may be placed over his body and covered with a sheet. Care must be taken that the sheet does not touch the bulb, since it might scorch and then become ignited.

In some hospitals the diapers from an infected infant are soaked in a disinfectant before being sent to the laundry, or they may be placed in a container marked for special care in the laundry.

For additional care of infants with diarrhea, see page 316.

## Umbilical Infection

**Etiology, Clinical Manifestations, Complications, Treatment, Prevention and Nursing Care.** Umbilical infection is usually due to *Escherichia coli* or staphylococci, but may be due to other pyogenic organisms. The *symptoms* are redness and moisture of the stump of the cord. These symptoms may be slight or severe, but in no case should they be disregarded. In severe cases there may be a characteristically foul odor from the stump. The condition may clear up without systemic effects. But if the causative organism is one of the pus-producing type, septicemia may develop. Infection by the tetanus bacillus is less common, but produces a higher mortality rate (see p. 193).

The *treatment* for a mild infection may be simply to touch the area with a silver nitrate stick and cover it with an alcohol sponge held in place by an abdominal band. For a more severe infection continuous warm wet compresses may be applied. Any antibiotic used will depend upon the causative organism.

*Prevention* of the infection is discussed on page 113.

This is another condition in which close, intelligent observation of the infant by the nurse is of the utmost importance. She is constantly with him and sees him nude when giving him his bath. The responsibility for noting the first signs of infection rests with her.

Early recognition and treatment may prevent serious, if not fatal, systemic complications. As with any infection, the infant should be isolated and, preferably, removed from the nursery.

### Sepsis Neonatorum

**Etiology, Clinical Manifestations and Treatment.** Sepsis neonatorum may be caused by any pathogenic organism which has entered the blood stream. The portal of entry may be through the skin, mucous membranes, respiratory or gastrointestinal tract, umbilicus, or circumcision or other wound. The infection may occur prenatally, during delivery or postnatally.

The *symptoms* and signs may appear suddenly after an insidious onset, the infant at first appearing only restless or listless with anorexia and poor weight gain. Later there is evidence of dehydration and emaciation. There may be vomiting and diarrhea. The infant's temperature and white blood cell count may be elevated, depressed or normal. Convulsions may or may not be present. Signs of jaundice may appear. On examination the spleen and the liver may be found enlarged. The majority of these symptoms are so variable that the diagnosis is made upon the general picture and the laboratory findings, particularly the blood culture and nasopharyngeal culture.

Immediate *treatment* consists in administration of large doses of antibiotics effective against a wide range of organisms. After the laboratory blood examination has proved the specific organism causing the septic condition the specific antibiotic is given. Symptomatic therapy is carried out from the onset of the disease. The infant is isolated. Fluids may be administered parenterally, and a blood transfusion may be necessary. Oxygen is given as the need for it arises.

**Prognosis and Course.** If the condition is recognized early and treatment is instituted at once, the mortality rate is low. The probability of death increases as the untreated condition becomes more severe. The nidus of the infection should be sought; it may be in the meninges, the perineum or elsewhere. The organism in the blood stream may cause secondary infection in almost any part of the body. If meningitis develops, convulsions may ensue. If the infant survives, hydrocephalus may result. Characteristic signs of damage to brain cells may be evident as the child grows older (mental retardation).

**Prevention and Nursing Care.** *Prevention* lies in aseptic technique during delivery and in the technique which has already been outlined for the prevention of infection among infants in the nursery. Personnel in the obstetric unit, delivery rooms and newborn nursery must be exceptionally conscientious in reporting any infection, however slight, in their own bodies. In a modern hospital where good technique prevails it is probable that bacteria in the nose and throat of some member of the hospital personnel who comes in close contact with the infants are the greatest potential source of danger to them. The shortage of physicians and nurses often results in personnel being on duty when they should not be in contact with maternity patients and newborn infants.

The preventive *nursing care* which has already been described in relation to infectious conditions applies in the care of infants suffering from sepsis neonatorum. Again, accurate observation and prompt reporting are of tremendous importance. From the discussion of signs and symptoms it is evident that the condition at the onset may easily be considered only a minor ailment and may go untreated until grave symptoms develop and the probability of complete cure is slight.

### Tetanus Neonatorum

**Etiology, Incidence and Incubation Period.** The causative organism is the tetanus bacillus (*Clostridium tetani*), an anaerobic, spore-forming, gram-positive bacillus. Entrance into the blood stream of the newborn is through the umbilical wound. Tetanus is most unlikely to occur in a well regulated hospital, since the natural environment of the organism is in the soil. In children and adults the organism enters the blood stream through a deep puncture of the skin and underlying tissue. Since infants and children today are receiving antitetanus injections with the other types of early immunization, the incidence of tetanus among them is low.

Tetanus cannot be transmitted through contact; it must enter the body through a break in the skin. It develops only where it is not exposed to the air. Thus a simple skin abrasion is not a portal of entry for the tetanus bacillus. Isolation of the infant is not necessary, but it may be carried out to protect the child from other infections.

Tetanus of the newborn is extremely rare in the United States, but occurs in other countries where the hands of the attendant at delivery (untrained midwife, neighbor or one of the family) are contaminated and a contaminated knife is used to cut the cord.

The *incubation period* is five days to five weeks. The shorter the period of incubation, the greater is the probability of a fatal outcome. In the average hospital in the United States an infant is not in the nursery more than five days, and if the condition were to occur, it would probably be after the infant had been sent home. Here again we see the need of follow-up of all infants who are not under the care of a private physician.

**Clinical Manifestations.** The symptoms which accompany tetanus neonatorum are produced by the toxic effects on the nervous system of the exotoxin of the tetanus bacillus. The infant is irritable and restless; he cannot open his mouth or suck because of *trismus* or tetanic spasm of the muscles of the jaw, and has great difficulty in swallowing. The facial expression is drawn and anxious, the exact opposite of that of the normal well infant. A symptom of diagnostic importance is stiffness of the neck. Pain-

ful muscular contractions or convulsions recur periodically. *Opisthotonos* with the head drawn back and the back arched, occurs during these muscular contractions. As a result of spasms of the facial muscles a fixed expression, or *risus sardonicus,* may be seen. Tactile or auditory stimuli may induce convulsions. The temperature may be elevated, rising to 104° F. (40° C.). The white blood cell count is 8000 to 12,000, and there is a slight increase in the cerebrospinal fluid pressure.

**Treatment, Prevention and Nursing Care.** Adequate *treatment* and nursing care cannot be given unless a nurse is with the child at all times. Tetanus antitoxin is given to neutralize the free toxin in the body and around the site of the infection. Before administration of the antitoxin the infant's sensitivity to horse serum should be tested in order to prevent a serum reaction.

Measures to control convulsions are essential. Large doses of sedatives are given to keep the infant relaxed and semiconscious. He should be in a quiet, semidarkened room, and stimulation of any sort, such as noise or unnecessary handling, should be reduced to a minimum.

*Nursing care* should be planned around the periods when medication or necessary treatment is given. Secretions in the nasopharynx should be aspirated. Oxygen administration may be necessary. Oxygen and carbon dioxide may be ordered to stimulate respirations. The equipment for tracheotomy should be ready for immediate use if needed. Since the infant is heavily sedated and unable to suck or swallow, it is necessary to gavage him. Fluids will probably be administered parenterally. An intake and output chart must be kept.

*Prevention* of tetanus neonatorum lies in the use of sterile instruments to cut the cord and adequate care of the cord during the neonatal period. For prevention of tetanus in the infant, see page 291.

**Prognosis.** The prognosis is very poor, the mortality rate being up to 50 per cent of the cases. Death is usually due to respiratory failure, exhaustion or a complicating aspiration pneumonia. If the infant survives, however, recovery is complete.

## REFERENCES

Adelson, L., and Kinney, E. R.: Sudden and Unexpected Death in Infancy and Childhood. Pediatrics: 17:663, 1956.

A H A's Recommendations on Prevention and Control of Staphylococcus Infections in Hospitals. Am. J. Nursing, 58:1099, 1958.

A N A Special Committee on Infections. Prevention and Control of Infection. Am. J. Nursing, 60:657, 1960.

Apgar, V., and others: Neonatal Anoxia. Pediatrics, 15:653, 1955.

Artificial Respiration for Infants and Small Children. Am. J. Nursing, 57:1324, 1957.

Bishop, H. C.: Factors Affecting Success and Failure in Neonatal Surgery. Pediat. Clin. North America, 6:945, 1959.

Callon, H.: How the Nurse Can Combat Staphylococcal Infections. Nursing World, 132:8, November, 1958.

Dill, D. B.: Introduction: Symposium on Mouth-to-Mouth Resuscitation. J.A.M.A., 167:317, 1958.

Gordon, A. S., and others: Mouth-to-mouth versus Manual Artificial Respiration for Children and Adults, J.A.M.A., 167:320, 1958.

Gross, R. E.: The Surgery of Infancy and Childhood. Philadelphia, W. B. Saunders Company, 1953.

Harder, H. I., and Panuska, M.: A Program to Control Staphylococcal Infections. Am. J. Nursing, 58:349, 1958.

Kiesewetter, W. B.: Pre and Postoperative Care in the Pediatric Surgical Patient. Chicago, Year Book Publishers, Inc., 1956.

Koop, C. E.: Emergency Surgery of the Newborn. Clinical Symposia. Ciba Pharmaceutical Products, Inc., Summit, New Jersey, 11:35, 1959.

Idem: Physiologic Considerations in the Surgery of Infants. S. Clin. North America, 35:1745, 1955.

Lank, B. E.: Anesthesia for the Newborn. Am. J. Nursing, 59:1255, 1959.

Linden, M. E.: Some Psychological Aspects of Rescue Breathing. Am. J. Nursing, 60:971, 1960.

Lynn, H. B.: Pediatric Surgery. Nursing Outlook, 6:272, 1958.

Mayer, D. M., and Swanker, W. A.: Anomalies of Infants and Children. New York, McGraw-Hill Book Company, Inc., 1958.

McCaskill, C. L.: Pediatric Surgical Nursing. Nursing Outlook, 6:274, 1958.

Medical Department of Bristol Laboratories, New York City: Staphcillin. Am. J. Nursing, 61:58, March, 1961.

Miller, A. L., and McDonald, E.: Staphylococcal Infections—A Community Problem. Nursing Outlook, 7:584, 1959.

Nelson, W. E. (editor): Textbook of Pediatrics. 7th ed. Philadelphia, W. B. Saunders Company, 1959.

Nyhan, W. L., and Fousek, M. D.: Septicemia of the Newborn. Pediatrics, 22:268, 1958.

Ochsner, A., and DeBakey, M. E. (editors): Christopher's Minor Surgery. 8th ed. Philadelphia, W. B. Saunders Company, 1959.

Paterson, D., and McCreary, J. F.: Pediatrics. Philadelphia, J. B. Lippincott Company, 1956.

Potts, W. J.: The Surgeon and the Child. Philadelphia, W. B. Saunders Company, 1959.

Rakich, J. H., and others: Nurses Are Asking about Staphylococcal Infections. Am. J. Nursing, 60:1766, 1960.

Ravenholt, R. T., and Ravenholt, O. H.: Staphylococcal Infections in the Hospital and Community, Am. J. Pub. Health, 48:277, 1958.

Rickham, P. P.: Diagnosis of Congenital Anomalies Incompatible with Life, but Amenable to Surgical Correction. Pediat. Clin. North America, 6:955, 1959.

Schaffer, A. J.: Diseases of the Newborn. Philadelphia, W. B. Saunders Company, 1960.

Shannon, V.: When Children Are Born with Defects. Children, 2:27, 1955.

Stanley-Brown, E. G.: Pediatric Surgery for Nurses. Philadelphia, W. B. Saunders Company, 1961.

Thompson, L. R.: Staphylococcus Aureus. Am. J. Nursing, 58:1098, 1958.

# Chapter 11

# Conditions of the

# Newborn Requiring Long-Term Care

## CONGENITAL DEFORMITIES

SEVERAL congenital anomalies require care over a period of weeks, months or years. For many of the anomalies discussed in this chapter surgery early in life is the treatment of choice. The risk to life must be considered in relation to the probable advantage to the child of operation. It is difficult for parents to be objective in making the decision for or against surgical treatment. Before operation is undertaken the parents should be convinced that their decision is right, that the probable benefit justifies the risk. Then, if the child should die, they do not blame themselves for permitting the operation.

Surgical correction may be necessary at a later date. The treatment and nursing care of some of these children will be discussed in chapters dealing with children of the age group in which correction of the anomaly is generally made.

**The Nurse's Feelings about Congenital**

**Abnormalities.** The nurse's feelings about congenital anomalies involve her attitude toward both the infant and his parents. She is influenced by her picture of the infant as he will be during childhood and adult life if operation is not performed, as compared with his condition if operation is successful. On the other hand, her attitude, particularly that of a young nurse wanting both a career in nursing and marriage, is complicated by a mental picture of how she would feel if the infant were her own.

Surgery for the newborn is a special field in which great advances are being made, but which is still more problematic than for older children or adults. To realize that the infant may live for months or years in his present condition, but may die tomorrow under operation, is anxiety-producing even if it is not the nurse who decides the question. Surgery, if recommended by a competent surgeon, is a calculated risk which the nurse knows should be taken. Since she is fully convinced of this herself, she is able to be of emotional support to the parents during their period of stress and indecision, and also if the child should die under operation.

It is difficult for even the physician and certainly impossible for the nurse to satisfy the parents' desire for information about the cause of the infant's condition. If the parents feel that in some way they are to blame, they may be reassured that it is in no way their fault and that science has not yet discovered all the many possible causes of congenital anomalies. The nurse, of course, should make no comment as to the outcome of the untreated condition or the probable results of surgery. Her attitude should be that the parents, after the physician has spoken to them frankly, make this important decision themselves, and that, if the operation is not successful, the result must be considered in relation to the handicapped life which the child would have led had operation not been attempted.

### SKIN LESIONS

#### Nevi

The nevi seen in the newborn are of two types: (*a*) the vascular group—nevi due to hyperplasia of blood or lymph vessels; (*b*) nonvascular nevi, caused by an overgrowth of connective or epidermal tissue. In either type the defect probably originates in the germ plasm. The hereditary factor is apparently important.

**Nevus Vasculosus.** The nevus vasculosus, commonly called a birthmark (although the mark may not appear until some time after birth), is composed entirely of blood vessels. These marks are likely to be flat and to appear on the back of the head. No treatment is required, since the majority disappear spontaneously.

The so-called *port-wine mark* is a flat, irregularly shaped mark often found on the side of the face. It is light pink in the newborn, but later becomes deep purple. It is due to a malformation of superficial capillaries and does not respond too well to local treatment. It may be removed by surgery or irradiation. The removal should be done only by an expert in this type of treatment. A small or faint lesion which appears to be similar to these marks on the face may appear on the nape of the neck, bridge of the nose or on the eyelids. These lesions, unlike those of the face, disappear without treatment.

The so-called *strawberry mark* is a slightly raised, bright red to deep purple nevus which may disappear spontaneously. These marks may be removed by applying carbon dioxide snow or dry ice over the area. Such treatments may be given at intervals of three to four weeks. After each treatment zinc oxide or other bland ointment should be applied to the area. The area should be covered with a dressing which should be changed daily. Radium therapy is also effective, but must be given only by an expert in this kind of treatment.

A *cavernous hemangioma* is formed by large sinus-like blood vessels. These lesions are cystic, deep-lying vascular anomalies that are blue or purple. Treatment is by irradiation (x-ray or radium), injection of a sclerosing solution, or surgery. Treatment should be begun

**Figure 64.** Nevus flammeus, or port-wine stain, present at birth. (Lewis: Practical Dermatology. 2nd ed.)

Figure 65. Vascular nevus (strawberry mark). (C. S. Wright in Nelson's Textbook of Pediatrics. 7th ed.)

Figure 67. Nevus pigmentosus. (C. S. Wright in Nelson's Textbook of Pediatrics. 7th ed.)

Figure 66. Cavernous hemangioma. (Pillsbury, Shelley and Kligman: Dermatology.)

early, since the lesions tend to grow larger as the child grows. There is also the possibility of severe hemorrhage if some trauma causes the lesion to bleed.

**Pigmented Nevi.** These lesions vary in size and color from harmless freckles to dark hairy nevi. Although such lesions are rarely malignant, the child should be kept from irritating the area. Although such nevi do not grow rapidly, they develop in proportion to the child's growth and therefore become increasingly more difficult to remove. If they are large, dark and on the face, they may cause both parents and child the emotional trauma likely to accompany any conspicuous disfigurement.

*Treatment.* The most satisfactory treatment of pigmented nevi is by surgical excision, including a portion of the nearby normal skin. Nevi on parts of the body where constant irritation of the skin occurs must be observed at regular intervals for changes in size or nature, and removed if such change occurs. Operation must be done if they appear to be growing at a disproportionately greater rate than the body skin. If only the cosmetic effect is the concern of the physician and the parents, the time for removal makes little difference. In general, however, it is advisable that operation be done during the first year of life or in the early school years.

### GASTROINTESTINAL SYSTEM

#### Cleft Lip and Cleft Palate

**Etiology, Pathology and Incidence.** The terms "cleft lip" and "cleft palate" describe the condition. The cause is a failure of union of the embryonic structures of the face. Fusion of the maxillary and premaxillary processes normally occurs between the fifth and eighth weeks of intrauterine life. The palatal processes fuse about one month later. Failure of fusion results in the typical cleft lip and cleft palate.

This partial or complete nonunion may involve more than the palatal bone and the upper lip. It may affect the maxilla, premaxilla and tissues of the soft palate and uvula. All these defects or any combination of them may occur. The abnormality appears to run in families and therefore to be influenced by heredity, but other factors may be involved. The condition is often one of several anomalies in the infant.

The *incidence* of cleft lip or cleft palate is about one in 800 of the population.

**Psychologic Trauma.** To learn that their newborn infant suffers this abnormality is a great shock to the parents—less so, however, if some relative on either side of the parental family lines has had a successful repair of the same condition. A sympathetic, tactful nurse can do a great deal to relieve their distress. With the infant in her arms she may speak of other infants on whom a successful repair has been done. The parents may be reassured that surgery for infants is safer today than formerly, since there have been great advances in

**Figure 68.** Harelip and cleft palate in a newborn infant. This congenital anomaly was successfully corrected by surgery. (Davis and Sheckler: DeLee's Obstetrics for Nurses. 16th ed.)

the administration of anesthesia to infants.

### Cleft Lip (Harelip)

**Incidence and Pathology.** Cleft lip is one of the most frequently occurring congenital anomalies. It is more common in males than in females.

As already noted, it is due to incomplete fusion of the central processes with one or both of the lateral processes from which the area around the upper jaw, lip and nose is formed. If the fissure is unilateral, it is generally below the center of one of the nostrils; if bilateral, beneath both nostrils. The extent of the defect varies from a slight indentation to an open cleft. The incomplete cleft may be little more than a notching of the vermilion border of the lip, but on the other hand may extend to the nostril. The complete cleft usually involves the alveolus to some degree, and the ala (the flap of flesh forming the side of the nostril) is displaced toward the side. The floor of the nares and even the gum in which the upper teeth are set may also be deformed.

**Treatment and Prognosis.** Plastic surgery should be done for the child's comfort as well as the cosmetic effect. In the mild incomplete type the child is not hampered by the deformity, and correction may be done at any time when he is in good condition. With complete cleft lip, repair should be made as soon as the child's condition permits, since the deformity interferes with feeding. The infant also becomes accustomed to breathing through his mouth, with the result that the mucous membrane becomes dry and cracked, and infection is more likely. In the rapidly growing structure of the infant's face the cleft prevents normal development. The psychological effect upon the parents, even if they try to be objective in their attitude toward the child's deformity, is likely to hinder the usual face-to-face cuddling which infants normally receive. If they show him to friends, he may not receive the warm greeting which adults normally give to perfect, healthy infants and which the

**Figure 69.** Appearance of a 2-month-old infant after repair of a cleft lip. A Band-aid is used to hold the suture line together. Elbow restraints prevent the infant from rubbing his face. The mother remained with this child throughout his hospitalization.

infant needs so as to develop his trust in others.

The *prognosis,* when repair is made by a competent plastic surgeon, is very good. The operation is usually done when the infant is one or two months old. At the time he should be free from infection and gaining weight. Postoperatively a Band-aid may be used to hold the suture line together. In many hospitals a Logan bar is used to prevent stretching of the wound postoperatively when the infant cries. (A Logan bar is a wire bow which is placed over the wound with each end taped to the cheek on which it rests.)

**Preoperative Nursing Care.** While the infant is at home the nurse should encourage the mother to treat him as if he were a normal infant. He should not be overprotected and certainly never rejected. The mother should not keep him from relatives and friends who will eventually accept him as a normal infant. She must realize, however, that the first impression of a child so disfigured is startling, and allow others to become accustomed to his appearance before expecting from them the normal reaction to an infant.

She should have explained to her that the infant's difficulty in feeding is due to the fact that he cannot create a vacuum in his mouth and so is unable to suck. A rubber-tipped medicine dropper is used to feed him, although in extreme cases gavage may be necessary. The mother can be taught both procedures. In feeding with the dropper the rubber tip should be put on the top and to the side of the tongue and as far back in the mouth as is practical. He should be bubbled frequently, for he swallows more air than does the infant nursing from the breast or the bottle.

The infant's hands should be restrained when he is not in his mother's arms, to prevent picking of the lips and to accustom him to arm restraint before the operation for repair of the lip. With a small infant it is usually sufficient to pull the sleeves of the shirt down over the hands and to pin the edge of each sleeve to the diaper. The older infant's hands may be restrained by using the clove hitch restraint (see p. 168), or elbow restraints may be used (see Fig. 69).

Because of mouth-breathing the lips are dry, and it is important to prevent cracks or fissures through which infection may enter. The area should be kept clean, and water should be given after feedings to rinse out the mouth. The mother or nurse should also watch for signs of respiratory distress or gastrointestinal disturbance. Every precaution should be taken to protect him from infection. The routine care of an infant must be taught the mother, since the infant will be at home until he is old enough for operation.

**Postoperative Nursing Care.**  The infant will require close observation to keep the airway open. He is accustomed to mouth-breathing, which is difficult with a Band-aid or a Logan bar in place. The nurse should note and report to the physician if the tissues of the tongue or mouth or the lining of the nostrils is swollen from surgery. A laryngoscope, endotracheal tube and suction apparatus should be ready for use if necessary.

A tray for cleaning the nostril and the incision should contain the solution ordered by the physician (usually a soap containing hexachlorophene, or hydrogen peroxide or physiologic saline solution), sterile gauze swabs (cotton is not used because wisps of the cotton cling to the sutures), forceps in alcohol, and a paper bag for soiled swabs. The nurse should cleanse the suture line frequently and with great care that the gauze does not catch upon and pull the sutures. The lip should be patted, not wiped. If a crust forms, a scar is likely to result, and if a suture is pulled or sloughs out, the suture line will not be even.

The infant should receive the routine good nursing care needed by all infants; he should be kept comfortable, warm and dry. He should be kept from crying, for even with the Band-aid or Logan bar crying brings some degree of strain on the suture line. He can be held and carried about. He should be given the feeding to which he is accustomed, either by medicine dropper or by nasal gavage. The medicine dropper should be inserted in the corner of the mouth so as not to touch the area about the suture line. He should be fed slowly and in a sitting position. He should be bubbled frequently both for relief of air which he has swallowed and for its general comforting effect. Water should be given to cleanse the mouth of milk after the feeding. As with any infant, water should be given between feedings.

Since the hands are restrained to prevent the infant from rubbing his face, normal movement is prevented. To improve the circulation and make the infant more comfortable, the arms should be released, first one and then the other, while he is held in his nurse's or mother's lap. (It is never safe to remove restraint of both arms at one time.) Since the infant cannot suck, he should be held and cuddled frequently to provide emotional satisfaction.

The infant should never be placed upon his abdomen, or even upon his side if there is a likelihood that he may roll over on his face. The lateral position has the advantage that he is less likely to aspirate mucus or regurgitated milk. His position should be changed frequently to lessen the danger of hypostatic pneumonia. If it is impossible to support him on his side, or if his position is changed and he lies upon his back, he may be held in the desired position by bands about the wrists fastened with the clove hitch restraint (see p. 168).

The adhesive anchoring the Band-aid or Logan bar should be kept clean and dry and be replaced if it loosens.

After two or three weeks, when the lip is completely healed, bottle or breast feeding may be resumed. Only an infant with an incomplete cleft can nurse, and therefore few of these infants are breast-fed satisfactorily. For a breast-fed infant, however, the mother should express her milk before and during the postoperative period when the infant is unable to suck.

### Cleft Palate

**Incidence, Etiology, Pathology and Clinical Manifestations.**  Unlike cleft lip, which occurs more frequently among boys than girls, cleft palate is more common in girls than in boys. Although it is often associated with cleft lip, the two anomalies are not always simultaneously present. Cleft palate is more serious than cleft lip. It interferes more with the infant's feeding and breathing and is far more difficult to repair.

The fissure may involve only the soft palate or may extend into the nose and also the hard palate. The cleft is in the midline of the soft palate and on one or both sides of the hard palate, and of course is longitudinal. The cleft forms a passage way between the nasopharynx and the nose. It is this passage way that causes part of the difficulty in feeding and is a factor in susceptibility to infection. Even if it is not accompanied by cleft lip, cleft palate is an obvious defect.

Since the infant is unable to suck (even when he is fed with a medicine dropper, part of the feeding may be expelled through the nose), it may be necessary to give him his formula by gavage.

If the cleft is not repaired before the child learns to talk, and if a dental speech appliance is not used, the gutteral tone produced by the deformity may become habitual and persist after repair of the cleft has made normal speech possible.

**Instructions to the Mother on Discharge of the Infant from the Nursery.** As with the infant with cleft lip, the parents of a child with cleft palate are apt either to overprotect him or emotionally reject him. While he is still in the nursery the mother should be taught how to care for him, and the infant should become accustomed to her feeding him.

The *nutritional problem* is immediate. An adequate fluid intake is necessary to prevent dehydration. The mother should be taught how to feed the infant with a rubber-tipped medicine dropper or a softened rubber nipple with a hole large enough to permit the milk to drop into the infant's mouth without suction. The infant should be held in an upright position in order to facilitate swallowing the feeding with-

out regurgitation through the nose or without aspirating it. He should be bubbled frequently. It may be necessary to gavage him. Later on, perhaps when he is several months old, he may be fed with a spoon or may learn to take his milk from a cup.

The infant's mouth is easily infected. Until he is old enough to cooperate, his arms must be restrained to prevent his sucking his fingers or otherwise irritating the cleft. Such restraints will become habitual to him, and he will not be disturbed by the arm restraints required postoperatively. Unless his condition is accompanied by cleft lip, elbow restraint is sufficient, even postoperatively, and his hands need not be tied. The mouth should be kept clean at all times, and for this purpose the physician may order a mild antiseptic. Feedings should be followed by a little water to rinse out the mouth.

Unless these infants are under the care of a private physician, it is essential that they report to a cleft palate clinic or a pediatric clinic at regular intervals in order to determine the proper time for operation. Repair may be attempted when the infant is as young as eighteen months or two years old, or may be postponed until he is five years old. The optimum time for operation depends upon the condition of the individual child. When operation is delayed, the surgeon may use to advantage the normal structural changes which take place in the palate during growth in the preschool years. On the other hand, if correction of the defect is not made before the child has learned to talk, he may retain his gutteral speech.

For the care of a toddler undergoing cleft palate repair, see page 463.

### CIRCULATORY SYSTEM

**Review of the Changes Occurring in the Circulatory System at Birth.** With the severing of the umbilical cord there is increased pressure from the incoming blood in the left side of the heart. This eventually causes the foramen ovale to close. In fetal life much of the pulmonary arterial blood passed through the ductus arteriosus to the aorta. At birth the muscles in the wall of the ductus arteriosus constrict, although complete closure may not occur until the second or third month of life. The heart has less work after than before birth, since placental circulation has been replaced by that of extrauterine life. In the normal newborn the pulse rate is variable, but at birth will probably be 150 to 180 beats per minute, dropping within the hour to 130 to 140. With varying degrees of activity of the infant it may normally range from 80 to 180 beats a minute. The blood pressure at birth, determined by auscultation, may be 80/46 mm. of mercury and at one day of age 85/40.

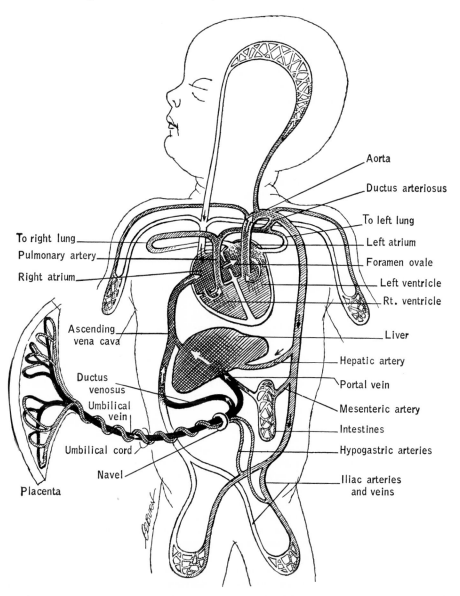

**Figure 70.** Diagrammatic illustration of fetal circulation. The degree of oxygen saturation is indicated by the blackness of the vessels.

## CONGENITAL HEART DISEASE

**Etiology, Diagnosis and Types of Cardiac Defects.** The heart is completely developed in the first eight weeks of intrauterine life. One or several anomalies may result from maldevelopment of the heart or great blood vessels leading to and from the heart with the result that the infant is born with congenital heart disease. Such defects may be hereditary, e.g. those caused by defects inherent in the genes or germ plasm. They may be caused by vitamin deficiency or viral infection such as rubella, or German measles, occurring during the first trimester of pregnancy. Anomalies of the bones, especially of the spine, may affect the development of the blood vessels in the embryo. Fetal intracardiac disease is possible. After birth there may be failure of obliteration of the ductus arteriosus or foramen ovale.

The *diagnosis* is made on the health history of the mother during pregnancy and on the characteristics of congenital heart disease in the infant. The signs and symptoms of congenital heart disease include abnormal murmurs, varying degrees of cyanosis and dyspnea, a generalized poor development and clubbing of the fingers and toes. The infant is weak and often irritable.

The diagnosis is confirmed when fluoroscopic examination shows divergence of the heart from its normal position and contour. Such an examination repeated at intervals of several months may reflect continued changes in the structure of the heart which occur as the infant's body develops. Examination with barium given by mouth may show indentation of the esophagus by the aorta and other vessels. *Aortography* is done by injecting radiopaque material into the left brachial artery so that any abnormal condition in the area about the branching of the left subclavian artery from the aorta can be seen. Such defects as coarctation (stenosis of the lumen) of the aorta or patent ductus arteriosus may be revealed. For *angiocardiography* the child is usually anesthetized, and radiopaque material is injected into the veins; its course through the heart chambers appears on a succession of x-ray pictures taken at rapid intervals. Abnormal communications between the chambers of the heart are also evident. By *electrocardiography* variations in the normal electrical potentials of the different parts of the heart can be noted. The electrocardiogram shows the condition of the muscular structure of the heart.

*Cardiac catheterization* is done under either general or local anesthesia. If local anesthesia is used, the infant should be under heavy sedation. The physician who catheterizes the heart must be supported by a well trained team of assistants accustomed to working with him. A small radiopaque catheter is inserted into a large vein of the arm or leg and pushed into the right atrium. With the tip of the catheter the physician can examine the heart minutely for anomalies of structure, often found in the right ventricle and the pulmonary artery. He is able to determine the blood pressure within the heart itself, and samples of blood can be taken to determine the exact degree of oxygenation.

Congenital defects in the structure of the heart may be classified in two groups: (1) *acyanotic* heart disease, in which the infant is not cyanotic, and (2) *cyanotic* heart disease, in which the infant shows varying degrees of cyanosis.

**General Treatment and Nursing Care.** For some years operation has been performed on the *outside* of the heart, but today operation is also performed on the *open heart*. Techniques developed to permit open-heart surgery include the following:

1. *Hypothermia.* In hypothermia the body temperature is lowered so that the metabolic rate is reduced. Reduction of the metabolic rate decreases the need for oxygen in the tissues of the body and so lessens the danger of anoxia.

2. *Heart-Lung Machine.* The heart-lung machine is interposed in the circulation, allowing blood flow to bypass the heart and lungs. Gaseous exchange occurs within the apparatus, and the

oxygenated blood is returned to the large arteries for systemic distribution. Since the machine carries on the functions of the heart and lungs, the surgeon is now able to open the bloodless heart and repair the defective structures.

*Preoperative Care.* The child should be admitted to the hospital several days before operation. Diagnostic tests are made during this time (see p. 204). Both the child and his parents need emotional preparation for these tests and for the operation which the child is to undergo. They regard surgery with an ambivalent attitude: of exaggerated fear because of the relative newness of heart surgery and of hope for the child's recovery. Parents should be told what to expect in the postoperative period, i.e. the use of chest tubes, oxygen and drug therapy, aspiration and other procedures, in terms of the specific operation to be performed.

If the child is old enough to understand (the child under two cannot understand), the purpose of the oxygen tent should be explained to him, and at any age he should be placed in the tent before operation in order to accustom him to the experience.

During the days before operation the nurse should observe the child closely for any sign of an upper respiratory tract infection, and he should be isolated from all possible sources of such infection.

Fluids are given as ordered by the physician.

*Postoperative Care.* After operation the child requires constant nursing care; a nurse who has had experience in heart surgery of children should be with him at all times, since his condition may suddenly worsen and remedial measures must be given at once. The nurse should observe his color and watch for evidence of restlessness and rapid respiration. The vital signs should be taken as ordered by the physician— pulse, respiration and blood pressure are usually determined at intervals of fifteen minutes to one hour. All these signs indicate how the lungs and heart are functioning and whether there is a hidden hemorrhage. Cyanosis indicates an immediate need for treatment; the physician should be notified at once. The temperature is taken frequently, since fever brings a strain upon the heart, and subnormal temperature in conjunction with other symptoms may indicate that the child is on the verge of shock.

The child should be placed on his back or right side, and his position should be changed frequently. He should not be allowed to change his position without help, since the exertion would be harmful. With the surgeon's approval he may be placed in a semisitting position.

The child should be encouraged to breathe deeply and to cough in order to aerate his lungs properly. The nasopharynx should be aspirated when necessary to maintain an open airway. The surgeon may aspirate the lower respiratory tract.

Oxygen is given by tent to infants and young children. Water-seal chest drainage to evacuate fluid from the chest may be used in some cases. The surgeon places a catheter in the lower part of the chest through a stab wound; the distal end of the extension on the catheter is placed under a fluid level. Excess air and fluid can drain from the pleural space, but nothing—neither fluid nor air—can re-enter the chest cavity. The drainage bottle must be fastened securely at the side of the bed. A clamp must be kept in readiness to close off the tube near the chest wall in case the tubing becomes disconnected or the suction bottle is moved. The nurse must observe the drainage bottle for excessive drainage of blood. If no drainage occurs, the nurse must report this finding promptly, because fluid may be accumulating in the thorax with resulting cardiac embarrassment.

Gastrointestinal suction may be necessary to relieve postoperative distention. Accurate intake and output records on all such patients are important. Intravenous therapy may be necessary after operation.

The diet is gradually increased from fluid to soft and then to solid as ordered by the physician. Antibiotics are routinely given postoperatively to prevent or counteract possible infection.

Convalescence is usually rapid. The child is allowed to lead as normal a life as is compatible with his condition. Unnecessary restriction causes psychologic trauma. Children soon learn how much exercise they can tolerate and tend to stay within their capacity; those in the younger age group do not continue activity which causes discomfort. A well balanced diet with additional vitamins and iron is given.

### ACYANOTIC TYPES OF CONGENITAL HEART DISEASE

In acyanotic congenital heart disease either there is no abnormal communica-tion between the pulmonary and systemic circulations or, if such a connection is present, the pressure forces the blood from the arterial side to the venous side. The peripheral blood is therefore oxygenated as in a normal infant, and cyanosis does not result. If the anomaly is such that venous blood eventually mixes with arterial blood when the heart weakens, cyanosis may result.

### Coarctation of the Aorta

**Types, Clinical Manifestations and Diag-nosis.** There are two types of coarcta-tion. In the *infantile* or *preductal* type there is a constriction between the sub-clavian artery and the ductus (see Fig. 71). This condition results in death.

Figure 71. Coarctation of the aorta. *A*, Preductal coarctation of the aorta with the ductus arteriosus, open or closed. *B*, Postduc-tal coarctation of the aorta with the ductus arteriosus closed. *C*, Longer areas of constriction, where anasto-mosis of aortic segments is not feasible, require the use of a graft to bridge the gap. (From Diagnosis of Con-genital Cardiac Defects in General Practice. Heart As-sociation of Southeastern Pennsylvania and Ameri-can Heart Association.)

The *postductal* type consists of a constriction at or distal to the ductus arteriosus. The symptoms in this type depend upon the degree of coarctation. Blood pressure is higher than normal in the upper part of the body with the result that epistaxis occurs. The older child complains of headache and dizziness, and may later have cerebrovascular accidents. Blood pressure in the legs is relatively low. The femoral pulse cannot be felt, and there is numbness of the legs.

The *diagnosis* is based on the reversal of normal blood pressure relations in the arms and legs and is confirmed by x-ray study. In older children the roentgenogram may show enlargement of the heart which was not evident during routine examination of the newborn, together with notching of the ribs due to enlarged collateral vessels. An aortogram may reveal the narrowed segment.

**Treatment and Prognosis.** Surgical repair consists in cutting out the narrowed portion of the aorta, with anastomoses of the ends. In some cases a graft of transplanted aorta is inserted where the narrowing is so extensive that removal with anastomosis is not practical.

If the infant's condition is such that the physician believes that he can live until he has reached the preferred age for surgical correction, operation is postponed until the child is from eight to twelve years old. Operation should be performed in preadolescence rather than during early childhood because the segment used as a graft will not grow as does the aorta. The shorter the time after operation before maximum growth of the child is reached, the less is the danger from difference in the rate of growth between the graft and the main structure of the aorta.

The *prognosis* is excellent if operation is successful; if not, cardiac failure may intervene.

### Patent Ductus Arteriosus

**Etiology, Incidence and Clinical Manifestations.** The ductus arteriosus (see Fig. 72) normally closes shortly after birth.

If the ductus remains open, blood u pressure from the aorta is shunted into the pulmonary artery, since the blood pressure in that vessel is less than in the systemic circulation. As a result, a small amount of oxygenated blood recirculates through the pulmonary circulation. This leads to increased vascular pressure in the pulmonary tree and diminished blood flow in the aorta.

Patent ductus arteriosus is one of the most common cardiac anomalies. It is frequently the only anomaly of the heart structure, but may occur in conjunction with other cardiac defects. It is almost twice as frequent in female infants as in male ones.

The *symptoms* of patent ductus arteriosus in the infant are usually so slight that the condition is not discovered at the initial examination, but is found during a routine examination when the child is brought for a check-up to a private physician or a clinic. As the child grows older and is more active, the characteristic symptoms appear. He is likely to show progressively greater dyspnea on exertion. Examination may reveal a malfunctioning left ventricle or congestive heart failure. Progression of the lesion is due to the strain upon the heart of pumping blood which passes a second time through the pulmonary circulation while at the same time supplying adequate systemic circulation for an active infant or child. It is easy to prevent overexertion in an infant, but far more difficult to limit the activities of a growing child without overprotecting him and building up the very qualities which may make for a handicapped child disliked by his playmates.

If the ductus is large and much blood from the aorta is shunted into the pulmonary circulation, there may be retardation in growth.

Physical signs include increased pulse pressure, sometimes felt when taking the radial pulse. Pulsations are of the water-hammer type. A cardiac thrill in the second left interspace is usually present; this may radiate over a larger area of the chest. There is the classic *machinery murmur*, continuous from systole into diastole. The electrocardio-

**Figure 72.** Patent ductus arteriosus. *A,* Relation of ductus arteriosus to great vessels. *B,* Ductus arteriosus transected (as shown here) or ligated. (From Diagnosis of Congenital Cardiac Defects in General Practice. Heart Association of Southeastern Pennsylvania and American Heart Association.)

gram usually shows no abnormality, but roentgenograms show a vigorously pulsating pulmonary artery and increased pulmonary vascularity. The heart may be normal in size, but is more likely to be enlarged.

**Diagnosis, Treatment and Prognosis.** The *diagnosis* is made on the clinical symptoms and signs of a machinery murmur of the heart and a low diastolic blood pressure. Cardiac catheterization (see p. 204) shows a normal or increased pressure, roentgenograms show the shadow of the pulmonary artery to be larger than is normal, and angiocardiography shows the ductus arteriosus.

The *treatment* is surgical, by division and ligation of the ductus, preferably when the child is from four to ten years of age. After the repair the heart becomes normal in size, murmurs disappear, and there is a general improvement in the child's condition.

With modern cardiac surgery done by a skilled specialist, the *prognosis* is excellent. The surgical mortality rate in the uncomplicated condition during childhood is only 1 or 2 per cent. Without repair subacute bacterial endocarditis or cardiac failure may develop as the child leads the less sheltered and more strenuous life of the school-age group.

### Dextrocardia

In this condition the heart is in the right side of the chest. This may occur with or without reversal of the position of the other organs. Although the heart may be normal, associated anomalies often complicate the condition. If no other anomalies are present, no treatment is necessary, and the prognosis is excellent.

### Double Aortic Arch

Infants and children with this defect may have respiratory symptoms or dysphagia, or both. These symptoms, beginning in the first year of life, arise from compression by the branches of the aorta on the trachea or esophagus, or both. This is due to the persistence of embryologic vascular precursors of the aorta and stem branches. The infant, in an effort to find relief, will hold his head in an extended position. The diagnosis is made on x-ray examination, which shows constriction of the esophagus by the aorta. Constriction or deviation of the trachea can also be seen. The treatment is surgical, and the prognosis is excellent.

### Interatrial Septal Defect

This is one of the more common congenital anomalies. The incidence is higher among girls than among boys. In this condition there is a communication between the left and right atria. Since oxygenated blood in the left atrium is under higher pressure, it is forced through the defect in the separating wall into the right atrium. Such an arterial-venous shunt does not produce cyanosis. Terminally, however, or with heart failure, if a reversal of flow occurs, then cyanosis may become evident.

The *diagnosis* is made on the basis of the roentgenogram and the electrocardiogram. The heart is enlarged, and there is congestion of the pulmonary circulation. On auscultation a loud murmur is heard in the area of the pulmonary artery.

The *treatment* is surgical repair of the defect. The edges of the opening are pulled together and sutured, or the opening is occluded by a plastic patch placed over the aperture. As this operation is perfected it is becoming increasingly successful. Without operation the life expectancy is only thirty-five years. Subacute bacterial endocarditis may develop at the site of the defect.

### Interventricular Septal Defect

This anomaly consists of an opening between the right and left ventricles. The condition may be slight or severe.

In the *mild form* the defect is so slight that only a small amount of oxygenated blood passes from the left to the right ventricle. It is a common congenital defect. The heart is seldom enlarged, and the only clinical finding is a murmur accompanying the heart beat. The treatment is by surgical closure of the opening, a procedure which is being developed at many research centers. The prognosis at present is not as good as could be desired, but will probably be far better in the futr Subacute bacterial endocarditis may develop at the site.

In the *severe form* there is a large opening in the septum, and oxygenated blood in greater amount passes from the left to the right ventricle. The result may be pulmonary hypertension. The symptoms include cardiac failure, a tendency to pneumonia and retarded growth. The diagnosis is made from the roentgenogram and the electrocardiogram. The treatment is by surgical closure of the defect. The heart is opened, and the edges of the septal opening are drawn together, or a plastic patch is placed over the opening. This type of operation involves the use of a cardiac bypass by means of the heart-lung machine. Without operation death is probable early in life.

### Aortic Valvular Stenosis and Pulmonic Stenosis

Although these constrictions may exist in newborn infants, symptoms may not be present for several years. Cardiac failure may occur, and the prognosis is generally poor. Treatment is surgical, by valvulotomy or mechanical dilatation of the passage through which blood must pass from the heart into the respective vessels.

#### CYANOTIC TYPES OF CONGENITAL HEART DISEASE

The common cause of the congenital cyanotic types of heart disease is a communication between the pulmonary and systemic circulations through which venous (unoxygenated) blood enters the systemic circulatory system. Cyanosis may be seen at birth or may not be apparent until later, commonly during the first year of life; it tends to increase as the child grows older.

*Polycythemia* (an increase in the number of red blood cells per milliliter of blood) results from the need of the tissues of the body for an adequate supply of oxygen. The symptoms vary in degree with the extent and nature of the anomaly. In general, there is clubbing of the fingers and toes, retarded growth and shortness of breath on exertion. If the blood, thickened by an abnormal concentration of red blood cells, clots in the blood vessels, further complications result.

### Tetralogy of Fallot

**Incidence and Pathology.** This is the most common type of cyanotic congenital heart disease which is compatible with continued existence into childhood. Pathologically, there are four associated anomalies: (1) funnel-like or valvular pulmonic stenosis, (2) interventricular septal defect, (3) dextroposition of the aorta, and (4) hypertrophy of the right ventricle.

Pulmonary stenosis restricts the flow of blood from the heart to the lungs for oxygenation. In addition, the hypertrophied right ventricle creates a venous-arterial shunt through the septal defect. Further, the aorta, straddling the defect, is the recipient of venous blood from the right ventricle and the venous-arterial mixture in the left ventricle. Since cyanosis is dependent upon the absolute concentration of reduced hemoglobin in the capillary circulation, it is evident that in the systemic circulation, containing a rich admixture of venous blood from the start, this value is almost invariably surpassed, and cyanosis is thus clinically manifest.

**Clinical Manifestations and Diagnosis.** The arterial blood is not normally saturated with oxygen, and as a result the skin is not the natural pink, but is instead of a bluish tint. The fingers and toes become clubbed and have a purplish hue, since the capillaries are distended with poorly oxygenated blood. The condition worsens during even the first year of life. The body's reaction to the inadequate supply of oxygen is an increased production of red blood cells (polycythemia).

The child's general condition is poor. His growth is retarded; exercise causes severe dyspnea. In order to relieve the strain of standing, he favors the *squatting position*. This behavior has diagnostic value. Although he may be of

**Figure 73.** Tetralogy of Fallot. Anomalies include (*1*) overriding aorta, (*2*) high ventricular septal defect, (*3a*) valvular pulmonary stenosis and (*3b*) infundibular pulmonary stenosis, and (*4*) hypertrophy of right ventricle. (From Diagnosis of Congenital Cardiac Defects in General Practice. Heart Association of Southeastern Pennsylvania and American Heart Association.)

normal intelligence, the poor supply of oxygen to the brain is likely to produce mental retardation, syncope or convulsions. The child is apt to be emotionally unstable, irritable and overdependent upon others. His parents, concerned over his physical condition, are likely to avoid discipline to prevent frustration, since they do not want him to become excited or cry. The result is that control, which would have been to his advantage, is not established. The child, on his part, attempts to avoid all exertion by being overdependent on others to meet all his wants. He realizes that if he cries, he will get his way and so is apt to become the typical spoiled child.

The *diagnosis*, based on the symptoms, is confirmed by fluoroscopic examination of the heart, which shows the enlarged chamber on the right side, the decrease in size of the pulmonary artery and reduced blood flow through the lungs. The unusual shape of the heart has led to its being called the wooden shoe or *boot-shaped heart*. The child should be allowed to handle the fluoroscope and x-ray machines before examination so that the procedures will be less frightening to him. If he is to take barium, the addition of chocolate to the mixture may make it look and taste like the chocolate milk to which he is accustomed. Laboratory findings show the decreased oxygen saturation of the blood, and exercise tolerance tests prove the child's tendency to extreme dyspnea.

**Instructions to the Mother.** On the mother rests the responsibility for giving the child good care until the time when operation is to be performed. Both physical and mental hygiene must be considered. Provision for normal growth and development is essential, but requires constant use of good judgment so that the child is neither overprotected nor allowed an independence in which he overtaxes his weakened heart. This program is easy to carry out while the infant is still so young that he accepts his mother's plan for all his activities of daily living.

During this period the infant becomes accustomed to limitation of activities without overdependence on others. He also learns to trust others to give him the help he needs. He should not be constantly checked in his activities, yet until he is old enough to understand the limits beyond which he should not go he should be kept from situations in which he is likely to overexert. Overfatigue should be avoided, and certainly he should never be urged to exertion beyond his tolerance. It may be difficult for the entire family and those adults he contacts outside the family circle to carry out such a regimen with a young child whose handicap is not visible, but it is in this period that the foundation for a strong, happy personality is made.

The child should never acquire the feeling of undue importance which is apt to develop in one who feels that his heart condition makes him a very special child who must always have his own way and be given first consideration. The influence upon the other children in the family must be considered. Although his needs may be more important than their pleasures, his pleas-

ure is not to be gained at the expense of their constant inconvenience. He should lead as normal a life as is compatible with his welfare, but learn to accept frustration and the inevitable restrictions which his condition imposes on his activity and social relations. He cannot do all that other children do.

The physician will discuss with the parents the influence of cyanosis upon the child's intelligence. If he is retarded, the parents are apt to attribute the retardation entirely to his physical condition, forgetting that low intelligence may be due to a number of factors. For him to lead as normal a life as is compatible with his condition is the best way to realize to the full his potential mental capacity. The experiences which develop the normal child, but in which he cannot participate, should be replaced by experiences of comparable learning value. His toys should be light and easily handled. He should learn that a ball rolls, though he may not be able to creep after it for any length of time. He may not creep up a flight of stairs, but he can go up one or two steps. He should be carried about more than the average child is and should be allowed to handle everything within the nursery. Picture books are valuable. He can pat-a-cake to slow music. Overexcitement is as taxing for him as overactivity. As he grows older he must learn not to compete in games requiring agility and strength. In fact, as a rule, competitive games are too exciting for these children. Even the very little child can learn that fun does not necessarily come through getting ahead of someone else.

If the mother proves her ability to give good care and to observe signs of a worsening in his condition, he may not need frequent visits to the physician. But if she is unable to judge his condition and to give him the care he requires, he should be seen regularly by the family physician or pediatrician. If he has been referred from the hospital to the children's clinic, he should be under the observation of the pediatrician there and should be visited by the public health nurse. He should be

**Figure 74.** Tetralogy of Fallot. *A*, Volume of blood to lungs increased by joining right subclavian to right pulmonary artery (end-to-side anastomosis—Blalock procedure). *B*, Volume of blood to lungs increased by creating stoma between left pulmonary artery and aorta (side-to-side anastomosis — Potts procedure). (From Diagnosis of Congenital Cardiac Defects in General Practice. Heart Association of Southeastern Pennsylvania and American Heart Association.)

seen by his physician before even minor surgery is done. The danger is not only from the anesthetic—often minor surgery would not require the use of an anesthetic—but also from the possibility of infection. Prophylactic antibiotic medication may be indicated.

**Treatment and Prognosis.** The treatment is surgical, and may be corrective or merely palliative. Without operation the life expectancy of the child is not more than twenty years. Operation is postponed as a rule until the child is three years of age or even older, but if his condition is critical, operation may be done upon the infant.

*Palliative* surgery does not correct the original deformity. An artificial ductus is made which connects the systemic circulation with the pulmonary artery. This allows for greater blood flow to the lungs, which in turn results in increased oxygenation of the blood in the left side of the heart and ultimately in the systemic circulation. In the Blalock-Taussig operation an anastomosis is made between the subclavian artery and the pulmonary artery. In the Potts operation a side-to-side anastomosis of the pulmonary artery and the aorta is made.

*Corrective* surgery is undertaken only by the most skillful surgeons. The heart must be stopped and exposed to direct vision. A pump oxygenator provides for both the circulation of the blood and its saturation with oxygen (see p. 566). The ventricular septal defect is closed and the pulmonary stenosis relieved. The risk to life is greater than in palliative surgery. There is an increasing number of research centers in which personnel are receiving training and experience in intricate cardiac surgery. In the future the operative risk will doubtless be less than it is today. As the risk decreases, the trend will be toward open-heart surgery.

Preoperative cardiac failure may be relieved by digitalis, diuretics, oxygen and complete bed rest.

The nursing care of a preschool child undergoing surgical correction is discussed on page 564.

### Eisenmenger Complex

**Clinical Manifestations, Treatment and Prognosis.** This condition is similar to the tetralogy of Fallot, though pulmonary hypertension with a reverse shunt is also present. No pulmonary stenosis exists. Dyspnea develops early in life. There is a systolic murmur, and also cyanosis which increases in late childhood. Surgery cannot relieve the defect. The child's activities must be restricted and cardiac failure be treated if it occurs.

### Pulmonic Stenosis with Patent Foramen Ovale

In this condition venous blood from the right atrium is shunted to the left atrium with resulting cyanosis. Clinically the condition is like the tetralogy of Fallot, but the cyanosis is not as severe. Treatment is by surgical valvulotomy of the stenosed pulmonary valve and closure of the septal defect. The prognosis after repair is good.

There are various other cardiac anomalies which are not compatible with life. No surgical procedure or treatment has been found which will bring relief to these children.

#### SUMMARY OF NURSING CARE IN CONGENITAL HEART DISEASE

The nursing care of infants and children with congenital anomalies of the heart and circulatory system is extremely important and has become a specialty in nursing which is attracting many graduate nurses. What is done for the child is, of course, dependent upon the treatment outlined by the physician and involves difficult procedures or nursing skills. The reason why the nursing care of these patients is called a special branch of pediatric nursing is that the nurse must be thoroughly familiar with the signs and symptoms of each condition. She must know what complications are likely to occur and must recognize the signs of impending danger so that she may notify the physician or carry out his standing orders.

The nurse should become familiar with the parents' reaction to being told that their child has a congenital cardiac condition, and she should learn how to reassure them without minimizing the danger of the defective heart. She should teach the parents how to care for the child in the interval between his leaving the newborn nursery and his re-entrance into the hospital for operation. What has been said about the care of the child with the tetralogy of Fallot may also be applied to other types of congenital heart disease.

### CENTRAL NERVOUS SYSTEM

#### Spina Bifida

**Incidence and Types.** Spina bifida is a malformation of the spine in which the posterior portion of the laminae of the vertebrae fails to close. Although it may occur in almost any area of the spine, it is most common in the lumbosacral region. It is the most common developmental defect of the central nervous system, occurring in about one out of 1000 newborn infants.

Three types are discussed: (1) spina bifida occulta, in which the spinal cord and meninges are normal, the defect being only of the vertebrae; (2) meningocele, in which the meninges protrude through the opening in the spinal canal; and (3) meningomyelocele, in which both the spinal cord and the meninges protrude through the defect in the bony rings of the spinal canal. Meningomyelocele is the most serious type.

#### Spina Bifida Occulta

**Clinical Manifestations, Diagnosis and Treatment.** The majority of patients have no symptoms. Some may have a dimple in the skin or a growth of hair over the malformed vertebra. If the condition is suspected from these signs or upon physical examination, a roentgenogram of the area will rule out or confirm the diagnosis. There is no need for treatment unless neurologic symptoms indicate that the defect is greater than was thought. If there is a possibility that the spinal cord may be involved in the defect, surgical treatment is indicated.

#### Meningocele

**Clinical Manifestations, Diagnosis, Treatment and Prognosis.** On examination the newborn infant is found to have a defect in the spinal column large enough for the meninges to protrude through

SPINA BIFIDA WITH CENTRAL CICATRIX

SPINA BIFIDA OCCULTA

MENINGOCELE

MENINGO-MYELOCELE

**Figure 75.** Diagrammatic representation of types of spina bifida, meningocele and meningo-myelocele, (Copyright, The Ciba Collection of Medical Illustrations, by Frank H. Netter, M.D.)

the opening. The defect is usually in the center line. There is generally no evidence of weakness of the legs, for the infant stretches and kicks in a normal manner, or of lack of sphincter control, although this is difficult to ascertain in the newborn.

The *prognosis* is excellent. Surgical correction is done on these defects. Hydrocephalus may be an associated finding or may be aggravated after operation for a meningocele.

### Meningomyelocele

**Clinical Manifestations, Diagnosis, Treatment and Prognosis.** In this condition an imperfectly developed segment of the spinal cord, as well as the meninges, protrudes through the spina bifida. The round, fluctuating bulge resembles that of the meningocele and is usually located in the lumbosacral region. There may be a minimal weakness to a com-

plete flaccid paralysis of the legs and absence of sensation in the feet. The feet may be clubbed. Bowel and bladder functioning require careful evaluation.

The objectives of *treatment* and nursing care are to prevent infection of the sac and to help restore function orthopedically and urologically.

Operation removes a cosmetically unacceptable deformity, prevents infection and in many instances improves the neurologic deficit, since traction is removed from the nerve pathways. Therapy may further improve function as the nervous system matures. If hydrocephalus is progressive, operation will be necessary.

Usually clinically silent, the *Arnold-Chiari syndrome* is a congenital malformation of the occipitocervical region, with displacement of the cerebellar tonsils and adjacent structures into a funnel-shaped enlargement of the upper cervical canal and swelling and displacement of the medulla against the upper portion of the spinal cord. The defect originates between the sixteenth and twentieth weeks of fetal life. This syndrome may occur in cases of lumbosacral spina bifida with meningomyelocele. The medulla and part of the cerebellum are pulled into the foramen magnum because the cord is attached at the site of the defect in the spine. The result may be an acute obstruction to the flow of cerebrospinal fluid, and hence hydrocephalus may follow repair of a meningomyelocele.

The symptoms are the result of complete or partial block of the flow of cerebrospinal fluid. In infants clinical manifestations include a running nose (sometimes confused with an upper respiratory tract infection) and crowing respirations. The nurse must observe these manifestations because immediate relief of pressure is indicated. In older children manifestations include stiff neck, headache and dizziness. When the child is old enough to walk or talk, his gait is unsteady and his speech impaired.

Surgery is the only known treatment for the Arnold-Chiari syndrome.

## Nursing Care in Meningocele and Meningomyelocele

**Preoperative Nursing Care.** Preoperative nursing care is that of a normal infant so far as it can be given while protecting the sac from pressure, injury or infection. To decrease the danger of infection of the area from urine and feces, the genitals and buttocks must be kept scrupulously clean. If the covering of the sac is infected or thin, some physicians order Varidase solution to drip on the area. The infant is placed in bed, and a meningocele apron is applied (see Fig. 76). It is customary in some hospitals to place the infant on a Bradford frame with the cover divided so that urine and stool may pass between the sections of the frame and the infant can easily be kept clean and dry.

*Use of a Bradford Frame.* The frame is covered as follows:

Canvas covers the head and foot areas of the frame, and foam rubber is placed between the covers. The open area between the covered head and foot sections of the frame is provided for the purpose of drainage of urine and feces away from the body. The covers are stretched tightly over the frame to prevent sagging from the weight of the infant's body. Plastic covers

**Figure 76.** Meningomyelocele. The meningocele apron is in place, and Varidase solution drips slowly onto the sac. (Courtesy of Dr. Eugene B. Spitz.)

are placed over the top and bottom sections of the divided canvas frame cover. A sheet is put tightly over each section of the frame. The frame is then placed on blocks to elevate it slightly from the bed.

Since the infant is incontinent, sheets of plastic are draped over the top and bottom edges of the opening in the frame cover to permit urine and feces to drain into a bedpan placed below the opening. Folded diapers are placed over the plastic and under the infant so that the plastic does not irritate the skin.

The buttocks and perineum must be washed frequently to protect the skin from irritation. The infant should never be diapered. Fixation in the correct position is important. Ankle restraints, using a clove hitch restraint, are applied. The child is not to be placed on his back, since such a position would cause pressure on the sac. If the surgeon permits, the child should be supported in the side position with a rolled blanket or pillow placed behind the head and the buttocks. The pillow or blanket behind the buttocks must be protected from fecal staining by a plastic cover. If the infant is unable to move his legs, foam rubber pads covered with soft cloth may be placed between the legs to prevent pressure on the skin of the knees and ankles. The infant's position should be checked at least every hour.

To prevent deformity of the feet, when the infant is placed on his abdomen, the ankles should be supported with foam rubber pads so that the toes do not rest upon the bed. To prevent injury from rubbing the skin of the elbows, face and knees, a mild ointment such as A & D ointment or zinc oxide may be used. To prevent chafing of the knees, ankles, toes and sides of the heels, should the infant move his legs back and forth on the sheet, it is a good plan to use long stockings, but since he has no diaper to which they may be pinned, it is difficult to keep them on his legs.

To change the frame covers or bed, the child may be placed on his abdomen or side in a baby carriage. If the physician permits, the nurse, aide or mother during visiting hours may hold the child to prevent complications arising from constant lying on the frame.

Antibiotics may be used if infection is suspected.

In addition to the danger of the sac becoming infected, the bladder of an infant having a meningomyelocele may also become infected. According to the urologist's evaluation the infant's bladder may need to be credéd if the sphincter is tight and urine is retained. The nurse in the hospital or the mother when the child is at home is responsible for emptying the infant's bladder every two hours during the day and once at night. Pressure should be applied firmly but gently, beginning in the umbilical area and slowly progressing under the symphysis pubis and toward the anus. The mother should be helped to learn this procedure as early as possible. She should practice under supervision until she feels secure. As the child grows, his urine may be expressed less frequently. By the time a child is seven to ten years of age he should be able to assume the responsibility for doing this procedure himself.

The infant may be transferred directly from the nursery to the pediatric unit. If he is taken home before his readmission to the hospital for operation, his parents will care for him. The father can make a substitute for the Bradford frame, and the mother can cover it as described above. She can carry out the essential features of nursing care and will have more time to hold the infant than do hospital personnel. Both parents should be shown how to hold him without causing pressure upon the sac.

The infant should be held for his feedings, if the physician permits, in order to have the feeling of being loved and secure, the benefit any infant receives from being held while feeding. He can be held on the shoulder, his mother's or the nurse's hands supporting him above and below the sac, while a second person, standing behind her, holds the bottle to his mouth. He cannot be bubbled like the normal infant, but the feeding should be stopped and the nipple withdrawn from his mouth several times during the feeding so that he may rest and air be expelled. If the lesion is in the lumbosacral area, he may be gently rubbed between the shoulders; this has a soothing effect and may aid in expulsion of air. These infants can also be fed lying on the side in the nurse's or mother's lap.

Contamination of the sac can be prevented by covering it with sterile gauze or a sterile towel when the infant is removed from bed.

If the physician believes that the infant should not be removed from the frame or bed for feeding, the restraints may be loosened and the infant turned slightly on the side. The nurse or mother should elevate his head slightly with her hand when feeding him.

One of the most essential functions of the nurse in the care of these infants is observation and accurate reporting of their behavior, as well as of signs and symptoms directly connected with their condition. She should record activity of the legs and the degree of continence, noting whether there is retention of urine or fecal impaction. All the vital signs should be taken and recorded with extreme care.

**Postoperative Nursing Care.** The goal of surgical treatment is closure of the surface defect while preserving all functioning nervous tissue.

The nurse is responsible for observing and reporting all signs and symptoms of the infant's condition. Temperature, pulse and respiration must be taken frequently. Symptoms of shock must be anticipated and an incubator be in readiness for use. If an incubator is not available, a heat cradle may be placed over the infant. Since he may have respiratory difficulty, oxygen should be kept near his bed. Abdominal distention caused by paralytic ileus or distention of the bladder follows most spinal cord surgery and should be reported immediately.

The physician may request that the circumference of the infant's head be measured frequently in order to determine whether hydrocephalus follows repair of the meningomyelocele.

The surgical dressing should be kept clean and dry. The child may be placed in bed or on a Bradford frame with an oblong piece of plastic sheeting taped (Scotch tape or masking tape may be used) below the dressing to cover the buttocks and shield the dressing from feces (see Fig. 76).

If casts have been applied to the child's lower extremities, they should be positioned properly and handled carefully (see p. 237).

Nutrition is important. The infant should be fed in a prone position unless the physician orders otherwise. While the infant is being fed his head should be slightly elevated either with the nurse's hand or by elevating the top end of the frame. The nipple should be withdrawn several times during the feeding so as to allow the infant to rest and to facilitate expulsion of air. Gavage feeding may be necessary (see p. 150).

All the foregoing suggestions for postoperative care are subject, of course, to the physician's orders.

**Postoperative Habilitation.** Habilitation of the child is necessary after operation. Functional improvement of the lower extremities and bowel and bladder function will require a long time and diligent care. Habilitation emphasizes constructive use of the normal parts of the body and minimizes the disabilities, making the child as self-helpful as is possible in the activities of daily living. Although the child is to be taught activities which render him less dependent on others, he must also learn to accept help which normal children do not need. Development of a pleasant personality is of the utmost importance.

Incontinence after infancy creates social problems. The child may need frequent suppositories or a special diet to avoid constipation. If he can achieve regularity of stool, he will be more socially acceptable. Regularity of urination is of even more importance. Mechanical means for making pressure on the urethra may be employed to prevent incontinence. If he cannot urinate, his bladder will need to be emptied by the Credé method (i.e. pressed upon periodically to expel urine), as it was prior to operation. A distended bladder must be prevented, since it is more subject to infection. For all these reasons a schedule of toileting should be instituted. Follow-up care by a urologist is necessary.

Although his legs are paralyzed, the infant can be taken about in a stroller and later can learn to use a wheelchair and possibly to walk with braces and crutches.

Care must be taken to prevent malnutrition and secondary contractions or other deformities. If the child is normal mentally, he can become a socially useful member of society.

### Encephalocele

An encephalocele is a protrusion of brain substance through a congenital defect in the skull. It occurs through a failure of the bones of the fetal skull to unite in the normal manner. It is commonly found in the midline and in the occipital or parietal area, although it may also be found in the frontal bone, the orbit of the eye or in the nose.

**Clinical Manifestations, Diagnosis, Treatment, Prognosis and Nursing Care.** The *symptoms* depend upon the degree of involvement of the nervous tissue and upon the location of the defect. The diagnostic evidence is a sac or hernia into which the meninges, cerebrospinal fluid or cerebral tissue has entered. Roentgenograms show the defect in the skull. Early surgical repair is indicated.

The *prognosis* depends upon the extent and location of the encephalocele. If it ruptures, there is danger of meningitis.

The *nursing care* is that of a normal infant, plus relief of symptoms and extreme caution in handling the infant. It is essential that no pressure be brought upon the sac and that it be not injured in any way.

### Hydrocephalus

Hydrocephalus is due to inadequate absorption of cerebrospinal fluid, with a corresponding increase of fluid under some degree of pressure within the intracranial cavity, or to obstruction within the ventricular system. To understand this process it would be well to review the formation, flow and absorption of cerebrospinal fluid.

Cerebrospinal fluid is formed by the choroid plexus of the four ventricles

|            |            |
|:----------:|:----------:|
| *A*        | *B*        |

**Figure 77.**  Encephalocele. *A*, Profile view. *B*, Diagrammatic representation. (Copyright, The Ciba Collection of Medical Illustrations, by Frank H. Netter, M.D.)

and by filtration from capillaries. It passes from the lateral ventricles by way of the foramina of Monro into the third ventricle. From the third ventricle it flows through the aqueduct of Sylvius into the fourth ventricle, and then into the cisterna of the subarachnoid space by way of the foramina of Luschka and the foramen of Magendie. From there it passes under the base of the brain and up over the convexity into the cortical sulci until it is finally absorbed into the venous sinuses by way of the arachnoid villi. It flows along the tissue spaces of the sheaths of all the cranial and spinal nerves and is taken up by the vascular system. Normally the amount absorbed equals that secreted (see Fig. 78).

**Etiology.** The obstruction in the flow of cerebrospinal fluid may be due to one of several causes. There may be congenital defective development of the ventricular foramina, neoplasm may be present, or a fibrous residue of meningitis may occlude the reabsorptive surfaces. Hemorrhage from trauma may cause hydrocephalus in the young infant.

In infancy the accumulation of fluid in the ventricles generally enlarges the child's skull, since the sutures are not closed and the bones are soft and yielding under pressure. The cranial enlargement tends to decrease the pressure upon the brain.

**Treatment** of hydrocephalic infants should be started as soon as the clinical manifestations are observed, before damage to the brain itself occurs. Several shunting procedures are now in use: e.g. ventriculovenostomy, ventriculoperitoneostomy, ventriculoureterostomy and lumbar subarachnoid peritoneostomy. The **prognosis** is dependent to a great extent on the promptness of treatment and the kind of operation performed.

## Communicating Hydrocephalus

**Etiology.** In communicating hydrocephalus there is a normal communication between the ventricles and the subarachnoid space at the base of the brain. There may, however, be adhesions between the meninges at the base of the brain, meningeal hemorrhage or a congenital defect in the brain, which prevents the absorption of cerebrospinal fluid. Hydrocephalus may occur after a successful operation for meningocele.

**Clinical Manifestations, Diagnosis and Treatment.**    The obvious *symptom* is an increase in size of the infant's head because of excessive amounts of cerebrospinal fluid. The fluid which is not absorbed in the subarachnoid space accumulates, compressing the brain and distending the cranial cavity. The sutures fail to close, and the bones of the skull become thin.

There is an excess of spinal fluid outside the brain. The convolutions of the brain are flattened and atrophied. Usually, however, the pressure of the fluid does not enlarge the head as much as in noncommunicating hydrocephalus, because the brain atrophies and this increases the space which the fluid may fill without enlargement of the skull. The fontanels are tense and widened. The child tends to be irritable.

The *diagnosis* is confirmed by puncture of the fontanels, and ventriculography may be used.

The *treatment* is surgical. Sometimes spontaneously a balance may rarely occur in the young child between the secretion of fluid and its absorption. Operation, however, should be performed as early as possible to prevent damage to the brain. Since the difficulty is mostly mechanical, corrective measures are aimed at forming an outlet for the surplus fluid.

## Noncommunicating Hydrocephalus

**Etiology and Pathology.**    In noncommunicating hydrocephalus, which is more important than the communicating type, there is a block between the ventricular and subarachnoid systems. Such a block may be partial or complete. It may have begun in the latter months of intrauterine life. Mechanical causes

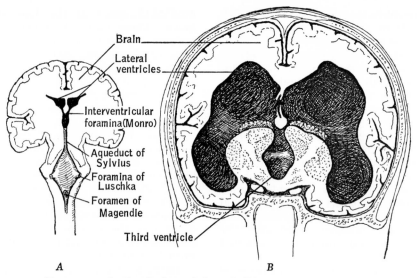

**Figure 78.** Noncommunicating hydrocephalus. *A,* Diagrammatic representation of brain showing sites of possible obstruction of cerebrospinal fluid. *B,* Diagrammatic representation of brain showing dilatation of lateral and third ventricles of brain.

**Figure 79.** Noncommunicating hydrocephalus. The infant is helpless and lethargic. Strabismus is present. The "sunset sign" of the eyes is obvious. The scalp veins are dilated. A covered pad of sponge rubber is kept under the infant's head. A blanket roll is kept under his shoulders.

include tumor, hemorrhages or anomalous development of the pathway. A mechanical block may result from absence of an aqueduct or stenosis or obstruction by exudate or a blood clot. The foramina of Magendie and Luschka may be occluded.

A varying amount of fluid distends the ventricles. There is a gradual thinning of the brain substance, which is compressed between the distended ventricles and the expanding skull. The bones of the cranium become thin, the fontanels large and the sutures separated.

**Clinical Manifestations and Diagnosis.** In the congenital type of noncommunicating hydrocephalus the infant may die in utero, or a cesarean section may be done to deliver the child.

After birth an increase in size of the head is noticeable. The fontanels widen instead of narrowing and are tense. Irritability, anorexia and vomiting occur. The infant becomes increasingly helpless and less able to raise his head. The neck muscles are underdeveloped from lack of use. Affect and normal infant responses may be diminished. Nystagmus or convergent strabismus may be present. There is possibly some interference with sight. The eyes seem to be pushed downward and protrude slightly. The sclerae are visible above the iris, since the upper lids are retracted by the taut skin over the bulging forehead. The scalp is shiny, and the veins are dilated.

The muscle tone of the extremities is frequently abnormal. As the child's condition deteriorates, his body becomes emaciated, often weighing less than the head. The cry is high-pitched and shrill. Convulsions may occur. These infants have little resistance to infection. Formerly many died of a concurrent infection whose lives now would be prolonged by the use of antibiotics.

Operation may be indicated to prevent further enlargement of the head and to facilitate nursing care of a child with massive head enlargement.

Symptoms in hydrocephalus due to infection, e.g. that resulting from meningeal inflammation, develop slowly or are clinically unrecognized. The bones yield to pressure as in the congenital type. The course of hydrocephalus is progressive.

*Diagnostic tests* are made to indicate the site of the obstruction. Daily measurements of the head are made to compare its growth with that of the normal child. By ventricular puncture the presence of excess fluid and the approximate thickness of the cortex are determined. Other tests include those using dye (i.e. phenolsulfonphthalein or indigo carmine) and the pneumoencephalogram.

*Pneumoencephalogram.* A roentgenogram of the skull is taken after the

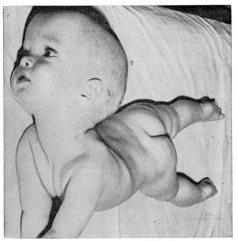

**Figure 80.** Opisthotonos resulting from meningitis in a hydrocephalic infant.

fluid filling the ventricles has been removed and replaced with air. This test is used only when the type of block cannot be identified with the dye test.

*Blackfan Test.* A ventricular tap is done (as modified by Dr. E. B. Spitz at The Children's Hospital of Philadelphia). Indigo carmine dye is injected. A ventricular tap is then done on the opposite side. If there is no obstruction, dye should be found. A delayed spinal tap is done; dye should be present in the spinal fluid. The dye should also appear in the urine. If the dye appears in the fluid obtained from the lumbar puncture, the hydrocephalus is of the communicating type; if not, it is of the noncommunicating type.

**Treatment and Prognosis.** Since the causes of noncommunicating hydrocephalus are mechanical, *treatment* must be surgical. At one time attempts were made to reduce the production of cerebrospinal fluid through dehydration diets, but these did not prove practicable. A former operation, now seldom used because it proved unsuccessful, was a plexectomy, in which part of the choroid plexus was removed in order to reduce the production of cerebrospinal fluid.

Modern surgery bypasses the point of obstruction by attempting to shunt the cerebrospinal fluid to the arachnoid villi or another area where it will be absorbed and finally excreted.

A ventriculojugular shunt can be made, using the internal jugular vein as the outlet for the cerebrospinal fluid. A valve has been invented which prevents blood from flowing back into the ventricles, but allows the cerebrospinal fluid, when under pressure, to enter the vein. As the child grows, the tube must be replaced at intervals. This operation has been perfected by Dr. E. B. Spitz and has proved successful in many cases.

In the ventriculoperitoneal shunt a tube is run from the ventricle to the peritoneum. An omentectomy is done to prevent blocking of the end of the tube.

In spinal ureterostomy the effectiveness of the tube is not influenced by the child's growth, but when a ventriculoureterostomy is done, longer tubes must be inserted as the child grows. In

**Figure 81.** A hydrocephalic infant on whom was done a ventriculoperitoneal shunt. Note the presence of the tube as it emerges from the skull and passes under the skin of the scalp and the chest.

both spinal ureterostomy and ventriculoureterostomy it is necessary to remove one kidney in order to insert the tube into the ureter.

A problem in the management of children having a ureterostomy is the loss of great quantities of salt in the fluid passed through the shunt. Massive sodium depletion may result. It is also possible that infections of the bladder may ascend the tube and cause meningitis. Infection reaching the cerebrospinal fluid by way of the shunt leading to the ureters is combated by the use of antibiotics.

In the Torkildsen operation (ventriculocisternostomy) a tube is run from the lateral ventricle to the cistern of the fourth ventricle.

The *prognosis* in the past was poor, but with newer surgical techniques excellent results have been obtained. If the brain is not seriously malformed at the time of operation, mental function may not be impaired. Motor function is retarded if the child cannot lift his head and move as a child would normally do. In many cases there is neurologic impairment. As in communicating hy-drocephalus, death may occur from extreme malnutrition or intercurrent infection.

**Nursing Care.** The hydrocephalic infant may be admitted to the hospital for diagnosis before operation is undertaken. The nursing care will include assisting with a number of tests. The basic care of the child admitted for diagnosis is that of the child admitted for operation.

*Preoperative Care.* With early diagnosis of the enlarging head treatment is given before the nursing care problem becomes difficult. The nurse is responsible for observing indications of irritability and changing vital signs. She must also provide care for the child when he exhibits the manifestations of anorexia and vomiting.

The nursing care of children with obviously enlarged heads presents many difficulties. The children may be unable to raise or even move the head, brain damage may have delayed their mental development, and malnutrition may have resulted from inadequate food intake and frequent vomiting.

These infants must be kept clean and

dry, especially in the area around the creases of the neck where perspiration and vomitus may collect.

To maintain nutrition, the feeding schedule should be arranged to avoid vomiting; i.e. the intervals between feedings should be those ordered by the physician, and all necessary care should be given *before* a feeding so as to avoid moving the infant after he has been fed. He should be held for his feedings. Since the head is heavy, the nurse should rest her arm upon a pad placed over the arm of her chair, or upon the mattress of the crib if it is low enough for her to do so. If the head is very large, the infant cannot be bubbled like a normal infant. The bottle should be taken from his lips several times during the feeding, and his head and shoulders should be slightly elevated (if the physician permits) while he is gently rubbed between the shoulders. When he is returned to his crib, he should be placed on his side to prevent aspiration of vomitus.

The infant's position should be changed frequently to prevent hypostatic pneumonia and to lessen the danger of pressure areas. These lesions are likely to appear on the head and ears unless every precaution is taken to prevent their occurrence. A pad of lamb's wool or sponge rubber should be placed under his head. A full-length sponge rubber mattress is excellent for these infants. If pressure areas develop, great care must be taken to prevent infection, which, in the infant's debilitated condition, might result in septicemia.

When the child is lifted from his crib, his head must be carefully supported in order to prevent trauma. In changing his position in bed, the weight of the head should be borne in the palm of the nurse's hand, thereby freeing her other hand to move the body. It is essential that head and body be rotated together, bringing no strain upon the neck. To lift the infant, the nurse leans over the crib, places her arm under his head and adjusts the head against her chest. She then raises him with her other arm supporting his body, as she would with a normal infant.

If a spinal puncture is to be done for diagnostic purposes, the nurse gives the usual assistance to the physician. The equipment needed to carry out a lumbar puncture on a child is the same as that needed to do the procedure on an adult. The nurse's most important responsibility in assisting with the procedure is restraint of the infant or child in such a way that his back is rounded and parallel with the side of the treatment table. With a small infant the nurse may place one hand behind his neck and the other hand over the buttocks and bend his back to the desired extent. To restrain an older infant or child, she may place one hand behind his neck or one arm around his neck and grasp his legs, and place her other arm around the buttocks and grasp his hands. By putting pressure on the neck and legs she can bend the child's body

**Figure 82.** A 6-year-old hydrocephalic boy whose ventriculojugular shunt has been functioning successfully for several years. He is normal mentally and attends school regularly. His motor functioning is that of the average child of his age.

**Figure 83.** Restraint of a child for a lumbar puncture. The nurse places one hand behind the child's neck and the other under his buttocks. By resting her body gently on the infant's body and by applying pressure on the neck and legs, she can thus round his back and keep it parallel with the side of the treatment table.

as necessary. An older child can be restrained with a sheet folded lengthwise in the same way as can an uncooperative adult.

The nurse's responsibilities in assisting with a ventricular tap are to apply a mummy restraint and to hold the head securely, because the needle is inserted through brain tissue. After the tap the nurse must observe for signs of shock and for leaking of fluid through the tap holes.

The parents should have constant contact with the neurosurgeon, since they are naturally apprehensive about operation on the infant. All diagnostic procedures should be explained to them, and they should be encouraged to help with the infant's care while he is in the hospital.

*Postoperative Care.* The temperature, pulse and respiration should be taken every fifteen minutes until the infant is reactive; blood pressure readings, if ordered, are taken at the same time (a small blood pressure cuff is needed). Signs of increased intracranial pressure are irritability, bulging of the fontanel, lethargy, vomiting, ele-

vated systolic blood pressure, widened pulse pressure, slowing and/or a change in nature of the pulse and respiration rates, or change in body temperature.

Recording of the vital signs may be ordered hourly for several days. If the temperature is elevated, alcohol sponging and aspirin may be ordered, and the infant should be clothed only in his diaper.

Intravenous fluids are given slowly in small quantities proportionate to the child's weight until the infant can be fed orally. If they are given too rapidly, there is danger of circulatory overload and cardiac failure.

Mucus from the nose and throat should be aspirated whenever necessary so as to prevent difficulty in breathing and the danger of aspiration of mucus. As always in the care of the hydrocephalic infant, there is danger of pressure areas developing on parts of the scalp which support the weight of the head. Cotton may be placed behind the ears, and over the ears under the head dressing. The child should be turned at least every two hours.

The elevation of the infant's head and his general position depend upon the amount of fluid draining through the tube used to shunt fluid from the ventricular system to another site— jugular vein, peritoneal cavity or ureter. The nurse should regularly record her observations of the bulging or tenseness of the fontanel. The physician will direct the elevation of the head and shoulders and the general position of the infant so as to increase or decrease the rate of drainage. If the fontanel becomes depressed too rapidly, a subdural hematoma may develop. If the anterior fontanel is depressed, the infant should be placed flat in bed with the head slightly lower than the body. When the tenseness of the anterior fontanel is normal, his head should be slightly elevated or flat.

If a spinal ureterostomy or ventriculo-ureterostomy has been done, a 24-hour urine specimen must be collected in order to determine the amount of fluid and electrolytes which are being excreted from the body. The technique is as follows:

For the male infant a plastic funnel-shaped tube is used. It is applied to the genitals by means of a binder with a hole through which the narrow end of the funnel protrudes. A flange around the rim of the appliance prevents it from slipping through the hole. If such a binder is not available, a finger cot can be attached to the collecting receptacle with adhesive tape, and the other end of the finger cot can be cut and attached to the penis and lower portion of the abdomen with adhesive tape (see Fig. 84). A plastic or rubber tube is attached to the open end of the funnel, which drains into a bottle attached to the bottom of the infant's crib.

For the female infant a specimen halter may be used to which is attached a plastic ring. Plastic tubing may be attached to the ring (see Fig. 85). The other end of the plastic tubing is placed in the drainage bottle attached to the bottom of the infant's crib.

The infant is restrained on the back by abdominal and ankle restraints. Such restraints (see Fig. 85) are made of double-thickness muslin with ties at both ends to tie on the springs of the bed. The abdominal restraint has a flap of double-thickness muslin stitched to the center of it. This flap may be pinned around the infant's abdomen. The ankle or extremity restraint has two smaller flaps sewn to it. These flaps may be pinned securely around either the ankles or the wrists. If this restraint is too large, a tuck can be pinned in the center of it (see Fig. 84).

The head of the crib should be slightly elevated if the infant's condition permits, to

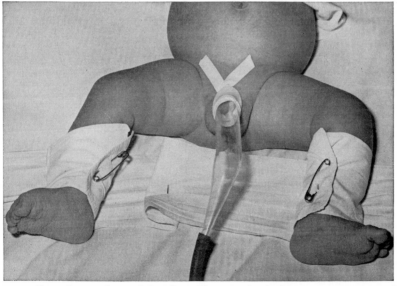

**Figure 84.** Procedure to be used for the collection of a 24-hour urine specimen from an infant boy. The collecting tube is held in place by adhesive tape. The ankle or extremity restraint is used to restrain the infant's legs. Note how the restraint is pinned in the middle in order to make it smaller.

**Figure 85.** Procedure to be used for the collection of a 24-hour urine specimen from an infant girl. A specimen halter to which is snapped a plastic ring and tubing is used. The other end of the plastic tubing is placed in the drainage bottle attached to the bottom of the infant's crib. The abdominal and extremity restraints are used to restrain the infant adequately.

prevent a backflow of urine. The genitals should be cleansed frequently to prevent excoriation. The restraints should be removed frequently, and passive exercise should be given to the legs and arms if the child cannot move himself. The nurse should not leave him until the restraints are again in position.

The physician usually orders sodium chloride to replace the amount lost through a ureteral shunt.

If a peritoneostomy (ventriculoperitoneal shunt) has been performed, the infant is given nothing by mouth. Abdominal distention is handled with a nasogastric tube which may be connected to mechanical suction. Irrigation of the tube may be necessary. The drainage is measured, and the amount and color are charted.

The infant's mouth becomes very dry, and mouth care is required four times a day. Clear fluids are given orally as soon as the child can tolerate them. The milk formula is introduced gradually, and later solid foods, suitable to the age of the infant, are given. A high protein diet should be offered.

The nurse should closely observe and report to the physician any of the following: signs of infection, tenseness of the anterior fontanel (an indication of inadequate drainage of the cerebrospinal fluid), vomiting (an indication of increased intracranial pressure or intolerance of diet), signs of dehydration such as loss of skin turgor, convulsions (duration, where initiated, all places of the body involved and the type of movements), nature of the vital signs, coldness or clamminess of the infant's body, pallor or mottled condition of the skin, the state of consciousness, movements or signs of paralysis, the type of drainage from the incision, and the degree of restlessness and irritability of the child.

**Teaching the Parent before Discharge of the Infant.** The importance of the mother's understanding the care she is to give her infant, and important conditions she should watch for and report to the physician, cannot be overestimated. She should be instructed in a way which will not increase her anxiety. She may be told of the success other mothers have had in caring for infants such as hers. This will help her to gain confidence in her ability to give the infant the care he needs. To understand the operation which was performed is a basis for understanding the reason for the care which she is taught and for following instructions exactly. She should understand the signs of increased intracranial pressure and of dehydration and their importance. With the surgeon's guidance the nurse may suggest exercises to the mother which will help to strengthen the infant's muscles so that he will learn to lift his head.

If the mother cared for the child before operation, she is probably skillful in handling him, but she must learn the problems which may arise in relation to the shunt. She should know the danger signals of too rapid drainage and should watch for them.

If the child is completely helpless and cannot move his body, there is always danger of pressure areas not only on the head, but also on the body. In hot weather the danger of such lesions is increased. Methods of prevention, such as have been described, can be taught to the mother. The infant should lead as normal a life as is possible. He should be given toys, and should be taken about in a baby carriage or stroller whenever possible.

### Microcephalia (Microcephaly)

**Etiology, Clinical Manifestations and Treatment.** Microcephalia is a relatively uncommon type of congenital anomaly. It is accompanied by mental deficiency. It is easily recognized at birth by the smallness of the skull. Growth of the skull is largely dependent upon development of the brain. Arrested brain growth in this type of mental deficiency is the cause of microcephalia. The condition of the brain may be due to hereditary factors, toxoplasmosis, German measles during pregnancy, or irradiation of the mother during the second or third month of pregnancy.

The *symptoms* are the small skull (less in volume and in circumference than normal when judged in relation to the body build of the infant) and severe mental retardation.

There is no *treatment* for the condition. Habilitation should be attempted to whatever extent is possible.

### Mongolism

**Incidence, Etiology, Clinical Manifestations, Treatment and Prognosis.** This condition occurs most frequently in the Caucasian race, although it sometimes appears among Negroes. The *incidence* is the same among all socio-economic classes and both sexes.

The *etiology* is not known, but research on the chromosomal count is in progress. The condition has its greatest incidence among infants born to women more than thirty-five years of age, although it has been found among the first-born of young mothers. There is a defect in the early embryologic development of the fetus.

The *signs* may be recognized at birth. The infant's physiognomy resembles that of an Oriental. The head is relatively small, the occiput flat and the face round. The eyes are set close together and slant slightly upward. The palpebral fissures (the openings between the eyelids) are narrow. The nose is flat, and the tongue protrudes. These children breathe through the mouth and may drool. Eruption of the teeth is delayed. The hands are short and thick, the little finger curved, and the creases of the palms are unlike those of a normal infant. There is a wide space between the first and second toes. The muscles are underdeveloped, the joints are loose, and the child can assume unusual positions. Growth and development are slow; mental development seldom reaches beyond that of the average child of five to seven years of age. Associated anomalies are frequent, among them congenital deformities of the heart.

These children are seldom destructive, but they are restless, inattentive, happy-go-lucky and difficult to train. They are often considered "cute" by strangers who do not understand their condition and are encouraged to show off their ability to assume unnatural positions.

Such children have little resistance to infection and usually die before puberty of an intercurrent infection. Modern drug therapy has prolonged their life expectancy to some extent.

Although there is no *treatment* for the condition, habilitation is important. If the child lives into adolescence, vocational training may be considered.

It is difficult for the parents to accept the child's condition. This is especially true if he is the only child of older

**Figure 86.** Mongolism. *A,* The child's physiognomy resembles that of an Oriental. *B,* The muscles are underdeveloped, the joints are loose, and the child can assume unusual positions comfortably for prolonged periods. (Courtesy of Dr. Ralph V. Platou and the American Academy of Pediatrics.)

**Figure 87.** Mongolism. The hands are short and thick, and the little finger is curved. (Courtesy of Dr. Ralph V. Platou and the American Academy of Pediatrics.)

parents. If the infant is the child of young parents, they may be afraid to have other children. In any event the parents need help in understanding the child's limitations and in planning his life to make the most of his capacities and to give him a happy childhood.

## GENITOURINARY SYSTEM

### Obstruction of the Urinary Tract

**Etiology, Clinical Manifestations and Diagnosis.** Obstruction to the flow of urine is important because of the back pressure produced above the level of the obstruction. The back pressure of accumulated urine causes the tract to become distended proximal to the point of obstruction. This may lead to stasis, hydroureter, hydronephrosis, possible infection and death due to renal insufficiency.

The *symptoms* are obstruction while voiding, dribbling, bladder distention or the presence of an abdominal mass. Infection of the urinary tract results in fever, chills, pyuria and convulsions. If there is eventual loss of kidney function with uremia, death results.

A number of tests are used to determine the location of the obstruction. It may be in the upper or lower urinary tract, above the bladder or below it. The symptoms are not always indicative of the site of the obstruction.

*Diagnostic tests* include catheterization immediately after voiding to determine the amount of residual urine. Intravenous urography is used to visualize the urinary tract and to measure renal excretory function. Cystoscopic examination and retrograde pyelography may be performed. The blood urea nitrogen level and phenolsulfonphthalein excretion rate may be determined to measure renal function.

### Obstruction of the Lower Urinary Tract

**Pathology and Clinical Manifestations.** Causes of lower urinary tract obstructions include urethral valves (filamentous valves that obstruct urinary flow are most commonly found in boys), ureteral diaphragm or congenital narrowing of the ureter, obstruction of the neck of the bladder (this is the most common site of obstruction), severe phimosis (obstructive phimosis is rare), neuromuscular dysfunction such as is found in association with cord injury and meningomyelocele, and meatal stricture.

All these obstructions result in dilatation and hypertrophy of the bladder. Residual urine is constantly present. The ureters dilate and become tortuous from the back pressure of urine which cannot pass into the distended bladder.

Later the pelves of the kidneys enlarge from pressure of urine which cannot pass down into the distended ureters. Destruction of kidney tissue inevitably results.

The *symptoms* are abnormalities of urination, a palpable, distended bladder and possibly distended ureters and kidneys. An important symptom is frequent infection of the bladder.

### Obstruction of the Upper Urinary Tract

Upper urinary tract obstructions are usually unilateral. The bladder is not involved. There is no problem of urination unless an infection occurs. Anomalies involving the ureters are the most common anomalies of the urinary tract.

The following *types* occur: obstruction or stricture of a ureter, congenital absence of one ureter, duplication of the ureter of one kidney, pressure of an aberrant blood vessel which blocks drainage through the ureter, neoplasm, calculi or an inflammatory stricture.

**Clinical Manifestations.** Often there are no symptoms, or there may be vague symptoms such as failure to grow normally, hypertension, fever, bacteriuria, pyuria or a mass in the abdomen.

**Treatment of Upper and Lower Obstructions.** The bladder is emptied by gradual decompression through an indwelling catheter. If the obstruction can be relieved by surgical means, operation is attempted in spite of the reduced renal function. Infections should be eradicated with appropriate chemotherapeutic medications. Little can be done for chronic renal insufficiency, manifested by progressive renal dysfunction. In the end death results from renal failure.

**Course and Prognosis.** Untreated obstruction results in renal insufficiency. If operation can remove the obstruction, improvement may result, and the child may live for many years.

### Patent Urachus

**Etiology and Pathology.** Patent urachus is due to persistence of the embryonic connection of the umbilicus

with the bladder. Occasionally the urachus may persist, and urine is discharged through the umbilicus after
birth. Often there is also an obstruction of the urinary tract below the bladder. Many times there is only a cyst at
the upper end of the tract, extraperi-
toneally under the umbilicus.

**Clinical Manifestations and Treatment.**
When the entire urachus is present,
urine dribbles from the umbilical region. When a urachal cyst is present,
there is a deep midline swelling below
the umbilicus. If the urachus is patent,
the tract should be obliterated surgically. Urachal cysts should be removed before they become infected. If
they do become infected, they should be
drained surgically before removal. Appropriate antibiotics are given for infection.

## Congenital Cystic (Polycystic) Kidneys

**Etiology, Pathology, Clinical Manifesta-
tions and Treatment.** The *etiology* is unknown. The infantile form is probably
transmitted as a mendelian recessive
trait. The renal tissue is filled with cysts
of varying sizes. The kidneys are enlarged and, when exposed at operation
or autopsy, have a spongy appearance.
The renal pelves and calyces are distorted because of the amount of surrounding tissue. The condition is rarely
unilateral. Other anomalies may also
occur, e.g. hydrocephalus, polydactyl-
ism or cardiac malformations.

The *clinical findings* depend upon the
location of the cysts. On palpation both
kidneys (less frequently only one) are
found to be enlarged. There is increasing renal insufficiency and, as a result,
hypertension and signs of congestive
cardiac failure. There may be severe
retardation in growth of the child. Laboratory findings show recurrent bacteriuria, hematuria, proteinuria and elevated blood nonprotein nitrogen levels.
X-ray films (urograms) show enlargement of the kidney and deformity of
the calyces and pelves.

There is no specific *treatment.* Supportive and palliative measures may be
used to combat renal acidosis and in-

sufficiency. Surgical drainage of large
cysts may be done when they interfere with renal function.

The *prognosis* depends upon the type
and severity of the interference with
function. In severe types the infant dies
in utero. Among infants living at birth
renal function decreases over the years.
In less severe cases, although the first
symptom may appear in childhood, the
condition may not become too evident
until adult life.

## Wilms's Tumor

**Incidence, Clinical Manifestations and Di-
agnosis.** Wilms's tumor is a highly
malignant embryonal adenosarcoma of
the kidney. It develops from abnormal
tissue in the embryo, beginning to grow
before or after the infant is born. It is
one of the most frequent types of neoplasm occurring in either sex during
infancy or the toddler age. It is commonly unilateral, but may be bilateral.
There are no early *symptoms* other
than malaise, pallor and possibly hematuria. A mass in the abdomen is usually discovered by the physician in a
routine examination of the child, or
the mother may notice the mass while
bathing him or changing his diaper.

After the diagnosis has been made
the mother must be careful not to palpate the infant's abdomen, since handling might favor metastasis. The
tumor extends through the kidney capsule or renal vein and then spreads to
other areas of the body by way of the
circulatory system. The late symptoms
are anemia and cachexia.

The *diagnosis* is confirmed by intravenous pyelography, which shows the
distortion and displacement of the
pelvis of the kidney.

**Prognosis, Treatment and Nursing Care.**
The condition without treatment is always fatal. The tumor tends to produce
pulmonary metastases via the renal
vein and venous circulation to the right
side of the heart and thence through
the pulmonary artery to the lungs.

The *treatment* is surgical extirpation
with x-ray irradiation before and/or
after surgery. Operation should be done

immediately after the diagnosis has been made unless irradiation is used to shrink the tumor before removal.

The *nursing care* is that of the normal infant, with special attention to nutrition. The specific danger in care is manipulating the abdominal wall inadvertently, as in bathing the infant or even when fondling him, and thereby increasing the danger of metastasis. The mother should be cautioned against

this, and in the hospital a sign should be placed on the infant's crib or on his abdomen—"Do not palpate abdomen."

### Exstrophy of the Bladder

**Pathology and Clinical Manifestations.** Complete exstrophy is an extensive anomaly. The entire lower urinary tract —i.e. the entire bladder to the external

*A*

*B*

**Figure 88.** Exstrophy of the bladder. *A,* Five-month-old infant with exstrophy of the bladder and bilateral indirect inguinal hernias. The association of these 2 conditions is common. (Gross: The Surgery of Infancy and Childhood.) *B,* Bulging everted bladder lying below the umbilicus. Beneath this a completely epispadiac penis is seen, while below this is a shallow, poorly developed scrotum devoid of testicles. (Schaffer: Diseases of the Newborn.)

urethral meatus—is exposed and may be without ventral covering. The defect in the male infant may be accompanied by a short penis, epispadias, undescended testes or an inguinal hernia. In the female infant the clitoris may be cleft, the labia separated and the vagina absent. In either sex the rectus muscles below the umbilicus are separated, and the pubic rami are not joined.

In complete exstrophy the posterior bladder lining is exposed and appears bright red through the fissure in the abdominal wall. The condition is more common in boys than in girls.

The *symptom* at birth is the obvious defect. Urine seeps onto the abdominal wall from the abnormal ureteral outlets. This causes a constant odor of urine and excoriation of the surrounding skin. There may be ulceration of the mucosa of the bladder. The separation of the pubic rami causes a waddling gait when the child learns to walk.

**Treatment, Complications and Prognosis.** If the exstrophy is not complete, the abdominal and bladder walls may be closed by plastic surgery. Recently even complete exstrophy has been corrected by plastic surgery with excellent results. The child then voids normally. In the majority of cases of complete exstrophy, however, the ureters are transplanted into the sigmoid (lower colon). Urine is then passed with stool from the anus. Plastic repair of the bladder, abdominal wall and external genitals may be done later. When the child is old enough to have control of his bowel movements, he learns to retain the urine in the colon by tightening the sphincter muscle. He is given antibiotics to combat infection. The waddling gait is improved by a brace which corrects the deformity of the pelvic girdle.

If the ureters are transplanted to the colon, hydronephrosis and hydroureter may result from back pressure originating at the site of the ureteral anastomosis. An ascending infection, usually caused by the colon bacillus, may result in pyelonephritis. Before operation there is danger of a skin infection around the area where the skin is constantly irritated by urine.

The *prognosis* depends upon the injury done to the kidneys by the back pressure of urine for which there is no adequate outlet, and upon whether the child has suffered severe or chronic infection of the urinary tract. Even if there is no infection of the kidney, these children may have a chronic disturbance of the body chemistry, since the bowel surface may absorb secretory products from the urine when the ureters are transplanted to the sigmoid.

**Parent Teaching before Discharge of the Infant from the Nursery.** It is important that the parents be taught the general care of these infants. Good hygiene is necessary in order for the infants to be in optimum condition to withstand an infection of the skin or kidney, and, later, surgical correction of the anomaly. The nurse should understand the mother's distress over her child's condition and appreciate that his care may be a task which she cannot immediately undertake. The nurse's acceptance of the child's condition is as important in teaching the mother as are the procedures in the care of the anomaly.

The mother may not have sufficient self-control to cleanse the area around the exposed bladder until she has become accustomed to the sight of the defect. If she is to be taught before she leaves the obstetrical unit, she should be fully recovered from giving birth to the infant. If she is not ready for his care, it would be better to keep him in the hospital for a few days and have the public health nurse instruct her in his care after he has been sent home. The mother should learn to keep the bladder area very clean and to apply sterile petrolatum gauze over it in order to prevent infection and possible ulceration. A bland ointment may be applied to the skin around the bladder area in order to protect the skin from draining urine. The diaper should be changed frequently for the infant's comfort and to prevent the odor of urine, which will embarrass the mother when she shows him to her friends. Stool should be removed immediately so that it does not contaminate the bladder mucosa. The infant's clothing should be light so as to avoid pressure on the exposed bladder.

**Nursing Care.** *Preoperative* nursing care includes the care which has been outlined above to be taught the mother. If the infant is not a newborn in the nursery, but an older infant admitted to the pediatric unit for tests or operation, the mother may be able to give good hints on his care. This will ensure the continuity of care which makes the transition from home to hospital less disturbing for the infant. If operation is to be done when the child is old enough to understand that he is to undergo surgery, he should be emotionally prepared for the experience. In any case the parents must be psychologically ready for operation to be done on the child before it is undertaken. It is helpful to both the parents and the child to allow the mother to help with his care in the children's unit.

If a urine specimen is needed, it is collected from the opening in the bladder with a medicine dropper, or the child may be held over an emesis basin in such a position as to allow urine to drip into the basin.

*Postoperative* care is that of any surgical patient. The dressings must be kept clean and dry. If the child is old enough to establish control of the anal sphincter muscle, he should be taught to hold the muscle tight to prevent seepage of urine. There will be some soiling of his clothes while he is acquiring this control. He should never be made to feel ashamed of "accidents." Control will be acquired more readily if he is not too anxious about his condition.

### Hypospadias

**Etiology, Treatment and Prognosis.** Hypospadias is a congenital malformation in which the urethra, in the male, opens on the lower surface of the penis just behind the glans, in the body of the penis or on the perineum; rarely, in the female, the urethra opens into the vagina. In the male associated congenital *chordee* is a cordlike anomaly which extends from the scrotum up the penis and pulls it downward in an arc. Urination with the penis in the normal elevated position is impossible.

The *treatment* is by plastic surgery. If the anomaly is slight, no treatment is given, since only severe forms interfere with procreation.

The child's parents are likely to be overconcerned about his condition. If it is severe, the anomaly should be repaired before the child is of school age so that he will not be embarrassed when voiding before his peers. This condition may rarely be seen in girls. In both sexes the problem is chiefly psychological.

A    B    C

**Figure 89.** Anomalies of the male genitals. *A*, Hypospadias, showing in one drawing a composite of the common locations of the deformity. *B*, Hypospadias of a severe degree in a false hermaphrodite. *C*, Epispadias. (From Arey: Developmental Anatomy. 6th ed.)

### Epispadias

In this anomaly the urethra in the male opens upon the dorsal surface of the penis. The urethra may lie just behind the glands or, in conjunction with exstrophy of the bladder, extend the whole length of the penis (see Fig. 89).

The only treatment is surgical. The emotional and psychological problems involved are the same as those in hypospadias.

### Hermaphroditism (Intersexuality)

Parents feel guilty about the birth of a child whose sex is not easily determined. Hermaphroditism is an extremely disturbing anomaly, although its influence on the child's physical health is slight. If there is any question about the sex of the child because of the lack of distinctive genitals, the newborn should have an exploratory examination to determine the gonadal sex. This should be done before the parents announce the child's sex to their friends and information for the birth certificate is given. The social role of the boy is different from that of the girl; clothing, activities and the pronominal references of speech all set off one sex from the other. It is psychologically harmful to both the parents and the child if the infant believed to be of one sex is later found to be of the other. All psychological identifications have been made in terms of the sex originally determined by the physician.

Parents, and the child when he is old enough, need to understand the anatomic problems involved and the treatment which should be given. They need support from professional people who consider the problem objectively, without the morbid curiosity and pity which friends and relatives may show. A child with such a problem needs help at school in adjustment to his peer group. It is advisable to have him/her under the supervision of the guidance clinic. Parents, even the most understanding parents, cannot judge the depth of such a child's emotional problems.

### Pseudohermaphroditism in the Female

**Etiology, Clinical Manifestations, Diagnosis and Treatment.** Female pseudohermaphroditism is the most common problem in sexual differentiation. It is due to congenital adrenal hyperplasia. Increased androgenic—i.e. producing male characteristics—steroid secretion by the fetal adrenal cortex causes masculinization of the external genitalia in the female infant. Recently more cases have been seen in infants born of mothers treated with steroids during pregnancy than have occurred spontaneously.

The *clinical findings* are enlargement of the phallus or clitoris, fusion of the labia resembling a bifid scrotum, and hypospadias. Such infants have a cervix and a uterus and the female chromosomal pattern.

The *diagnosis* may be made by exploration and biopsy of the gonads during the neonatal period or by assay of steroid excretion products in the urine.

In spite of the anomalous external genitalia, these children should definitely be reared as girls. Infants with congenital adrenal hyperplasia should be treated by administration of cortisone or hydrocortisone, which will inhibit excessive production of adrenal androgens. Infants who do not have adrenal hyperplasia require no treatment other than corrective plastic surgery. Correction should be undertaken between the ages of eighteen months and four years.

If the diagnosis is made in infancy and plastic surgery is performed in the toddler or preschool age, the *prognosis* is very good.

### Pseudohermaphroditism in the Male

**Etiology and Treatment.** There are several types of this condition, but all such infants are chromosomal males. One type is caused by gonadal dysgenesis. These are infants whose testes were

*A*                                                    *B*

**Figure 90.**   Pseudohermaphroditism in the male. *A*, View of torso of 1-month-old infant showing normal female configuration. A swelling can be seen in the right inguinal region. At operation this proved to be a testis which had herniated into the inguinal canal. *B*, Closeup of external genitals, which appear to be made up of completely normal female labia, clitoris, vulva and vagina. Skin biopsy revealed the male chromosomal pattern. At laparotomy no female internal organs were found. (Gaspar, Kimber and Berkaw, in A.M.A. J. Dis. Child., Vol. 91, with the permission of the authors.)

damaged early in fetal life, resulting in feminization of the fetus. Another type is characterized by normal female external genitals, but testes, not ovaries, internally. In this type the testes should be removed and the child reared as a girl. At the usual time for puberty the child should be given estrogens to compensate for those normally produced by the ovaries of the female. In still another type the genitals are predominantly masculine or ambiguous. Such children masculinize at puberty. Any structures not of the male sex should be removed surgically.

### True Hermaphroditism

True hermaphroditism is rare. The clinical findings show both ovarian and testicular tissue in the same infant. The chromosomal sex may be male or female. True hermaphroditism must be excluded in all infants showing inter-

sexuality except those with congenital adrenal hyperplasia. The treatment is the same as for male pseudohermaphroditism.

### ORTHOPEDIC ANOMALIES

As recently as ten years ago children with minor orthopedic deformities were treated on an inpatient basis, remaining in the hospital for months. Today, with the recognition of the psychologic importance of the separation of the child from his mother, such children are treated largely on an outpatient basis. They are admitted to the hospital only for application of a cast or for operation and are cared for at home between admissions. This places increased responsibility upon the nurse to help the mother understand the care of the child.

Two important orthopedic congenital anomalies which can be recognized at birth or shortly thereafter are clubfoot and dislocated hip.

### Clubfoot

Clubfoot is a foot which has been twisted out of shape or position in utero and cannot be moved to an overcorrected position. An infant may appear to have this deformity because of the fetal position of comfort in utero. Unlike true clubfoot, however, his foot can be moved to a correct or even overcorrected position and made normal by simple exercises. In such a case before the mother is given the infant to nurse or fondle she should be told that the defect is only temporary.

**Incidence, Etiology, Diagnosis, Pathology and Types.** True clubfoot is one of the most common orthopedic deformities. Several theories have been advanced to explain the *etiology*. The condition may be due to a defect in the ovum, a familial tendency or arrested growth. It may be a paralytic deformity occurring in conjunction with meningomyelocele. Not all cases of clubfoot seen in older children are congenital in origin. The defect may have been caused by injury or anterior poliomyelitis.

The *diagnosis* of the specific type of clubfoot (several types are recognized) depends upon the anomaly in the individual child. The *pathology* varies from slight changes in the structure of the foot to abnormalities in the bones of both the foot and the leg.

The two most common types of clubfoot are talipes equinovarus and talipes calcaneovalgus. Both types are usually bilateral. In *talipes equinovarus* the foot is fixed in plantar flexion and deviates medially; i.e. the heel is elevated. The child walks on the toes and outer border of the foot. More than 95 per cent of the cases of congenital clubfoot are of this type. In *talipes calcaneovalgus* the foot is dorsiflexed and deviates laterally; i.e. the heel is turned outward, and the anterior part of the foot is elevated on the outer border. The child walks on the outwardly turned heel and the inner border of the foot.

**Figure 91.** Congenital bilateral club feet in an infant. (Courtesy of R. Pullen: Applied Physical Diagnosis.)

**Treatment and Nursing Care.** *Treatment* should be started as soon as possible. Delay makes correction more difficult, since the bones and muscles of the leg develop abnormally, and the tendons will be shortened. In infancy, treatment is usually conservative. It may consist of manipulation, the application of a cast to hold the foot in a corrected position, or use of a wedged cast. The advantage of this type of cast is that a position of greater correction can be achieved by means of the wedge and that the cast need not be changed. A Denis Browne splint is often used for infants under one year of age. The appliance is made of two foot plates attached to a cross bar. When the splint is fitted to the shoes, varying positions of angulation of the feet may be maintained by set screws. As the child kicks, he automatically forces his feet into a corrected position.

If conservative measures fail to correct the deformity, forcible correction may be done under anesthesia and a cast applied. Surgery on the tendons and bones may be done in early childhood, and the leg and foot placed in a cast.

The *nursing care* of these children is

difficult. Both physical and psychologic problems are numerous. The usual method of applying a cast is followed. A plaster of Paris bandage is closely fitted over stockinet or wadding extending from below the knee to the toes. In the Kite method of correction the cast is wedged. When the child returns to the pediatric unit after application of a cast, the nurse should observe for areas of pressure and should note the condition of the skin around the edges of the cast, the circulation in the toes as shown by color and temperature, the child's ability to move his toes, and any sign of discomfort. If pressure areas develop or if the circulation is impaired, the cast is split to relieve the pressure or is removed. The nurse may put adhesive petals

A. Strip of adhesive tape 1" in width.

B. Strip of adhesive folded in half with the adhesive side out. Cuts are made as indicated by the broken lines approximately every 2-1/2" to 3" apart. Petals may be longer depending on the thickness of the cast.

C. Completed petal. Petals are placed over the edge of the cast as shown in the figure below.

Bilateral talipes equinovarus before and after application of the plaster casts. Adhesive petals have been placed around the ends of the casts.

**Figure 92.** Method of applying adhesive petals around the edges of a cast to prevent **the** plaster from irritating the skin.

around the edges of the cast to prevent the plaster from irritating the skin.

Children are mischievous and are likely to slip small particles of food, or anything else which they can reach, under the edge of the cast. It requires close observation to prevent the child from doing this, but prevention is essential, since such particles may cause irritation and possibly infection. No powder or oil should be put on the skin beneath the cast. Neither will add to the child's comfort, and both may cause irritation.

If forcible manipulation under anesthesia is used to place the foot in a corrected position and a cast is applied, the child should remain in bed for twenty-four hours with the leg and the foot elevated on pillows or in a sling which supports the cast evenly. Elevation prevents swelling of the foot and leg and also constriction of the circulation.

If the child has undergone operation and a cast has been applied, upon his return to the pediatric unit the nurse must observe for evidence of bleeding, i.e. for discoloration of the cast over the wound. If this occurs, she should circle the area of discoloration with gentian violet or other suitable material for marking, and watch for further bleeding as shown by a spread in the area of discoloration. Thereby the approximate amount of bleeding can be estimated. After operation it is necessary to change the cast approximately every three weeks in order to bring the foot gradually into normal position and ensure permanent correction. When the cast is no longer needed, exercises and special orthopedic shoes may be required.

**Instructions to the Mother.** Before the infant is discharged from the nursery the nurse should discuss with the mother the necessity of taking the infant regularly to the clinic or to her private physician. Mothers are naturally distressed at the discomfort of corrective measures. They may need encouragement to follow treatment through until all possible correction has been made and the surgeon has discharged

the child. If the mother is to manipulate the foot, she should be taught by the physician and supervised in her practice until she can do so correctly.

If the child is sent home from the pediatric unit in a cast, the mother should understand that after the position of the foot has been corrected, as shown by roentgenograms, the cast will be removed and the foot manipulated. If she has not already been taught how to do this, the physician will show her the procedure, and she should practice under his supervision or that of the nurse. The mother should be told that eventually the child will be fitted with shoes designed to correct a clubfoot and will learn to walk, but that it may be necessary for him to wear a splint on the leg and the foot at night.

After forcible manipulation or surgery and the application of a cast the mother should be told that it will be necessary for the child to be brought back to the surgeon for examination over a period of months. Often parents believe that operation will correct the condition without further ado.

If the family is financially unable to bear the expense of frequent change of the cast, special shoes and possibly surgery, the parents should be referred to the medical social worker. Often an apparent lack of interest in returning for necessary treatment of the child may be due to financial difficulty in meeting the cost of his care.

**Prognosis.** The prognosis depends to a great extent upon the age of the child when treatment was begun. If the deformity is corrected in infancy, there is usually a good functional result, although the shape of the foot is not always normal in severe cases.

### Dislocated Hip

**Etiology, Incidence and Diagnosis.** Congenital dislocations of the hip are believed to be due to lack of embryonic development of the joint. Although this seems to be true, the *etiology* is not entirely clear. It has been suggested that heredity is a factor.

Newborn infants seldom have a con

plete dislocation of the hip. Rather, the head of the femur does not lie entirely within the shallow acetabulum. When the child begins to walk, weight bearing may convert this condition to a true dislocation.

The anomaly is more frequent among girls than among boys, the ratio being eight to one.

The initial *diagnosis* is based upon the following symptoms, which become apparent during the first or second month of life. The first and most reliable sign is limitation in abduction of the leg on the affected side. When the infant is lying on his back with knees and hips flexed, the normal hip joint permits the femur to be abducted until the knee almost touches the table at an angle of 90 degrees. With dislocation abduction on the affected side is limited to no more than 45 degrees.

**Pathology, Clinical Manifestations of Complete Dislocation, and Treatment.** The early sign of dislocation of the hip is a shallow and extremely oblique acetabulum. The head of the femur on the affected side tends to be smaller than normal, and the ossification centers are delayed in appearance. Evidence of true dislocation is found on the roentgenogram, which shows lateral and upward dislocation of the head of the femur in relation to the acetabulum.

*Signs and symptoms* of complete dislocation are shortening of the leg and prominence of the soft tissue of the gluteal folds on the affected side, limited ability to abduct the leg and, when the child begins to walk, a characteristic limp. *Trendelenburg's sign* is present: lowering of the normal hip when the child is stood upon the affected leg and raises the normal leg.

If the child has bilateral dislocation, his gait will be waddling and lordosis will be evident. Naturally, he is likely to be late in walking.

*Treatment* should be started as soon as the diagnosis is made. Delay prolongs treatment and may result in conversion of a partial to a complete dislocation. The objective of treatment is to place the head of the femur within the acetabulum and by constant pressure to enlarge and deepen the socket with ultimate correction of the dislocation. This is achieved in the young infant by placing a pillow between his thighs, thereby keeping the knees in a froglike position. The pillow should be protected by a plastic covering over the infant's diaper or under the cotton pillow cover. The Frejka splint is a more elegant modification and is easier to maintain in position. With the older child a stiff, shell-like cast may be used which spreads his legs apart and forces the head of the femur into the acetabulum. Complete casts are not used during the first few months of life, but, when applied, will be maintained for six to nine months.

If operation is performed, an open reduction of the dislocation and/or repair of the defect in the acetabular shelf is done. A cast is applied after operation to hold the head of the femur in the corrected position, i.e. fitted into the socket of the acetabulum.

**Nursing Care.** This is one of the congenital anomalies which may not be discovered in the neonate, but may be found during the regular monthly ex-

**Figure 93.** Limitation of abduction is an early sign of congenital dysplasia of the hip. (C. C. Chapple and J. R. Moore, in Nelson's Textbook of Pediatrics. 7th ed.)

**Figure 94.** Bilateral congenital dislocation of the hip. Note extreme lumbar lordosis. (Courtesy of R. Pullen: Applied Physical Diagnosis.)

aminations which every infant should have. The earlier the diagnosis is made and treatment begun, the more successful will be the outcome.

In general a child is admitted to the hospital for application of a cast. If a cast is used, it encircles the waist and extends down to the toes. The cast holds the leg in an abducted position. In bilateral dislocation both legs are abducted and held in position by the cast. The nurse caring for the child should watch closely for signs of impaired circulation such as discoloration or cyanosis, impaired movement, loss of sensation, edema or temperature change in the toes. She should observe for any evidence of discomfort. These indications of poor circulation are gen-

erally caused by pressure of a cast which fits too closely over some areas of the extremity.

The skin around the edge of the cast is in danger of becoming excoriated. To prevent this the edges should be smoothed or lined with adhesive tape (see p. 237). The skin should be kept dry and clean. The greatest danger is in the area around the opening which exposes the genitals and makes it possible for urine and feces to be expelled without soiling the cast. The perineum should be kept clean. The nurse should wash the skin under the edge of the cast whenever necessary and dry it *thoroughly*. Neither oil nor powder should be used on the skin under the cast.

If operation has been done, the nurse should watch for bleeding, and if there is evidence of hemorrhage, she should follow the procedure outlined under nursing care for clubfoot (p. 238).

The little child who has nothing else to entertain him is likely to put bits of food or small articles under the cast. The nurse should give him toys which are too large to be used in this way and should watch him closely when he has food in his hands. She should also investigate the area under the cast to make certain that no excoriations or foreign material is present.

After application of the cast the child is placed on a Bradford frame (see p. 215). This helps to keep the cast clean. If ponies or blocks are used under the head of the frame, they should be placed under the child's shoulders, never directly under the head. Lower blocks should balance the ponies, and the corners of the frame should be tied to the bed to prevent its slipping. Pillows should be placed at the sides of the frame to support the child's arms. A restraining jacket and ankle restraints are used to maintain the child's position and to prevent his falling. In unilateral dislocations the cast on the unaffected side extends only to the knee, and the leg is not abducted. In order to turn the child upon his abdomen, space should be left at the foot of the frame so that the toes of the leg which is not abducted hang over the edge of the frame, or the ankle may be supported on a sandbag or small pillow.

Much can be done to keep the child comfortable in his cast, but careless nursing leads to a soiled cast and excoriated skin. Suggestions for care of the child include the following: the use of "petals" of waterproof adhesive tape around the openings of the cast to protect the plaster and the stockinet lining from soiling and to prevent bits of plaster from cracking off and slipping under the cast. The opening around the buttocks and genitals should be covered with plastic material. If the child is taken off the frame for any reason and a diaper is necessary, it should be small and changed as soon as it is soiled.

If the child is old enough to use a bedpan, a Bradford frame is unnecessary. To give the bedpan, the child is placed upon his back with a pillow under his shoulders so that the upper part of his body is higher than the buttocks. A piece of plastic is tucked under the front and back edges of the opening around the buttocks and genitals. The bedpan is then slipped beneath the buttocks with the ends of the plastic strips hanging into the pan. For urination unaccompanied by stool, a male or female urinal is more convenient and comfortable than the bedpan.

A hospital for acutely ill patients may have a special unit for convalescent and chronically ill children. If the child cannot be sent home, he may be placed here. Every effort should be made to give children who are not sent home as normal a life as is possible in an institution. Many of the suggestions outlined below for the mother to follow are applicable to the care of the institutionalized child. Carts built for crippled children, adult wheelchairs with the back dropped and the foot raised level with the seat or Kiddy-Kars may be provided for children able to use them.

**Guidance of the Mother after the Child's Discharge from the Hospital.** Children with long-continued disabilities should lead as normal a life as is possible. They should be given the means to help themselves in habilitation in all the daily life activities. A large plaster cast which holds the legs in frog position is unsightly and difficult to fit into clothing, furniture or equipment made for normal children. Practical suggestions which have been tried out and are in use in many convalescent units will help the mother in caring for her child. Wide flaring pants extending down to the ankles may be used to cover the cast. These are made of attractive material and worn with a jacket of the same or a contrasting color. In such an outfit the child feels dressed up.

A home-made substitute for the Bradford frame serves the same purpose as the type used in the hospital. It will resemble a sling in which the child's legs can extend over the edges. The canvas sling is suspended from a wooden frame. Another appliance which can be used is a stroller made of wood with openings for the legs on either side. The base must be large so that the stroller does not tip. Casters are put at the corners and should be large enough to permit pushing the stroller easily.

There is on the market a wooden cart often used in hospitals and convalescent units. It resembles a long wooden box mounted on a chassis which has large wheels at the top and small wheels, which pivot, at the bottom. The cart can be pushed like a baby carriage, and the child can turn the cart so that he can look this way or that by revolving the large wheels. It turns readily, since the wheels at the foot pivot. The cart will hold a Bradford frame the width of the child's body, but support must be provided for the legs, which extend over the side of the cart. If the child has control of urination and defecation, he may be laid upon a mattress in the cart rather than upon a Bradford frame.

Plaster soaks up urine readily and causes an odor. Excoriation of the skin is also likely. The following is suggested for keeping the cast clean. The opening around the buttocks and genitals may be coated with waterproof adhesive "petals." Plastic may be used in the same way, but requires adhesive to attach it to the cast (a firm quality must be used). The cast may be painted with white shoe polish or shellac.

Any appliance made by the parents or any technique used in his care should be checked by the physician to ensure the child's safety and to protect the cast from cracking.

These are long-drawn out cases, and the final result is uncertain. All that has been said previously about the psychologic management of handicapped children should be applied in the care of these children, whether at home, in a convalescent unit or in a hospital. Since the child will be readmitted to the hospital many times during the course of treatment, a good working relation between nurses and parents is essential or, in the clinic situation, among the parents, hospital and public health nurses and medical social service worker.

## CLINICAL SITUATIONS

Mr. and Mrs. Jamison had moved into a moderately low-income housing area a short time before their first child, Joan, was born. Mr. Jamison planned to attend college while nineteen-year-old Mrs. Jamison looked forward to caring for her infant. Since Mrs. Jamison knew few people in her new community and since she had no previous experience with children, the public health nurse was asked to visit Mrs. Jamison and her five-day-old infant on their first day home from the hospital. Mrs. Jamison asked several questions.

1. "I have read about 'demand feedings' for babies. Why are these important?"
   a. "The more often you feed Joan, the better will be her nutritional status."
   b. "If you give Joan feedings every four hours, she will quickly learn correct eating habits."
   c. "If you feed Joan when she is hungry, you will be meeting her own individual needs."
   d. "If you feed Joan frequently, you will not have to adhere to a rigid schedule and to plan your other household responsibilities around it."

2. "I am concerned because Joan's breasts are swollen a little even though the doctor said this was normal. What could I do about this?"
   a. "All newborn infant girls have breast changes to a degree. It is nothing to worry about."
   b. "Be certain to ask your doctor again about these changes. They may be important."
   c. "Some newborn infants respond in this way because of hormone activity originating from the mother. No treatment is necessary."

   d. "Fortunately few infants have this congenital condition. Be certain that you express the secretion from the breasts so that the swelling is reduced."
3. "Sometimes when I feed Joan her bottle, she has 'air on her stomach' and vomits a little formula when I place her in her crib. How can I prevent this?"
   a. "Do not give her all the formula the doctor recommended because she is obviously eating too much."
   b. "Bubble her frequently during her feeding and especially after she has finished eating. Then place her in bed on her right side."
   c. "Bubble her frequently during her feeding and especially after she has finished eating. Then place her in bed on her left side."
   d. "Bubble her frequently during her feeding and prop her against a pillow in the corner of her crib so that it will be mechanically more difficult for her to vomit."

4. "I am concerned about Joan's bowel movements. Do you think they are normal?" The nurse should know that the stool of a normal six-day-old formula-fed baby should be
   a. Greenish-black in color, sticky in consistency, and odorless.
   b. Hard in consistency, almost white in color, and having a very unpleasant odor.
   c. Yellow in color, putty-like to hard in consistency and having an unpleasant odor.
   d. Yellow in color, soft in consistency, and having a not unpleasant odor.

5. The nurse should know in discussing infant feeding with mothers that breast milk in comparison with cow's milk per volume contains
   a. More carbohydrate, less protein.
   b. More carbohydrate, more fat.
   c. More carbohydrate, more protein.
   d. More calories per ounce.

6. When the nurse was examining Joan, she realized that the infant should be referred to the physician if she had the following manifestations:
   a. Positive rooting reflex and positive sucking reflex.
   b. Positive grasping reflex and negative Chvostek's sign.
   c. Negative startle reflex and negative tonic neck reflex.
   d. Positive tonic neck reflex and positive swallowing reflex.

7. The nurse tested Joan's Moro reflex. A normal baby would respond by
   a. Sudden, generalized, symmetrical movement with the arms thrown outward in an embrace position and the legs drawn up together.
   b. Rapid movement of the arm and leg on the side where the nurse stimulated her.
   c. Slow generalized random activity of the whole body followed by a rigid positioning of the extremities.

d. Rapid movement of all the extremities, but with no fixed pattern.

Mr. and Mrs. Basito had a five-year-old daughter, Dolores, when Juan was born prematurely in the emergency room of their local hospital. Since both parents had to work because of financial problems, Mrs. Basito had not had time to visit the clinic for prenatal care. At birth Juan weighed 4 pounds 1 ounce. He was admitted to the pediatric unit and placed in an incubator.

8. The nurse regulated the temperature of the incubator on the basis of
   a. The environmental temperature of the unit.
   b. The temperature of the infant's extremities.
   c. The set temperature of 88° F. for all prematures.
   d. The individual infant's body temperature.

9. Juan had a period of apnea about three hours after delivery. The nurse, in order to stimulate his respirations since no mechanical resuscitator had been brought to his unit,
   a. Held him up by his ankles with his head down and spanked him.
   b. Plunged the infant alternately into a bath basin of warm, then a basin of cool water.
   c. Carefully suctioned the infant, then gently carried out mouth-to-mouth insufflation.
   d. Gently suctioned the infant, then applied rhythmic pressure to his chest.

10. Oxygen was ordered for Juan in the usual concentration. The nurse should realize that in order to prevent retrolental fibroplasia she should
   a. Maintain a constant level of oxygen concentration less than 40 per cent in the incubator.
   b. Give at least 70 per cent oxygen to prevent this condition.
   c. Open the arm holes of the incubator in order to mix the oxygen with room air to prevent too high a concentration.
   d. Use an oxygen analyzer once a day to check the concentration of oxygen in the incubator.

11. A few hours after delivery Juan's skin began to be increasingly jaundiced. His bilirubin level was found to be near the critical level. A diagnosis of erythroblastosis fetalis was made. The nurse should realize that
   a. His mother was Rh positive, his father, Rh negative.
   b. Both parents were Rh negative.
   c. Both parents were Rh positive.
   d. His mother was Rh negative, his father Rh positive.

12. An important reason why one or more exchange transfusions are done on an infant having erythroblastosis fetalis is to prevent
   a. Hemorrhagic disease of the newborn.
   b. Kernicterus.
   c. Ophthalmia neonatorum.
   d. Toxoplasmosis.

13. When Mrs. Basito was discharged from the hospital, she came to the pediatric unit to visit her son. She became emotionally disturbed when she saw the nurse gavaging Juan even though the physician had told her he was doing well. The nurse could explain the reason for this procedure and reassure her by saying
   a. "I am feeding Juan this way in order to prevent infecting his mouth with a rubber nipple, since he has very little resistance to infection."
   b. "Although Juan is gaining weight well, we do not want to tire him by having him suck on a nipple."
   c. "Juan is more likely to vomit and inhale his formula if we feed him by nipple."
   d. "I am very busy. This is the quickest way I can feed Juan and be certain that he gets all his formula."

14. When Juan weighed 7 pounds, the physician discharged him from the hospital. Before discharge the nurse demonstrated the physical care which he would need at home. In view of the total family situation, which comment by the mother should alert the nurse to the mother's need for further guidance?
   a. "Dolores, his sister, is so anxious to help me take care of the baby."
   b. "Poor Juan. I have caused him so much trouble. I will never let anything happen to him again."
   c. "He is such a beautiful baby! All my neighbors will want him when they see him."
   d. "My husband wanted a son so much. He has prayed each night that he would live."

Tommy Walker, who had a unilateral cleft lip, was admitted to the pediatric unit from the newborn nursery because his mother was emotionally unable to care for him at home. Mrs. Walker had previously had two infants who died at birth. Both she and her husband were distraught over Tommy's obvious defect.

15. The nurse could best help Tommy's parents adjust to their situation on admission by
   a. Placing him in a crib where other parents and children could not see him.
   b. Explaining that Tommy's deformity is really mild in comparison with others she has seen.
   c. Agreeing with the parents that Tommy's deformity is difficult for her to accept also.
   d. Treating Tommy as a normal infant and at the same time accepting the parent's feelings of disappointment.

16. After operation on the cleft lip Tommy's parents were delighted with the results. On his tenth postoperative day his mother asked for permission to hold her baby and to try to feed him. The nurse explained that
   a. The mother could hold Tommy on her lap and feed him with a rubber-tipped medicine dropper if she did not touch the area around the suture line.

b. Tommy should lie flat in bed during his feeding because of the possibility of injury to his lip.

c. Only nurses were permitted to feed babies while they were hospitalized.

d. Tommy would have to be gavaged for at least a few more days and that the mother would have to wait until the baby was discharged to care for him.

17. Tommy's mother asked several questions about the skin of a newborn infant. The nurse should realize that only one of the following characteristics is found in all normal infants.

a. Mongolian spots.

b. Miliaria.

c. Intertrigo.

d. Good turgor.

18. Since Tommy was Mrs. Walker's first living infant, she asked the nurse several questions about his care after discharge from the hospital. She asked, "Should Tommy's mouth be wiped out each morning when I bathe him?"

a. "Yes, in order to clean away milk curds."

b. "No, you will probably gag the baby and cause vomiting."

c. "Yes, cleanse the mouth with a cotton swab moistened with boric acid solution in order to prevent thrush."

d. "No, a baby's mouth should not be cleansed except by rinsing after feedings with boiled water."

19. "How can diaper rash be prevented?"

a. "Powder the buttocks thoroughly, particularly in the creases, when you change Tommy's diaper."

b. "Wash his buttocks with a mild soap and water and dry thoroughly whenever you change his diaper."

c. "Wipe the buttocks with a dry swab and oil well when he is soiled."

d. "When you change his diaper, wipe the buttocks with oil and powder in the creases well."

## GUIDES FOR FURTHER STUDY

1. Make a list of questions asked by mothers of newborns who have been admitted to the pediatric unit for treatment of congenital anomalies. Discuss your answers to these questions in seminar.

2. List the specific differences between fetal circulation and circulation after birth. If expected changes do not occur at or after birth, which congenital heart lesions would result? What clinical manifestations of these conditions could you observe?

3. Observe a group of normal newborns for common traits and for individual differences in relation to sleep, i.e. bodily movements, facial grimaces, sucking activity and reactions to hunger. Discuss your observations in seminar.

4. Discuss in seminar differences in practices of various religious and cultural groups in relation to the care of newborns.

5. Help an individual mother plan a 24-hour program of care for a normal newborn infant. What difficulties were encountered?

6. A newborn having a meningomyelocele is being discharged from the nursery. He will be admitted to the pediatric unit of another hospital in two weeks for operation. Help the mother plan a program of care for this infant at home. During your discussion note the mother's attitude toward this infant. What could you do or recommend in addition to helping her plan for his physical care that would assist her in adjusting emotionally to this situation?

## TEACHING AIDS AND OTHER INFORMATION*

*American Cancer Society*
A Cancer Source Book for Nurses. Reprinted 1959.

*American Heart Association*
Gluck, R.: Diagnosis of Congenital Cardiac Defects in General Practice, 1958.

*American Public Health Association*
Cleft Lip and Cleft Palate, 1955.

*The Children's Medical Center, Boston, Mass.*
Harelip and Cleft Palate.

*U.S. Department of Health, Education, and Welfare*
The Mongoloid Baby.
The Child with a Cleft Palate, 1953.

## REFERENCES

Ansell, J. S.: Nephrectomy and Nephrostomy. Am. J. Nursing, 58:1394, 1958.

Association for the Aid of Crippled Children: Proceedings of the Second Scientific Conference. Mechanisms of Congenital Malformation. New York, Association for the Aid of Crippled Children, 1955.

Bailey, C. P.: Surgery of the Heart. Clinical Symposia. Ciba Pharmaceutical Products, Inc., Summit, New Jersey, 10:131, 1958.

Blain, I.: The Nurse in the Orthopedists' Office. Am. J. Nursing, 61:62, Jan., 1961.

Bluestone, S. S., and Deaver, G. G.: Habilitation of the Child with Spina Bifida and Myelomeningocele. J.A.M.A., 161:1248, 1956.

Carter, W. N.: The Child with Congenital Heart Disease and the Office Nurse. Am. J. Nursing, 59:199, 1959.

Cooley, D. A.: Open Heart Surgery in Children. Am. J. Nursing, 58:200, 1958.

Craig, W. A., Hamra, M. L., McDermott, I., and Nicholson, E.: Congenital Dysplasia and Dislocation of the Hips. Am. J. Nursing, 56:1274, 1956.

Creevy, C. D.: Ileac Diversion of the Urine. Am. J. Nursing, 59:530, 1959.

Gilson, M., and Matson, D. D.: Care of a Child after an Arachnoid-Ureteral Shunt. Am. J. Nursing, 56:1424, 1956.

* Complete addresses are given in the Appendix.

Graves, N.: Nursing during Prolonged Hypothermia. Am. J. Nursing, 60:969, 1960.

Gross, R. E.: The Surgery of Infancy and Childhood. Philadelphia, W. B. Saunders Company, 1953.

Kiesewetter, W. B.: Pre and Postoperative Care in the Pediatric Surgical Patient. Chicago, Year Book Publishers, Inc., 1956.

Larson, C. B., and Gould, M.: Calderwood's Orthopedic Nursing, 4th ed. St. Louis, C. V. Mosby Company, 1957.

Lewis, G. M.: Practical Dermatology. 2nd ed. Philadelphia, W. B. Saunders Company, 1959.

MacCaskill, C. L.: Pediatric Surgical Nursing. Nursing Outlook, 6:274, 1958.

MacCollum, D. W., and Richardson, S. O.: Care of the Child with Cleft Lip and Palate. Am. J. Nursing, 58:211, 1958.

Idem: Management of the Patient with Cleft Lip and Cleft Palate. Pediatrics, 20:573, 1957.

Mayer, D. M., and Swanker, W. A.: Anomalies of Infants and Children. New York, McGraw-Hill Book Company, Inc., 1958.

Nelson, W. E. (editor): Textbook of Pediatrics. 7th ed. Philadelphia, W. B. Saunders Company, 1959.

Nugent, G. R.: Prolonged Hypothermia. Am. J. Nursing, 60:967, 1960.

Ochsner, A., and DeBakey, M. E. (editors): Christopher's Minor Surgery. 8th ed. Philadelphia, W. B. Saunders Company, 1959.

Paterson, D., and McCreary, J. F.: Pediatrics. Philadelphia, J. B. Lippincott Company, 1956.

Pillsbury, D. M., Shelley, W. B., and Kligman, A. M.: Dermatology, Philadelphia, W. B. Saunders Company, 1956.

Potts, W. J.: The Surgeon and the Child. Philadelphia, W. B. Saunders Company, 1959.

Prinzing, D. M.: Cleft Palate Rehabilitation. Nursing Outlook, 7:577, 1959.

Reed, S. C.: Counseling in Medical Genetics. Philadelphia, W. B. Saunders Company, 1955.

Schaffer, A. J.: Diseases of the Newborn. Philadelphia, W. B. Saunders Company, 1960.

Silver, H. K., Kempe, C. H., and Bruyn, H. B.: Handbook of Pediatrics. 3rd ed. Los Altos, California, Lange Medical Publications, 1959.

Sweetser, T. H., and others: Care of the Child with Exstrophy of the Bladder. Am. J. Nursing, 58:1115, 1958.

Tollefson, D. M.: Nursing Care of the Patient with an Ileac Diversion of the Urine. Am. J. Nursing, 59:534, 1959.

Warkany, J.: Etiology of Mongolism. J. Pediat., 56:412, 1960.

Warkany, J. (Guest editor): Congenital Malformations. Papers presented at a Conference on Teratology, January 12 and 13, 1956. Pediatrics, 19:719, 1957.

Willman, V. L.: Anatomy and Physiology of the Heart in Congenital Heart Disease. Am. J. Nursing, 60:190, 1960.

Wortham, E. D., and Ritchie, G.: Nursing Care of Children after Open Heart Surgery. Am. J. Nursing, 58:203, 1958.

# The Infant

# Chapter 12

# The Normal Infant:

# Growth, Development

# and Care during the First Year

THE CARE and development of the infant, after the neonatal period, throughout the first year of life will be considered in this unit. As with the newborn, we will study his emotional and physical status and his needs in health and in sickness.

In discussing the care of the infant, stress must be placed on the fact that spontaneity and enjoyment of the infant by the adult are probably of greater significance than the specific procedures used in his care. Neither the parents nor the nurse should feel so pressured that they lose their enjoyment in the care of the child. If they are particularly harassed and overburdened, their care of the infant will not be beneficial for him. At such times some kindly support or temporary relief from the pressure may be necessary.

## OVERVIEW OF THE INFANT'S EMOTIONAL DEVELOPMENT

The nurse should understand a child's developmental needs and should know how to respond to them so that he may continue to grow emotionally and physically while he is in the hospital as he would if he were at home. This is particularly important with infants and young children because separation from their parents, in itself, produces problems with which they need help.

### Sense of Trust

As was stated earlier (see p. 21), different components of the healthy personality develop at various periods in the process of growing up. The first of these, and probably the most impor-

249

**Figure 95.** The foundation of the sense of trust is laid in infancy. (H. Armstrong Roberts.)

tant, is the *sense of trust*, which normally develops in the first year of life. It is, of course, strengthened or weakened by experiences after that age, but the foundation is laid in infancy. If this sense of trust in others is not learned, the reverse, a *sense of mistrust*, is acquired. This tendency will be increasingly difficult to change as the infant enters childhood. A distrustful child is not friendly, and his attitude evokes a similar response in adults and other children.

During the first year the infant is completely dependent upon his mother or someone who is a substitute for her. The modern infant, however, may be cared for by his father, siblings, baby sitters and probably grandmother. He seems to accept their care as he does his mother's. They all appear as mother-substitutes to him. By the time he is several months old he has learned that each gives a different kind of satisfaction, and he turns from one to another. Nevertheless, unless his mother is employed outside the home, his preference will be for her.

The infant's earliest approach to life is *incorporative,* as shown in his want-

ing to put everything in his mouth, to make it a part of himself. If this need is satisfied, he has laid the foundation for *giving* as well as *receiving*.

Turning to his mother or her substitute for comfort and love is the first evidence of an infant's desire to *turn outward* for pleasure. His interest is no longer solely in physical sensations which he himself produces (sucking his fingers, sucking at the breast or on the nipple of his bottle, kicking, stretching, and the like) or which someone provides for him (the comfort of having his diaper changed or his warm bath). The newborn infant is self-centered, and the growing infant learns very slowly that *people* give care which he enjoys and so learns to turn to them for relief of tensions.

The sense of trust does not develop independently of other aspects of growth. It is an integral part of his total development. An infant learns to trust others through the relief of his basic needs; i.e. he learns to trust those people who give him pleasant sensations. The young infant does not differentiate his body from that of others who handle him. He likes the warm feeding in his mouth, but does not differentiate his mother's hand upon the bottle from his own fingers. Later, when he has learned the limits of his body and knows in a vague way that he is a separate organism, he will respond to his mother's presence. *He has learned to associate her care and caresses with her.* He smiles and coos when he sees her, for he knows that something pleasant will happen to him. He has learned to trust his mother and has laid the foundation for trusting other people.

If, however, someone speaks to him in a harsh tone or is sudden and spasmodic in his movements, the infant is frightened. He has received his first lesson in *mistrusting* others. If this happens often, he is likely to grow uneasy and apprehensive when strangers come near him.

During the first six months of life the infant wants to *receive all* that has to him a connotation of pleasure. He is not ready to give or even forego pleasure. When at six weeks of age he smiles at his mother, it is not to give her pleasure, but because he feels comfortable. He smiles in his sleep and when alone. In imitation of his mother he smiles when she smiles. Later he learns that she smiles when he smiles and coos and that a smiling mother does pleasant things for him.

During the second six months the infant learns to *bite*. The first teeth erupt between the fifth and seventh months, and he quickly learns to use them. A crisis occurs at this time, for he is no longer a passive recipient of attention from other people; he is becoming an active person in his social environment and is also seeking control over his physical environment. Now his playful putting of everything available into his mouth becomes a drive to have something between his gums on which he can bite. Fists, toys, blankets, the nipple of his bottle are all used to satisfy his need to bring pressure on his gums.

As he develops he becomes increasingly aware of himself as a separate organism. His mother, thinking that he is now more sturdy and less dependent upon her, is likely to leave him more to himself while she resumes activities which she enjoyed before his birth. This is natural if she and her husband plan to have other children and she expects to be pregnant again before many months have passed. If she intends to continue with a profession or employment outside the home, she wants to accustom the infant gradually to her absence. She leaves him alone while she does her housework. Although she has always done this, the infant while very young slept the greater part of the time, but now is awake and alone. If she can afford it, she frequently employs a baby sitter to care for him when she goes out.

The crisis develops around the adjustment which mother and infant make to their changed relations. The infant's successful adjustment depends less on the amount of time his mother now spends with him than on the *quality* of their relations during his first six months and while the crisis is being resolved. Another factor in his adjustment is the continuity of care from other members of the family which formerly supplemented that of his mother.

## NEEDS DURING THE FIRST YEAR

Although the infant's need to put everything in his mouth and later to bite was given priority among his essential needs because of its great psychologic importance, he has four other needs which must be met if he is to learn to trust the people about him. These needs are for feeding, sucking pleasure, warmth and comfort, and both love and security.

### Need for Feeding

The infant's world is small. He has no sense of time and lives entirely in the moment. The only rhythms he knows are those set up by his physiologic mechanism. He experiences hunger, which produces tension. He soon learns that people around him can satisfy this need and reduce his tension—make him comfortable—and that this is done with varying emotional attitudes on their part. This is a time for showing him love and affection.

Nurses are often criticized for the professionally emotionless attitude they show when feeding hospitalized infants. This is unfortunate, indeed, since infants sense a lack of warmth and spontaneity. We have also noted that breast feeding is more emotionally satisfying for the infant than bottle feeding if the mother sincerely desires to breast-feed her infant. The mother's attitude or that of her substitute is expressed in voice, touch and handling the infant while he is nursing. He associates this attitude with being fed and later on with food. Unfortunately even the mother's attitude is not always one of pleasure in caring for the child she loves. She may be busy with housework and the needs of the older children.

She may find that the feeding time conflicts with duties and pleasures outside the home and be irritated at having to feed him. If she employs someone else to care for him, he will probably be kindly treated, but no one else would be likely to show the affection which a loving mother would give and which the infant needs. Today, when many young mothers want a career outside the home, affectionate infant feeding is one of the major problems of child care.

### Need for Sucking Pleasure

The infant's habit of putting fingers and toys in his mouth is closely allied to his pleasure in sucking. The need for sucking, however, is quite apart from the need for food. He thoroughly enjoys the act of sucking, and if he does not have the opportunity to suck, tension results. Giving him something to suck on relieves the tension, and he promptly relaxes. Being put to the breast or held lovingly with the nipple of his bottle between his lips and the warm milk in his mouth is his first experience of love and comfort. The intensity of the sucking urge varies and is an example of individual differences in children.

During the second six months he may bite upon the nipple. If he is at the breast, this hurts his mother even if his teeth have not erupted. She may think of weaning him. If this is done and he is taught to drink from a cup before he has outgrown the need for sucking, he will suck upon toys, the end of a blanket, his fingers or anything else he can use for the purpose. If he wants to bite, he should be given a piece of toast or a suitable toy. He may, however, continue to bite the nipple. The mother may use a shield for protection, but generally, unless the infant's teeth are erupting, she will not need it. He will release the nipple immediately if his attention is distracted by a caress. The intensity of the urge to find satisfaction through sucking and biting gradually decreases as other gratifications become available.

### Need for Warmth and Comfort

An infant enjoys the warmth and softness of his mother's body when held in her arms. He has a real hunger for this pleasant experience. He enjoys rhythmical rocking, being handled and the comfort of having his position changed.

### Need for Love and Security

Just as the infant becomes hungry, is fed and becomes relaxed, repeating the rhythm over and over, so he needs a rhythm of attention shown in bathing him, riding in the stroller, being played with, being cuddled close to his mother's body and being put to sleep. Throughout these activities of daily living he needs a feeling of security, of being wanted and loved. Infants do not consciously feel apprehension about the future, but their daily care is the basis for either serenity or a tenseness which in an adult we would call apprehension or a state of generalized anxiety.

### METHODS OF MEETING THE NEEDS

Meeting the infant's needs is an interrelated process which begins immediately after birth. The infant's communication with the outside world is normally through his mother. Herein lies the importance of the newborn's rooming-in with his mother.

Breast feeding meets many needs simultaneously. The infant is held close to his mother and has the comfort of feeding in the normal manner, taking as little or as much as he wants of the natural infant food. Many physicians believe that the breast can be given to comfort the infant even if he is not hungry.

If the infant is bottle-fed, he should be held in the same position as the infant at the breast. If the mother accepts the idea of a self-demand schedule (see p. 135), the infant will establish his own feeding rhythm. The holes in the nipple should be of such a size that two or more hours of sucking a day are required for him to take his entire feeding. Bottles should never be propped, because propping does not fulfill the basic needs of an infant.

If his basic needs are met, an infant cannot be spoiled in early infancy. His mother should go to him if he is uncomfortable—wet, cold or tired of lying in the same position. Spoiling does not result from his being kept comfortable, and he needs pleasant experiences in order to learn to trust others.

When the infant has developed to the stage at which he identifies his mother and others who care for him as separate beings, he does not want to be left alone. He needs to have someone look into his room and speak to him frequently until he learns that temporary absence does not mean that the friends in whose presence he feels secure are permanently gone. If he has to endure long periods of separation, he may become chronically afraid that he will be left alone. (The family dog is a poor substitute for human companionship, but better than inanimate toys.) During this period the infant may become very shy and appear insecure and afraid of the world. Sympathetic adults must accept this lack of friendliness and, without forcing their attentions upon him, win his trust in them.

In early infancy the child cannot express his wants, and his mother must anticipate his needs. Later he will convey his wants through movements and sounds. Development of speech is primarily determined by his stage of mental growth and his need to communicate with others. But an important factor, often overlooked, is his mother's response to his coos and babbling. The smiling and cooing of the infant are enormously rewarding to the mother. If she responds by talking to him, showing her appreciation of his achievement in one way or another, he will continue to vocalize and will speak at an early age.

Although the very young infant needs maximum pleasure and minimum discomfort, the older infant needs small doses of anxiety to learn how to handle frustrations and be prepared for the usual problems which every child must meet. If he has not been overprotected, everyday experiences are likely to provide all the frustration he requires to build up his ability to handle successfully the activities of daily living.

## FRUSTRATION OF NEEDS

Some infantile responses persist in adult life, but are modified by the culture of the group. Probably the adult fondness for biting into crisp food and for chewing gum is an infantile pleasure carried over into adult life.

If the child's need for food in infancy is not met, he may exhibit anxiety about eating shown by overeating or not eating enough.

If his need for love and security is not met, the child may doubt his own ability to influence his environment and become insecure in his personal world. He may not be able to take the next steps in personality development. If he does not learn to trust others, he does not merely remain neutral toward them, but rather is likely to be unable to make and hold friends, for he mistrusts them as he learned to mistrust those who cared for him in his early infancy.

## OVERVIEW OF PHYSICAL GROWTH AND DEVELOPMENT

### Principles of Growth and Development

Chapter 2 dealt with the general principles of growth and development. These might be summarized as follows.

1. Development of the human organism is a *continuous process* which begins before birth, each stage of development being dependent upon the preceding stages. A specific example of this would be the development of human dentition (see Fig. 96).

The term *developmental sequence* means that these changes are specific, progressive and orderly and lead eventually to maturity. Each child progresses through similar steps, but the age at which each child achieves these steps varies, since achievement depends upon his inherent maturational capacity interacting with his physical and social environment. It is especially important for nurses to observe *individual differences* in the children under their care in order to meet adequately the needs of each child.

2. The different areas of growth are *interrelated.* By this is meant that all types of growth and development—physical, mental, emotional, social and spiritual—proceed together and in various ways affect each other in the normal advance toward maturity.

Three principles should be stressed in motor development. (*a*) Muscular development is *cephalocaudal,** i.e. proceeding from the head to the feet. The result is that the child acquires the ability to control his neck muscles before those of his legs and feet. (*b*) The development of muscular control is also from *proximal to distal;* i.e. development begins near the body and progresses outward to the extremities. (*c*) The two preceding principles operate in conjunction with development from *general to specific* movement. Muscles controlling gross movements are in general the large muscles proximal to the body. The child uses the larger muscles of the upper arms and legs before he has control of the muscles of the hands and feet, fingers and toes. The infant waves his arms and kicks long before he is able to control the muscles of his fingers in handling anything. Children hold their toys, roll over and sit up before they are able to pick up a crumb as an adult would do.

Tests of motor ability are used as intelligence tests in the young infant, since a child of subnormal mentality is late in sitting, standing, walking and achieving control of the arms and hands in any but gross movements.

* From *kephalos,* Greek for head, and *cauda,* Latin for tail, so called because of the location of the nerve cells of the central nervous system which control muscular activity. Tail is here the equivalent of the lower part of the spinal cord. The feet of an infant having a meningomyelocele in the lumbar region may be paralyzed.

## Basic Factors in Development

Development results from two basic factors—maturation and learning.

*Maturation* refers to the inborn, genetically transmitted capacity for development. This capacity normally covers all areas of development.

*Learning* is the result of experience, experimentation and training. The test of learning is whether it changes the child's behavior. The ability to learn is highly dependent upon the inborn capacity for mental development. If the potential capacity for learning is poor, i.e. if the child has a low intelligence rating or quotient (I.Q.), he will find learning difficult. The child learns from experience that the floor is hard when he falls upon it and that strained fruit tastes good when he is given a spoonful. Later on he learns by experimentation to open and close the door and the easiest way to creep up stairs and back down.

When he has matured to a higher level, he will learn partially from the experience of others, both by observing them and by listening to what they tell him. He has learned that adults know much more than he does and that what they say—in earnest, not in jest—is true. When his mother tells him that the stove is hot and will burn his hand if he touches it, he believes her and usually does not experiment to find out. From a child who describes his stay in a hospital he learns what that child believes hospitalization to be like. When he goes to school, he will learn from the experience of men since man was first upon this earth.

Maturation and learning are interrelated. No learning takes place unless the child is mature enough to be able to understand, and change his behavior. If the child is forced beyond his capacity to learn, unfavorable attitudes may be established which may later retard learning in that area. The child who is not given opportunity to learn by experience and from others at the optimum time—that period in his development when he is best able to learn the particular task—is hindered

**Figure 96.** The development of human dentition is a continuous process from the fifth month in utero to maturity. The deciduous or primary teeth are the darker ones in the illustration. Note the displacement of the deciduous teeth by succedaneous permanent teeth. (Adapted from I. Schour and M. Massler, University of Illinois College of Dentistry.)

Table 2.  *Average Achievement Levels of Infants, 1 Month to 1 Year*

---

### 1 Month

---

*Physical*
  Weight: 8 pounds. Gains about 5 to 7 ounces weekly during first 6 months of life
  Height: Gains approximately 1 inch a month for the first 6 months
  Pulse: 120–150
  Respirations: 30–60

*Motor Control (Figs. 97, 98)*
  Head sags when supported. May lift head from time to time when he is held against his mother's
    shoulder
  Makes crawling movements when prone on a flat surface
  Lifts head intermittently, though unsteadily, when in prone position. Cervical curve begins to develop
    as the infant learns to hold his head erect
  Can turn his head to the side when prone
  Can push with feet against a hard surface to move himself forward
  Has "dance" reflex when held upright with feet touching the bed or examining table
  Shows a well developed tonic neck reflex (head turned to one side, the arm extended on the same side,
    and the other arm flexed to his shoulder)
  Holds hands in fists. Does not reach with hands. Can grasp an object placed in his hand, but drops
    it immediately

*Vision*
  Stares indefinitely at his surroundings and apparently notices faces and bright objects, but only if
    they are in his line of vision. Activity diminishes when he regards a human face
  Can follow an object to the midline of vision

*Vocalization and Socialization*
  Utters small throaty sounds
  Smiles indefinitely
  Shows a vague and indirect regard of faces and bright objects
  Cries when hungry or uncomfortable. Much or all of his crying is tearless

---

in the learning process. An adult in charge of a child for even a short period should consider his interest in learning, his perseverance in carrying out the activity over a period of time, and the progress he makes.

For example, if a mother places her one-month-old infant in a sitting position in a corner of the crib, he will probably fall over because he has not yet matured to the stage at which his muscles can support him in that position. He may be thoroughly frightened by the experience of having lost his balance and fallen. If, however, a mother observes her older infant repeatedly trying to pull himself to a sitting position even though he falls over many times, she should recognize his eagerness to learn and should help him until he is able to sit without support. Thereby she will have helped him in his development by assisting him at the right time and in the right way.

In summary, we may say that the effectiveness of teaching or learning depends upon the child's maturity. His maturity, on the other hand, when tested by his behavior, will be greatly influenced by his opportunities to learn.

### LEVELS AND ACHIEVEMENTS IN GROWTH AND DEVELOPMENT

It is important for the student to review the over-all principles of emotional and physical development in order to understand the specific growth levels and range of achievements typical of infants during their development month by month.

The behavior of infants as it changes with development has been the subject of much research. Developmental schedules (see Table 2 and Figures 97 to 109 on pages 256 to 269) have been derived by taking the average age at which infants achieve certain specific activities. These schedules will probably not be typical of many infants whom the student knows, because they are *aver-*

**Figure 97.** The one-month-old infant. *A*, Shows random, generalized activity in response to stimulation. *B*, Makes crawling movements when prone on a flat surface. Pushes with toes. Holds hands in fists. *C*, Lifts head from the bed a short distance. Can turn head to the side when prone. *D*, Has a well developed tonic neck reflex.

**Figure 98.** The one-month-old infant has a "dance" reflex when held upright with feet touching the bed or examining table.

### 2 Months

*Physical*
  Tears appear
  Posterior fontanel closed
*Motor Control (Fig. 99)*
  Can hold head erect in midposition. Can lift head and chest a short distance above bed or table when lying on his abdomen
  Tonic neck reflex is fading
  Can turn from side to back
  Can hold a rattle for a brief time
*Vision*
  Can follow a moving light or object with his eyes
*Vocalization and Socialization*
  Shows a "social smile" in response to another's smile. This is the beginning of social behavior. It may not appear until the third month
  Has learned that by crying he will get attention. His crying becomes differentiated; the sound of his crying varies with the reason for crying—for instance, hunger, sleepiness or pain
  Pays attention to the speaking voice

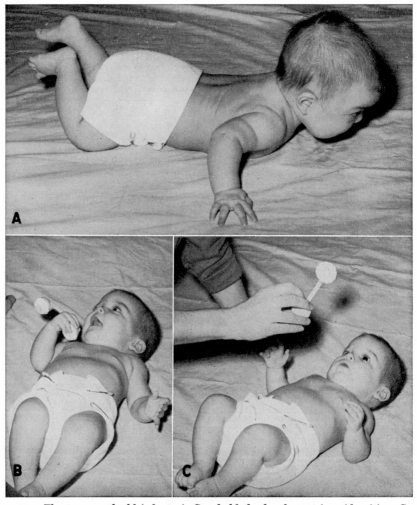

**Figure 99.** The two-month-old infant. *A,* Can hold the head erect in midposition. Can lift the head and chest a short distance above the bed or table when lying on abdomen. *B,* Can hold a rattle for a brief period. *C,* Can follow a moving object with eyes.

**3 Months**

*Physical*
   Weight: 12–13 pounds
*Motor Control (Fig. 100)*
   Holds his hands up in front of him and stares at them
   Plays with hands and fingers
   Reaches for shiny objects, but misses them
   Can carry hand or object to mouth at will
   Holds head erect and steady. Raises chest, usually supported on forearms
   Has lost the walking or dancing reflex
   Grasping reflex has weakened
   Sits, back rounded, knees flexed when supported
*Vision*
   Shows binocular coordination (vertical and horizontal vision) when an object is moved from right
      to left and up and down in front of his face
   Turns eyes to an object in his marginal field of vision
   Voluntarily winks at objects which threaten his eyes
*Vocalization and Socialization*
   Laughs aloud and shows pleasure in making sounds
   Cries less
   Smiles in response to mother's face

**Figure 100.**   The three-month-old infant. *A,* Holds hands up in front and plays with fingers.
*B,* Reaches for a shiny object, but misses it. *C,* Sits with support, back rounded, knees flexed.
*D,* Smiles in response to mother's face and laughs aloud.

**259**

*Table 2.* *Average Achievement Levels of Infants, 1 Month to 1 Year (Continued)*

| 4 Months |
|---|

*Physical*
  Weight: Between 13 and 14 pounds
  Drools between 3 and 4 months of age. This indicates the appearance of saliva. He does not know
    how to swallow saliva, which therefore runs from his mouth
*Motor Control* (*Fig. 101*)
  Symmetrical body postures predominate
  Holds head steady when in sitting position
  Lifts head and shoulders at a 90-degree angle when on abdomen and looks around
  Tries to roll over. Can turn from back to side
  Thumb apposition in grasping occurs between third and fourth months
  Holds hands predominantly open. Activates arms at sight of preferred toy
  Sits with adequate support and enjoys being propped up
  Tonic neck reflex has disappeared
  Sustains portion of own weight
*Vision*
  Recognizes familiar objects
  Stares at rattle placed in his hand and takes it to his mouth
  Follows moving objects well. Even the most difficult types of eye movements are present
  Arms are activated on sight of dangling toy
*Vocalization and Socialization*
  Laughs aloud and smiles in response to smiles of others.
    Initiates social play by smiling
  Vocalizes socially; i.e. he coos and gurgles when talked to.
    He does not cry when scolded. He is very "talkative."
    "Talking" and crying follow each other quickly
  Shows evidence of wanting social attention and of increasing interest in other members of the family.
    Enjoys having people with him

*ages* and therefore do not necessarily apply to any one infant. Few infants are the average for their age in all areas covered by these schedules. Furthermore, there are great individual differences among infants. These schedules will, however, provide a kind of yardstick with which the student can determine in a general way whether individual infants she is caring for are developing according to the usual pattern.

## PLAY

**Purpose.** Infants learn many things through play. In play they practice motor skills, acquire control of the body, gain in general coordination of movements and specific coordination of hand-eye movements. Infants learn to relate to objects and to people, to express their feelings and to work off frustrations through play. Play, then, is all-important in the development of the child's personality; it occupies almost all his waking hours.

Learning to play with things and to amuse himself with his own movements and the sounds he can make begins in infancy. Later on in childhood he learns to play with other children. This, it is said, lays the foundation for adult ability to work well with others.

Although the general purposes of play are the same for all infants, each infant discovers how to use a particular toy or game for his own purposes. Thus play is an individual matter. Not all children learn in the same way from playing, because each infant's or little child's play is a result of his own need at the time. For this reason, play should be self-directed. Adults, through their interest in a child's development, are apt to overdirect his play activity.

**Selection of Play Materials.** The variety of toys generally listed as suitable for children of any age group is based on the assumption of normal growth and

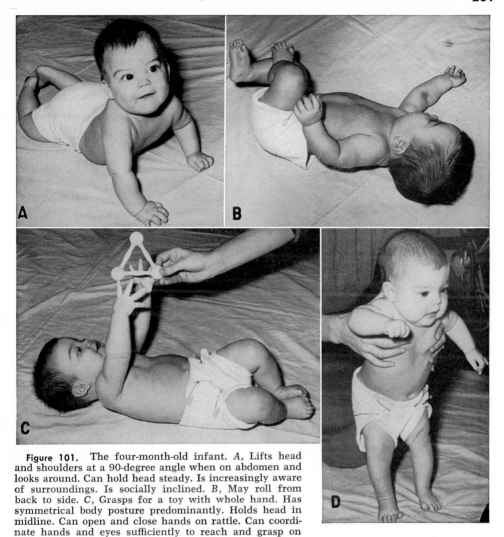

**Figure 101.** The four-month-old infant. *A,* Lifts head and shoulders at a 90-degree angle when on abdomen and looks around. Can hold head steady. Is increasingly aware of surroundings. Is socially inclined. *B,* May roll from back to side. *C,* Grasps for a toy with whole hand. Has symmetrical body posture predominantly. Holds head in midline. Can open and close hands on rattle. Can coordinate hands and eyes sufficiently to reach and grasp on sight. *D,* Sustains part of own weight when held.

development in the child to whom the toy is to be given. The nurse, knowing the characteristics of growth and development of each age level, will select from the toys suitable for the age group the ones best adapted to a particular child's needs, for he may be advanced or retarded for his age.

Selection is important, for toys have many functions; i.e. toys help children to learn different things in different ways. An essential factor in the selection of a toy is that it be safe for the child's use. This, in general, depends on his level of growth and development, but varies with his physical condition and other individual characteristics. Some children are more cautious than others. This may be due to slow or rapid development, but also to specific experiences from which a child has learned to be careful when trying out a new use for toys. It is never safe to give toys designed for older children to infants. For instance, the small plastic parts which (*text continued on page* 270)

**Table 2.** *Average Achievement Levels of Infants, 1 Month to 1 Year (Continued)*

---

### 5 Months

*Physical*
  Weight: Twice the birth weight (15–16 pounds)
*Motor Control (Fig. 102)*
  Sits with slight support. Holds back straight when pulled to sitting position
  Can use thumb in partial apposition to fingers more skilfully
  Can balance head well
  Reaches for objects which are beyond his grasp. Grasps objects independently of direct stimulation
    of the palm of the hand (partial grasp). Grasps with the whole hand. Accepts an object handed
    to him
  Has completely lost the Moro reflex
*Vocalization and Socialization*
  Vocalizes his displeasure when a desired object is taken from him

---

**Figure 102.** The five-month-old infant. *A,* Reaches and grasps objects with the whole hand and carries them to mouth. *B,* Holds back straight when pulled to a sitting position. Continues to drool.

---

### 6 Months

*Physical*
  Gains about 3 to 5 ounces weekly during the second 6 months of life
  Grows about ½ inch a month
  Is teething. Teeth begin to grow in the jaw in the fifth prenatal month. The first of the 20 temporary
    or deciduous teeth erupt between the fifth and eighth months of life. These are usually lower in-
    cisors. (As a rule the lower incisors erupt before the upper ones.) Teething may incite irritability
    and anorexia, but not an elevation of temperature or convulsions
*Motor Control (Fig. 103)*
  Sits momentarily without support if placed in a favorable leaning position
  Grasps with simultaneous flexion of fingers
  Retains transient hold on 2 blocks, one in either hand
  Pulls himself up to a sitting position
  Completely turns over from stomach to stomach with rest periods during the complete turn. This
    ability is important in protecting him from falling out of bed
  Springs up and down when sitting
  Bangs with object held in his hand, rattle or spoon
  Hitches. Hitching is locomotion backward when in a sitting position. Movement of the body is aided
    by use of his arms and hands. This ability is usually present by the sixth month

*Vocalization and Socialization*

Babbles from the third to the eighth month

Vocalizes several well defined syllables. Actively vocalizes pleasure with crowing or cooing. Babbling is not linked with specific objects, people or situations

Cries easily on slight provocation (change of position or withdrawal of a toy)

Thrashes arms and legs when frustrated

Begins to recognize strangers (fifth to sixth month)

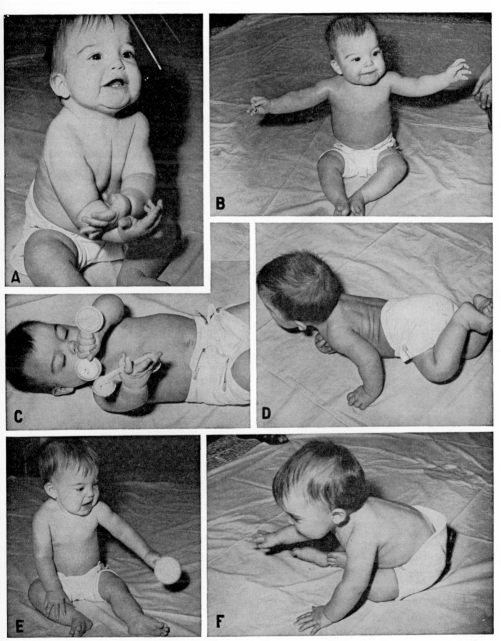

**Figure 103.** The six-month-old infant. *A*, Has 2 lower central incisors. *B*, Sits momentarily without support. Holds arms out for balance. *C*, Retains transient hold on 2 objects. Grasps with flexion of fingers. *D*, Turns completely over. *E*, Bangs with a rattle held in hand. Balances well by leaning forward slightly on one or both hands. *F*, Can hitch. Moves backward in a sitting position by using arms and hands to push.

*Table 2.    Average Achievement Levels of Infants, 1 Month to 1 Year (Continued)*

| 7 Months |
| --- |

*Motor Control (Fig. 104)*
> When lying down, lifts head as if he were trying to sit up
> Sits briefly, leaning forward on his hands. Control of trunk is more advanced
> Plays with his feet and puts them in his mouth
> Bounces actively when held in a standing position
> Can approach a toy and grasp it with one hand
> Can transfer a toy from one hand to the other with varying degrees of success
> Rolls more easily from back to stomach

*Vocalization and Socialization*
> Vocalizes his eagerness
> Vocalizes "m-m-m" when crying
> Makes polysyllabic vowel sounds
> Emotional development, 7 to 8 months: Shows fear of strangers.
> Emotional instability shown by easy and quick changes from crying to laughing

**Figure 104.**   The seven-month-old infant. *A*, Bounces actively when held in standing position. Can support a larger portion of own weight for a longer time. *B*, Can approach a toy and grasp it with one hand.

**Table 2.    Average Achievement Levels of Infants, 1 Month to 1 Year (Continued)**

### 8 Months

*Motor Control* (*Fig. 105*)
    Sits alone steadily
    Complete thumb apposition *prhension*
    Hand-eye coordination is perfected to the point that random reaching and grasping no longer persist
*Vocalization and Socialization*
    Greets strangers with coy or bashful behavior, turning away, hanging his head, crying or even scream-
        ing, and refuses to play with strangers or even accept toys from them
    Shows nervousness with strangers
    Emotional development: "Eight months' anxiety" is to be distinguished from anaclitic depression (see
        p. 272 ). "Eight months' anxiety" occurs between the sixth and eighth months as a result of the
        child's increased capacity for discriminating between friend and stranger
    Affection or love of family group appears
        Emotional instability still shown by easy changes from laughing to crying
        Stretches arm to loved adult as in invitation to come

**Figure 105.**    The eight-month-old infant. *A,* Sits alone steadily. Has increased interest in activity in environment. *B,* "Eight months' anxiety." Greets stranger by turning away and crying.

**Table 2.   Average Achievement Levels of Infants, 1 Month to 1 Year (Continued)**

**9 Months**

*Motor Control (Fig. 106)*

Shows good coordination and sits alone

Holds his bottle with good hand-mouth coordination. Can put the nipple in and out of his mouth at will

Preference for the use of one hand is marked

Crawls instead of hitching. Crawling may be seen as early as the fourth month; the average age is about nine months. In crawling the infant is prone, his abdomen touching the floor, his head and shoulders supported with the weight borne on the elbows. The body is pulled along by the movement of the arms while the legs drag. The leg movements may resemble swimming or kicking movements

Creeps. This is a more advanced type of locomotion than crawling. The trunk is carried above the floor, but parallel to it. The infant uses both his hands and knees in propelling himself forward. Not all infants follow this pattern of hitching, crawling and creeping. Different children stress different means of locomotion and may even skip a stage. (This is particularly likely to occur if an infant is sick or for some other reason is unable to practice moving about)

Raises himself to a sitting position. Requires help to pull self to feet

*Vocalization and Socialization*

Shows the beginning of imitative expression. Sounds stand for things to him. Says "Da-da" or some such expression

Responds to adult anger. Cries when scolded

**Figure 106.**   The nine-month-old infant. *A*, Holds own bottle with good hand-mouth coordination. Can put the nipple in and out of mouth at will. *B*, Can creep. Carries trunk above the floor, but parallel to it. Uses both hands and knees in propelling self forward. *C*, Can pull self to feet if assisted.

*Motor Control* (*Fig. 107*)

Sits steadily for an indefinite time. Does not enjoy lying down unless he is sleepy

Makes early stepping movements when held

Pulls himself to his feet, holding to the crib rail or similar support. (This is a good time to begin the use of the play pen or yard)

Creeps and cruises about very well. (Cruising is walking sideways while holding on to a supporting object with both hands)

Can pick up objects fairly well and pokes them with his fingers

Feeds himself a cracker or some such food which he can hold in his hand

Is able crudely to release a toy

Can bring his hands together

*Vocalization and Socialization*

Says one or two words and imitates an adult's inflection

Pays attention to his name

Plays simple games as bye-bye and pat-a-cake (motor control is such that he can bring his hands together) and peek-a-boo

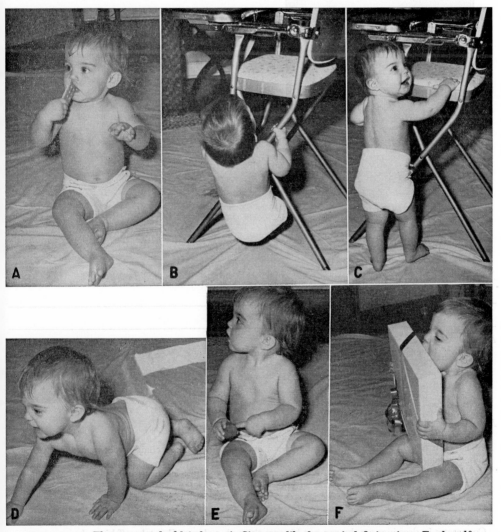

**Figure 107.** The ten-month-old infant. *A*, Sits steadily for an indefinite time. Feeds self a cracker. *B*, Pulls self to feet, holding on to legs of chair or similar support. *C*, Cruises or walks sideways around furniture while holding on to supporting object with both hands. *D*, Creeps well. *E*, Can pick up objects fairly well and pokes them with finger. *F*, Plays peek-a-boo over top of box.

**11 Months**

*Motor Control* (*Fig. 108*)
    Stands erect with the help of his mother's hand or supporting himself by holding on to some object as the side of his play yard

**Figure 108.** The eleven-month-old infant stands erect with the help of mother's hand.

**12 Months**

*Physical*
    Weight: Three times his birth weight (21–22 pounds)
    Height: 29 inches
    Head and chest are equal in circumference
    Has six teeth
    Pulse: 100–140 per minute
    Respirations: 20–40 per minute
*Motor Control* (*Fig. 109*)
    Stands for a moment alone, or possibly longer
    Walks with help. Cruises, walking sideways around chairs or from chair to chair, holding on with one hand
    Lumbar curve and the compensating dorsal curve develop as he learns to walk
    Can sit down from standing position without help
    Holds a crayon adaptively to make a stroke and can mark on a piece of paper
    Can pick up small bits of food and transfer them to his mouth. Can drink from a cup and eat from a spoon, but requires help. He likes to eat with his fingers
    Cooperates in dressing; e.g. he can put his arm through a sleeve. Can take off his socks

*Vocalization and Socialization*
Can say two words besides "Mama" and "Dada"
Slow vocabulary growth, as a rule, owing to his interest in walking
Knows his own name
Uses expressive jargon. Communicates with himself and those around him
Inhibits simple acts on command. Recognizes the meaning of "No, no"
Shows jealousy, affection, anger and other emotions. He may cry for affection. He loves an audience,
    and will repeat a performance which brings a response. Crying is more often associated with irri-
    tation or frustration than it formerly was. Stiffens in resistance
Loves rhythms
Still egocentric, concerned only with himself

**Figure 109.** The twelve-month-old infant. *A*, Stands alone for a moment or possibly longer.
*B*, Walks with help. *C*, Holds a crayon adaptively to make a stroke and can mark on a piece of
paper. *D*, Cooperates in dressing. Puts arm through sleeve.

an older boy uses in building a toy car would not be suitable for an infant, for he would put them in his mouth and might easily swallow or even aspirate them.

Toys should be washable, durable, easily handled, not too heavy, and smooth with rounded edges and no sharp points. Children enjoy gaily colored toys. If the toy is painted, it should be with nonlead paint. The size of the toy should be appropriate to the use the child will make of it. An infant's toy should be well constructed even though it will cost more than the ten-cent-store type. For instance, a rattle should be one the infant cannot break when he bangs it against the rail of his crib or on the tray of his chair. If it broke, he might pick up and swallow some of the pebbles it contained.

A toy should be one which has many uses for the individual child. It is difficult to predict to what uses he may put it, and his creative ability should be encouraged. But safety factors must be considered. Blocks are meant for building, but the infant may throw them. For this reason they should be made of some rubberlike substance so that he can hurt neither himself nor another child. These he can place together, clap together or toss as he happens to fancy. Cuddly toys can be used in many ways besides being cuddled at bedtime. They can be dropped, dragged along or sat upon. Many adults do not understand that the infant may use a toy for its express purpose and also for whatever other use he desires. They bring pressure upon the child to use a toy as an older child would do or even to watch them use it, withholding the toy if the child grasps for it.

**Play Responses during Infancy.** Toys to be used during the first year must be very simple. The infant's attention span is short. They must be easy to handle, not too large, yet large enough so that the infant cannot swallow or aspirate them, since he puts toys of all kinds in his mouth.

*Birth to Five Months.* An early type of motor play is for exercise, but it is also thoroughly enjoyable to the infant.

He reaches for objects and attempts to turn from back to side. He kicks, wiggles and plays with his hands.

*Five to Eight Months.* At this age the infant still finds pleasure in motor activity for its own sake. He plays with his feet, bounces his body, shakes his head, leans against objects when learning to sit, grasps at anything he can reach and moves on the floor or in his play yard by hitching. He usually plays contentedly by himself during the first six months. By seven months he enjoys company, but is still happy when playing alone with his toys. He likes to explore his hands and feet and talks to himself. He enjoys his bath when he is free from the restraint of clothing and can move his body easily. He happily responds to his mother's movements.

*Eight to Ten Months.* Motor activity is still the infant's chief source of play. He kicks his legs. Now that he can sit alone he likes to lean over the side of his carriage or the arm of his chair. He plays with his toes and rolls with ease. He crawls, creeps or pulls himself into a sitting position and stretches to get toys which are out of his reach. He transfers a toy from one hand to the other and puts the toy in his mouth. He has learned where the toy goes when he drops it over the edge of the crib or the tray when he is sitting in his high chair, and looks down at it.

*Ten to Eleven Months.* The child still plays alone for relatively long periods, but lets the family know when he wants their company or the stimulus of having another toy. His play is becoming more highly developed. He plays in a sitting position, creeps about, pokes objects with his fingers and enjoys pulling himself up to a standing position.

*Twelve Months.* Now the child plays with several toys, picking them up and dropping them. He can play simple games such as grasping a ball and letting it go, and will take or give a toy on request or gesture. He greatly enjoys walking with help.

**Toys for Infants.** Suggested toys include large wooden beads and spools

**Figure 110.** The one-year-old child plays simple games such as grasping a ball and letting it go.

strung on a cord or shoe string, rattles, soft toys (not fuzzy) of different shapes, balls and large or small blocks.

## EFFECTS OF SEPARATION FROM PARENTS

**Factors in Development of the Child.** It may be said that the kind of person the infant will become depends in part upon the characteristics of his parents, their relations to each other and the emotional atmosphere of the home in general. Their attitude toward the infant is of fundamental importance. He may receive from them a feeling of love and peace, or they may communicate to him their own feelings of anxiety and insecurity. Another important factor is the infant's place in the family—whether he is an only child or the youngest child, the middle child or one of the middle children or the eldest child.

The socio-economic and cultural backgrounds of the family influence his development through their effects upon his physical and social environment. The physical histories of the family and of the child himself are also important.

Among the significant developments in psychiatry in recent years has been the increasing awareness that the kind of parental care given during infancy and early childhood is of great importance to the child's future mental and physical health.

During infancy and early childhood he should have an intimate, warm and continuous relationship with his mother or permanent mother-substitute in whom he finds happiness. In such a situation the basis for mental ill health characterized by excessive anxiety and feelings of guilt is not likely to develop.

**Maternal Deprivation.** Maternal deprivation is the term used for an infant's lack of this warm relationship. The condition occurs (1) when the mother cannot give loving care even though the infant lives with her or (2) when the child is removed from his mother's care, is hospitalized or institutionalized, or remains in the home while she is absent.

There are various degrees of deprivation. In a situation of *incomplete* or *partial deprivation* the infant or young child may show acute anxiety, a feeling of wanting to strike back or revenge himself, at the same time experiencing an excessive need for love and affection. Later in childhood, as a result of his experience, he may show depression or evidence a feeling similar to an adult's feeling of guilt because of his revengeful and attacking attitude in infancy. In *complete* or *total deprivation* the infant may become permanently incapable of forming normal relations with others.

Since the infant learns to know his mother as a person when five or six months old and to recognize and fear strangers when seven to eight months old, he should have his mother or a permanent substitute to care for him and be near him during the first year of life.

If a child is deprived of a mother's care, his personality structure will be underdeveloped. He will not have had an opportunity to identify with a loving person. He will be under severe emotional stress with or without physical stress.

Although deprivation is serious at any time during infancy, the effects of deprivation differ if it occurs in the first or the second half of the first year. The first period is from birth to six months of age. Deprivation is one of the greatest problems in the care of infants in foundling homes or during long-term hospitalization. The second period is during the last six months of his first year. Since the infant has learned to recognize his mother as a person and has become apprehensive in the presence of strangers, the results of maternal deprivation can be seen especially in infants hospitalized for long periods of time.

*Deprivation in the First Six Months.* Infants of this age have inadequate psychic and physical development to adjust to an impersonal sort of care given by a succession of kindly, competent persons who do not love him as they would their own infants. Infants deprived of maternal care by their own mothers or by an adequate mother-substitute lack all that goes with love and seldom receive sufficient stimulation to promote normal development. In foundling homes they become emotionally isolated from adults, and their activity is likely to be restricted. They generally show signs of retarded mental development even if they receive the best possible physical care.

The result of such care in foundling homes is evident in the infant's behavior. The young infant may cry a great deal. He may not gain weight as he should, and his motor development is likely to be poor, since he is seldom handled or taken from his crib. Gradually he will refuse contact with adults. He will lose weight, and his sleep pattern will be altered. He will develop a rigid facial expression. He has poor resistance and is liable to contract infections readily. After a few months he will become completely passive and eventually appear retarded. He may make bizarre finger movements. The incidence of marasmus and the death rate are relatively high among these children.

Prevention of maternal deprivation in foundling homes is almost impossible. Foster home care should be provided in the earliest months of infancy, and the child should remain in the same home with his loving, permanent mother-substitute. If foster home care is impossible—it is difficult to find enough homes for these infants—a permanent mother-substitute should be provided in the foundling home. She should be chosen from among the nursing personnel and should have a limited number of infants to care for so that she can give them individual attention. She must communicate to each child that he is loved and wanted.

An infant hospitalized because of a congenital deformity or illness may exhibit the same symptoms as the infant in a foundling home if warm, affectionate care is not provided by a substitute mother. Such care is often more difficult to provide in a hospital than in a foundling home because of the constant change in the nursing personnel (both student nurses and auxiliary personnel) and also because the more acutely ill infants need more than their proportionate share of attention. An adequate, stable graduate nurse staff is essential on the pediatric unit if these children are to receive continuous loving care. Volunteers may serve successfully as mother-substitutes, but the time they can spend with each infant is generally limited.

*Deprivation during the Second Six Months.* This is the period when *anaclitic depression* occurs. It results from a change in the infant's life, from the warm relations with his mother and family to a situation in which he is one of a group of infants who do not receive continuous loving care from their mothers or a mother-substitute.

The result is that the infants become

depressed, cry a great deal and look sad, and are withdrawn in their relations with adults caring for them. This is in decided contrast to their previous happy, outgoing behavior. They may refuse to eat. If deprivation continues more than three months, the constant crying subsides. Their sad expression is replaced by a rigid facial expression. They may suffer anorexia and sleep disturbances. It may become difficult and eventually almost impossible for nurses to establish contact with them.

If the child is restored to his mother within three months, recovery may be rapid, although psychic recovery may never be complete. If deprivation continues, recovery becomes increasingly difficult and less likely to be complete.

*Treatment to Prevent Anaclitic Depression.* After six months of age the normal infant takes the initiative and seeks adult contact. He needs a room where he can creep and cruise around unrestrainedly. In institutions, if such a room is provided, it will probably be overcrowded. Infants of this age like to see other infants, but are not sufficiently mature to enjoy active interaction with each other, and so they gain very little from the experience. They need space for motor activity and for investigation of their environment. Above all, they need the continuous warm affection of a mother-substitute who gives them individual attention. If these two requirements are fulfilled, they may continue to be essentially normal infants, but if these requirements are not fulfilled, the infants will probably become depressed and unloving.

**Summary and Conclusions.** Although the probable results of extreme deprivation are those which have just been described, some infants who have lacked their mother's love for any of a number of reasons appear to suffer little permanent personality damage. The reason for this is not clearly understood. It must be remembered that each infant's environment is influenced by his characteristics. It is likely that the environment of infants in a hospital differs from that in a foundling home, and in many homes even more so. Though it should not be so, a pretty child who was friendly before separation from his mother and is shy, but not afraid, among strangers is apt to evoke a warm relation from those who care for him. His life is likely to be different from that of the child who, on entrance to the institution, was withdrawn from the personnel, not making friends or responding to their friendly advances. The personnel of an institution, whether for foundlings or for sick infants, are human and likely to be very different in their treatment of the likable and unlikable infants.

To fulfill the function of her profession, every nurse should provide for all children under her care the kind of warm, loving care which children need to prevent them from suffering the extreme effects of maternal deprivation.

**Foundlings and Adoptions.** In the foregoing discussion the term "foundling home" was used. A *foundling* is an infant abandoned by its parents and found by others. In former years, when infants eligible for adoption far exceeded the number of adoptions, many foundlings remained in institutions under the auspices of religious, public or charitable organizations for long periods. Today such infants in general are adopted, since the demand for infants eligible for adoption exceeds the supply. Although time must elapse between the finding of an infant and his legal adoption, he may be given temporarily to the future adoptive parents through a legally approved organization. Adoptive parents, as a rule, want to take the infant when he is only a few weeks old. Thus few foundlings, if they are normal infants, remain in institutions.

Homes for infants retain the word "foundling," since they were incorporated when in fact they did care for foundlings and because they still receive infants deserted by their parents and care for them until adopted. In general, the infants and children in these homes today are illegitimate children whose mothers surrendered them to the institutions at birth and who are there only until adopted. Today infants who are in a children's home for a long time are those whose parents are unable to care for them or are not considered by the court to provide a suitable home for them. Such children generally come from homes where both the physical and the social conditions are poor, though the mothers might have had loving relations with the infants. It is these infants, rather than foundlings, who constitute the great problem of the institutionalized child.

Aid for dependent children under the Social Security Act has resulted in relatively few infants and children being institutionalized because of the death of one or both parents.

## INFANT CARE

### Planning Daily Care of the Infant

Every infant is an individual with his own needs, and each member of the family—mother, father and siblings—has his individual needs. The plan for the infant's care must take into consideration ways of adjusting all these common and conflicting needs. Parents should not feel that they must compulsively give up their whole lives for their infant. If they do, their care of the child may ultimately lack spontaneity and warmth.

The natural rhythms of a normal infant and of the particular infant must be considered—whether he is to be on a self-demand schedule or on one which is planned for him.

These rhythms will change as the infant grows older. His pattern of sleeping and waking and his periods of playful exercise will alter. The parents have schedules which their activities require them to follow and with which the infant's schedule is interrelated. Both parents should plan to spend some time with the infant in the evening, and this requires a corresponding arrangement of his periods of sleep.

If the mother does her own housework and is not employed outside the home, she is able to spend considerable time with the baby, at periods which best fit into her schedule. But if she works outside the home, it may be necessary to adapt his schedule to the hours when she is free to be with him. If there are siblings in the home, her activities must be adapted to their needs also. She and her husband should spend some time with the siblings without the infant being present to distract the parents' attention from the other children. This is important in the prevention of sibling jealousy of the infant and in their acceptance of their status as older than he. Older siblings should realize that they are given prerogatives which he does not receive, just as he receives attentions which are not given them.

As the infant shifts to having three meals a day with nourishment such as orange juice between meals, he may gradually be included in the family group at meal times.

It is important to remember that there is no set pattern of daily care for all infants, since their needs vary from month to month, and the family situation of each differs from that of the others.

### Carrying the Infant

The technique of carrying the infant is based on his anatomic structure and motor ability. His head is large in proportion to his body, and he is unable to hold his head erect without support until he is about three months old. The shoulders and back must be supported at first because of weakness. If the student remembers these two facts, lifting and carrying the infant will be comfortable and safe for him and easy for her. Different techniques for carrying infants have been given descriptive titles, such as the cradle technique—holding the infant to the nurse's or mother's shoulder—and the football hold. Each technique has its special use.

The *cradle technique* is commonly used in lifting, turning and carrying the little infant. The nurse or mother grasps the child's feet with her right hand (in order not to press the ankle bones together she keeps her index finger between the ankles), slides her left hand and arm under the infant's back, giving support to the buttocks, back and head. She then releases the feet and brings her right hand up and under the buttocks, while she moves her left arm and hand up to give greater support to the head, shoulders and back. She then raises the infant so that he is cradled in her arms, his body against her chest.

If the nurse or mother holds him in an upright position, on her shoulder, her left forearm is under his buttocks, his body pressed against her chest and shoulder and his cheek resting slightly over her shoulder. Support for his back and head is given with her other hand. If for a moment she must use her right hand, as in opening a door, she should bend her body backward so that his body is pressed against hers by gravity and he lies there without a sense of loss of support.

Fig. 111                    Fig. 112

Figure 111.   A modified cradle position. The young infant's head and back must be supported adequately.

Figure 112.   The infant may be held upright against the shoulder. The head must be supported until the infant is able to do so by himself.

Figure 113.   Football hold. A, Front view. B, Side view.

The *football hold* is useful in washing the infant's head over a basin or making the crib while holding the infant. His hips are supported in the bend of the nurse's or mother's arm, with the forearm and hand supporting his back and head. This frees her other hand and is therefore a convenient way of carrying an infant.

### Bathing

The purpose of the bath is not only cleanliness, but also to give the infant a chance to exercise without clothing and, if he is put in a tub of water, to kick and splash. It is a time for mother or nurse to talk to him and play with him. It provides her with an opportunity to note his growth and development and to observe his body for evidence of rash or chafing.

The time when the bath is given makes little difference and can be whenever the mother or nurse finds it most convenient. The bath should not be given within one hour after the infant has been fed, however. It should have a regular place in the day's schedule of care and should never be given when the mother is tired or the infant fretful. The modern father bathes the infant now and then in order to learn to know him better and to give him the same sense of being loved and cared for by his father that he has from his mother.

For the procedure of the bath, see page 136. The infant may have a sponge bath in bed or be bathed in a tub. A tub-stand combination constructed for the purpose of infant bathing may be used if the parents can afford it. The tub cover has straps which buckle over the infant's chest so that the mother can change the infant's diaper and wash his buttocks without fear of his falling. When using this equipment, the mother may have difficulty in transferring the infant from the table to the tub. The equipment for bathing the infant should be conveniently near and everything required in readiness so that the mother will not have to leave him.

Safety factors must be kept in mind when bathing the growing infant; precautions to safeguard him and to avoid fear are necesary. It is important, also, that the infant learn to like his bath. If he is immersed in the tub too quickly or does not feel that he is held securely, he may stiffen and appear startled. If this happens, he may acquire an adverse attitude toward his bath. The nurse or mother should place him in the tub very gently. She should hold him with his head and shoulders on her forearm and her hand grasping his opposite arm. He should not be soaped too liberally, since it is then difficult to retain a firm hold upon his body and limbs. He would be frightened if he were allowed to slip or if his face were covered with water.

An infant or little child should never be left alone in a tub of water even if he is old enough to sit up and hold on to the sides of the tub. It is not safe to give him a powder can to play with even if it appears to be empty, for he may inhale a little of the powder left in the bottom of the can if he shakes it vigorously.

### Clothing

Various kinds of sleeping garments are used for infants. Many mothers like to put a nightgown on the infant when he is old enough to kick the covers off. If the gown is open at the bottom and all down the back, the sides should be folded so that he does not lie upon the gown and wet it when he voids. If there is a drawstring through the hem and the gown is partially closed at the back, the drawstring can be tightened so that the gown covers his feet, but there must be room for him to kick unrestrainedly. As the infant grows older and becomes more active, he needs pajamas or sleepers with feet. The two-piece type saves laundry and time, since it is necessary to change only the lower half when he soils the garment.

A sleeping bag or garment made of blanket material like a loose, long, full-sleeved kimona with the bottom sewed up and closed with a zipper in front is useful for keeping the infant covered.

It should be large enough for him to move freely within it. The neck should be loose so as not to bind the infant when he turns.

When the infant learns to creep or move around freely, his clothes should be loose in the crotch and the arm-holes. Overalls will protect his legs when he creeps. They should be open in the crotch so that the diaper may be easily changed. Sunsuits are excellent in summer weather.

Shoes should be soft until the child walks. They are needed only to protect his feet when he crawls and, later, creeps. If the floor covering is warm, smooth and clean, he should be allowed to go barefoot. Crawling and creeping exercise the foot muscles. Socks are generally worn under the shoes and should be at least ½ inch longer than the infant's feet. Infants' feet grow quickly, and unless the socks are ample in size when bought, they will soon be too small. They should not be used if they cramp the child's toes.

## Fresh Air and Sunshine

The infant should be outdoors as much as possible. He should be dressed according to the weather. When the day is warm enough, an infant of three or four weeks may be given a brief sun bath. Such baths are desirable even if he is outdoors a great deal and is kept in a sunny room when indoors, since ultraviolet rays are destroyed by window glass, clothing and the dust and smoke in the atmosphere. The infant's first exposure to the sun should be for only three to five minutes, and only the face and hands should be exposed. Both the time of exposure and the area exposed are gradually increased until the skin of the body and limbs is pig-mented. Sun baths should be given before 11 a.m. or after 3 p.m. The in-fant should be placed with his feet away from the sun and his eyes and head protected from the glare. Deep burning is harmful to the child. The objective of sun baths is to acquire an even tan. While having his sun baths

he should continue to take vitamin D in a standard vitamin preparation.

## Exercise

An infant gets exercise in a number of ways. He is active at bath time when he kicks and squirms without the re-straint of clothing. Mere change of posi-tion is a form of exercise. When he is old enough to turn over—and later play in his play yard—his clothes should not restrict his movements. He should have toys which encourage movement.

## Sleep

The greater part of a young infant's time is spent in sleep. He needs rest for his rapid growth and his energy output. The amount of sleep he takes depends upon his needs, which vary from day to day. If he is given the opportunity, he will develop his own schedule.

The position in which an infant is placed for sleep is important. As soon as he can move his head from side to side to prevent his nose from being pressed against the surface on which he lies, it is safe to place him on either his back or his abdomen. The danger of sleeping on his back is that he may vomit and aspirate fluid. In general, ly-ing on his side is preferred for comfort and safety.

Signs of increasing maturity in rela-tion to sleep are a reduction in the total sleeping time and longer intervals between sleeping periods. Although each infant varies from any standard or norm, eighteen to twenty hours of sleep a day is typical during the first few months of life. At 3 months the usual amount of sleep in a 24-hour period is about 16 hours. He will often sleep throughout the night. At six months the average amount of sleep is about twelve hours at night and three to four hours during the day. The num-ber of naps and their length vary with the individual infant. At one year of age he sleeps about fourteen hours out of the twenty-four. At this age he is fear-ful of leaving his mother and of being deserted by her. He should not be put to bed and immediately left alone in the dark. A soft light is often used to make the situation more familiar. A child of this age should have one or two naps a day.

**Promotion of Sleep and Care after Wakening.** Overstimulation should be avoided before bedtime. The infant should be dry and comfortable. All his toys should be removed. Quieting activities should be provided, such as rocking him or singing to him.

The environment should be suited to his needs, one of which is a room of his own. Twilight is preferable to either a bright light or darkness. The light, even if dimmed, should not shine directly in his eyes.

The temperature of the room should be such that the infant is neither chilled nor overheated. A suitable temperature in the day would be 70 to 75° F. and at night 60 to 65° F. The room should be well ventilated, but there must be no drafts. Screens should be used to cut off unavoidable drafts, but blankets should not be hung over the sides of the crib, since they may fall over the infant and smother him.

The mattress should be firm and completely covered with heavy plastic material. A small piece of light plastic material should not be used under the sheet. Should the infant pull the sheet from the bed, he might be covered with the plastic, which could cut off his supply of air. Pillows are not used, since there is danger of the infant's burying his face in a pillow or having it fall on his face. In either case he might be suffocated. He should lie on a flat surface, since this is best for his bone development.

Since an infant is not old enough to tell how he feels, his mother should observe for signs and symptoms of discomfort and illness. The infant's color is a good indication of his condition. His eyes should be clear and bright. When tired, he should fall asleep without fretting.

After the infant has wakened the window shades should be pulled so that the room is light, and he should be given a toy. The older infant should have his face washed to give him a feeling of freshness.

*Safety Measures*

**Importance of Accident Prevention.** Since accidents are a major cause of death of infants and children of all ages, great emphasis should be placed on accident prevention. Nurses and mothers must consider the child's interests and the hazards resulting from the activities into which his interests lead him. The protection and education needed by each sex and age group are then adapted to the prevention of accidents to which they are most liable. Health education given during the prenatal period and while mothers are in the obstetrical unit should not frighten them. Rather it should be constructive, not listing all possible dangers to which a child might be subjected, but emphasizing reasonable precautions against the hazards he is likely to encounter in the near future. Accident prevention education should be given slowly to parents and to children.

It may sound ridiculous to speak of teaching accident prevention to an infant. What is meant, of course, is merely that he becomes accustomed to the safety measures which he is taught, and learns what he may not do through such simple injunctions as "No, no." As he passes from the toddler into the preschool age simple explanations can be given. He should learn to exercise caution, because he may be hurt if he does not. A certain degree of fear of being hurt is normal and is the logical reason for caution. Health hazards tend to lessen as the child goes to school and later enters adolescence, but accident hazards increase. Accident prevention is taught in the schoolroom and on playgrounds. Accidents common to each age group will be mentioned in this text in their appropriate place.

**Specific Safety Measures.** Safety factors during the bath, in relation to toys or clothes and in the selection of furniture have already been discussed.

The infant's bed should not be placed near a radiator, since he may burn his hand if he touches it when reaching through the bars of his crib. Safety pins should always be closed and removed from the crib; they should never be stuck in the mattress or left in a receptacle or cake of soap (soap is sometimes used to lubricate the point of a safety pin so that it goes through the thick layers of diaper more readily).

Since an infant puts everything within his reach into his mouth, small articles should not be left in his crib or close to his chair. Articles which frequently are aspirated are beads, coins, peanuts, and the like. Even an infant too young to roll may move himself upward by pushing with his feet. For this reason he should never be left unprotected on a bed or a stand. If the mother or nurse must reach for some equipment, she must keep one hand on the infant.

All toys and infant furniture should carry a guarantee that no paint containing lead or other poisonous substance was used. The infant would ingest such substances when he licked and chewed his toys or the bars of his play yard or crib.

When the infant is old enough to creep on the floor, all electrical outlets which he can reach should be covered. Tablecloths which hang over the edge of the table should not be used, since the toddler or even the infant who creeps about will pull on them. This will carry anything on the table—hot foods, for example—over the edge, spilling the contents on the floor and possibly upon the child, or hitting him as they fall. Adults with a baby in arms should not walk on a slippery floor or where toys or other small articles have been left on the floor. It is difficult to regain balance after stumbling with an infant in one's arms.

## INFANT FEEDING AND NUTRITION

Feeding of the newborn was discussed in Chapter 7. The infant will continue to feed from the breast or bottle until he is weaned, at which time he will learn to drink from a cup. Mothers who breast-feed their infants may want to give them experience in the use of a bottle, giving them water, a formula or orange juice in this way. If an emergency arises and breast feeding must be discontinued, his acceptance of the bottle is helpful both to him and to those who care for him.

Table 3 gives the nutritional requirements of infants under one year of age.

### Addition of Other Foods and Substances to the Diet

When the infant is two weeks old, he is ready for other foods to be added to his milk diet. The reasons for this are that (1) he needs a nutritionally complete diet, and (2) he should become accustomed at an early age to various tastes and textures of food. Infants under five or six months of age accept new foods easily, but after that age they may begin to resist new tastes and textures. For this reason it is well to offer the infant a wide variety of new foods.

**Figure 114.** The mother may want to give her infant experience in sucking from a bottle even though it is usually breast fed.

Table 3. Recommended Daily Dietary Allowances for Infants 1 to 12 Months of Age*

|  | 1–6 Months | 7–12 Months |
|---|---|---|
| Calories | Kg. × 120 | Kg. × 100 |
| Protein | Not given | Not given |
| Calcium | 0.6 gm. | 0.8 gm. |
| Iron | 5 mg. | 7 mg. |
| Vitamin A | 1500 I.U. | 1500 I.U. |
| Thiamine | 0.4 mg. | 0.5 mg. |
| Riboflavin | 0.5 mg. | 0.8 mg. |
| Niacin equivalents | 6 mg. | 7 mg. |
| Ascorbic acid | 30 mg. | 30 mg. |
| Vitamin D | 400 I.U. | 400 I.U. |

From the Food and Nutrition Board, National Research Council: Recommended Daily Dietary Allowances (1958).

* Human milk is the natural food for infants from birth to one month and is the desired feeding for them during the first months of life. No specific daily dietary allowances are stated, therefore, for the first month of life.

Specific substances to be added early are water, vitamin C and vitamin D.

**Water.** Newborn infants learn to drink water—boiled for safety—from a bottle. This is given them between feedings because they need more fluid than is supplied in either breast milk or their formula. The infant's thirst should determine the amount of water he takes. In the home the mother should prepare freshly boiled water daily (this is done routinely in the hospital). The water is put in 4-ounce sterile nursing bottles. These may be warmed and given to the infant between feedings. When the infant is about five months old, some of the daily supply of boiled water should be kept in a sterile covered container and may be offered to the infant from a cup; this, however, is supplementary to the use of the bottle until he learns to drink from the cup.

**Vitamin C.** The infant requires a minimum of 30 mg. of vitamin C daily to prevent scurvy. The addition of vitamin C is particularly important for the bottle-fed infant, since this vitamin is destroyed by heating the milk in the infant's formula. Vitamin C is usually given also to breast-fed infants to as-

sure an adequate supply (the mother's intake of this vitamin may be insufficient, in which case the infant will not receive enough to meet his needs).

In general, infants are given orange juice, which is rich in vitamin C, beginning by about two weeks of age. It is customary to begin with ½ tablespoonful of strained fresh juice diluted with an equal quantity of water. This is increased slowly until 2 or 3 ounces of juice and a small amount of water are given daily at 2 months of age. Frozen orange juice may be used and diluted with boiled, cooled water according to the directions on the can.

In teaching mothers how to give orange juice to their infants the following precautions should be stressed: (1) the orange juice should not be boiled or have hot water added to it, since vitamin C is easily destroyed by heat. It is also destroyed through prolonged contact with the air or a utensil containing copper (e.g. a bowl). (2) To mothers of a low socio-economic group and possibly to those of low intelligence it should be explained that orange-flavored drinks (orange soda and the like) usually contain no fresh orange juice and may contain ingredients harmful to the infant. It is also necessary to stress the need for cleanliness throughout the procedure of preparing and giving the orange juice.

If the mother prefers to use *tomato juice,* the infant must be given twice the amount as of fresh orange juice prescribed by the physician. The tomato juice should be given in an equal amount of water. Since a small infant cannot take much fluid in addition to his formula, tomato juice is not given until he is five or six months old.

*Ascorbic acid* in tablet form may be given in addition to the orange juice until the infant is old enough to take willingly the required amount a day, or the physician may order it if an infant cannot tolerate orange juice. Ascorbic acid tablets must be crushed and dissolved in boiled, cooled water before being given to the infant.

**Vitamin D.** This vitamin is added to the diet when the infant is about 2 weeks old; in general, 400 International units are required per day. Vitamin D helps the infant to make use of the calcium he receives in his milk; in this respect it is a substitute for sunshine or is needed in addition to sunshine. Many preparations are available, such as cod liver oil and concentrates, other fish liver oil concentrates, and vitamin D-supplemented evaporated or fresh milk. The amount of these substances to be given to the infant depends on the physician's order. Vitamin D preparations vary so much in potency that the physician's order should be followed carefully.

Plain cod liver oil is used less frequently than formerly. Usually ¼ teaspoonful is given at first and increased to 1 or 2 teaspoonfuls.

The way in which it is given is important. It is given cold. The mouth of the bottle should be wiped to remove all the old oil. No displeasure or disgust should be shown while giving this medication, since the infant will copy the attitude toward the oil from the adult who gives it. The infant's head should be elevated and the infant should be held in a sitting position when he is given the medication by dropper or spoon, in order to prevent aspiration (see p. 307). Preparations containing oil should never be given while the infant is crying.

The usual dose of vitamin D concentrates is 5 to 10 drops a day.

Some vitamin D preparations can be given in milk, but the infant may not take all the milk and therefore will not ingest the full dose of the vitamin. It is not feasible to put any oily substance into the formula because (1) the oil adheres to the glass, and (2) since oil rises to the top when the feeding bottle is inverted, the infant sucks the oil through the nipple only at the close of the feeding. Often he does not suck long enough to receive the full dose.

Mothers should be cautioned against increasing the amount of vitamin ordered. Hypervitaminosis may result.

### Addition of Solid Foods

**Foods Which Infants Like.** If we remember the kinds of solid foods infants prefer, we can help an infant under our care to take solid foods more readily by offering these to him. In general, infants like bland foods which are *slightly* sweet, sour or salty. They do not like bitter foods or those strongly sour or salty. An infant's preference for texture and consistency of food varies according to his age. Naturally the newborn infant likes only liquid food. An infant a few weeks old likes food which feels smooth (puréed food). When his teeth are coming through, he likes foods on which he can chew, such as teething biscuits, zwieback or chopped foods. The shift from puréed to chopped foods should be a gradual one. Chopped foods ("junior foods") can be started from six to nine months, depending upon the infant's ability to chew.

Infants prefer food at moderate temperatures. Just as they like their formulas to be lukewarm, so they like their food. An infant may be frightened by food either too hot or too cold and may refuse it when it is offered him again.

**Method of Introduction.** The infant's reaction to his first solid food is to make sucking movements and then to push the food out of his mouth because of the new taste and consistency. The nurse should explain to the young mother that this reaction is to be expected.

An infant's introduction to solid food should be a pleasant experience. The infant should be held securely in the same position as for taking his formula from the bottle, but his head and shoulders should be raised slightly more than in bottle feeding. A bib is necessary, since he will spit out the food and make his fingers sticky by putting them in his mouth. The food should be smooth and thin. Cereal should be diluted with the formula; fruit or a vegetable with boiled water. The food should be lukewarm.

A small serving (1 teaspoonful) is all that an infant will take at first. A small spoon should be used. (Do not use a spoon with a curved handle; it is awkward in an adult's hand.) The food should be placed on the back of the infant's tongue, but no pressure should be exerted, since that would cause him

Fig. 115              Fig. 116

**Figure 115.** The infant's reaction to his first solid foods is to make sucking movements, but with practice he is able to take food from a spoon more easily.
**Figure 116.** The infant will learn to drink from a cup when he is ready to give up the bottle. At first he will make no attempt to hold it for himself.

to gag. New foods should be introduced one at a time. A new food should be offered before his formula or a food to which he is accustomed. The infant should not be hurried, coaxed or allowed to linger. Thirty minutes is long enough for a feeding. If he has not taken the food at the end of that time, the feeding should be discontinued and another attempt made the next day. Medication should not be mixed with the food unless the physician specifically orders that this be done.

Many mothers and nurses become anxious when teaching an infant to take solid food. The feeder should be calm, patient, gentle, and pleasant in her approach to the infant. He is then more likely to take the food than if he is scolded or coaxed. He should never be held tightly in an effort to control his hands, nor be forced to eat. Such measures make him antagonistic to the feeding process. If the nurse or mother is giving the infant foods which are distasteful to her, she should not show any evidence of her dislike. The infant is likely to imitate her reaction to the food. If he wants to touch the food, he should be allowed to do so. Touching is one of his methods of learning. His hands, of course, should be washed both before and after his feeding.

Physicians vary as to the time when they order solid foods to be added to the diet. Many physicians order cereal, puréed fruits or other foods for an infant as early as a few weeks of age; others wait until he is three months old. As the child grows older he can take a greater variety of solid foods. He needs additional nourishment because he is more active and uses more calories in energy output.

Just as physicians vary as to the time for starting solid foods, so they vary as to which food should be given first. Traditionally, cereal has been the first food to be given.

**Cereal.** Early administration of cereal was formerly advised because it contains iron. A young infant needs iron since he does not receive a sufficient quantity of it in breast milk or his formula. But cereal does not contain as much iron as some puréed foods, and for this reason many physicians order other foods before cereal is started.

Cereals which are ready-prepared for infant use may be given, or the infant's portion may be taken from that prepared for the family breakfast. Dry cereals, however, are not suitable for infants. The cereals especially prepared for infants are more finely divided and easily digested than those for the family table. If the cereal cooked for the family is to be used for the infant, his serving should be cooked longer in order to break the starch or polysaccharide down to the simpler forms of carbohydrate—disaccharide or monosaccharide—which the infant can more readily digest. (It is best to use a double boiler to cook cereals so that the cereal does not stick to the bottom of the pan.) Cereals prepared for the infant should not be sweetened.

A variety of cereals should be given so that the infant may learn to accept a variety of tastes. It is well to begin with a teaspoonful of cereal once a day. This may be increased gradually until at 6 or 7 months he will take from 2 to 5 tablespoonfuls a day.

As the infant grows older he may be given a baked or boiled potato in place of his cereal. The potato can be mashed with a fork and moistened with a little boiled milk or water.

**Fruits.** Some physicians, as we noted, prefer to give the infant other puréed foods before cereal. Fresh fruits (apples, peaches, apricots, and the like) should be stewed and put through a sieve. No sugar should be added. Banana can be given raw, mashed to a pulp with a spoon. The fruit should be thoroughly ripe.

The giving of fruits should be started with 1 teaspoonful, and the amount gradually increased until the infant is getting 3 or 4 tablespoonfuls a day. Several kinds of fruit should be tried so that he learns to like a variety.

**Vegetables.** As with fruit, the infant should be given only a teaspoonful at first, with an increase until he is taking 2 to 4 tablespoonfuls. The vegetables should be steamed or cooked in as little water as possible in order to retain their mineral and vitamin content. Vegetables, when first introduced, should be put through a sieve. The infant should be given green and yellow vegetables which have a bland

taste and contain necessary vitamins. Later, in the second half of the first year when he is teething, he should be given coarsely mashed or chopped vegetables. Peas, carrots or string beans may be included in the diet, and should be cooked until soft so that they can be readily chopped, mashed or crushed with a fork.

**Eggs.** Many physicians suggest that egg yolk be given the infant when he is from three to five months old. They also suggest that egg white not be given until toward the end of the first year, because infants may be allergic to egg albumen. Egg yolk contains iron and riboflavin as well as protein. It should be hard-cooked, mashed with a fork and fed in small amounts until the infant has become accustomed to it and then gradually increased. It can be given alone or mixed with milk or cereal. When egg white is added to the diet, the egg may be boiled (hard or soft) or poached. Only small amounts of egg white should be given until it is evident that the infant is not allergic to the protein it contains; then the entire egg may be given.

**Meat.** Many physicians add strained meats to the diet early in the first year. Meat, like eggs and milk, provides protein. Meat especially prepared for infant feeding can be bought in small-sized cans. It can also be prepared by scraping raw meat—liver or beef—with a knife; the scraped meat is then formed into a patty and cooked in a custard cup set in a pan of boiling water. When the meat is thoroughly cooked, the patty will be brown.

At first the infant is given only a teaspoonful of meat prepared in this way, but it is soon increased to 2 tablespoonfuls a day. Liver is especially valuable because of its high content of iron, vitamin A and vitamin B complex. Chicken and lamb are added to the diet later. The infant should not be given fatty meats because fat requires more time for digestion and is therefore less easily utilized. When he is able to chew, his meat may be finely ground rather than scraped.

**Fish.** Near the end of the first year

fish can be substituted for meat or egg several times a week. The fish should be boiled, baked or steamed, but not fried, because of the increase in the fat content. The fish must be finely divided in order to be certain that it does not contain small particles of bones.

**Bread.** Dried bread or zwieback may be added to the diet when the infant is about six months old and his teeth are coming through the gums. If he is permitted to hold the bread, he will learn in an easy way to carry food to his mouth. This is the first step in acquiring the ability to feed himself. He will also get exercise for his jaws through chewing the dried bread.

**Whole Milk.** If the infant is not breast-fed, his formula is discontinued by about six months, and he is given whole boiled milk. By that time his digestive system can tolerate the protein in cow's milk without dilution. Since he is receiving carbohydrate in his cereal and other foods, he does not need sugar added to the milk. By the time he is old enough to take milk from a cup easily (about one year of age) he is able to digest the curds of pasteurized milk, and it is unnecessary to boil the milk. He has also developed sufficient resistance to the nonpathogenic bacteria in pasteurized milk, which is therefore safe for him to take.

**Desserts.** Desserts are given in the latter part of the first year. Those suited to the infant's needs are fruits, gelatin, milk puddings, junkets and custards.

### Home or Commercial Preparation of Infants' Foods

Mothers may prepare the infant's foods at home or buy inexpensive, ready-prepared foods; some may want to can food for his use.* Such foods must be thoroughly cooked without seasoning and strained for infant feeding purposes.

Mothers can buy precooked cereal at their local grocery stores. These pow-

* Directions for canning fresh foods may be obtained from the United States Department of Agriculture, Washington, D.C., or from a state College of Agriculture.

dered cereals can be made into a liquid or paste by the addition of boiled water or the infant's formula. Vegetables, fruits, meats and egg yolk can also be obtained in cans or jars in puréed or chopped form for infant feeding. These containers can be safely refrigerated for two or three days after being opened. It is good practice to remove from the container only one serving at a time. The remainder in the jar or can may be safely covered and refrigerated. The original container was sterilized in processing and is the safest receptacle for the food. The advantages of prepared infant foods are variety, convenience, high retention of nutrients, year-round availability, uniform quality and consistency, and sterility.

### Development of Eating Habits

The mother is generally responsible if her child develops poor eating habits. If she makes the feeding period a happy one for him, he is likely to continue to enjoy his food. But if he learns to associate discomfort of any sort with the taking of his formula, feeding problems are likely to develop either then or later. It is easier to make a good start in feeding than to correct a bad habit when the infant is older. Because he is very much interested in eating and eating is one of his chief pleasures, his eating habits develop rapidly.

By *one month*, when the physician usually orders solid food, the infant is able to take food from a spoon. At *five to six months* the average infant begins to use his fingers in eating (finger-feeding), taking zwieback or dry, thin toast in his hand and learning to carry it to his mouth. At *eight to nine months* he has acquired the skill of holding a spoon and playing with it. At *nine months* the average infant can hold his own bottle and seems to prefer doing so. The *twelve-month-old* child drinks from a cup, although he may want his bottle at bedtime for the comfort of sucking. He should be allowed the bottle at bedtime until he voluntarily gives it up.

During the first year the infant's appetite will be good because of his increasing activity and rapid body growth. At the end of the first year his appetite will decrease because of his slower rate of growth and his corresponding decreased need for food. This is a normal occurrence and should never be a signal for the mother or nurse to force him to eat or to become anxious lest he starve. Encouraging him to eat too much food at this time often results in feeding problems during the toddler period.

## Colic

Colic is most common during the first three or four months of life. By colic is meant paroxysmal intestinal cramps due to accumulation of excessive gas. This causes discomfort and pain. The infant may pass gas from the anus or belch it up from the stomach. In reaction to his pain the infant cries loudly, draws up his arms and legs and becomes red in the face. His abdomen feels hard to the mother's or nurse's hand while he is having intestinal muscular contractions.

**Etiology, Treatment and Prognosis.** The causative factors in colic are not known with certainty, but are held to be (1) excessive swallowing of air, (2) too much excitement, (3) excessive intake of carbohydrates which cause fermentation and gas, (4) too rapid feeding or overfeeding, and (5) an anxious, disturbed or easily excited mother or nurse who communicates her tenseness to the infant. The tenseness causes intestinal cramps.

The *treatment* is to bubble the infant gently and frequently, holding him in an upright position to help him get rid of the air in the intestinal tract. Sometimes giving him a drink of warm water will help him to expel the gas. He may be turned upon the abdomen, because the pressure upon the abdomen tends to aid in the expulsion of gas. To relieve his tenseness he needs loving care, to be held and soothed by his mother or nurse. The physician may recommend a small warm enema or feel that a change in formula is advisable.

Colic is not a serious condition, and infants often gain weight in spite of the periods of pain.

### Weaning

**Psychological Background.** Weaning from the breast or bottle to drinking from a cup has a psychological significance quite apart from pleasure in the new activity and from the mere motor ability to drink rather than to suck. It is the end of an infant's receiving his major pleasure reactions from an object through the use of his mouth and sucking.

An infant usually indicates his readiness for advance in behavior when the old technique is no longer needed and its limitations frustrate him in his desire for new experiences and control of his environment. In his journey toward maturity he must experience a certain amount of frustration at his inability to control his physical and social environment in order to be stimulated to try to achieve this control.

During the second half of the first year the infant both wants and needs more freedom to move about and to acquire increasing control of his body and knowledge of his environment. It is no longer necessary to hold him closely to communicate to him a feeling of love and protection. In fact, he is likely to resist such restraint. He now gains a feeling of trust in others through their smiling faces and through their words spoken in a tone of voice which he has always associated with pleasant experiences. He wants to leave his infant way of taking nourishment—sucking from the breast or bottle—and try to drink from a cup (see Fig. 116).

In all learning there is an optimum stage of development when a new activity is learned most readily. This is the time when the opportunity for experimentation should be given the infant, under conditions which favor his success. He should not be hurried to drop the old pattern of behavior while he is learning the new. By six months or so he has learned that good things to eat come from dishes and cups and is ready to try milk from a cup when it is presented to him. He shows his readiness to drink from a cup by sitting up and reaching for it. He then looks to the adult for help in the technique of this new way of taking milk. If he fails to take it, the nurse or mother should wait a few weeks and then try again. The old and the new techniques will overlap.

**Time for Weaning.** The best time for weaning depends upon the individual infant, but is generally in the second half of the first year. Although some infants learn to drink from a cup at five months, they seldom show pleasure in it and should not be forced to give up sucking pleasure until they are ready to do so. We have already noted that many infants who find pleasure in drinking from a cup during the day want their bottle when going to sleep in the evening or at nap time.

Infants may be weaned from breast to formula feedings before six months of age if the mother's milk is diminishing in quantity or if it is necessary that she return to work outside the home. If some breast milk is available, this should be given to the infant and supplemented with a formula. The feeding should be given by bottle and not by cup, since a little infant needs the comfort of sucking.

Pregnancy and illness are other reasons for weaning before six months. It is a strain on a pregnant woman's physical strength to supply enough of the essential food elements for two infants and at the same time meet her own physical needs. Chronic illness in the mother, such as cancer and diseases of the kidneys, heart or blood, may necessitate weaning the infant. Severe, long-lasting infections in the mother are also a cause for weaning. Pulmonary tuberculosis in the mother is a contraindication to breast feeding, since the infant would be contaminated from such close contact with his mother.

**Methods of Weaning.** The infant should be weaned gradually so that he is less likely to be frustrated by the change from sucking to drinking. If he shows no interest in the cup, it is well to give him the bottle and try the cup again in a few days.

The milk in the cup should be warm, so that the fluid in his mouth has the same temperature he has known in the past. As soon as he drinks well from the cup the number of breast or bottle feedings can be slowly reduced. Some breast-fed infants change to taking their milk from a bottle before learning to drink from a cup. It is an individual matter whether to use the bottle feeding as an intermediate step between breast feeding and drinking from a cup. It is a good plan to let the infant learn to like the taste of cow's milk before breast feeding is discontinued completely.

Weaning should never be undertaken when the infant is sick for any but a compelling reason, for he is already under a physical and emotional strain from his illness.

**Reaction to Weaning.** When the complete process of weaning is too abrupt, the infant may show signs of discomfort (anxiety, sleeplessness and irritability). He may cry a great deal. He is likely to suck his thumb excessively.

If the infant receives extra attention during and after the period of weaning, he will find many other pleasant experiences to compensate for the lost satisfaction of ingesting milk through sucking and will have little or no reaction to the weaning process.

## Elimination

As different kinds of food are added to the infant's diet, the color as well as the consistency of the stools will change. For example, if beets are given, the stools will have a reddish tinge. Gradually, as a variety of foods is taken in the daily diet, the stools will be formed, and their predominant color will be brown.

## HEALTH PROTECTION: CHILD HEALTH CONFERENCE

The Child Health Conference is part of a continuous program of health supervision which should start in the prenatal period and continue throughout childhood and into adult life. The family is studied in the Child Health Conference so that the personnel can help the family to make the most of their resources in the care of the individual child.

### Family Approach

Consideration must be given to adjustments of general principles for application to the individual family. It is essential that parents have an easy self-confidence in their ability to fulfill their parental roles. The physician, social worker, counselor or public health nurse must know the socio-economic status and cultural background of the family when making recommendations, and should make no recommendation which the family will be unable to carry out.

It is difficult for many mothers to measure a child's development in terms of his individual capacities; they tend to compare growth, development and abilities of one child with those of others. This is a matter in which the Child Health Conference is particularly useful, since it keeps a continuous record of the child's progress.

If the personnel of the Conference work as a team and show an intense interest in the children brought to them for health supervision and guidance, the mothers will follow advice and instructions to the best of their ability. Not too much advice should be given at one time, since this might lead to confusion.

### Purposes of the Child Health Conference

**Over-All Purposes.** The main purpose of the Child Health Conference is to provide health supervision for infants and young children who would not otherwise receive this service. Some children are not directly under the supervision of any physician, either in private practice or in a clinic; others may be taken to a private physician or to a clinic only when they are sick. The Child Health Conference does not displace the services of the private physi-

cian, but supplements them by giving a kind of service which some children would not otherwise receive.

A secondary purpose of the Conference is to educate parents in better ways of caring for children and to give them an understanding of growth and development.

The Conference personnel should strive to meet the individual mother's needs and to increase her confidence in providing care for her children. Personnel must not be autocratic or judgmental in their approach, but rather should be interested and understanding. Many mothers are confused by the conflicting ideas of child rearing gathered from relatives, friends and magazine and newspaper articles. They should be helped to learn the best concepts of child care and feel secure in their ability to adapt these concepts to their particular needs and then put them into practice without doubts and misgivings.

Although direct teaching is one responsibility of the personnel, it is equally important that they accept the mother as she is. If she is suffering from feelings of anxiety or is fearful and possibly has feelings of guilt, the personnel should help her to understand the basis for these attitudes, so that the energy wasted in combating her frustration can be used in loving and working for the children.

**Specific Purposes.** The broad aims of the Conference are implemented through specific aims: (1) to help mothers understand the physical growth and emotional development of their children and to show them how serious problems can be averted if parents know what to expect of a child at various ages; (2) to recognize physical defects or illness through a complete examination and to inform parents of the sources in the community, such as a private physician or a clinic, where these conditions can be treated; (3) to provide protection against certain communicable diseases by immunization procedures; (4) to offer advice about the specific nutrition of the child and to give general assistance with budgeting for the whole family diet; (5) to help establish sound child-physician-mother relations and attitudes toward medical treatment; and (6) to provide assistance with behavior problems and to help the family in their total relations with the child.

The physician in some instances may refer a child to a social worker, psychologist or psychiatrist. The nurse will help the mother to understand and accept the need for such service. This is best done by allowing the mother to express her fears and work through the problem with the emotional support of the nurse. The nurse should also help her to extend the constructive relations she has had with the Conference personnel to the new friends in other professions who can provide the service the child needs.

**Concomitant Outcomes.** Records on the physical and developmental progress of children and on parental reactions to their roles are kept in the Child Health Conference. These records are of potential value in future care of the child. In some cities children are given physical examinations in the Conference, and the completed records of their health histories are sent to school with them.

### Mothers and the Child Health Conference

A mother may learn of Child Health Conferences while receiving prenatal care or in the hospital after the birth of her child. In some areas the public health nurse who delivers the birth certificate may inform the mother if she has not already been told of the availability of the Conference. Any nurse, whether working in a hospital, clinic or public health service, should know of the facilities the town or city offers for child health supervision and should explain these to the mothers with whom she works. Any infant whose mother does not have a private physician should be taken to such a conference.

Many mothers come to the Child Health Conference to find out whether they are doing a good job in bringing up a child. They want reassurance that their judgment is sound and that the

child is responding normally to their care. Some mothers come because they feel discouraged and inadequate or want to be relieved of a sense of guilt. All come seeking information and to have their children examined by the physician and given the customary immunizations. Some come because their friends come, and they consider it a pleasant social gathering. Such mothers dress their children to be admired by other mothers and by the clinic personnel. Their attendance should not be discouraged, though obviously they need to take a more serious view of child care.

### THE CHILD HEALTH CONFERENCE

**Personnel.** The minimal personnel required to meet the needs of the mother who brings her child to them includes the physician and at least one nurse. If there is a full staff, a social worker, a child guidance worker, a nutritionist and a dental hygienist are available for consultation or treatment. The physician should be a pediatrician or should have had extensive experience with mothers and children. The nurse in charge of the Conference should have had public health experience and have worked successfully with children. In an ideal situation the mother and the child should both see the physician and the nurse at each visit.

Students may be present to have the responsibilities and goals of the Child Health Conference explained to them. Volunteers may have an important part in the Conference, doing many things to help the nurses.

### Administration and Procedures

The Child Health Conference may be a voluntary organization and under private support, or it may be under public auspices and supported through public funds. Private physicians in the community are requested to support and to help plan and conduct the Conference.

If possible, the Conference should be held in a place convenient for the parents of the children who will be brought there. In large cities many are located in housing projects or health centers. In rural areas the Conference may travel from community to community; some organization within the community to be visited makes all the necessary arrangements. These Conferences are highly successful and have done much to improve the health of children living in rural areas.

The physical setup requires three or four rooms. One room is used as a reception or waiting room and should be large enough to accommodate the mothers and children without crowding. Posters and exhibits can be placed in this room. A small room is required for weighing and measuring the children. The physician's consultation room should be equipped for examining the child and should have a comfortable chair for the mother in which she can hold her infant while she talks to the physician. There should also be a separate room in which the mother and the nurse or nutritionist may consult about any problems the mother may have.

If such space is not available, one or two rooms may be divided by screens so that the work of the clinic may be carried on. Ideally, room should be available for taking the child's history, for undressing and examining the child, for comfortable seating of mothers and children while waiting to be seen, and for play among older children. The play area should have small chairs and washable toys for the children. A volunteer worker may be available who will supervise the children. The area where immunizations are given should be away from the room where the children and their mothers are waiting, so that they do not hear a child cry when he receives an injection.

**Conducting the Conference.** The nurse in charge is responsible for the conduct of the clinic. She may have one or more nurses to assist her. The nursing personnel should strive to create an atmosphere of friendliness and dignity. The nurses should thoroughly understand the purposes of the Conference and the recommendations made by the physician for each child so that they may feel secure in conferences with the mothers. Nurses cannot impart a feeling of confidence in the clinic if they themselves are uncertain of the objectives and of the specific recommendations given by the physician for the individual child.

The services offered by the Child Health Conference include the following:

1. Keeping a complete health history of the child
2. Recording the child's height and weight and taking his temperature
3. Giving a complete physical examination
4. Guidance for the regulation of feeding and general care of the child
5. Immunization according to the best medical practice
6. Anticipatory guidance and advice on behavior problems
7. Appraisal of the child's physical and emotional status
8. Nursing interpretation of the physician's advice
9. Referral to private or clinic physicians for illness or correction of physical defects or to a psychiatrist for emotional problems.

*Health History.* A careful and complete history is of extreme importance in order to give the clinic personnel a picture of the whole child and to help them establish friendly relations with the mother. The history should not be taken hurriedly. The mother should have time to discuss her problems and those of her child or other family members who are constantly in contact with him. If the nurse takes the child's history, she should utilize opportunities for health teaching and should explain to the mother the purpose of the Conference. In this way she prepares the mother for her consultation with the physician.

*Height, Weight and Temperature.* Recording height and weight and taking temperatures are the nurse's responsibility, though these are often done by a volunteer under her supervision. The undressed child should be observed for rashes or other signs of illness. Demonstrations can be made to the mother of the procedures of weighing the infant and taking his temperature. As she observes the nurse the mother learns how to utilize safety measures in handling the child.

PROCEDURE FOR WEIGHING THE INFANT. The *purpose* is to determine the exact weight of the infant. The infant's weight provides a way of evaluating the infant's progress or lack of it in his physical status and in growth. Accuracy is therefore essential.

The *equipment* includes infant weighing scales (placed with the head end toward the wall), scale paper, an infant blanket, pencil and paper on which to record the weight, and a paper square with which to handle the scale weight.

The procedure should be done with care for the infant's safety and for the prevention of cross-contamination. The nurse or volunteer should note the infant's weight on the previous visit, undress the infant, wrap him in a blanket and carry him to the scales. To avoid contaminating the scales she should place a piece of scale paper on the scoop and handle the weight of the scale with the paper square. The infant is then placed gently in the center of the scoop with his head to the wall so that he will not fall if he kicks or pushes with his legs. The volunteer or nurse should hold her left hand over the infant while he is weighed to prevent his falling if he tries to sit up. The difficulty in weighing an infant is to keep him still, for if he moves, the weight is not accurate. The mother should stand beside the scale table and speak to him and show him a toy to divert his attention; in this way he will be quiet, and the exact weight can be read. The scale paper is then removed and disposed of in the receptacle for contaminated paper. The infant is wrapped in his blanket and given to his mother to hold until the physician is ready to examine him. The exact weight is then recorded.

PROCEDURE FOR MEASURING AN INFANT'S LENGTH. The *purpose* is to determine the length of the infant.

The *equipment* includes a metal tape measure or a ruled area on the paper-covered table and a pencil and paper for recording the length.

The nurse or volunteer should place the infant's head against a board or wall at one end of the table. The infant should be stretched lengthwise with his knees flat on the table. A mark may be put at his feet. When the infant is removed, his length can be measured from the board or wall at his head to the mark made at his feet. The length is then recorded.

*Physical Examination.* Physical examination of an infant should be made as often as necessary, but the number of examinations given at various age levels and what is included in the examinations vary in different clinics. In general the schedule is for the infant to be seen by the physician each month during the first year of life, every three months during the second and third years, and every six months during the fourth and fifth years.

Complete examination at each visit is not necessary. A thorough examination is made when the infant is first brought to the clinic and when he is six and twelve months old. After that once a year is considered sufficient. This is not, of course, a set rule. An infant should be examined whenever the physician thinks it necessary. The need for a complete examination is determined by a limited examination made at each visit or by the mother's report of signs or symptoms of disease, abnormality or lack of normal development.

In general a limited examination is directed toward finding abnormal conditions commonly connected with the stage of development reached by the infant—e.g. conditions of the feet, legs or back when he is learning to walk. The physician's examination, even if limited, consists in noting the mother-child relations, the general growth and development, state of nutrition, general health and evidence of disease or abnormality. A urine test for phenylketone bodies should also be done. The physical examination should precede immunization procedures, which are likely to make the infant cry and be uncooperative.

*Guidance for Feeding and General Care.* The entire personnel of the Conference give guidance. The physician prescribes the formula and the addition of solid foods to the infant's diet. The nurse should help the mother to understand the recommendations given by the physician, and her own suggestions for his care should be carefully explained. She should be sure that the mother understands in detail *what* is to be done and *how* it is to be done.

The nurse must know enough of the home situation to be sure that the plan of infant care made by the clinic personnel is practical and will fit into the cultural complex of the family. If the plan does not meet these criteria, it should be remade; otherwise the service of the clinic is of little value. If the plan is not suitable, it is not likely to be carried out, or it may cause friction within the family which will adversely influence the mother-child relations.

*Immunization.*   Prevention of disease is one of the most important goals in child care. During infancy and early childhood preventive measures can be carried out against certain infectious diseases. Immunization is given at the ages indicated by research and by common practice. Immunization of infants against diphtheria, pertussis, tetanus, smallpox and poliomyelitis should be carried out initially during the first year of life, with booster doses during subsequent years.

DIPHTHERIA, PERTUSSIS AND TETANUS.   Active immunization against these 3 diseases can be accomplished at the same time through the administration of 0.5 ml. of combined alum-precipitated or aluminum hydroxide-adsorbed diphtheria and tetanus toxoids and pertussis vaccine, commonly known as D.P.T. A minimum of three intramuscular injections of this combined toxoid-vaccine mixture should be given at intervals of four weeks, beginning at one or two months of age.

To reduce the possibility of occasional local or general reactions, the material should be given with a 1-inch needle inserted deeply into the gluteal or lateral thigh muscles. In older children it may be given in the deltoid or triceps muscles. After the injections reactions of irritability, fever, and swelling and redness at the site of injection may occur. Such reactions should be reported to the physician.

Booster doses of D.P.T. should be given at eighteen months and two years later, at three to four years. Booster doses of 0.1 to 0.25 ml. of combined diphtheria-tetanus toxoids should be given at 6 to 7 and again at 9 to 10 years of age. Pertussis vaccine is not necessary for children over six years, since this disease is most severe in infancy. Additional booster doses of diphtheria-tetanus toxoids should be given every three years after the age of ten years.

An acutely ill child should not be given immunization materials. Pertussis vaccine should not be given to any infant or child who has a history of convulsions.

SMALLPOX.   An infant should receive smallpox vaccination by the multiple pressure or puncture method by about five months of age. Revaccination should be done once every five years. Smallpox vaccination should not be given to anyone who has eczema or other open skin lesions, nor should it be given if another person in the child's family has eczema and has not been vaccinated. In the latter instance the infant could be vaccinated if he were separated from the other person until his vaccination healed. These precautions are necessary to prevent secondary vaccination or generalized vaccinia. Smallpox vaccination should not be given to any child who is acutely ill.

POLIOMYELITIS.   Immunization against poliomyelitis may be started at 3 months of age, when 1.0 ml. of poliomyelitis vaccine is given at a different site from the injection of D.P.T. Recently a commercial preparation has been produced which combines diphtheria and tetanus toxoids with pertussis and poliomyelitis vaccines. A second poliomyelitis immunization should be given at four months, and a third seven months later. Greater protection is gained if a fourth injection is given one year after the third one.

OTHER IMMUNIZATIONS.   If the parents plan to travel to other states or to foreign countries, further information about other immunizations which might be necessary can be obtained from health departments or the Public Health Service, Washington, D.C.

*Anticipatory Guidance and Advice on Behavior Problems.*   These are the responsibility of both the physician and the nurse. The mother can be stimulated to ask questions by mentioning a few of the problems most likely to occur in infants the same age as hers. If the physician is able to spend an adequate amount of time on each mother's problems, it is unnecessary for the nurse to interpret or supplement his recommendations by a thorough nurse-mother conference. But the physician seldom has time to give the mother all the attention she needs, and therefore the nurse-mother conference is commonly held before the mother leaves the clinic. The nurse should be thoroughly familiar with the physician's recommendations so that she does not confuse the mother or alter the physician's plan of care for the infant by giving conflicting directions.

*Appraisal of the Child's Physical and Emotional Status.* Such appraisal is made by both the physician and the nurse of the Child Health Conference, as well as by the public health nurse who visits in the home. In planning care of the infant or little child such factors as the history of transmissible defects or diseases, the mother's condition during pregnancy, and the natal and postnatal health history of the infant should be viewed in relation to the socio-economic background of the family.

All nurses working with children— particularly the public health nurse— should know the norms of infant and child growth and development so that they can recognize and evaluate deviations from the normal condition. This is true also of students observing or assisting in the Child Health Conference. Experience in the Conference is of little value to them unless they have a mental picture of the general course of growth and development of infants and children.

*Nursing Interpretation of the Physician's Advice.* This means more than a nurse interpreting what the physician has said; it means that the mother carries over into the nursing care she will give her child the *medical advice* given by the physician, including preventive medicine and mental hygiene. Nurses often fail to realize that nursing has something to contribute to the child care program which medicine cannot give. Their recommendations to the mother are based on the physician's or-

ders and on the body of knowledge which belongs to the profession of nursing.

*Referral to Private or Clinic Physicians.* Referral of an infant or little child to a private or clinic physician for illness or correction of physical defects, or to a psychiatrist for emotional problems, is certainly a necessary function of the clinic, for it is not prepared to handle such problems. Case finding and referral are some of the main functions of the Conference. The referral is sometimes made by the nurse under the physician's direction, or it can be made by the social worker with his approval.

### Functions of the Nurse

In the general management of the Conference the atmosphere should be such as to reduce the strain on the mother and the child and to make them feel at ease. The nurse should greet them pleasantly and introduce them to other mothers. If it is the mother's first visit, the nurse should explain each step of the routine to her. Facilities for privacy should be provided during the mother's conferences with the physician, nurse or other personnel. The nurse takes the social history of the newly admitted children and talks with the mother before the mother sees the physician. The nurse screens patients and mothers on the basis of their different needs and problems, and it is desirable that the same nurse discuss with the mother the physician's recommendations after her conference with him. The nurse who admits the infants and children to the clinic observes them for signs of illness when they enter in order to isolate any child whose condition may be infectious or to refer him immediately to the appropriate agency or the physician.

The nurse should have adequate time for both individual and group teaching. This will be possible only if a systematic plan of work is in operation and the Conference is running smoothly. The appointment system is essential. Each patient's name should be registered in order of arrival, and all patients should be seen in order of appointment. If a mother brings her child without an appointment, however, it is customary for the physician to see the child if he appears sick or if the mother is anxious about his condition. The appointment system is a good check on the regularity of the infant's visits to the clinic. Before the mother leaves, the date and time of the next appointment should be given her in writing and should be entered in the appointment book.

**Parental Education.** Parental education is of little value unless the parents are motivated to receive suggestions from the personnel of the health team. Without motivation they are not likely to put into practice what they are taught. Motivation is increased if teaching has reference to their individual child and is specific and not general.

Instructions should be simple and should cover the essential information. Excess information is apt to be confusing. Completeness of instruction is not measured by textbook standards, but by the degree in which parents make suggestions and think through their own problems. Self-direction is more effective than direction by others.

Visual aids are valuable in clarifying the application of theory to the child in the home situation. Visual impression is lasting. The parents' understanding of the content covered in parental education should be checked by asking the parents questions. What and how much can be taught parents at any time depends on their social level (i.e. their financial status, living situation) and their intelligence level (how much knowledge they can absorb at one time). Literature in the form of folders or pamphlets should be provided for the parents; it is most effective if given in answer to specific questions and if it is reviewed with them.

The motivation of the parents is their desire to keep their child well. If they are indifferent to his health, they are not likely to profit from instruction.

The child's daily routine should be planned in sufficient detail to make it of practical value to the mother. Suggestions for guidance of the young child may be given. The feeding of the infant or young child is extremely important and is a matter on which there is a great deal of advice from miscellaneous sources. Some of this advice is good, but there are likely to be confusion and conflicts between what is good and what is biased or actually harmful.

The purpose and need for regular visits for health checks should be stressed, for parents are likely to feel that these are unnecessary if the child appears well. It is the mother, constantly with the child, who is in a position to observe the early signs of illness. It is imperative that she know these signs and realize the importance of reporting her observations and securing early treatment for the infant or child when he is ill.

Group instruction may be given to mothers on pertinent topics of common interest, such as the kind of clothing suitable to the weather and home conditions, routine immunizations carried out on all children, general principles of feeding and the management of minor behavior problems.

**Home Visits.** A visit to the home should be made after a child has been brought to the clinic, in order to observe the home environment, to teach the mother and to inspect the child. Ideally, this visit is made by the nurse in charge of the clinic, but if this is not possible, the public health nurse makes the visit and sends a report to the clinic. During the home visit the nurse should observe the socio-economic status, sanitary conditions, housing, and recreational facilities, which are important not only to the infant's health, but also to that of the entire family. In the home the nurse can observe the parent-child relation better than in the more or less formal atmosphere of the Child Health Conference. If the mother feels that she is understood and recognized as a person, she will profit by her contact with the clinic personnel.

**The Nurse and Volunteer Workers.** The work of volunteers is valuable, for they help the nurses to serve as an important means of communication with the public. The nurse should teach the volunteers how to perform nonprofessional duties in the clinic. If it is well done, their work may have a warmth and personal interest which are often lacking in professional service.

The following is a list of functions performed by volunteer workers in many clinics:

Check ventilation and light
Assist in setting up the clinic
Greet each mother and register the children
Bring to the attention of the nurse the fact that a child does not appear well
Begin the admission record
Take the child's weight and height and record the findings on the chart
Talk with the mother about educational material and interest her in it
Supervise the play of the preschool children
Assist with any additional duties given her.

### Need for Expansion

An increasing number of cities and rural areas have organized or are organizing Child Health Conferences. As the number of them grows they become a factor in reducing the morbidity and mortality of children in the area in which they serve. There is, however, still a great need for such facilities in many areas. Nurses must use their influence to secure such services for as many children as possible and encourage attendance at those Conferences which are already in existence. Nurses may exert their influence as a body through their state nurses' associations and through united action in bringing pressure upon the city, county and state legislatures and councils to provide more Child Health Conferences under public auspices. As individuals, nurses can help the public to know about the value of such conferences. Nurses are assuming their professional and civic responsibilities by helping to procure clinic services for all children not fully cared for by private physicians.

### TEACHING AIDS AND OTHER INFORMATION*

*Bureau of Publications, Teachers College, Columbia University*
Baruch, D. W.: Understanding Young Children.
*Child Study Association of America*

* Complete addresses are given in the Appendix.

Wolf, K. M., and Auerbach, A. B.: As Your Child Grows: The First Eighteen Months.
*Eli Lilly and Company*
Elements of Biologicals.
*John Hancock Mutual Life Insurance Company*
You and Your Baby.
*National Association for Mental Health*
Grossman, J. S.: You Don't Have to be Perfect (Even If You Are a Parent).
*Public Affairs Pamphlets*
Hymes, J. L.: Enjoy Your Child—Ages 1, 2 and 3.
Neisser, W., and Neisser, E.: Making the Grade as Dad.
*Ross Laboratories*
How to Be a Parent—and Like It.
The First and Second Years of Life.
Your Baby, Your Doctor, and You.
*U.S. Department of Health, Education, and Welfare*
A Healthy Personality for Your Child, 1952.
Infant Care, 1955.
Your Children's Feet and Footwear, 1957.
Your Well Baby, 1949.

### REFERENCES

Amann, A., and Williams, A. M.: A Study of Child Health Problems. Nursing Outlook, 4:109, 1956.
American Public Health Association: Health Supervision of Young Children. New York, American Public Health Association, 1955.
Bakwin, H.: Emotional Deprivation in Infants. J. Pediat., 35:512, 1949.
Batson, R., and others: Response of the Young Infant to Poliomyelitis Vaccine Given Separately and Combined with Other Antigens. Pediatrics, 21:1, 1958.
Bender, L.: There Is No Substitute for Family Life. Child Study, 23:74, April, 1946.
Bowlby, J.: Maternal Care and Mental Health. Geneva, World Health Organization, 1952.
Cooper, L. F., Barber, E. M., Mitchell, H. S., and Rynbergen, H. J.: Nutrition in Health and Disease. 13th ed. Philadelphia, J. B. Lippincott Company, 1958.
Elmer, E.: Failure to Thrive: Role of the Mother. Pediatrics, 25:717, 1960.
Erikson, E. H.: Childhood and Society. New York, W. W. Norton and Co., 1950.
Fineberg, H., and Jones, E. C.: Babies Draw Affection from "Mother Bank." The Modern Hospital, 89:60, July, 1957.
Fischer, C. C., and Whitman, M. A.: Simplified Method of Infant Feeding: Bacteriologic and Clinical Study. J. Pediat., 55:116, 1959.
Fraiberg, S. H.: The Magic Years. New York, Charles Scribner's Sons, 1959.
Gesell, A.: How a Baby Grows, A Story in Pictures. New York, Harper and Brothers, 1945.

Gesell, A., and others: The First Five Years of Life. New York, Harper and Brothers, 1940.

Gesell, A., and Amatruda, C. S.: Developmental Diagnosis. 2nd ed. New York, Harper and Brothers, 1947.

Glaser, K., and Eisenberg, L.: Maternal Deprivation. Pediatrics, *18*:626, 1956.

György, P.: Trends and Advances in Infant Nutrition. Nursing Outlook, 6:516, 1958.

Hanlon, J. J.: Principles of Public Health Administration. 3rd ed. St. Louis, C. V. Mosby Company, 1960.

Hurlock, E. B.: Child Development. 3rd ed. New York, McGraw-Hill Book Company, Inc., 1956.

Jensen, A.: A Community Survey to Determine the Need for a Child Health Conference. Am. J. Pub. Health, 48:765, 1958.

Josselyn, I. M.: The Happy Child. New York, Random House, 1955.

Krause, M. V.: Food, Nutrition and Diet Therapy. 2nd ed. Philadelphia, W. B. Saunders Company, 1957.

Lewis, M. M.: How Children Learn to Speak. New York, Basic Books, Inc., 1959.

Matthews, P. N., and Rhodes, W. C.: Combatting Maternal Deprivation. Children, 4:54, 1957.

McFadden, D., and Walsh, E.: The Nurse's Conference in a Child Health Station. Nursing Outlook, 4:392, 1956.

Mustard, H. S., and Stebbins, E. L.: An Introduction to Public Health. 4th ed. New York, Macmillan Company, 1959.

Nelson, W. E. (editor): Textbook of Pediatrics. 7th ed. Philadelphia, W. B. Saunders Company, 1959.

Recommended Dietary Allowances. Washington, D.C., National Academy of Sciences, National Research Council, Revised 1958.

Report of Committee on Nutrition: On The Feeding of Solid Foods to Infants. Pediatrics, *21*:685, 1958.

Spock, B. M.: Baby and Child Care. 3rd ed. New York, Duell, Sloan and Pearce, Inc., 1957.

Spock, B., and Lowenberg, M. E.: Feeding Your Baby and Child. New York, Duell, Sloan and Pearce, Inc., 1955.

Spock, B., Reinhart, J., and Miller, W.: A Baby's First Year. New York, Duell, Sloan and Pearce, Inc., 1955.

Stuart, H. C., and Prugh, D. G., (Editors): The Healthy Child. Cambridge, Harvard University Press, 1960.

Wallace, H. M., and others: Health Problems of Infants and Pre-School Children. Report of a Study. Am. J. Pub. Health, 48:1145, 1958.

Watson, E. H., and Lowrey, G. H.: Growth and Development of Children. 3rd ed. Chicago, Year Book Publishers, Inc., 1958.

Wilkes, E. T.: What To Do for a Colicky Baby. Parents' Magazine, *31*:32, July, 1956.

Winnicott, D. W.: Mother and Child. New York, Basic Books, Inc., 1957.

Wishik, S. M.: Attitudes and Reactions of the Public to Health Programs. Am. J. Pub. Health, 48:139, 1958.

Witmer, H. L., and Kotinsky, R.: Personality in the Making: The Fact-Finding Report of the Midcentury White House Conference on Children and Youth. New York, Harper and Brothers, 1952.

# Conditions of Infants Requiring

# Immediate or Short-Term Care

HOSPITALIZATION during infancy is often a totally new experience for both mother and child. Since the mother is anxious, the infant also becomes infected with this emotion. The mother should be encouraged to verbalize her fears about the child's welfare, thereby relieving some of her anxiety.

When an infant becomes ill for even a short time, both his physical and emotional well-being are threatened. This is especially true if the infant is hospitalized and deprived of his mother's love at a time when he is in pain, restrained for treatment or not permitted to suck.

After a comparatively brief period of hospitalization the infant usually will have no residual effects from his experience, particularly if his mother has visited him frequently or has been encouraged to remain with him throughout the day.

## EAR, NOSE AND THROAT

### Otitis Media

**Etiology and Incidence.** Otitis media is an infection of the middle ear. It is usually secondary to a respiratory infection and for that reason occurs in the colder months of the year. It may also occur as a sequel to measles or scarlet fever.

Bacteria causing the condition are generally the hemolytic streptococcus and pneumococcus, though other organisms, such as those causing diphtheria and tuberculosis, may be involved. In older children infected adenoid tissue around the opening of the eustachian tube may be responsible for recurring otitis media.

Otitis media is most common in infancy because the eustachian tube, lying between the pharynx and the middle ear, is shorter, wider and straighter than in the older child. A contributing factor is that the infant lies flat in bed during the greater part of the day, and so infected material is carried more readily through the canal.

**Clinical Manifestations, Diagnosis, Course and Complications.** The first stage of otitis media is due to swelling of the mucous membrane and consequent closing of the eustachian tube. Congestion, serous exudation and infection of the middle ear follow.

The *symptoms* are rhinopharyngitis (inflammation of the nasopharynx) with pain, which is augmented as exudation occurs and fluid pressure increases in the middle ear.

The *diagnosis* is made by examination of the ear drum with the otoscope. The drum appears bulging and lacks its normal luster. Later the bony landmarks and cone of light are obliterated. If the tympanic membrane has ruptured, a culture may be taken from the drainage from the middle ear.

The older child will complain of severe, sharp pain in the ear, but the infant often has no great discomfort and may cry very little. He is likely to tug at his ear, however, as if something there annoyed him.

The *course* of the infection is rapid. There is fever, commonly up to 104° F., with possible convulsions in the infant and chills in the older child. The little child is restless and fretful and suffers from gastrointestinal disturbance and anorexia. Fever and pain continue until the inflammation is reduced by adequate treatment, possibly including myringotomy, or the ear drum ruptures spontaneously and the exudate is released.

*Complications* are rare and may result from insufficient therapy. They include chronic otitis media, meningitis, mastoiditis, brain abscess, lateral sinus thrombophlebitis or thrombosis, and septicemia. A chronic condition with a perforated ear drum may lead to impaired hearing or deafness in the affected ear (see p. 483). If mastoiditis

occurs, a complete mastoidectomy should be done.

**Treatment.** Nose drops are used to shrink the mucous membrane and provide drainage from the blocked eustachian tube. Measures for immediate relief of pain include the application of dry heat to the ear, instillation of warm glycerin or oil into the ear (but preferably not before the physician has inspected the ear, so as not to interfere with his obtaining a clear view of the ear drum) and the giving of aspirin. *Myringotomy,* i.e. a clean elliptical incision of the tympanic membrane, or aspiration of the middle ear may be performed to relieve pressure and prevent the ragged opening made by spontaneous rupture. After a myringotomy, puncture or spontaneous rupture of the drum the physician will probably order irrigations of the ear with hydrogen peroxide. If congestion of the drum is visible so that an early diagnosis can be made, antibacterial therapy appropriate to the organism will clear up the infection in the early stage. If a myringotomy is done or the drum has ruptured, antibacterial therapy is necessary in full dosage and long enough for complete cure. Cultures of the organism will determine the appropriate antibiotic to use.

**Nursing Care.** Nursing care is based on both the characteristics of little children and the plan of treatment ordered by the physician. The general local treatments which the nurse will probably be asked to give include the following.

*Instillation of Warm Glycerin or Oil.* The nurse places the infant with his head turned so that he lies upon the unaffected ear, and the ear into which the drops—warmed—are to be instilled in a position for the drops to run down the external canal onto the ear drum. It may be necessary for a second nurse to hold his head and restrain his hands, or a mummy restraint may be used.

*Ear Irrigations.* For these treatments it is necessary to "mummy" the infant unless his mother or another nurse is available to hold him. If the

child is under three years of age, the
auricle is pulled down and back—if
over three years, up and back—in order
to facilitate the passage of the fluid onto
the ear drum.

*Local Heat.* A hot-water bottle (the
water temperature not above 115° F.
and the bottle encased in a cotton
flannel bag) or a suitably covered electric pad may be placed under the affected ear and the child kept upon
the affected side.

*Cleanliness of the Ear Canal.* The
nurse should wash her hands before
touching the ear in order to prevent a
mixed infection resulting from her carrying bacteria into the canal. If myringotomy is done or spontaneous rupture of the drum occurs, the purulent
material from the external auditory
canal is removed by cotton cones or
pledgets moistened with physiologic
saline solution or hydrogen peroxide.
The area is then wiped dry with sterile
cotton.

*Care of the Skin.* If the discharge is
profuse, the skin of the face around
the ear should be covered with cold
cream or zinc oxide to prevent impetigo or irritation. If the skin itches,
the child's hands should be restrained
to prevent scratching and spread of the
infection.

*Use of an Ear Wick.* If an ear wick
is used, it should be small, inserted
loosely and changed frequently. If cotton is packed into the ear too tightly,
free drainage cannot occur, and infected material may be forced into the
mastoid area. If the infant is placed
on the affected side, drainage will be
promoted.

*Observation for Complications.* The
nurse should watch for symptoms of
complications such as continued fever
after free drainage has been established, evidence of continued pain and
especially tenderness in the mastoid
area, or evidence of the less common
complications listed above.

**Prevention.** The most important
means of preventing otitis media is in
the prevention and treatment of the
common cold (see p. 299). In older
children it may be necessary to remove

hypertrophied and infected adenoid tissue.

## RESPIRATORY CONDITIONS

*Control of Respiration.* Respiration
is controlled by the respiratory center
in the brain stem. Changes in the carbon dioxide tension affect the respiratory center, which is stimulated by lack
of oxygen. Certain drugs (anesthetic
agents, opiates, barbiturates), brain injury and hypothermia depress the
respiratory center.

*Muscles of Respiration.* In normal
breathing only the inspiratory muscles
of respiration are used, mostly the
diaphragm. When these muscles relax,
expiration occurs. But when breathing
is difficult, the intercostal, spinal extensor and neck muscles are brought
into use. In forced expiration, as in
coughing, the abdominal muscles are
used. If these are weak, the child will
find it difficult to cough. The nurse can
help the older child to cough by ex-
erting manual pressure over the abdomen after he has taken a deep breath.

*The Infant's Respiratory Tract.* Naturally the respiratory tract of the infant
or little child is very small. This is one
reason why any obstruction in the airway to the lungs is extremely serious.
Obstruction may be due to edema or
may be in the form of mucus or an
aspirated foreign body. Depending on
the position and extent of the obstruction, the air supply may be cut off to
an entire lung or to only part of a
lung. If the obstruction is extensive
and high in the respiratory tract, the
whole lung is affected; if it is in the
lower part of the tract, only tissue
below the obstruction is involved.

**Incidence.** Respiratory disturbances
as a group constitute one of the greatest
problems in the care of children. The
patient's age is important in the kind
of disease from which he is likely to
suffer and in its clinical picture.

Although respiratory infections are
common in young children, it is difficult to identify them as separate clinical entities. The reason for this is that

the tissues of the respiratory tract are continuous from the nose, pharynx and larynx to the tracheobronchial tree and also to the paranasal sinuses and the middle ear. Often an infection beginning in the upper respiratory tract will proceed downward to the lower respiratory tract during the course of an illness.

**Epidemiology.** Infecting organisms are passed from person to person through the air. As an infant or little child breathes, he draws into his lungs organisms carried on minute droplets of water or particles of dust. These organisms multiply rapidly in the mucous membranes, and the newly infected infant becomes a source of infection to others and of further infection to himself.

These pathogenic organisms die quickly in outdoor air, owing to the action of ultraviolet light from the sun and a temperature unfavorable to their growth. This is the reason why in summer, when infants and children are outdoors and houses are better ventilated, colds are few. In winter, when children are kept indoors—the younger ones at home and the older ones at school—cross-contamination is apt to occur, and colds spread through the family, play group or class. Children during the first few years at school are likely to have more upper respiratory tract infections because they are more frequently exposed and have not built up resistance to infection as has the healthy older child. Infected preschool-age and school children thus become a source of infection for smaller siblings at home.

**Etiology.** Infection is the most common etiologic factor in respiratory conditions occurring after the neonatal period. The infant, however, may aspirate foreign bodies or irritating substances containing oil or zinc stearate.

Acute respiratory conditions are generally contracted from members of the family. Chronic respiratory problems are more frequently the result of conditions within the child's body, such as abnormalities of the nasopharynx, allergy or increased susceptibility to infection.

Acute infection may be caused by viruses mostly or by some bacteria. The influenza virus has been recognized for many years as one of the organisms causing such infections. During recent years several other viruses have also been recognized, such as the adenoviruses, the Coxsackie viruses and the ECHO (enteric cytopathogenic human orphan) viruses.

### Acute Nasopharyngitis (Common Cold)

This is the most common respiratory infection in infants and children. The nasal accessory sinuses and the nasopharynx are involved. The difficulty in caring for such children is that the infection spreads quickly, and serious complications may result. The clinical pattern in infants and small children is different from that in adults.

**Etiology.** The common cold is caused by a filtrable virus or a group of viruses causing an acute catarrhal inflammation of the upper respiratory tract. Bacteria are the cause of the purulent, second stage of the cold; these may be pneumococci, hemolytic streptococci and/or staphylococci.

Although bacteria may be disseminated during the second stage of a cold, the actual infective period of acute nasopharyngitis is only a few hours before and a day or two after the onset of the beginning infection.

*Contributing Factors.* Infants and children vary in their susceptibility to colds. Age and state of nutrition are factors in the danger of complications and in the severity of the cold. Chilling of the body reduces the temperature of the nasal mucous membrane with resulting loss of resistance in the tissue. This produces symptoms of nasopharyngitis in susceptible persons. Resistance may also be lowered if the infant or child is emotionally disturbed or fatigued.

**Immunity.** There is universal susceptibility to the common cold. Children have little resistance to infection and therefore must be protected from exposure. Serious complications may result, particularly among infants in infants' homes, in a children's hospital or in children's units of a general hospital.

**Pathology.** The initial lesion is an edema of the submucosa followed by infiltration with leukocytes. There is separation of epithelial cells and destruction of nasal epithelium.

**Clinical Manifestations.** The child is fretful, irritable and restless. He sneezes and has a nasal discharge which at first is thin and later purulent. The discharge may irritate the edge of the nostril and the upper lip.

Respiration is difficult, owing to congestion of the mucous membrane of the nostrils. The throat is sore, and the cervical lymph nodes are swollen. Gastrointestinal disturbances such as vomiting and diarrhea are common. Fever of 102 to 104° F. is prominent in patients up to 2 to 3 years of age. The temperature in older children is not likely to be over 102° F., and the school child and the adult may have little or no elevation of temperature. Anorexia, cough and general malaise are common. In the small infant obstruction of the nostrils may interfere with sucking, since he cannot breathe and swallow at the same time.

**Differential Diagnosis.** One of the problems in the diagnosis of the common cold in little children is that its onset resembles that of a number of infectious diseases, e.g. measles, pertussis, poliomyelitis or congenital syphilis (the "snuffles" of lues are part of the general pathology of the disease, but resemble the "sniffles" characteristic of the common cold). The nasal discharge in allergic rhinitis may appear to be the first sign of nasopharyngitis; it does not progress to a purulent stage, however, as does a cold. Also, in allergy the nasal mucous membranes are pale, whereas in the cold they are inflamed.

**Complications.** Serious complications are more common in infancy than in childhood and are caused by extension of the infection from the nose to the sinuses, ears, mastoids, throat, larynx, bronchi and lungs. The common cold, then, may result in sinusitis, otitis media, mastoiditis, brain abscess (due to extension of infection from the mastoids), tracheitis, bronchitis, pneumonia, pleurisy or empyema.

**Treatment.** The treatment is largely symptomatic. In the hospital the child is isolated in his cubicle. It is important to maintain his nutritional state with a suitable diet and adequate vitamins. The fluid intake should be increased. The child should be kept in bed during the febrile stage. Nasal congestion, especially in infants, should be alleviated so that the infant may suck properly. Nose drops should be used in an aqueous solution. Neo-Synephrine Hydrochloride (0.25 per cent) or ephedrine (0.5 to 1 per cent) are frequently used. Whatever the drug, in general one half to one quarter of the adult strength is used for infants and young children. Oily nose drops should never be used because of the danger of lipoid pneumonia. Medication such as aspirin reduces the child's temperature. The dose is generally figured as 60 mg. (1 grain) of aspirin per year of age up to 5 years, given 2 or 3 times a day; the dose for older children is 0.3 gm. (5 grains) given at the same intervals. Medication should be used only during the first day or two of the cold. Overuse of salicylates may result in salicylate poisoning. Sulfonamides and antibiotics should not be used routinely for the treatment of colds, but are indicated for complications or prolonged infections. Nasal drainage must be carried out, since infants cannot blow their noses.

**Nursing Care.** *Rest.* Since rest is important in the acute stages of this disease, the infant must be spared from many of the ordinary day-to-day noises in the home and from the excitement of family visitors or the activities of siblings.

*Fluid Intake.* Water should be offered frequently, since the infant cannot take large amounts at a time. He has great difficulty in sucking and breathing at the same time and should be allowed to rest frequently while taking his formula or water. The breast-fed infant may find sucking even more difficult than the bottle-fed infant does, since the breast is likely to partly cover his nose. The mother should support the breast with her fingers so as not to impede his breathing. The child who is old enough to drink from a cup needs increased amounts of fluid; small amounts may be given frequently. Little glasses, pretty cups with pictures on the bottom and gaily colored straws make the taking of fluids more interesting to the small child. For children of nursery school age a little pitcher from which a cup can be refilled encourages a greater fluid intake. With a group of children of this age or older an achievement chart may be kept where all can see it. Such a chart shows graphically the fluid intake of each child, and they compete in the race to get ahead of the others.

*Humidity.* The humidity of the room should be kept at 80 to 90 per cent in order to liquefy the secretions in the respiratory tract and reduce the cough. Excellent mechanical devices to increase the humidity of the atmosphere are on the market. If none is available, a long shallow pan of water may be placed on the radiator. But unless the radiator is very hot, evaporation is slow, and the moisture in the air is not sufficiently increased. The temperature of the room should be about 70° F.

*Nasal Drainage.* Drainage is facilitated by placing the infant on his abdomen and raising the foot of the bed. A nasal suction apparatus may be used, but with great care, since there is danger of injuring the infant.

*Nose Drops.* Drops should be given only when obstruction is present, not more frequently than every three hours and only for the first two or three days. The therapeutic effect is to shrink the mucous membrane, to relieve the stuffed feeling so characteristic of colds, and to reduce the excessive nasal discharge. The drops are given fifteen to twenty minutes before feedings and at bedtime. The nurse must be certain that the infant's nose is cleared of mucus before feeding and when the infant is put to bed.

Because of the danger of cross-infection, each child should have his own bottle of nose drops and medicine dropper. The dropper is kept in the bottle and serves as a stopper. The dropper has a smooth bulblike tip or is tipped with rubber tubing so that the infant's nose may not be injured. If one bottle must be used for several children, a separate dropper must be provided for each child and never replaced in the bottle after use. The bottle must at all times be kept out of the infant's reach. If an individual bottle is used, it is kept in the infant's cubicle or in the treatment closet.

Before instilling the drops, drainage must be secured. To give the drops, the infant is laid upon his back, his head over the side of the mattress or his neck extended over a blanket roll. His face is held by the nurse's left hand encircling his chin and cheeks, while she inserts the drops with her right hand. If such restraint is not sufficient and a second nurse is not available to assist in the procedure, it may be necessary to "mummy" him. After the drops have been instilled the infant's head is kept below the level of his shoulders and held in that position for one or two minutes. The nurse or mother may hold the infant in her lap in any way which is comfortable for him, so long as the head is thrown back.

*Prevention of Excoriation of the Lip.* Excoriation of the upper lip with subsequent infection is caused by the irritating nasal discharge. This may be prevented by applying cold cream or petrolatum to the area.

*Medications.* These are rather difficult to give to little children. Pills and tablets should be crushed into a powder and mixed with water or syrup, or both. They should be given from a spoon.

*Position.* The child's position should be changed frequently. The infant should be propped first on one side and then on the other, with his back supported by a rolled blanket.

*Cleansing the Nasal Passages.* As soon as the little child is old enough to understand, he should be taught the therapeutic way of clearing the nasal passages. He should learn to keep his mouth open and blow the secretions from both nostrils at the same time. He should never be told, as many adults

**Figure 117.** Diffuse impetiginous dermatitis following acute nasopharyngitis with excoriation and infection of the upper lip. (From Pillsbury, Shelley and Kligman: Dermatology.)

do tell children, to "Close the mouth and blow hard."

*Care by Noninfected Nurses.* Infected nurses are a serious problem in the pediatric unit. They contract colds from the little children who are too young to cooperate in the prevention of spread of infection. A nurse with a cold carries the risk of infecting the infants even though her technique is good. Isolation technique should be maintained as long as a child is infectious. When he is no longer infectious, there is danger of his contracting a secondary infection from organisms carried by nurses or other children.

*Medical Aseptic Technique.* The technique is the same whether we are speaking of the nursing care of an infant with a cold or with a contagious disease such as measles or diphtheria which can also be spread by discharges from the respiratory tract (see p. 53).

Medical aseptic technique *in the home* is difficult to carry out. If possible, the isolation unit should include a bathroom. Members of the family other than the mother should not enter the room. She should use the same technique the nurse uses, making any nec-

essary adaptations to the home environment. The person providing care in such a situation is responsible for cleaning the sick room and for concurrent and terminal disinfection.

**Prevention.** All patients having infections of the respiratory tract should be isolated so that contact between them and well children will be avoided. A child in good nutritional state is not so likely to catch cold. In older children tonsillectomy and adenoidectomy may be indicated. Vaccines are of questionable value in preventing a common cold. Children acquire resistance to infections upon exposure to them by building up protective antibodies. For this reason the older the child, the more likely is he to be able to resist infection.

### Acute Bronchiolitis and Interstitial Pneumonitis

These two terms are used interchangeably, especially in speaking of the disease in infants and small children. It is difficult to think of a pure bronchiolitis without involvement also of interstitial tissue. In bronchiolitis, expulsion of air from the air sacs is blocked; the result is overdistention of the lung, dyspnea and cyanosis.

**Incidence, Epidemiology and Etiology.** The majority of infections occur in the first six months of life and are not often seen in children more than two years of age.

The condition occurs most frequently in winter and early spring. Many cases occur sporadically, but there is an increase in the number of infants who contract acute bronchiolitis when there is an epidemic of upper respiratory tract infections among school children and adults. Sex and race do not influence susceptibility to bronchiolitis.

No one organism is responsible for the disease. A virus would appear to be the causative agent, since the condition cannot be treated with sulfonamides or antibiotics, but a specific virus has not been found.

**Clinical Manifestations, Diagnosis and Differential Diagnosis.** *Symptoms* of bronchiolitis occur several days after an infection of the upper respiratory tract and vary in severity. Respiratory symptoms are more severe than those of toxicity. The infant has a dry, persistent cough with increasing dyspnea. There is widespread inflammation of the bronchial mucous membrane. The mucosa swells, and a thick exudate is produced. Since air can enter the alveoli on inspiration, but is not expelled on expiration, it is trapped in the lungs each time the infant breathes, and the chest becomes overdistended. There is retraction on inspiration, but the chest collapses poorly on expiration.

The elevation of temperature is variable, ranging probably between 100 and 101° F. There is no relation between fever and the clinical severity of the disease.

Vomiting and diarrhea are not likely to be severe, but since dyspnea interferes with sucking, feeding may be a problem. The infant is alert, but appears irritable and anxious. The respirations are rapid and shallow and have a characteristic expiratory grunt. The accessory muscles of respiration are used, and there is suprasternal and subcostal indrawing with inspiration. As the lungs become more distended, the alveoli can no longer aerate the blood. Cyanosis may be severe, or the infant may be pale. Rales may not be present or may be scattered and fine, owing to small areas of pneumonia. Chest sounds, termed "wheezing," are common. Dehydration may be severe because of the infant's failure to take fluids and because of loss of water through hyperventilation.

Fluoroscopic and roentgenographic examinations show obstructive emphysema of varying degrees with or without scattered parenchymal infiltration. The white blood cell count is within normal limits. No specific organisms are cultured from the nasopharynx.

The disease has many symptoms which make it difficult to differentiate it from a number of other diseases, among which are asthma, cystic fibrosis of the pancreas with pulmonary changes, miliary tuberculosis, pertussis,

aspiration of irritating substances and salicylate poisoning.

**Prognosis and Complications.** The *prognosis* is usually good if the child has received adequate, prompt supportive therapy. The mortality rate is low, but death may occur because of exhaustion and anoxia.

*Complications* which may follow the acute condition are bacterial bronchopneumonia, otitis media, pulmonary atelectasis with abscess, and cardiac failure.

**Treatment.** The treatment is symptomatic. The child requires an atmosphere of high humidity. (Cold vapor is better than hot steam.) This liquefies the secretions and makes it easier for the child to cough up the mucus which fills the air passages. Oxygen therapy should be given to infants with even moderately severe dyspnea before cyanosis appears. Bronchoscopic aspiration may be done if the exudate has accumulated in the tracheobronchial tree. The infant's head and chest should be slightly elevated. In this position respirations are easier because the abdominal organs do not press against the diaphragm. Broad-spectrum antibiotics are given. Large amounts of sedatives or opiates are dangerous since they tend to depress the cough reflex and respiratory centers. Small amounts of sedatives, however (e.g. phenobarbital), may be given to quiet a child in a Croupette. The fluid intake should be increased, orally or parenterally, or both. Water-soluble vitamins should be given.

**Nursing Care.** In planning the nursing care of the acutely ill child his physical and emotional status must be considered. In addition, the emotional reaction of his parents and his nurses cannot be disregarded. Let us draw a mental picture of just what this means in regard to an infant acutely ill with bronchiolitis.

The infant's parents are anxious and fearful and possibly blame themselves for the child's condition. They feel helpless because of their lack of knowledge of the disease, its treatment and nursing care. They may be fearful be-

**Figure 118.** Croupette. The trough at the back of the Croupette is filled with ice and tap water to the level indicated. (From Air-Shields, Inc., Hatboro, Pa.)

cause of separation from the infant and the financial problem of his hospitalization. They need to have the plan of treatment explained to them and to receive both emotional support and reassurance.

The student nurse may be anxious when caring for an infant who is seriously ill, and fearful about handling equipment and carrying out procedures which are new to her. She should remember that she is one of the nursing team who work together in caring for the patient. By working with competent graduate nurses and under the supervision of her instructor she will lose her feeling of anxiety and incompetence and will contribute her full share in the care of the infant.

*Specific Care.* A Croupette is extremely useful in the care of these little patients. It provides high humidity and oxygen, if oxygen is used. The Croupette aids the child's breathing through the higher oxygen content and liquefies secretions in the bronchioles, making coughing less distressing to the child. Air under pressure may be used to provide increased humidity if oxygen is not necessary.

The equipment needed is as follows: a Croupette, including a canopy and a jar containing distilled water; ice, chopped or in cubes; a Croupette gauge; water to fill the container at the back of the Croupette; three blankets; a bucket; and a small towel.

If the child is old enough to understand, the procedure is explained to him.

The blanket is placed over the sheet to absorb the increased moisture from the water vapor in the Croupette. A mackintosh or plastic mattress cover is placed under the sheet to prevent the loss of oxygen, since it is heavier than air.

The trough at the back of the Croupette is filled with ice and tap water to a depth of about 10 inches or to the level indicated.

The jar into which oxygen or air under pressure flows is three quarters filled with distilled water. This is the source of water vapor.

The canopy is snapped on the back of the Croupette and draped over the frame. It is tucked under the frame on both sides.

The oxygen is turned on to the liter flow ordered by the physician.

The child is then placed in the Croupette and made comfortable. A favorite toy may be given him. His head is protected from the humidity by a small towel. A sheet or blanket is placed over the child.

If the child's head and chest are to be elevated, a hard rubber or plastic-covered pillow should be used for support. The knees should be supported by a sandbag rolled in a sheet lengthwise. The ends of the sheet are tucked under the mattress at the sides to prevent the bag from rolling out of position.

The canopy is sealed at the end with a folded sheet or blanket tucked loosely under the mattress at the sides of the bed so that carbon dioxide can escape.

The disk at the top of the steam outlet is turned to provide the needed amount of water vapor.

The condensation shelf must be checked to see whether it is draining properly. The melting ice is drained off through the drainage tube at the side of the Croupette trough into the bucket.

The blankets and the child's clothing must be changed when they become damp so that he may not become chilled. This should be done with as little disturbance as possible, and the time should be planned to fit into his schedule of feeding and medication.

Complete *charting* of the procedure is important. The date and the time when the child was put into the Croupette and when taken out should be recorded, as well as the amount of oxygen concentration used. It is important to record the infant's response to this therapy as shown in his color, the nature of his respirations and the degree of his restlessness.

Any secretion in the nostrils should be removed. Secretions tend to force the infant to breathe through his mouth. Cotton cones should be used for this procedure.

The fluid intake should be increased through offering water between feedings. If the infant cannot be taken from the Croupette, the nurse should support his head and back with one hand while she holds his bottle with the other. The hole in the nipple should be large enough so that the infant will not have to suck vigorously to get his feeding, but should not be so large that there is danger of his aspirating for-

**Figure 119.** Croupette. Air under pressure instead of oxygen may be used to produce water vapor. (From Air-Shields, Inc., Hatboro, Pa.)

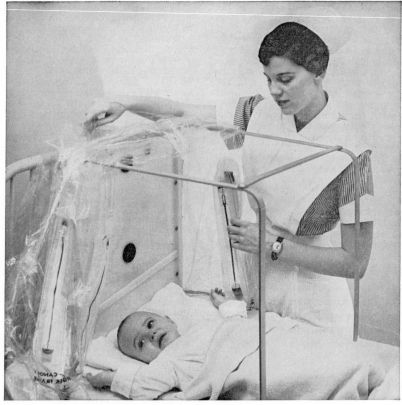

Figure 120.    Croupette. The child is covered with a sheet or blanket and made comfortable. (From Air-Shields, Inc., Hatboro, Pa.)

mula coming too rapidly into his mouth.

Water-soluble vitamins, antibiotics and sedatives are given as ordered by the physician. The nurse should remember that the infant's breathing is labored and should give medications very slowly, raising the infant's head as they are given.

### Aspiration of Foreign Bodies

**Etiology, Pathology, Clinical Manifestations and X-ray Findings.**    Small objects which an infant puts into his mouth may be aspirated. Such objects include safety pins, peanuts, beads, and parts of toys, such as the button eyes or squeakers of stuffed animals. Carelessness of mothers and nurses in leaving small objects within an infant's reach or giving him toys unsuited to his stage of development is most often the cause of such accidents.

Some objects are radiopaque, others nonopaque. If they can be located by x-ray study, removal is facilitated.

The *pathology* resulting from aspiration depends upon the nature of the object and upon the degree of obstruction of the air passages it causes. Very small objects may cause little difficulty if they do not obstruct the larynx or a bronchus. Yet an obstructive object may produce atelectasis, bronchiectasis, pulmonary abscess or empyema.

A particle of food, such as a peanut, may lodge in the bronchus and cause an obstructive inflammatory condition involving eventually the distal respiratory tract. In that case the infant would have a cough, fever and continued dyspnea.

The *clinical findings* may be given meaning by the parents' telling of the infant's playing with a small object which later could not be located. X-ray studies may prove the nature and location of the object.

The immediate symptoms are choking, gagging, coughing and inspiratory stridor. The signs are laryngeal and tracheal in origin. The child may have stridor, dyspnea and hoarseness. If the foreign body is large enough to cause obstruction, cyanosis may occur.

**Course.** Bronchial obstruction has serious consequences. A foreign body lodged in a bronchus must be removed promptly. If it is allowed to remain more than five days, it will cause a local purulent infection and a pulmonary abscess. Eventually atelectasis, emphysema and diminished breath sounds will occur. There will be unequal motion of the sides of the chest on respiration. If the foreign body is radiopaque, its location and form can be identified by the shadow it casts on a roentgenogram; the location of a foreign body not radiopaque can be identified by the effects it produces in the trachea or bronchus.

**Treatment.** Immediate treatment is to hold the child head down by his feet, shake him and hit him upon the back. If such measures do not cause the object to fall from his mouth, laryngoscopy or bronchoscopy, or both, if done in time, will permit removal of the foreign body. If the object has lodged in the larynx or trachea, an emergency tracheotomy may be necessary to keep the airway open until further treatment can be given.

If a secondary infection occurs, it should be treated with antimicrobial agents according to the laboratory sensitivity tests done on specimens of the organism involved.

**Prognosis.** The prognosis is good if there is prompt diagnosis and removal of the object. Nevertheless serious conditions or death may result.

**Prophylaxis.** Prophylaxis is evident. Keep small objects out of infants' reach. Keep safety pins closed and out of reach, and do not give a little child peanuts or other nuts. Toys with small movable parts are not safe for little children. Older children should not give an infant food which he may put into his mouth in such large quantities that he chokes upon it, or objects which may be aspirated if they cannot be eaten. It is not safe for little children to play with the baby unless the mother is there to supervise them. Adults should not set a bad example by putting pins or other objects in their mouths, for small children tend to imitate people about them and will do likewise.

### Lipoid Pneumonia

**Incidence, Etiology and Clinical Manifestations.** Lipoid pneumonia occurs most frequently in weak and debilitated infants. The condition is caused by aspiration of oils or any lipoid material. Vegetable oils are less irritating than animal oils. When oily nose drops are used or when the infant is given such substances as cod liver oil while crying, there is danger of aspiration. A child with a defect in his ability to swallow —e.g. a cleft palate—or a child lying flat in bed without his shoulders and head elevated by a pillow or the nurse's arm is liable to aspirate formula or food while feeding. If this contains lipoid material, lipoid pneumonia may result.

The onset is insidious. There is first an interstitial proliferative inflammation, followed by a chronic proliferative fibrosis. In the last stage there are multiple localized nodules in the lungs.

The *clinical manifestations* are not characteristic of this condition alone, thereby making diagnosis difficult. The infant has a cough which is dry and nonproductive, his respirations are rapid, and he is dyspneic. Unless there is a superimposed infection, he has no fever or leukocytosis. Bronchopneumonia is a common complication, however.

The roentgenogram shows characteristic features of this condition.

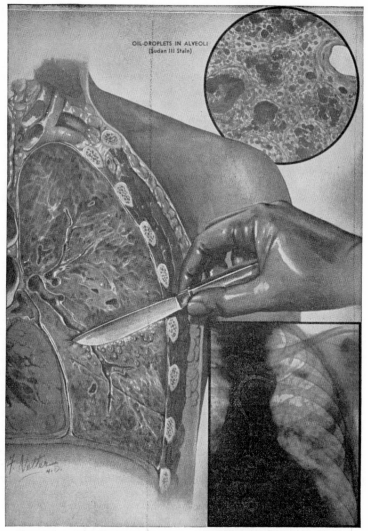

OIL-DROPLETS IN ALVEOLI
(Sudan III Stain)

Figure 121.   Lipoid (oil aspiration) pneumonia. (Copyright, The Ciba Collection of Medical Illustrations, by Frank H. Netter, M.D.)

**Treatment, Nursing Care, Prognosis and Prevention.**   There is no specific remedy for lipoid pneumonia, and a mild form of the disease may persist for several months before the child recovers.

Since there is no specific treatment, *nursing care* is all the more important. The child's position should be changed frequently to prevent hypostatic pneumonia. The child should be isolated to prevent his contracting a secondary infection from other children or adults.

The *prognosis* depends on the degree

of pulmonary damage and on the severity of any secondary infection.

*Prevention* is negative rather than positive. Intranasal medication with an oil base is not to be used. The child should receive concentrated vitamin preparations with a water-miscible vehicle. No mineral oil or castor oil should be given.

If the infant is apt to vomit or regurgitate, he should be placed on his side or abdomen after being fed to prevent aspiration of fluid.

## GASTROINTESTINAL CONDITIONS

### Foreign Bodies in the Gastrointestinal Tract

**Etiology.** An infant still in the oral phase of development enjoys putting objects in his mouth. As he sucks upon a small object, he may swallow it. Objects which do not stick in the esophagus, but reach the stomach, will generally pass through the intestinal tract. Some objects, however, do not pass through the pylorus and around the bends of the intestine, but become lodged at some point. Sharp objects—needles, bobby pins, hairpins, open safety pins, and the like—may perforate the intestine. Objects within the stomach can usually be removed gastroscopically.

**Treatment.** There is no specific treatment if gastroscopic removal of the object is not done. A normal diet is continued; neither a "cotton diet" nor laxatives are used today. Roentgenograms are taken daily. If the object is shown to be moving along in the intestine, perforation is not likely; but if the object is shown to be stationary for more than twenty-four hours, operation may be indicated because of the dangers of ulceration and perforation of the bowel. The nurse should observe closely for signs of perforation—nausea, vomiting, blood in the stools, rigidity, tenderness of the abdomen or evidence of pain. If the physician believes that perforation has occurred, operation is done at once.

**Nursing Care.** There is no specific nursing care other than close observation of the child for signs of perforation and observation of the stools. The stool should be placed in a fine-meshed sieve and water run with force upon it until the fecal matter disintegrates and an object, if present, is easily seen.

**Figure 122.** Some foreign bodies which failed to pass spontaneously and had to be removed by laparotomy, mostly from the stomach and duodenum. (Gross: The Surgery of Infancy and Childhood.)

## Vomiting and Diarrhea

Vomiting and diarrhea are clinical manifestations of a variety of disorders of infants and young children. These two conditions are together one of the major causes of morbidity among infants and children in many countries where sanitation and hygiene are poor and children are treated with folk remedies rather than with scientific medicine.

Unsanitary and unhygienic conditions have more serious consequences in infancy than in childhood because of the greater susceptibility to, and lesser ability to combat, infection.

In the infant vomiting and diarrhea cause a serious water loss with resulting electrolyte disturbance. If death results, it is most often due to the effects of dehydration and to acid-base imbalance.

Before the student can understand the seriousness of these effects it is important to review certain fundamental concepts of fluid and electrolyte equilibrium and the causes and effect upon the infant of imbalance.

**Fluid and Electrolytes.** Each body cell is bathed in tissue fluid. The water and electrolyte composition of this fluid has a vital influence on the activity of the cell. The importance of water to all life is well known, but often forgotten in the hygiene and the bedside care of the sick.

*Water.* An adequate and continuous supply of water is a requirement for life in all human beings. Dehydration in the infant is more serious than in the adult, however. About 53 per cent of the body weight of the adult male is made up of water. Infants have an even higher proportion of water, that of the newborn being 70 to 83 per cent. But in the first six months of life the proportion of water to body weight declines rapidly. Since fat essentially contains no water, there is a greater proportion of water to body weight in the thin person, whether an adult or an infant.

Water within the body is held in compartments separated by semipermeable membranes. These compartments are of three types, according to the kind of fluid they contain: (1) cellular or *intracellular* fluid (water within the cells), (2) *extracellular* fluid (water within the blood vessels or intravascular water contained in plasma), and (3) *interstitial* fluid (water in the tissues between vascular spaces and cells, which is similar to plasma in composition except that it is practically devoid of protein).

Depending upon the age of the person, water is distributed between cellular and extracellular compartments in different proportions. During adult life about one third of body water is outside the cells; during infancy and early childhood about half of the body water is extracellular.

SOURCE. The main source of water is through ingestion of fluids and some solid food as vegetables and meats which contain large amounts of water. A second source is through metabolism. When foodstuffs are broken down into simpler elements, water of oxidation is formed.

WATER LOSSES. Water in the normal healthy person is continually lost through (1) the gastrointestinal tract in stools and saliva; (2) the skin and lungs, since body heat is removed by the vaporization of water—this volume of water varies to a great extent, depending on the person's activity, the temperature of the environment and individual make-up; and (3) the kidneys, whose excretion contains urea and other products of metabolism in combination with water.

In disease these losses may be increased, owing to fever, greater urinary output, diarrhea and vomiting. If, at the same time, a child ingests insufficient water, he will show signs of dehydration such as thick secretions, dryness of the mouth, loss of skin turgor, sunken eyes, loss of weight and concentrated urine.

Besides the difference in the proportion of total body water in cellular and extracellular compartments between infants and adults, there is a further difference. The infant takes in and excretes more water than the adult when these amounts are expressed in milliliters per kilogram of body weight. There are two reasons for these differences: (1) the basal heat production per kilogram is twice as high in infants as in adults. Because of this and because he has a greater body surface area in proportion to his size, the infant loses twice as much water per kilogram as does the adult. (2) Because of the infant's greater metabolic rate, there is an increase in production of waste materials. Water must be used to eliminate these in greater urinary excretion.

Since the daily turnover of water in the infant is about half of his extracellular fluid volume, any fluid loss or lack of fluid intake depletes his extracellular fluid supply rapidly.

*Electrolytes.* It is easier for the student to understand the scientific basis of fluid balance in the body than the electrolyte balance. The following explanation is simplified so that the student may understand the therapy ordered for her patients.

Chemical compounds in solution may either remain intact or may dissociate. Examples of those whose molecules remain intact are dextrose, creatinine and urea. These are nonelectrolytes.

Those that dissociate in solution break down into separate particles known as *ions*. Compounds which behave in this manner are known as electrolytes. They have gone through the process of ionization and have an important function in maintaining acid-base balance. Each of the dissociated particles, or ions, of an electrolyte carries an electrical charge. Sodium ions ($Na^+$) carry a positive charge; chloride ions ($Cl^-$) carry a negative charge. Water molecules are attracted to and surround the ions, preventing positively charged pairs from coming together.

*Cations*, or positively charged ions in body fluid, include sodium ($Na^+$), potassium ($K^+$), calcium ($Ca^{++}$) and magnesium ($Mg^{++}$). *Anions*, or negatively charged ions in body fluid, include chloride ($Cl^-$), bicarbonate ($HCO_3^-$), phosphate ($HPO_4^{--}$), sulfate ($SO_4^{--}$) and ions of organic acids and many proteins.

Each water compartment (see p. 310) has its own electrolyte composition which differs from that of the others. *Milliequivalents* (mEq.) indicate the number of ionic charges or electrovalent bonds in the ionized solution in each compartment. Although the electrolyte composition of the fluid in each of the compartments is known, in treat-

**Figure 123.** Poor skin turgor. The skin has lost its elasticity, owing to severe dehydration. (Courtesy of Dr. Ralph V. Platou and the American Academy of Pediatrics.)

ment of a particular patient measurement is made of electrolytes within the intravascular compartment, because blood samples are more readily obtainable for analysis. This does not give a true measurement of the electrolytes in the cellular space itself.

SODIUM. Most of the sodium in the body is outside the cells, only a small amount being within the cells. The average daily intake of sodium equals the output. The average diet meets normal sodium requirements, but if additional amounts are required in therapy, isotonic sodium chloride solution in 0.85 to 0.9 per cent solutions and whole blood from the blood bank may be given.

Some sodium is excreted through the skin in perspiration. It is excreted in large amounts when the temperature surrounding the body is relatively high, and during bodily exercise, fever or emotional stress. Loss of sodium through the skin does not regulate sodium excretion; it is simply a byproduct of temperature regulation of the body. Normally most of the sodium excretion is through the kidneys, which are the chief regulators of body sodium.

Hormones have a definite effect on sodium excretion. The pituitary antidiuretic hormone tends to promote sodium excretion from the kidneys and to encourage water resorption from the distal tubules. The adrenal cortical hormones decrease urine sodium concentration by sodium resorption in the renal tubules, and thus tend to raise serum sodium concentration.

Water exchange in the infant into and out of the cell is three to four times more rapid than in the adult. Since the sodium exchange is equally rapid, there are special problems in maintenance of a sodium balance in the infant.

POTASSIUM. The major portion of potassium which is exchangeable lies within the cells. The serum potassium ranges between 4.5 and 7.3 mEq. per liter in the infant, a range higher than that of the adult. The daily turnover, intake and output of potassium are balanced, however. The average diet meets the potassium requirements of the body.

Potassium balance may be maintained at a low intake. Renal excretion of potassium, however, is accelerated by ACTH, desoxycorticosterone and cortisone.

The activity of all cells is influenced by the potassium concentration in the fluid around them. A high serum concentration of potassium produces a clinical effect on the heart muscle. A low extracellular potassium level may produce complaints in the patient of lassitude and weakness, and a loss of tone of both smooth and striated muscle may occur. Circulatory failure may be seen over a period of time.

Potassium should not be given to a patient until his renal function is adequate; otherwise the serum potassium may be raised to high levels. The main contraindications to potassium therapy are adrenal insufficiency and renal failure which have not been relieved by treatment.

**Acid-Base Equilibrium.** One of the most important considerations in fluid and electrolyte therapy is the acid-base equilibrium or balance. Whether a solution is acid or alkaline depends on the concentration of hydrogen ions $(H+)$. If the concentration of hydrogen ions is increased, the solution becomes more acid; if the concentration is decreased, it becomes more alkaline. The amount of ionized hydrogen in solution is indicated by the concept of pH. A solution having a pH 7 is neutral, since at that concentration the number of hydrogen ions is exactly balanced by the number of $OH^-$ ions present. As the hydrogen ion concentration falls, the pH value rises. In other words, an acid solution has a pH value under 7, and an alkaline solution a pH value greater than 7.

The extracellular body fluid normally is slightly alkaline, having a pH from 7.35 to 7.45. If the pH rises higher than this, a state of *alkalosis* exists; if the pH drops below, a state of *acidosis* exists. In acidosis the body fluid may still be considered alkaline, although less alkaline than normal. If the pH of body fluid rises above 7.7 or falls below 7.0, the patient's life is in danger.

Normal function of the kidneys and lungs is important in maintenance of the acid-base equilibrium. The kidneys tend to excrete surplus ions and other substances so that acid products of metabolism are lost from the body. The lungs may vary the rate at which carbon dioxide is lost from the body. If the plasma is too alkaline, the respiratory rate will decrease; if the plasma is too acid, the lungs will expel the carbon dioxide, which is slightly acid, more quickly.

Another important concept is that of *buffer solutions*. A buffer solution is one which tends to soak up surplus hydrogen ions or to release them as necessary. They are therefore important in regulating the acid-base equilibrium in the body fluid.

There are several buffer systems in the body. Probably the most important one in the extracellular fluid is the carbonic acid⇌sodium bicarbonate system. A disturbance of acid-base equilibrium can be considered to be the result of imbalance in the carbonic acid⇌sodium (or some other base) bicarbonate system. These bicarbonates are found in the extracellular fluid in a ratio of one part of carbonic acid to twenty parts of base bicarbonate. The acid-base equilibrium and the normal pH of the body fluid are changed when this ratio is disturbed.

In a clinical situation a measurement of the blood concentration of bicarbonate will indicate the severity of the acid-base imbalance. The values of the carbon dioxide content or carbon dioxide-combining power of plasma are therefore determined. The normal carbon dioxide content for an infant or child is approximately 18 to 27 mEq. per liter. The normal carbon dioxide-combining power for an infant or child is approximately 40 to 60 volumes per 100 cc. Acidosis is present when these values are below the levels given; alkalosis when the values are above the levels given. In certain cases of acid-base disturbance these relations may be reversed.

*Purposes of Fluid and Electrolyte Therapy.* The physician may order fluid and electrolyte therapy for one or more of the following reasons: to provide for the basic nutrition of the patient, for maintenance requirements, to replace previous losses or to meet concurrent losses.

*Route of Administration of Fluids.* Size must always be considered when giving fluids to infants and children. If insufficient fluids are given, dehydration may continue and the child's condition may remain unimproved. If too much fluid is administered by any route, the circulatory system may be overburdened and collapse may occur. In such a situation the child's heart may not pump fluid at the normal rate, and fluid will ooze from the vascular system to produce edema of the subcutaneous tissues or the lungs.

The giving of fluids by mouth is preferred, though they may be given intravenously or subcutaneously.

Fluid and electrolyte therapy is extremely important in the treatment of vomiting and diarrhea.

### Diarrhea

**Incidence.** Diarrhea is a symptom of a variety of conditions which together constitute one of the main causes of morbidity and mortality among infants and young children throughout the world. The incidence of diarrhea has decreased wherever people use modern concepts of refrigeration, cleanliness and the proper preparation of milk and other foods for infant feeding. Contaminated infant foods form a favorable medium for bacterial growth. In countries where the standard of living is low the infant death rate from diarrheal disorders is likely to be high. Breast feeding safeguards the infant from the main source of infection—contaminated milk. Although these general causes of diarrhea are known, the specific cause in any case is proved only by laboratory studies.

**Etiology.** In many cases of diarrhea the etiologic factor is difficult to determine. The following are generally recognized causes of an infectious or noninfectious diarrhea.

Faulty preparation of the infant's formula or other food and/or the technique of feeding the infant may cause diarrhea. Among such factors are overfeeding, an unbalanced diet (unsuitable combination of protein, fats and carbohydrates—excessive sugar causes diarrhea) and spoiled food, often because of the lack of refrigeration and unsterile or unclean technique in the preparation of the formula or other infant foods.

Socio-economic causes are difficult to determine. The incidence of contaminated milk and other foods as a cause of diarrhea is highest in the lowest socio-economic group. In the higher socio-economic groups the cause is more likely to be an infection by direct or indirect contact with someone who has the organism that causes diarrhea in the child. Causative organisms are pathogenic serotypes of *Escherichia coli* and various viruses, some of which cause respiratory illnesses in older children and adults. *Staphylococcus aureus* also causes diarrheal diseases, though sometimes the diarrhea occurs in connection with infections from this organism elsewhere in the body. Other organisms—the Shigella (Shiga, Flexner, Sonne-Duval and others), typhoid and Salmonella groups of bacteria—may be causative agents. Sometimes diarrhea results from administration of antibiotics to the child. Other organisms may overgrow in the intestinal tract because of a change in the normal intestinal flora as a result of antibiotic therapy. Such infectious agents include Proteus and Pseudomonas.

Other causes of diarrhea include allergy to certain foods, emotional excitement and fatigue or the unwise use of laxatives in infancy.

**Diagnosis, Clinical Manifestations and Treatment.** The *diagnosis* of diarrhea is made from the history and clinical evaluation. The causative factor may be learned from bacteriologic culture from rectal swabs taken at eight- to twelve-hour intervals and from bacteriologic cultures of stools. The laboratory studies usually done consist in determining the carbon dioxide content or carbon dioxide-combining power, and the hemoglobin, hematocrit, pH, sodium, chloride, potassium and nonprotein nitrogen values of the blood.

The *clinical manifestations* of mild diarrhea are different from those of severe diarrhea. Severe diarrhea is of two types, that with a gradual onset and that with an abrupt onset.

*Mild Diarrhea.* The clinical manifestations are a low-grade fever, possibly vomiting, irritability and disturbed sleep. The warning that these symptoms are due to diarrhea is an increase in the number of stools (two to ten a day) and a change in the nature of the stools, tending to looseness and even fluid consistency. At this stage acidosis and dehydration are not severe, though 10 per cent of the body weight may be lost. Weight loss exceeding this is an indication of severe dehydration.

Treatment is by a reduction in the formula feedings, especially in fat and carbohydrate, in order to put less strain on the gastrointestinal tract. The fluid offered by mouth is increased. Five per cent glucose in saline solution may be given orally every three to four hours. In some cases the physician orders a brief period of starvation (twelve to twenty-four hours) followed by giving glucose in saline solution and, later, half-strength skimmed milk or skimmed lactic acid milk.

*Severe Diarrhea.* The clinical manifestations of severe diarrhea with a gradual onset are elevation of temperature, with vomiting, anorexia and abdominal cramps. Diarrhea develops, the stools becoming greenish because of unchanged bile content, containing mucus and possibly tinged with blood. The stools become more frequent—two to twenty a day—and are expelled with force. The infant may be stuporous, have periods of irritability and may have convulsions. Because of dehydration the skin becomes dry and loses its turgor, the pulse is rapid and weak, the fontanels and eyes are sunken, the output of urine is decreased, and the weight loss may be as great as 25 per cent of the infant's former weight. These signs of dehydration are due chiefly to loss of interstitial fluid.

In acidosis the carbon dioxide level may be less than 10 volumes per milliliter. When the amount of urine is decreased and renal function is lost, acidosis is increased, since the kidneys fail to excrete acid-producing metabolites. The depth of respirations increases, while the rate may decrease or increase. In severe diarrhea with rapid onset the temperature ranges from 104 to 106° F. The infant is in extreme prostration; he vomits, and toxic symptoms appear. He is irritable and restless and may have convulsions. Respirations are rapid and hyperpneic. The diarrhea is not as severe as that with gradual onset, but acidosis is present. Collapse is due to loss of intracellular water and shrinkage of plasma volume. Signs of collapse in the infant are pallor and a flaccid state. The death rate in this kind of diarrhea is high.

The objective of treatment in severe diarrhea is first to replace the water loss and restore the electrolyte balance. By comparing the child's weight with that before he became ill the approximate amount of water loss is ascertained. Laboratory studies will show electrolyte imbalance and the level of kidney function. Specifically, the objective of this initial therapy is restoration of renal function by means of a hydrating solution, without potassium, provision of fluid maintenance needs and making up for previous fluid loss by giving a balanced solution. During the initial therapy the infant may be starved for a period of possibly up to forty-eight hours.

Fluids may be given into the peritoneal cavity if the infant is moribund on admission to the hospital. This will assist in hydrating the infant quickly. Sterile technique must be used to prevent infection of the abdominal cavity.

Continuous intravenous therapy is used with the very sick infant because fluid will not be absorbed from subcutaneous spaces. Blood transfusions are not given until the infant has been hydrated because of the greater concentration of blood during the state of dehydration.

When the infant is on the road to better hydration, subcutaneous fluids may be used. Hypertonic solutions should not be given, since they draw fluid into the area of clysis and may precipitate circulatory collapse. Hypotonic or isotonic solutions may be used, and hyaluronidase may be given into the site to promote absorption.

When the number of stools lessens and vomiting ceases, glucose and electrolyte mixtures may be started by mouth. Gradually, if no more diarrhea occurs, the concentration of fluids taken by mouth may be increased and fat and protein may be included until the dietary intake is normal within six to eight days. Diluted skimmed milk, lactic acid milk or breast milk may be used initially and gradually concentrated as the infant improves.

Specific chemotherapy is given as soon as the organism causing the diarrhea has been determined. If dysentery or salmonella organisms are present, sulfonamides or chloramphenicol may be given. Neomycin may be given orally for pathogenic strains of *Escherichia coli*. If the diarrhea is accompanied by a parenteral infection, this condition must also be treated.

If the child has fever, a tepid sponge bath may be ordered to reduce the temperature and prevent convulsions. No sedatives or cathartics are given, since they may obscure or distort symptoms indicative of the child's condition.

**Prevention.** Breast feeding is probably the most important preventive of diarrhea, particularly among the lower socio-economic group where other preventive measures are difficult to maintain. The proper method for making, storing and giving infant formulas should be taught all mothers, and the nurse should help the mother in making the necessary adaptations to the equipment in the home. In hot weather the infant should be offered water frequently, but the food intake is temporarily reduced. The infant should be dressed according to the temperature and not the season of the year. In summer he should be kept as cool as possible, but dressed warmly if the weather turns cool.

The child should be kept from contact, direct or indirect, with adults or children having infections, particularly of the alimentary tract, and an infant sick with diarrhea should be isolated to prevent the spread of infection.

Public health measures have a great deal to do with the incidence of diarrhea among infants. Safe sewage disposal, pure water and control of insects and pests are all part of good sanitation. The mother should be taught to make the best use of what she has in protecting the infant from health hazards in the environment which she cannot control. For instance, she should boil all water given to the infant, carefully cover his food to prevent contamination from flies, and place a mosquito netting over the infant during the seasons when flies and other insects are prevalent.

**Nursing Care.** *Needs as a Basis for Care.* When an acutely ill infant is admitted to the hospital, the nurse must be aware of the needs of the infant, of the family and especially of the mother. She should also be aware of her own needs in fulfilling her responsibilities in the care of the patient and his family.

The *needs of the infant* are paramount to all others; they are also more intimately within the nurse-child relationship. The infant must be given the means to satisfy his sucking needs, since feeding by mouth has been discontinued. He may be given a pacifier. If so, he should be bubbled in order to help him expel air which he may have swallowed. He will need to be comforted when his mother is unable to visit him. The infant of seven months is becoming aware of his mother as someone different from other women and may be afraid of strangers who handle him or even approach his bed.

He will need comforting because of restraints necessary during intravenous therapy. An infant just learning to sit up and move about may find restraint very frustrating. Many of the treatments given him will be painful, and he will need the reassurance of his mother's presence and of her caresses. If she is not able to stay with him, one of the nursing personnel—an aide or practical nurse if his own nurse is not available—should give him the affection and attention he needs, temporarily taking the place of his mother.

If nothing is given by mouth, his lips and tongue become very dry, and he will need mouth care. As long as he is dehydrated he will require special skin care to prevent lesions. He will need to have his position changed frequently, and passive exercise should be given, if possible, during periods of restraint.

The *needs of the mother and the family* cannot be listed in the order of their importance—all are important. The mother needs reassurance if she feels that the child's sickness is in some way her fault. She may feel that she has not been as careful as she should have been in preparing the feeding or in keeping the infant away from other children who had some infection. When she comes to visit the child or telephones to ask about his condition, she should be told of his progress. If his condition becomes worse, the physician should tell her this and take time to answer her questions and to help her accept the child's slight chance of recovery. The mother may be worried over nonessential matters such as shaving the infant's head for intravenous therapy. Such procedures and the need for the treatment should be explained to her.

The mother may be worried about her ability to pay the hospital bill. If so, she may be referred to the social service department or the credit department of the hospital.

The nurse must think of the other children in the home and whether one of them may have the same infection as the infant.

The *needs of the nurse* are also important. She must maintain her own health at the optimum level so that she can adequately meet her responsibilities as a nurse and in her personal life.

The nurse will need factual information about diarrhea and its treatment so that she can give intelligent care both when following the physician's orders and when giving care which promotes the aim of therapy, but is not prescribed by the physician.

*Assisting with Venipuncture.* The nurse will assist with venipuncture to obtain specimens for blood chemistries. Since infants do not have large veins in the antecubital fossa, blood must be obtained from the external or internal jugular vein, femoral vein or, uncommonly, the superior longitudinal sinus. A sterile syringe must be used for this procedure because of the risk of reinjection of blood into the vein. A no. 20 or 22 needle may be used even though the smaller the bore of the needle, the greater is the risk of clotting of the blood. If the specimen must be obtained under oil, sterile mineral oil may be used.

If the jugular vein is to be used for obtaining blood, the nurse is responsible for positioning the infant so that blood can be drawn with the least difficulty for the physician and the least discomfort for the child. The infant may be restrained by a mummy restraint (see Fig. 41). The infant's head is turned to one side and his neck extended over the edge of a small pillow, blanket roll or table edge so that the sternocleidomastoid muscle is stretched. The nurse should place one hand on the infant's occiput and the other over his face, leaving room, however, for him to breathe easily (see Fig. 12). The external jugular vein will be visible during crying, and crying during the procedure will facilitate the drawing of blood from the vein. The internal jugular vein is not visible, but accurate puncture will ensure easy removal of blood.

If the femoral vein is to be used, the infant's arms must be restrained with a blanket and the groin exposed, the legs being held in a frog-like position away from the body (see Fig. 13). The physician can palpate the femoral artery as it emerges from the abdomen. The femoral vein, which runs medially to it, is easily punctured. *Firm pressure should be applied to the jugular or femoral vein after the needle has been withdrawn.*

*Assisting with Intravenous Fluids.* If the infant has been vomiting, is unconscious or has anorexia or electrolyte imbalance, or if the physician wants to rest the gastrointestinal tract, intravenous therapy may be necessary. The fluids used for such therapy must be sterile, and have a neutral or nearly neutral chemical reaction and the same isotonicity as the interstitial fluid.

When fluids are given by this route, the physician must take great care to calculate both the amount and the rate of flow. If the circulation is overloaded by too rapid administration or by too much fluid, fatal cardiac embarrassment may occur. With continuous intravenous therapy up to 150 cc. per kilogram a day can be given. The nurse must keep an accurate record, at least every hour, of the kind and amount of fluid given, the amount absorbed, the rate of flow or number of drops per minute and the amount remaining in the bottle. She must regulate the number of drops given so that too much is not given too quickly. The regulation of drops should be done when the infant is resting quietly. If it is done when he is crying, the tenseness of his muscles will constrict the blood vessels and cause the fluid to run slowly. Then, when he quiets down, the rate of flow will increase.

The nurse who assists the physician in starting intravenous fluids is responsible for restraining the infant so that whatever site is to be used is immobilized. Because an infant's veins are very small, it is usual to select one over the temporal region of the skull. In that case the scalp must be shaved over the area and the infant restrained with a mummy restraint. The nurse must hold his head turned to one side as for puncture of the jugular vein. If she presses her fingers against the bony skull and the prominences of the infant's face, she will be more successful than if she puts pressure only on the soft tissue. The head may then be pressed against the pad on the table or bed. Care must be taken to avoid interfering with the infant's breathing while restraining him.

After the physician has inserted the needle it may be supported with folded gauze and taped in place. The infant's head may be mobilized by placing a sandbag on either side; these are held in place by 2-inch strips of adhesive tape. The mummy restraint may be removed and the infant's arms restrained with arm restraints (see Fig. 126) or clove hitch restraints (see Fig. 51).

Other veins in addition to those in the scalp

# INTRAVENOUS SCHEDULE
## 7 a.m. to 7 p.m.

PATIENT___MARSHA  A·  DAIR___          DATE__MAY 22, 1960

### SPECIAL INSTRUCTIONS TO DOCTORS

1- Write fluid orders for 24-hr. period ending 7 a.m. or portion thereof.
2- Write for various solutions in order of their uses.
3- Specify both drops per minute and number of cc. per hr. to be absorbed.
4- Provide a small rate latitude so that a lag in schedule may be overcome, e.g. 'run a 15-25 gtts. per min. and 60cc. per hr. Rate schedule is in back of your order book.'

### TO NURSES

1- Use this record whenever I.V. fluids are ordered.
2- Check I.V. hourly and record.
3- Do not discontinue I.V. or let it dry out.
4- Notify doctor if unable to maintain schedule for two successive hours.
5- Notify doctor if I.V. infiltrates.
6- Give solutions in same order as written for.
7- Do not run I.V. at greater than maximum rate.

| Amount to be absorbed by: | Amount Absorbed | Solution Now Running | Cc's Left in Bottle Now Running | Drops per Minute | Checked by: |
|---|---|---|---|---|---|
| 7a.m. | | | | | |
| 8a.m. | | | | | |
| 9a.m. | | | | | |
| 10a.m. | | | | | |
| 11a.m.  0 | 0 | 150cc 5% Dextrose/½P.S.S. | 150 | 15 | P.T. |
| 12a.m.  20 | 20 | " | 130 | 14 | P.T. |
| 1p.m.  40 | 35 | " | 115 | 16 | F.M. |
| 2p.m.  60 | 60 | " | 90 | 14 | PT |
| 3p.m.  80 | 80 | " | 70 | 14 (70cc Discarded) | P.T. |
| 4p.m.  100 | 90 | 100 cc Whole Blood | 90 | 10 | L.C. |
| 5p.m.  120 | 105 | " | 75 | 12 | L.C |
| 6p.m.  140 | 115 | " | 65 | 12 | B.K. |
| 7p.m.  160 | 130 | " | 50 | 14 | L.C. |
| 8p.m.  180 | 150 | " | 30 | 14 | L.C |
| 9p.m.  200 | 160 | " | 20 | 14 | L.C. |
| 10p.m.  220 | 180 | " | 0 | 15 | L.C |
|  | | 150cc 5% Dextrose/½P.S.S | 150 | | |
| 11p.m.  240 | 205 | | 125 | 15 | L.C |
| 12p.m.  260 | 225 | ' | 105 | 15 | S.D |
| 1a.m.  280 | 240 | " | 90 | 14 | S.D. |
| 2a.m.  300 | 260 | " | 70 | 16 | 2.R |
| 3a.m.  320 | 285 | " | 45 | 14 | S.D. |
| 4a.m.  340 | 305 | " | 25 | 14 | S.D. |
|  | | 100 cc 5% Dextrose/water | 15 | (15cc Discarded) | |
| 5a.m.  360 | 315 | +50cc m/6 Lactate | 150 | 15 | S.D |
| 6a.m.  380 | 335 | " | 130 | 15 | S.D. |
| 7a.m.  400 | 355 | " | 110 | 14 | S.D. |

Left margin notes:

400 c c. — Total of all fluids ordered until 7a.m.

Run at 12 16 gtts. per minute

Rate of flow per hour 20 c c.

**Figure 124.** Record the nurse should keep on every child receiving intravenous therapy. On this record is recorded the amount of fluid absorbed, the type of solution, the amount of fluid remaining and the drops per minute.

may be used for giving intravenous fluids to infants. Veins in the hands (see Fig. 136), feet, ankles or the antecubital fossa are used. In the last two areas it is often necessary to expose the veins by surgical dissection. A length of sterile plastic tubing is then inserted into the vein and tied in place. The plastic tubing is connected with the infusion apparatus (see Fig. 126).

If the flow of fluid during continuous intravenous therapy is stopped for any reason, another vein will probably have to be used when it is started again. Since this involves repeating the entire procedure, the nurse responsible for checking should report any slowing in the flow to the physician, who may be able to establish a free flow again by flushing the needle. Air bubbles should never be allowed in the tubing between the dropper and the needle. If there is swelling or if the older child complains of pain at the site of insertion of the needle, the problem is usually one of the needle's slipping from the vein. The nurse should report to the physician the presence of air bubbles, which are potentially dangerous, in the lower tubing or any swelling of the area of insertion.

Sometimes the physician may order oral feedings to be started while the infant is still receiving intravenous fluids. If the needle is in a scalp vein and the infant's head is restrained, it is

**Figure 125.**    Arrangement for long-continued drip of intravenous fluids to a baby. *1,* The child is mummied. Small needle, carrying a soft rubber connector, being inserted into vein. *2,* Needle in vein. *3,* Needle strapped into place with adhesive tape. *4,* The rubber connector attached to the infusion apparatus. With an arrangement of this sort, infusion can be continued for many hours. When the child is put back in his crib, sandbags can be placed in front of the forehead and behind the occiput to limit movements of the head. With this sort of continuous infusion in the scalp the baby should not be fed by mouth. There is too much danger of vomiting and aspiration, since the child cannot move his head adequately to clear the throat. (Gross: The Surgery of Infancy and Childhood.)

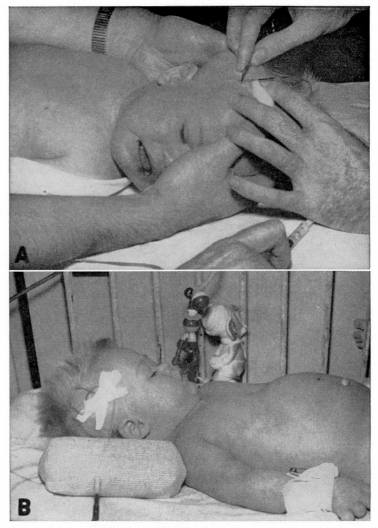

**Figure 126.** Venous cannulation. When the need for fluid administration is urgent and superficial veins are inaccessible, a vein must be cannulated with polyethylene tubing. *A*, Insertion of the polyethylene tubing. *B*, Sandbags placed on both sides of the infant's head, and extremity restraint used to prevent the child's moving and dislodging the tubing. (R. Kaye, J. D. Bridgers and D. M. Picou: Solutions for and Techniques of Parenteral, Oral and Rectal Administration. Pediat. Clin. North America, Vol. 6.)

important that only clear feedings be given. There is serious danger, since the infant's head cannot be raised, that the infant might aspirate a little of a milk formula, with the possibility of lipoid pneumonia resulting.

*Subcutaneous Infusion.* When ordering fluids to be given by subcutaneous infusion or clysis, the physician orders the total quantity of an isotonic solution on the basis of the child's size and bodily needs. The rate of flow is not ordered specifically as it is in intravenous therapy, because the flow is determined by the rate of absorption from the subcutaneous tissues. In order to facilitate absorption of such fluids, hyaluronidase may be injected into the area.

Various sites may be used for subcutaneous injection. In the infant the tissues of the pectoral region, the back, the lower part of the abdomen or the thighs are used. If the pectoral region is used, the mummy restraint which exposes the entire chest may be used to immobilize the child (see Fig. 42). The needles are inserted lateral to and below the nipples. If the subcutaneous tissue of the back is used, the needles are inserted in the upper portion of the back and the fluid is injected from a large syringe. Fluids may be injected into the lower part of the abdomen if the infant is not to have abdominal surgery (such surgery is extremely un-

A

B

Figure 127. Hypodermoclysis into (*A*) tissues of back of a small baby, given with a needle and syringe. *B*, Common method of giving hypodermoclysis in thighs of babies. The ankles are restrained. Needles are inserted and strapped to each thigh. (Gross: The Surgery of Infancy and Childhood.)

likely in a child with severe diarrhea). The most frequent sites for subcutaneous injection are the anterolateral aspects of the thighs. The infant's arms and legs must be restrained with the clove hitch (see Fig. 127) or extremity restraint (see Fig. 84). Sterile technique must be observed throughout the procedure. Subcutaneous abscesses have sometimes developed after such treatments. The needle point should not be inserted near the femoral or saphenous vessels and should lie between the skin and muscle layers.

Whatever site is used, gentle massage will help to diffuse the fluid into the tissues. If the center of the injected area becomes pale, the position of the needle should be changed.

When an infant is receiving fluids by either the intravenous or subcutaneous route, it is imperative that the nurse recognize his needs for sucking pleasure and for love and attention. A pacifier, unless it is contraindicated, should be used for the satisfaction of the infant's sucking need. The infant should be bubbled in order to relieve him of swallowed air. This attention, as well as talking to him and playing with him, will relieve his distress so far as is possible during this treatment.

*Oral Fluids.* If the infant has a mild diarrhea or is recovering from a severe one, oral fluids may be ordered. The amount of fluid varies with the size and needs of the child. Infants should receive in excess of 125 cc. per kilogram of body weight if their current need and deficit are to be met.

A nurse who is skillful, patient and kind in caring for infants can usually encourage them to take adequate amounts of fluid if they are physiologically well enough to do so. The nurse should offer at frequent intervals whatever formula or fluid is ordered. An infant who is able to take small amounts frequently will probably retain more than the infant who is encouraged to take too much at a time. Forcing fluids is to be discouraged, because such action too frequently leads to vomiting of all fluid taken.

Before giving the formula the nurse should check the physician's order in case the type of formula has been changed. The formula or fluid should be warmed to approximately body temperature as for a well infant. After the infant has taken the fluid or formula the nurse should chart the following: type of feeding, amount taken, degree of appetite, occurrence of vomiting.

*Change of Position.* Change of position and passive exercise are necessary if the infant is restrained for long periods or is too ill to move himself. These measures not only increase his comfort, but also reduce the possibility of intercurrent infection.

*Skin Care.* If vomiting occurs, the skin of the infant's neck and face should be cleansed and carefully dried to prevent excoriation. The skin of the buttocks should be cleansed after changing the diaper to reduce the danger of irritation and a breakdown of the skin. Oil or a bland ointment may be applied after the cleansing of the skin. If the skin does become excoriated, the infant should be placed on his abdomen and his buttocks exposed to the air. The nurse must observe a very debilitated infant frequently so as to prevent suffocation when he is lying in this position.

Besides exposing the buttocks to the air, a light treatment may be given. All oil should be removed from the skin before the treatment. A 25-watt bulb should be put in a gooseneck lamp clamped to the bed. The lamp should be about 1 foot above the patient, and the buttocks are exposed to the heat for 30 minutes several times a day according to the infant's condition. Care must be taken that the bulb does not touch the bed linen and set fire to it.

*Body Temperature Control.* The infant's temperature should be taken by axilla to prevent undue stimulation of the intestines through irritation of the rectum.

If the infant has a fever, a tepid sponge bath may be necessary. If his temperature is subnormal, additional blankets should be placed over him and tucked in about his body. A hot-water bottle (water temperature 115° F.)

properly covered may be applied. The hot-water bottle should be examined for leaks before being used. A small infant may be placed in an incubator.

*Stool Collection and Culture.* The physician may request that the infant's stools be kept for his inspection. The nurse should wrap the most recently soiled diaper in newspaper or place it in a container for this purpose, discarding the previous specimen. She should always chart the following characteristics of each stool: color, size, consistency, presence of blood or pus, and odor. If a stool culture is ordered, depending on the custom of the hospital, a culture of the freshly passed stool or from the rectal area is taken. In either case a sterile applicator should be used, and the specimen placed in a sterile test tube and sent to the laboratory immediately.

The *frequency of voiding* should also be recorded. Although the amount cannot be measured, it can be estimated.

*Care of the Lips.* Since the lips are dry, owing to the dehydration, cold cream should be applied.

*Isolation Technique.* Isolation technique, including gown technique, should be followed if the diarrhea is infectious and is spread by fecal contamination. Strict isolation is necessary to protect the other children in the area and the personnel. All persons coming in contact with the patient should wear a gown. All equipment used frequently, such as a thermometer or baby oil, should be isolated with the infant. In the majority of hospitals the laundry is equipped to handle contaminated linen, but if the nurses are to sterilize it, the common procedure is to boil it for ten to fifteen minutes. Feces, urine, vomitus and liquid food waste may be emptied into the sewage in communities with adequate sanitary disposal. In a rural neighborhood or other area where such facilities are impossible contaminated material should be mixed thoroughly with equal volumes of 10 per cent formalin solution or chlorinate of lime, or phenol or cresol in 5 per cent solution, and allowed to stand for at least an hour. Nursing

bottles and nipples must be boiled after use. There should be netting over the infant's bed, and screens on doors and windows during fly season.

If the mother cares for the infant, she must be cautioned to keep her fingernails short so that she will be less likely to carry pathogenic organisms on her hands, and should wash her hands thoroughly after caring for the infant. Nurses should teach the mother the elements of isolation technique so that she can follow the necessary precautions when she visits the infant and avoid carrying infection to the children at home (see p. 53).

*Prevention of Infection of the Nurse.* The nurse must remember that she herself may become infected through a break in her technique when caring for the child or his equipment. She must keep her own nails short and clean and wash her hands thoroughly after caring for him.

### Vomiting

One of the most common symptoms occurring in infancy and early childhood is vomiting. No attention need be paid to the occasional vomiting of the healthy infant, but an infant who vomits frequently requires medical attention. Persistent vomiting may be serious not only because of its etiologic significance, but also because it results in dehydration and electrolyte imbalance leading to alkalosis. Convulsions and tetany may occur in infants and young children if alkalosis is severe. Alkalosis resulting from severe vomiting is due to a loss of chlorides and potassium. The intracellular fluid has gained sodium ions and lost potassium ions. Potassium ions must be provided in adequate amounts if the normal balance within the cell is to be regained. As soon as renal function and hydration are assured, potassium must be given.

Ultimately, if the infant is not treated and fails to retain any fluid, he may show signs of the ketosis of starvation. Because of the serious consequences of vomiting, every effort should be made to find the cause and to institute immediate treatment.

**Etiology and Treatment.** Faulty feeding technique is the cause of vomiting in healthy, contented infants. Overfeeding leads to gastric distention, which in turn results in regurgitation of the excess formula. *Regurgitation* is the type of vomiting in which the formula comes up in small amounts and drools from the infant's mouth.

The *treatment* for infants who cannot take and retain a large amount of formula is to concentrate the formula so that the stomach will not be overdistended, and yet the infant will ingest the needed calories. If the infant is on a self-demand schedule and takes too much too frequently, reduction of the frequency of feeding tends to reduce vomiting. If he swallows the feeding too rapidly, so that none leaves the stomach before all is taken, overdistention may result. These infants should be fed from a nipple with a smaller hole so that the feeding may pass slowly from the stomach into the intestines while they are nursing. If an infant swallows air in large amounts, the stomach will be overdistended and vomiting will result. The infant should be bubbled frequently to expel air during the feeding. After he has taken all his formula he should be placed on his abdomen or right side so that formula may pass from the stomach into the intestines and air may more readily escape; thereby the eructed air will be less likely to force milk before it through the esophagus and out of the mouth. Air forced ahead of the milk into the intestines will cause abdominal distention and pain.

Sometimes young infants will vomit because of mucus collected in the back of the throat. A preventive measure is aspiration of the nasopharynx before offering the feeding.

Some vomiting is voluntary, as in *rumination*. Rumination is the voluntary bringing up of small amounts of food from the stomach within a short time after feeding. The food is brought back into the mouth by manipulating the tongue or putting the fingers far back into the mouth. The food may be reswallowed, but is more likely to drool from the mouth.

The causes of rumination are not known. It may be that the infant dislikes the food or the person feeding him. Rumination may be due to tension in the environment that prevents the feeding process from being satisfying to the infant. This may indicate disturbed parent-infant relations in which the infant lacks affection and probably attention. Whatever the cause, the habit of rumination may lead to death from starvation.

No treatment has been successful in all cases. Thickened feedings have been tried, since they are more difficult to regurgitate than the usual formula or serving of infant food. Arm restraints were used in the past to prevent the child from putting his fingers in his mouth, but this usually resulted in his learning to ruminate by maneuvering his tongue. Some hospitals used a cap which extended under the chin and prevented the infant from opening his mouth. Neither of these mechanical preventives proved successful.

The treatment suggested at present lies in psychotherapy for the mother and increasing the amount of affection shown the infant. Playing quietly with him for some time after his feeding has often proved helpful. Fortunately it is a habit which he will drop if it can be prevented for a few weeks and the conditions which produced it are changed through a general improvement in his care.

*Improper feeding leading to irritation of the stomach* is a common cause of vomiting. Irritation of the stomach may result from a formula which contains too much carbohydrate or fat. Excessive fat slows emptying of the stomach; fermentation takes place, and this leads to irritation. Prevention and treatment of the condition are by giving the infant a formula better suited to his nutritional needs.

Foods to which the infant is allergic or which are too highly seasoned, new foods or even lumps in the food, if he is unaccustomed to them, may cause him to vomit.

*Vomiting associated with infections or conditions outside the intestinal tract* is common. Among these are infections of the respiratory tract, ear and pharynx. To these should be added acute communicable diseases; for example, vomiting often accompanies an attack of coughing in pertussis (whooping cough). When the infectious condition is cured, vomiting ceases. Infections of the gastrointestinal tract which produce diarrhea are likely to be accompanied by vomiting. Such vomiting ceases when the infection is treated successfully.

Conditions other than infections may produce vomiting because of increased intracranial pressure—e.g. hydrocephalus, intracranial hemorrhage, encephalitis or meningitis. Vomiting due to intracranial pressure is not associated with the feeding time, but is closely related to periods of increased intracranial pressure. The only treatment for this type of vomiting is reducing the cause—intracranial pressure.

*Vomiting may be due to obstruction of the gastrointestinal tract.* In the newborn period vomiting may be due to congenital obstruction (see p. 183) of the intestines or bile ducts. Later, pyloric stenosis (see p. 326), intussusception (see p. 331), volvulus (see p. 183) and strangulated umbilical or inguinal hernia (see pp. 337, 333) may cause intestinal obstruction and vomiting. Treatment of the intestinal obstruction will cause this type of vomiting to cease.

Vomiting is a symptom, and *treatment* should be directed toward correction of the cause. In addition to correcting the immediate cause of vomiting, parenteral fluid and electrolyte therapy may be indicated to correct dehydration and alkalosis.

In order to determine the degree of renal function and dehydration, the nurse should chart whenever the infant voids, giving the exact time and estimating the amount of urine voided.

Only after the amount and frequency of voiding have been ascertained may potassium be given.

If the vomiting is persistent, drugs of the phenothiazine group may be given in the form of rectal suppositories. Commonly used among these drugs are promazine (Sparine) and chlorpromazine (Thorazine). To give a rectal suppository the nurse must lubricate it, insert it gently into the rectum and hold the infant's buttocks together until the tendency to expel it has passed.

**Nursing Care.** The nurse must make friends with the infant so that he feels secure in her care and is relaxed while feeding. Treatments should never be given at feeding time.

The feeding technique should be followed with care. The correct position for feeding is that which resembles the position when feeding at the breast. The infant's head and shoulders should be elevated while his body is cradled in the nurse's arms. Affection is shown by the gentle pressure of his body against hers. If the infant cannot be moved from the crib, his head and shoulders should be raised, if his condition permits, supported by the palm of her hand or her forearm. He should be fed slowly and bubbled frequently if he is in the nurse's lap. If he is fed in bed, he should be bubbled if possible, or allowed frequent intervals of rest. He will probably expel gas before the nipple is again inserted into his mouth. Elevating the head of the bed after feeding mechanically minimizes the tendency to vomit. The infant should be handled as little as possible after feeding, since rest inhibits or lessens the probability of expelling the feeding.

It is important to prevent aspiration of vomitus. The infant's head should be turned to the side so that the vomitus may run from the mouth. If the infant is placed on his right side or on his abdomen after feeding, his head is, of course, turned.

Care of the skin is important. The face should be cleansed and dried after the infant has vomited. Particular attention should be given to the folds of the neck and the skin behind the ears.

The charting of vomiting must be accurate. The nurse should chart the time in relation to feeding, the amount (estimated), odor, type, color and consistency of the vomitus, whether the infant appeared nauseated before vomiting, and the act of vomiting—whether rumination, regurgitation, vomiting without force or projectile vomiting.

It is clearly the nurse's responsibility to prevent vomiting due to inadequate sucking time and lack of affection.

### Pyloric Stenosis (Congenital Hypertrophic Pyloric Stenosis)

**Incidence and Pathology.** This is the most common surgical condition of the intestinal tract in infancy. It occurs most frequently in some family strains, in first-born infants and in males. It is uncommon among Negro infants. The symptoms appear in infants two to four weeks old, and only then can the congenital condition be diagnosed.

Pathologically, there is an increase in the size of the circular musculature of the pylorus. The enlargement is usually about the size and shape of an olive. The musculature is greatly thickened, and the resulting tumor-like mass constricts the lumen of the pyloric canal. This impedes emptying of the stomach. The musculature of the stomach then hypertrophies, owing to the effort required to force the formula through the constricted pylorus.

**Clinical Manifestations and X-ray and Laboratory Findings.** The initial *symptom* of pyloric stenosis is vomiting, which usually begins when the infant is about two weeks old. It occurs both during and after feedings. The vomiting is at first mild, but it becomes progressively more forceful until it is projectile. The vomitus does not contain bile, but may contain mucus and streaks of blood.

Since little of the feeding is retained, the infant is always hungry. He will take formula immediately after vomiting, only to vomit again. There is either failure to gain or loss of weight.

The normal, soft, rounded outline of infancy is lost, and the infant acquires the typical appearance of the starved child—he looks like a little old man. Because little food passes through the pylorus, the bowel movements decrease in frequency and amount. In some cases, however, a starvation type of diarrhea occurs.

The *signs* of pyloric stenosis are dehydration with poor skin turgor, distention of the epigastrium (in badly malnourished infants the outline of the distended stomach and peristaltic waves passing from left to right may be seen during and after feeding) (see Fig. 128) and an olive-shaped mass, located by palpation, in the right upper quadrant of the abdomen.

Metabolic alkalosis occurs, owing to loss of hydrochloric acid and potassium depletion. There is an increase in the carbon dioxide content of the plasma and in pH, and a decrease in serum chloride.

If barium is added to the feeding, an *x-ray* film of the stomach will show the enlargement and the narrowing and elongation of the pylorus, increased peristaltic waves and an abnormal retention of the barium in the stomach. A film taken several hours after feeding shows that little food has left the stomach.

*Laboratory findings* show an alkaline, concentrated urine. Hemoconcentration is shown by elevated hematocrit and hemoglobin values.

**Diagnosis and Complications.** The *diagnosis* is generally made without difficulty; however, pyloric stenosis may be confused with pylorospasm. In *pylorospasm* there is no structural defect of the pylorus. The spasm occurs in hyperactive infants, causing them to vomit frequently and often projectively as in pyloric stenosis. Such vomiting may cease when the infant is fed with the proper technique.

The treatment of pyloric spasm is by institution of proper feeding technique and administration of antispasmodic drugs such as atropine. Sedation is helpful, and phenobarbital may be used. Some physicians may order the feedings to be thickened or small-curd feedings to be given (see below).

The most common *complication* of pyloric stenosis is tetanic seizures resulting from metabolic alkalosis and a reduction in the free serum calcium.

**Treatment.** Few physicians recommend medical treatment for pyloric stenosis. If it is not successful, the infant's condition worsens and the danger from operation increases. If operation is performed early, however, the prognosis is excellent. But if medical

treatment is carried out (it is not attempted in breast-fed infants), it is an extension of that already given for pyloric spasm.

*Medical Treatment.* THICKENED FEEDINGS. These are mechanically more difficult to vomit than liquid feedings. Cereal or barley flour can be used to thicken the milk formula. A precooked cereal should be used, since the polysaccharides in it are broken down into simpler sugars. The feedings can be made in any desired degree of thickness. When the infant vomits directly after

HYPERTROPHY
OF PYLORIC
MUSCLE

EXTERNAL VIEW OF
HYPERTROPHIC
PYLORUS

OCCLUSION OF PYLORIC
LUMEN IN CROSS SECTION

VISIBLE PERISTALSIS,
DEHYDRATION AND WEIGHT LOSS

**Figure 128.** Pyloric Stenosis (Copyright, The Ciba Collection of Medical Illustrations, by Frank H. Netter, M.D.)

being fed, he should be refed. Some physicians order small-curd feedings such as those made with lactic acid solution added to whole milk.

LAVAGE. When there is gastric distention, lavage may be ordered to prevent further distention with subsequent vomiting (see also p. 329).

DRUGS. Antispasmodic drugs such as atropine or Eumydrin may be ordered to relax the smooth muscle of the pylorus. These drugs are given fifteen to twenty minutes before feeding. If atropine is ordered, a freshly prepared solution should be given. Most infants have a relatively high tolerance for this drug, though some may show signs of idiosyncrasy. The initial dose of atropine should be small and must be carefully measured to avoid overdosage. The initial dose is gradually increased until vomiting ceases, when it is gradually decreased. If the drug must be temporarily discontinued, a smaller dose is given when it is again administered. If flushing of the face, dilation of the pupils or fever occurs, the physician should be notified. He will probably discontinue the medication or reduce the dose.

Phenobarbital may be ordered for its sedative effect upon hyperactive infants. If heavy sedation or excessive drowsiness occurs, the dose should be decreased.

Medical treatment is seldom prolonged unless there is definite evidence of improvement in the infant's condition.

*Surgical Treatment.* Surgery consists in performing the Fredet-Ramstedt operation, or pyloromyotomy. This involves a longitudinal splitting of the hypertrophied circular muscle of the pylorus without incising the mucous membrane. When the lumen has been enlarged by this procedure, food can more readily pass through. If the operation is done with skill, the pyloric mucosa is not incised. If the mucosa is punctured, there is danger of peritonitis due to the leaking of stomach secretions into the peritoneal cavity.

PREOPERATIVE PREPARATION. The fluid and electrolyte balance must be restored, since a dehydrated infant is a poor surgical risk. If fluid deficiency, electrolyte imbalance and blood losses are not corrected, shock may occur during operation. Replacement of fluid and electrolyte deficits should be made two or three days before operation. After the infant has been hydrated whole blood is given as needed. Vitamins B, C and K are given parenterally.

Just before operation a catheter is passed through the nose and into the stomach. Removal of stomach secretions and swallowed air ensures a deflated stomach during operation and reduces postoperative vomiting.

**Nursing Care.** *Preoperative Examination.* The nurse assists the physician in examination of the infant to determine the presence of gastric peristaltic waves visible through the abdominal wall. The equipment needed is a bottle of sterile water, a bib and a flashlight. The procedure is simple. The infant is placed on his back with his face toward his left side. The abdomen is exposed. The bib is placed under his face. While the nurse gives the infant water the physician will hold the flashlight over the infant's abdomen from the left side. He stands on the right side of the infant and observes at the level of the abdomen. If peristaltic waves are present, they will be clearly visible.

*Preparation and Types of Formulas.* THICKENED FEEDINGS. The formula should be appropriate for the age of the infant. To it should be added varying amounts of precooked cereal. The consistency of the thickened formula may be thin or such that it will not drop from a spoon. The physician will order the precise degree of thickening. A very thick formula may be fed from a teaspoon or may be pressed through a nipple with a large hole, or one from which the tip has been cut, with the bowl of the spoon or a tongue blade.

FINE-CURD MILK. Milk containing a very fine curd is usually prepared by adding acid, or less frequently by fermentation through bacterial action. In fine-curd milk the casein is so altered that a softer and smaller curd is formed in the stomach. Such a curd is easier to digest and can more readily pass through a constricted pylorus. Lactic acid, U.S.P., may be added to a previously boiled cow's milk formula. The amount of acid ordered varies with the fat content; milk having a higher fat concentration requires more acid. Milk containing 3.5 to 4.0 per cent fat requires 6 cc. (1½ fluid drams) to the quart. Both the ingredients and the equipment must be cold to prevent too rapid curd formation. The acid should be diluted with a small amount of sterile water and added to the milk slowly with constant stirring. Commercial preparations of dried lactic acid milk may be purchased instead of preparing it in this way.

*Method of Feeding.* The infant should be fed slowly and bubbled frequently to prevent vomiting. He should also be bubbled before feedings to eliminate gas bubbles in the stomach. After feeding he should be handled as little as possible and moved very gently. He should be placed on his right side or abdomen, and the head of the bed raised slightly. If he vomits after the feeding, he should be refed, if the physician so orders.

Charting of the feeding is important. His apparent hunger, whether he vomits—including the type and amount,—the presence of peristaltic waves and whether he cries before or after vomiting should all be charted.

*Lavage.* Lavage may be ordered once or twice a day before feeding to cleanse the stomach of formula remaining from previous feedings.

For lavage the infant should be placed in a mummy restraint. A basin or pail should be placed on the chair beside the bed. A sterile catheter (size 10 to 12 French) is used, and is connected to the funnel by 2 feet of rubber tubing. The catheter is lubricated with sterile water and passed rapidly through the infant's mouth into the stomach to a distance of 9 or 10 inches, i.e. the distance from the tip of the nose to the tip of the sternum. If the catheter should pass into the larynx instead of the stomach, the infant would cough, breathing would become irregular and difficult, and cyanosis would occur. In such event the catheter should be withdrawn immediately. The

nurse can be certain that the catheter is in the stomach if gastric contents appear in the tube and if the infant breathes normally.

Turn the infant on his left side and syphon off the stomach contents into the basin. Turn the infant on his back and pour an amount of physiologic saline solution or sterile water, a little less than that syphoned off, into the funnel. If the fluid does not flow, owing to air in the tube, "milk" the tube gently. Turn the infant on his left side, invert the funnel over the receptacle, holding it lower than the infant's head, and allow the fluid to drain off. Repeat the procedure until the returning fluid is clear. Usually 500 to 1000 cc. of fluid is used. Upon completion of the procedure, pinch the catheter tightly to prevent fluid from dripping into the pharynx as the catheter is removed.

Lavage is a trying procedure for the infant, and he will need to be held, cuddled and reassured before he is fed.

*Other Procedures.* If drugs are given, the nurse should watch for evidence of overdosage. All symptoms should be carefully charted on the record. If the infant has a fever, the physician should be notified at once.

The nurse may be asked to assist the physician with administration of parenteral fluids (see p. 317).

The infant should be weighed daily at the same time in the day's schedule. Accuracy is essential, for the weight roughly indicates the degree of dehydration and of malnutrition.

The infant must be protected from infection, since he is unable to withstand an intercurrent infection. Unless all other children with infection are isolated in the pediatric unit, the patient should be isolated for his own protection. Nurses and visitors with any infection should not come in contact with him.

The infant's position must be changed frequently to prevent hypostatic pneumonia. The infant must be kept warm, with blankets and hot-water bottles if necessary.

The charting of output is important and includes the color, frequency and estimated amount of voiding and the type and number of stools.

*Postoperative Care.* Intravenous fluids may be given for the first few days after operation to meet the daily fluid requirements.

The infant's position is important.

The infant should be kept on his right side or on his abdomen; this position aids digestion of fluids or formula because the pylorus is on the right side of the abdomen, and also prevents the infant from aspirating if he vomits. After the immediate danger of vomiting has passed, placing the infant in a fairly upright sitting position tends to prevent vomiting by making it mechanically difficult. His position should be changed frequently, without disturbing him.

The nurse should note the indications of shock: rapid, weak pulse, cool skin, pallor and restlessness. If symptoms of shock appear, the foot of the crib should be elevated and additional warmth provided. It is important to observe the abdomen for distention. Distention might be due to air which the infant has swallowed, but it might also be caused by infection of the peritoneum.

Physicians vary in regard to details of the postoperative feeding ordered for these infants. Some physicians prefer a modified Down's regimen (Table 4), in which feedings are started four to six hours after operation. The infant is given small amounts of 5 per cent glucose and water orally at frequent inter-

**Table 4. Down's Regimen**

Name _____     Date _____

| No. | Time of Feeding | | Type of Feeding | Remarks |
|---|---|---|---|---|
| 1. | | at_____ | Give 30 minims of glucose water | _____ |
| 2. | 30 min. later | at_____ | Give 1 dram of glucose water | _____ |
| 3. | 30 min. later | at_____ | Give 2 drams of glucose water | _____ |
| 4. | 30 min. later | at_____ | Give 2 drams of glucose water | _____ |
| 5. | 30 min. later | at_____ | Give 2 drams of glucose water and 1 dram of milk* | _____ |
| 6. | 1 hr. later | at_____ | Give 3 drams of glucose water | _____ |
| 7. | 1½ hrs. later | at_____ | Give 2 drams of glucose water and 2 drams of milk | _____ |
| 8. | 1½ hrs. later | at_____ | Give 4 drams of glucose water | _____ |
| 9. | 1½ hrs. later | at_____ | Give 2 drams of glucose water and 3 drams of milk | _____ |
| 10. | 1½ hrs. later | at_____ | Give 5 drams of glucose water | _____ |
| 11. | 1½ hrs. later | at_____ | Give 1 dram of glucose water and 5 drams of milk | _____ |
| 12. | 1½ hrs. later | at_____ | Give 6 drams of glucose water | _____ |
| 13. | 1½ hrs. later | at_____ | Give 1 dram of glucose water and 6 drams of milk | _____ |
| 14. | 1½ hrs. later | at_____ | Give 7 drams of glucose water | _____ |
| 15. | 1½ hrs. later | at_____ | Give 1 dram of glucose water and 7 drams of milk | _____ |
| 16. | 1½ hrs. later | at_____ | Give 1 ounce of glucose water | _____ |
| 17. | 1½ hrs. later | at_____ | Give 1 dram of glucose water and 1 ounce of milk | _____ |
| 18. | 1½ hrs. later | at_____ | Give 9 drams of glucose water | _____ |
| 19. | 2 hrs. later | at_____ | Give 1 dram of glucose water and 9 drams of milk | _____ |

Then give 1 ounce of skim milk every 3 hours plus not more than 1 ounce of glucose water between feedings.

*Skimmed milk.

vals. This may be increased gradually. A dilute formula of half skimmed milk and water may be substituted for the glucose solution. The formula may be gradually increased in amount and thickened in consistency until the infant is taking the normal quantity. If he vomits, a more gradual increase in volume or a temporary reduction in oral intake should be made.

If the infant was breast-fed before operation, the mother's milk should be expressed and given as soon as he can tolerate it. He should be able to feed at the breast three to four days after operation.

The method of feeding is similar to that used preoperatively. A medicine dropper with a rubber tip may be used for the initial feedings, but the bottle or breast should be given when warranted, because they will satisfy the infant's sucking need. The bottle-fed infant should be held in the nurse's lap and cuddled before feeding as soon postoperatively as it is safe to handle him. The breast-fed infant should be held as usual, for he derives pleasure from this while satisfying his hunger and his need for sucking.

Prevention of infection of the wound is extremely important if a waterproof dressing has not been used. The diaper should be placed low over the abdomen so as not to come in contact with the incision. If the penis is large enough, it may be taped to the thigh so that contamination of the incision does not occur when the infant voids.

**Prognosis.** The prognosis is excellent. Complete relief follows successful surgical repair. The mortality rate is low, provided operation is undertaken before the infant has become too dehydrated and malnourished.

## Intussusception

**Incidence and Etiology.** Intussusception is an invagination of one portion of intestine into another. Intussusception and incarcerated inguinal hernia are two of the most frequently occurring acquired types of mechanical intestinal obstruction in infancy. More than half of the cases of intussusception occur in the first year of life. Most of the remaining cases occur in the second year and in male infants who were previously healthy.

The *etiology* is questionable. Often no cause is found. Hyperperistalsis of infancy may be responsible. Also the intestinal tract of the infant is freely movable, especially the cecum and ileum, making it easier for one portion to invaginate into another. The immediate cause may be diarrhea, constipation, polyps of the intestinal tract which act as a foreign body, or swelling of intestinal lymphatic tissue. Intussusception may at times occur around a Meckel's diverticulum (see p. 632).

**Pathology and Clinical Manifestations.** Usually the upper part of the intestine invaginates into the lower. This may occur at any point in the intestinal tract. Intussusception is classified according to its location. The majority of cases occur at the ileocecal valve.

The mesentery is carried into the lumen of the intestine, and the blood supply is cut off to the invaginated bowel. Edema of the part results. In some cases reduction is spontaneous, but generally necrosis occurs at the site of invagination and of the invaginated part. The strangulated portion may perforate, thereby causing peritonitis and death.

The *clinical manifestations* result from the acute intestinal obstruction. The onset in a healthy infant is sudden. The extent and severity of abnormal physical findings depend on the duration of the symptoms. There is paroxysmal pain in the abdomen, shown by the infant's kicking his legs and drawing them up upon his abdomen. The infant screams. At first, between pains, the infant may be comfortable. But the pain becomes progressively more severe. Vomiting occurs, first of the contents of the stomach; then it becomes bile-stained. This may be followed by fecal vomitus, depending on the site of intussusception. There are one or two loose stools followed by a discharge of mixed blood and mucus

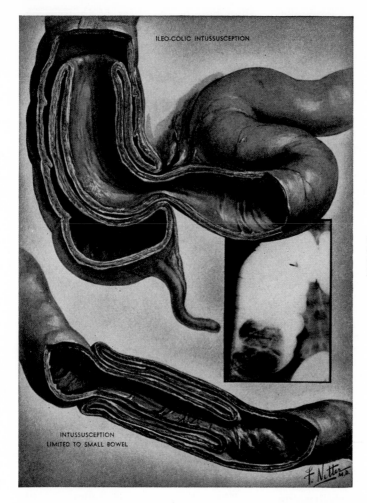

ILEO-COLIC INTUSSUSCEPTION

INTUSSUSCEPTION
LIMITED TO SMALL BOWEL

**Figure 129.** Intussusception. (Copyright, The Ciba Collection of Medical Illustrations, by Frank H. Netter, M.D.)

(currant jelly stools) about twelve hours after the onset. No more fecal matter is passed.

The infant is first restless and then prostrated. His temperature may go up to 106 to 108° F. Shock and dehydration occur. A tumor mass may be felt at the site of intussusception; it is usually sausage-shaped. The abdomen is at first soft and then distended or tender. The ring of intestine may be felt on rectal examination if the intussusception is of the ileocecal type. The infant will strain when the intussusception reaches the rectum.

**Diagnosis and Treatment.** The *diagnosis* is usually easy if there is sudden tenesmus, abdominal pain, vomiting, blood and mucus from the rectum, abdominal tumor and prostration. After a barium enema a roentgenogram may show the intussusception, which is seen as an inverted cap and an obstruction to further progress of the barium.

*Medical treatment* is seldom given in the United States, but is used to a great extent in other countries. Medical reduction is carried out by a surgeon under fluoroscopic observation after a large barium enema has been given the infant. The intussusception is reduced by hydrostatic pressure. The abdomen is not touched during the process. If the intussusception is reduced, the small intestine will fill with barium and the mass will disappear; if not, operation is performed.

*Surgical relief* is more commonly accomplished in this country without first attempting medical measures. The infant is prepared for operation by measures to prevent shock and to correct fluid and electrolyte imbalance. Operation is performed as soon as possible. If gangrene or an irreducible mass is present, the involved segment is resected. Usually all that is necessary is reduction of the intussusception. Surgical intervention is preferred in this country because it is certain to reduce the intussusception and allows inspection to seek for a polyp or other cause of difficulty.

**Nursing Care.** *Preoperative Care.* Good hydration is necessary preoperatively. The nurse assists in giving parenteral fluids and electrolytes, and whole blood if that is needed to combat shock. Deflation of the stomach by constant gastric suction is necessary. The nurse must observe whether drainage is constant and must measure the amount of drainage accurately. Prophylactic chemotherapy may be ordered. Antibiotics in proper dosage must be given so that the blood level of the agents will be adequate at the time of operation.

*Postoperative Care.* Nursing care after a simple reduction is largely symptomatic. Parenteral fluid therapy may be continued until feedings can be resumed. Usually clear fluid feedings are given soon after peristaltic activity has been heard in the abdomen and after distention and vomiting have ceased. It is absolutely necessary to keep the operative area clean and dry. The diaper should be placed low over the abdomen.

If bowel resection was necessary, parenteral fluids are given for several days, and gastrointestinal suction is necessary to prevent distention. Accurate measurement of drainage is important, since whatever fluids and electrolytes are lost must be replaced. In all cases the nurse must note symptoms of postoperative shock or peritonitis.

Changes in vital signs, color, presence of abdominal distention or odor from the incision should all be charted and reported.

Since intussusception may occur during the second half of the first year —an age when the little child not only misses his mother, but also is afraid of strangers—the importance of his mother's frequent visits must be stressed. These infants are physically uncomfortable and psychologically hesitant to relate to strangers in the hospital situation. Since intussusception is an emergency, the mother will need an opportunity to verbalize her feelings, her shock on learning of the child's condition, and her self-reproach if she did not immediately take him to a physician at the first signs of his pain and the change in nature of his stools.

**Prognosis.** The prognosis is good if operation is performed at once. The chances of recovery are directly related to the number of hours of illness before operation is done. After twenty-four hours a high mortality rate is expected. Death in untreated cases results from exhaustion in about three to five days after the onset. Spontaneous reduction may occur in some cases. Recurrences of intussusception are uncommon after operation.

### Inguinal Hernia

**Incidence, Etiology and Pathology.** Inguinal hernias occur much more frequently in boys than in girls. Such hernias may be present at birth or may occur at any age. They may be unilateral or bilateral.

As the testis descends retroperitoneally from the genital ridge during embryonic life, a sac of peritoneum precedes it into the scrotum, forming a tube. After descent of the testis the tube normally atrophies. If it does not close completely, intestine or peritoneal fluid may descend into it and produce a hernia. The hernia may vary in size, depending on whether it extends through the external inguinal ring or into the scrotum.

Although a hernial sac is present at

**Figure 130.** Inguinal hernia, strangulated. (Copyright, The Ciba Collection of Medical Illustrations, by Frank H. Netter, M.D.)

birth, the hernia may not appear until the infant is two or three months old. At this time he has a lusty cry, which increases the intra-abdominal pressure sufficiently to open the sac and force peritoneal fluid or intestine into it. As a result a bulge appears in the inguinal region or the scrotum.

In female infants an ovary may descend into a hernial sac as a result of increased intra-abdominal pressure.

**Clinical Manifestations.** When the hernial sac is empty, there are no symptoms. When abdominal contents are in the sac, incomplete bowel obstruction occurs. The infant expresses his discomfort and pain in fretfulness. Constipation and anorexia may occur.

If a loop of intestine is incarcerated or caught in the sac, all the symptoms of intestinal obstruction appear. There is danger of strangulation of the bowel with cutting off of the blood supply and ultimately gangrene. Incarceration occurs most frequently in the first six weeks of life. The symptom of an incarcerated hernia is the appearance of a firm, irreducible swelling below the external inguinal ring. The infant may vomit, and he becomes highly irritable. Later there is cessation of bowel movements, abdominal distention, increased vomiting, leukocytosis and fever.

The physician may be able to reduce the incarcerated hernia within twelve hours after it has occurred. If it cannot be reduced, emergency operation must be done. In severe cases bowel resection may be necessary.

If strangulation occurs before operation, the infant has severe pain and symptoms of complete obstruction. Immediate operation is necessary to relieve the condition.

**Diagnosis and Treatment.** The *diagnosis* is based on the history of intermittent appearance of a mass in the inguinal region and, on physical examination, the finding of a sac which fills when the infant cries or strains or which can be reduced easily.

Healthy infants are best *treated* by surgical repair as soon as the condition is diagnosed. Operation involves removing the hernial sac and transfixing the neck at the internal ring. Infants tolerate this operation very well. After operation, in the majority of cases, the danger of strangulation and of edema and gangrene is removed.

If incarceration occurs before operation, an ice bag should be applied over the area to reduce the edema. The foot of the bed should be elevated to prevent more abdominal contents from going through the inguinal ring. If manual reduction under sedation is not successful, operation is necessary immediately.

For temporary treatment trusses may be used. They are difficult to keep clean since they are close to both the genital and the anal areas, and are difficult to apply. If improperly applied, they may, because of pressure, cause testicular atrophy. A truss made of knitting yarn may be used. It is simple and effective and can be made by the mother.

To make the truss, one fifth to a quarter of a skein of white knitting yarn is wound into a smaller skein, the length of which should be

Figure 131. Method of applying a yarn truss to a baby for inguinal hernia. *1*, The hernia has been reduced and is held back with the finger as shown. *2*, The wool truss has been threaded through the first loop. This makes a lump which is brought to rest over the inguinal ring. *3*, The yarn presses down over the inguinal canal and is passed up over the buttocks to be tied posteriorly. It must be tied near the midline posteriorly to prevent the truss from slipping when the thigh is flexed. (Gross: The Surgery of Infancy and Childhood.)

Figure 132. Stiles's dressing for postoperative herniorrhaphy in an infant or small child. The cradle keeps bed clothing off the body. A diaper is suspended from the lower end of the cradle to catch any urine which is passed. The incision is therefore kept dry. The arms and legs are restrained with clove hitch restraints. (Gross: The Surgery of Infancy and Childhood.)

approximately three times the circumference of the infant's abdomen. Tie the strands together at each end.

Commercially made trusses can also be purchased.

**Nursing Care.** To apply a yarn truss, double the skein in half and place it under the infant's waist at the back. Slip the free end through the folded end and place the knot over the inguinal hernia, first making certain that the hernia is completely reduced. Bring the free ends under the groin on the side of the hernia and attach them to the yarn waist band in the back.

Besides learning how to reduce the hernia and apply a truss, the mother should be taught to make several of these trusses so that a fresh one may be applied as often as is necessary.

A reduced hernia should be kept in place constantly. To ensure this when changing the truss, one person should hold the hernia in place while another applies the fresh truss. If the hernia slips out of place when the truss has been adjusted, the hernia should be reduced again and the truss reapplied snugly at once.

A yarn truss should be laundered in lukewarm water with a mild soap and should be thoroughly rinsed and fluffed before drying completely so as to retain the softness and elasticity of new yarn.

The skin under the truss should be kept clean and dry in order to prevent excoriation, and the truss should be changed whenever it becomes soiled with urine or feces.

As far as is possible, the infant should be kept happy and tranquil so that he will not cry. The stools should be regulated, since either a constipated or an irritating loose stool will cause the infant to strain. Both crying and straining tend to raise the intra-abdominal pressure and so produce the hernia.

*Postoperative Care.* After an inguinal herniorrhaphy the major nursing problem is prevention of contamination of the wound. This is accomplished by keeping the area clean and dry. The diaper should be placed very low on the infant's abdomen, only the genitals being covered. Another way of accomplishing the same purpose is to tie a piece of string from one side of the bed to the other at the level of the infant's waist and to pin a diaper to the string. The other end of the diaper is spread under the infant's buttocks. When the male infant voids, the diaper will become wet, but the incision will be kept dry.

Figure 132 shows still another method which can be used to accomplish the same purpose.

Feedings are generally resumed a few hours postoperatively unless a bowel resection was done. The infant should be held for feedings and cuddled while being fed. After a simple hernia repair the older child may be as active as he desires to be.

### Umbilical Hernia

**Etiology, Incidence and Clinical Manifestations.** An umbilical hernia is due to imperfect closure or weakness of the umbilical ring. These hernias occur in all races, but are more common in Negro children.

The *clinical manifestations* are a swelling at the umbilicus which is covered with skin. This protrudes when the infant cries or strains. It can be easily reduced by gentle pressure over the fibrous ring at the umbilicus. The contents of the hernia are small intestine and omentum (see Fig. 133). The size varies from less than a centimeter to 5 cm. in diameter.

**Prognosis, Treatment and Nursing Care.** Most small umbilical hernias disappear without treatment, but large ones require operation. If the hernia is only 1 or 2 cm. in diameter, it is strapped for 6 or 7 months, by which time it will probably have disappeared. These hernias rarely cause incarceration or strangulation of the bowel.

For taping, the hernia is first reduced by gently pushing the abdominal contents back through the umbilical ring. The sides of the adjacent abdominal wall can be brought together in the midline to make a pleat of skin. The area to be taped should be painted with tincture of benzoin to protect the skin and to cause the adhesive to adhere to the skin. A 2-inch strip of adhesive can be applied to the abdomen when the

**Figure 133.** Diagrammatic representation of an umbilical hernia. (Copyright, The Ciba Collection of Medical Illustrations, by Frank H. Netter, M.D.)

**Figure 134.** Side view of infant with an umbilical hernia.

tincture of benzoin is dry, from the far bed line, over the pleat of skin, to the near bed line, covering the umbilical hernia. It should be pulled tightly across the pleat.

Years ago a penny or button was placed under the adhesive and over the hernia, to give added pressure and so hold the reduced hernia in place. This was a mistaken concept, and such a procedure should never be done, because the button or coin tends to prevent approximation of the edges of the hernial orifice.

If strapping does not eliminate the hernia, operation should be delayed until the surgeon believes it necessary.

Postoperative *nursing care* requires no special technique. The child may be as active as he desires to be. A normal diet and fluids are given. Pressure dressings, applied at the time of operation, must be kept clean and dry to prevent wound contamination.

## GENITOURINARY CONDITIONS

### Hydrocele

A hydrocele is an accumulation of fluid around the testicle or along the spermatic cord. It may be a congenital condition or may occur during infancy. In diagnosis a hydrocele causing a swelling of the scrotum must be differentiated from an inguinal hernia. A hydrocele appears as a fluctuant, oval, translucent, tense sac. Fluid may grad-

ually absorb during infancy, but if it does not, surgical correction is necessary.

### Pyelonephritis (Pyelitis)

**Incidence and Etiology.** Pyelitis is an infection of the renal pelvis. Pyelonephritis is an infection of the renal pelvis and renal parenchyma plus, in most cases, inflammation of the ureters and the bladder. Since infections in infants and children are rarely limited to one part of the urinary tract, the term "pyelonephritis" is probably more applicable than "pyelitis."

The condition is relatively common in pediatric practice and is the most common renal disease in childhood. The *incidence* is greatest between two months and two years, the period when diapers are worn. The condition occurs more frequently in girls than in boys.

The female urethra is shorter than the male urethra. Infection entering the urinary tract from the stool in a soiled diaper contaminates the urethra and may be carried to the bladder, causing cystitis. Infection may enter the urinary tract not only through the urethra, but also by way of the blood stream or the lymphatics. Congenital anomalies causing obstruction of urine are predisposing factors because urinary stasis is associated with chronic urinary tract infections.

Organisms causing acute infection are the colon bacilli—responsible for

Figure 135. Bilateral hydrocele in an infant. (Davis and Sheckler: De-Lee's Obstetrics for Nurses. 16th ed.)

more than three quarters of the cases —and staphylococci, hemolytic streptococci and *Streptococcus faecalis.* Chronic infections are often caused by multiple types of bacteria. Proteus and Pyocyaneus may also be causative organisms.

**Pathology, Clinical Manifestations and Laboratory Findings.** There are inflammatory changes in the renal pelvis and throughout the kidney. In the majority of cases there are changes also in the ureters and the bladder. The kidney may be large and swollen. Clumps of bacteria may be present. In chronic pyelonephritis there is loss of function because of scarring of the kidney parenchyma. Eventually the kidney becomes small; kidney tissue is destroyed, and renal function fails.

The *clinical findings* are variable. Symptoms related to the urinary tract may or may not be present. The onset may be gradual or abrupt. Fever may be moderate or as high as 104.5° F. (40.3° C.). Prostration, pallor and anorexia appear. Vomiting and diarrhea occur; dehydration may result. Urinary urgency and frequency with dysuria are distressing symptoms. The child is irritable, of course, and convulsions may occur.

It is possible that the infant may show none of the symptoms of localizing of the infection to the urinary tract.

Pain and tenderness in the kidney are signs of the condition. If the infection is chronic, it may continue for months and years, causing anemia and failure of growth and development. Eventually renal failure and hypertension result.

*Laboratory findings* include pyuria, pathologic organisms in the urine, and leukocytosis. Slight or moderate hematuria may occur, and casts may be present.

**Diagnosis and Treatment.** The *diagnosis* is made on the basis of pus and bacteria in the urine. A catheterized specimen must be obtained. If there is recurring or persistent pyuria, intravenous or retrograde urography should be resorted to. There may be neurologic or structural abnormalities which cause

stasis and continued infection. The cystogram is useful for examining the child for ureteral dilatation.

General *treatment* during the febrile period includes rest; analgesic drugs are given if needed. Specific chemotherapy or antibiotic therapy is given to shorten the course of the illness and to avoid possible progressive renal damage. Sulfonamides are most widely used against urinary tract infections. Mandelic acid acidifies the urine. The effectiveness of this acid when used as a urinary antiseptic depends on maintaining a *very acid* urine. Acid-forming salts may be given to achieve this result. Nitrofurantoin (Furadantin) is a bacteriostatic and bactericidal agent against most of the urinary tract pathogens.

During the acute stage the child should be encouraged to take more than normal amounts of fluid to dilute the concentration of urine. If anemia is present, transfusions may be indicated. If there are obstructive lesions, surgical correction may be attempted. Surgical removal is not always possible, however.

**Nursing Care.** Clean specimens of urine should be obtained (for collection of specimens, see p. 58). The genitals must be thoroughly cleansed with green soap solution and cotton pledgets before the specimen is collected. The area is rinsed with sterile water. If a little girl is old enough to use a bedpan, it should be sterilized before use. If a little boy can control himself during urination, a midstream specimen may be obtained. This means that he voids a small amount, stops, and then voids into a sterile receptable for the specimen. Laboratory examination of a clean specimen of urine gives a rough estimate of the number of bacteria present.

For bacterial culture only a catheterized specimen should be used. The equipment for catheterization is the same as for the procedure in the adult, with the exception of the size of the catheter used. For children size 8 or 10 French is used. Two catheters should be in readiness, since the first to be used may be accidentally contaminated. Various solutions are used for cleansing the genitals.

The procedure for catheterization of the older child is the same as that for the adult and should be explained to the child. The child should be given an opportunity to handle the equipment and should be completely relaxed if catheterization is to be done successfully. The nurse may ask the child to breathe deeply through the mouth in order to promote relaxation while the catheter is being inserted into the bladder. For the younger child two nurses are necessary, one to assist the child in cooperating and the other to carry out the procedure.

The following points are stressed: (1) thorough cleansing of the genitals. This is done with cotton balls dipped in the cleansing solution. *One ball is used for each stroke.* Strokes should be from above downward toward the anus, to prevent organisms from the anus from being carried up over the urethral meatus.

2. The tip of the sterile catheter should be lubricated with sterile saline solution before insertion into the urethral meatus.

3. The anatomy of the infant or small child is different from that of the adult, and this makes catheterization more difficult for the nurse. The bladder in the infant lies more anteriorly and higher over the symphysis than in the adult, and the urethra lies under and around the symphysis. The meatus in the small child may be exceedingly difficult to locate because of its small size. Because of these anatomic differences it is essential that the light be good so that the meatus can be seen by inspection without causing the infant unnecessary discomfort by probing with the tip of the catheter. Such probing also contaminates the catheter and necessitates use of the second catheter. The catheter is introduced gently, directed downward and inserted along the rounded path to the bladder, lying above the symphysis.

The fluid intake is important. If fluids are ordered in quantity greater than normal, they should be offered between feedings or between meals.

## TEACHING AIDS AND OTHER INFORMATION*

*Abbott Laboratories*
   Fluid and Electrolytes, Some Practical Guides to Clinical Use, 1957.

### REFERENCES

Anthony, C. P.: What Makes Fluids Flow? Am. J. Nursing, 56:1256, 1956.

Barness, L. A. (Consulting Editor): Fluid and Electrolyte Problems. Pediat. Clin. North America, 1959, Vol. 6, pp. 1–328.

Clatworthy, H. W., and Stewart, M. M.: Intravenous Therapy for Infants and Children. Am. J. Nursing, 57:630, 1957.

Cooper, M. L. and others: Epidemic Diarrhea among Infants Associated with the Isolation of a New Serotype of Escherichia Coli: E. Coli 0127:B8. Pediatrics, 16:215, 1955.

Gross, R. E.: The Surgery of Infancy and Childhood. Philadelphia, W. B. Saunders Company, 1953.

Hansen, D. E.: Abdominal Hernias. Am. J. Nursing, 61:102, March, 1961.

Hemmendinger, M.: ℞: 'Admit Parents at All Times.' Child Study, 34:No. 1, 3, 1956.

Kiesewetter, W. B.: Pre- and Postoperative Care in the Pediatric Surgical Patient. Chicago, Year Book Publishers, Inc., 1956.

Koop, C. E.: Inguinal Herniorrhaphy in Infants and Children. S. Clin. North America, 37:1675, 1957.

Lowe, C. U. Principles of Parenteral Fluid Therapy. Am. J. Nursing, 53:963, 1953.

McCaskill, C. L.: Pediatric Surgical Nursing. Nursing Outlook, 6:274, 1958.

Mellish, R. W. P.: Timing in Pediatric Surgery. Pediat. Clin. North America, 6:987, 1959.

Nelson, W. E. (editor): Textbook of Pediatrics. 7th ed. Philadelphia, W. B. Saunders Company, 1959.

Paterson, D., and McCreary, J. F.: Pediatrics. Philadelphia, J. B. Lippincott Company, 1956.

Robertson, J.: Young Children in Hospitals. New York, Basic Books, Inc., 1958.

Silver, H. K., Kempe, C. H., and Bruyn, H. B.: Handbook of Pediatrics. 3rd ed. Los Altos, California, Lange Medical Publications, 1959.

Snively, W. D., and Brown, B. J.: In the Balance. Am. J. Nursing, 58:55, 1958.

Snively, W. D., and others: Systematic Approach to Fluid Balance. GP, 13:74, January, 1956.

Swenson, O.: Pediatric Surgery. New York, Appleton-Century-Crofts, Inc., 1958.

* Complete addresses are given in the Appendix.

# Chapter 14

# Conditions of Infants

# Requiring Long-Term

# Care

LONG-TERM illness brings with it problems of personality adjustment different from those produced by acute, short-term illness. Long-term illness may follow an acute condition or may have a slow, insidious development. Some conditions are congenital. Many of them have periods of exacerbation and of remission. Although some may be relieved by surgical or medical treatment, others result in early death. Whatever the disease, when a child has been ill for a long time, his nutritional status declines, and this adversely influences his growth and development. He may appear to be considerably younger than his age. He is particularly in need of tender, loving care. If he is separated from his mother for long periods, he suffers from maternal deprivation, which severely injures his personality.

Infancy covers only a short time. An illness of even a few months may retard an infant in accomplishing the developmental tasks of infancy. One of the most important of these tasks is to learn to trust other people. It is essential that the hospitalized infant keep his trust in his mother's loving protection and learn that others give him physical care and affection. The mother should be allowed to spend all the time she can spare from other duties with her child.

The mother's reaction to her child's long-term illness depends, naturally, on the seriousness of his condition. Many long-term illnesses begin as dangerous, acute conditions whose prognosis is doubtful. If the critical period can be passed, as well as such other crises as may occur, there is always hope that some new drug or treatment may be discovered which will cure or mitigate the severity of the disease. Parents may be told of this possibility, but should not be led to believe that such discoveries are sure to be made.

If the illness is severe and the prognosis doubtful, the mother is under a prolonged emotional strain. Her reaction may be to overprotect her baby. The infant may respond to this with a lack of normal attempts to try out new muscular activities in an infant's way of self-help and self-amusement. Even an infant is likely to compensate for a lack of control over his environment by a control over adults who will give him what he wants and do for him what he has not yet learned he can do for himself.

The nurse should understand clearly what activity the physician allows and within that range give the infant opportunity for habilitation. This applies not only to physical activity, but also to psychologic and emotional growth.

The mother should be allowed to verbalize her feelings and thereby relieve to some extent the emotional strain under which she labors. This is not only for her sake, but also because of her influence upon the infant. Unlimited visiting hours in the pediatric unit will give her an opportunity to observe the nurses' care of her child and to discuss with them the technique of his habilitation, whether it is letting him attempt new physical activities or playing by himself without expecting constant attention.

The mother may become overdependent upon the nurse for emotional support. But as she sees the nurse's care of the infant and his response, she will join the health team and cease to cast her responsibilities upon the other members of the team. When she herself is a member of the team, she loses her sense of frustration at others being able to give the child more and better care than she can, and will understand that they excel in professional service, but that she excels in meeting the child's need for affection and security in the love of one person, who will be with him throughout childhood.

## NUTRITIONAL DISORDERS (DEFICIENCY DISEASES)

The diets of infants and young children may be deficient in nutriment, i.e. in the total amount of any of the three main food constituents—protein, fat or carbohydrate—or in essential vitamins or minerals. Although several factors may contribute to the production of deficiency diseases, the basic problem is usually a lack of intake, though sometimes there may be poor absorption of one or more components of food after ingestion.

Deficiency diseases are especially harmful during infancy because this is the period when growth is most rapid, and the human organism needs adequate supplies of all essential food elements. The deficiency may be of a single food element or of several elements.

### Malnutrition (Athrepsia, Marasmus)

**Incidence, Etiology and Diagnosis.** Malnutrition is less prevalent in the United States and Europe than it was a generation ago. The level of living is higher, and the nutritional needs of infants are better understood and practiced. But in India, China and among primitive peoples malnutrition of children is one of the problems in which the World Health Organization is vitally interested.

Malnutrition should be considered secondary to the condition causing it. It is a general term indicating undernutrition. Specific vitamin deficiencies are likely in malnourished infants.

The fundamental cause is that the infant does not receive an adequate diet or is unable to assimilate sufficient nutriment for the metabolic needs of his body, with the result that reserve food elements in the tissues are used. The specific cause may be (1) an inadequate intake or a badly balanced diet, (2) poor feeding habits due to improper training, (3) a physical defect such as cleft lip or cleft palate, or cardiac abnormalities which prevent the infant's taking an adequate diet, (4) diseases which interfere with the assimilation of food (these are generally chronic diseases such as cystic fibrosis of the pancreas), (5) infections which produce anorexia and decrease the infant's ability to digest his food, and yet at the same time increase his need for food, (6) loss of food through vomiting and diarrhea, or (7) emotional disturbances such as disturbed mother-child relations.

The *diagnosis* of malnutrition may be determined by the obvious symptoms found on physical examination, by failure of growth or by measurement of the blood constituents. Dietary surveys establish the probability of malnutrition in children of any group.

**Clinical Manifestations and Laboratory Studies.** Failure to gain weight followed by loss of weight is only one manifestation of deficiency diseases. Growth of the skeleton and of the brain continues, with the result that the body is long and the head large in proportion to the weight. To maintain metabolism, the body uses its own fat and protein. The subcutaneous fat disappears, but the sucking pads of the cheeks remain, giving the face a factitious roundness. The fat of the abdominal wall decreases. The skin becomes wrinkled, and the eyes are sunken. The features have a drawn appearance, and when at last the fat pads have been absorbed, the face takes on an aged look. Skin turgor is lost, and the skin lies in loose folds on the body. The bones are prominent. The infant is no longer active, his muscles are flabby and relaxed, and his cry is weak and shrill. Finally he ceases to be hungry, hunger movements disappear, and he shows all the signs of exhaustion and emaciation.

As his blood volume diminishes and he becomes anemic, his color becomes ashen gray. His temperature is subnormal, the pulse is slow, and the basal metabolism tends to be reduced. His digestive capacity decreases, and his appetite is poor. He may have constipation or starvation diarrhea, in which the stools contain mucus and bile. He is subject to infections and has poor resistance. There may be evidence of a specific deficiency disease such as rickets, scurvy, tetany or nutritional anemia, and nutritional edema may also be present.

The *laboratory findings* show severe hypochromic anemia. The plasma protein level is usually lowered unless hemoconcentration is present. In that case the serum level may be within the normal range.

**Complications.** Intercurrent infections are frequent and are located in different systems of the body. The most common infections are oral thrush (gastrointestinal tract), pyelitis (genitourinary tract) and bronchitis or upper

**Figure 136.** Malnutrition due to inability to assimilate food. Subcutaneous fat has disappeared. The infant's skin is wrinkled, especially in the groins. The bones are prominent. Note the arm restrained for intravenous therapy.

respiratory tract infections (respiratory tract). Skin infections such as furunculosis occur, as well as infected bed sores over the bony prominences, e.g. the occiput, heels and knees. Nutritional anemia due to a low iron intake may develop. Nutritional edema results when the body, lacking sufficient protein obtained from food, has burnt its own tissues and destroyed the protein in the plasma. When the level of plasma albumin becomes low, nutritional edema occurs. Nutritional edema is seen in infants who have been malnourished for several months. When sufficient protein is given and the infant has recovered so that the body is able to absorb the necessary amount of protein, the edema disappears.

Kwashiorkor, a condition seen among the underprivileged in tropical and subtropical countries, is a type of malnutrition due to a deficiency of protein and other nutrients. Prevention of kwashiorkor lies in giving an adequate diet after the infant has been weaned.

**Treatment and Prognosis.** The basic *treatment* is through diet. The initial feedings should be low in quantity and in calories, because the digestive capacity is poor. If too much feeding is given too quickly, the infant will probably suffer diarrhea and vomiting. The initial feeding should be diluted breast milk or, if that is not available, skimmed lactic acid milk. The amount of protein and carbohydrate in the formula is slowly increased, but kept within the infant's ability to tolerate these important constituents of a normal diet. It is necessary to increase the fat content more slowly than the carbohydrate, since fat is more difficult to digest. Evaporated or dried milk may be given within a few days, since the curd is smaller than that of fresh milk. Food requirements for such infants may be as high as 75 to 100 calories per pound each day before they gain weight. They must receive increased protein to build body tissue.

If the infant is dehydrated or shows evidence of electrolyte imbalance, parenteral fluids are given. Depleted reserves of electrolytes must be restored gradually.

Small but frequent blood transfusions may be necessary to correct the anemia and to increase the infant's resistance to infection. Medications are aimed at correction of the dietary deficiencies. Intramuscular injections of crude liver extract may be given every two or three days for several weeks, and vitamins A, B, C and D may be given in usual or increased amounts.

Complications such as concurrent infections or skin conditions are treated as they occur.

The *prognosis* depends on the severity of the condition, its length and on whether infection is present. Severely malnourished infants may go into a state of collapse and die suddenly. This is most likely to happen in infants who have continued to lose weight after institution of treatment and have experienced a sudden drop in temperature accompanied with a slow pulse and evidence of a circulatory crisis. Such infants may have acquired a severe, overwhelming infection against which they have no resistance.

**Nursing Care.** The body temperature must be maintained. If the infant has a subnormal temperature, he should be placed in an incubator or given extra clothing and covered with blankets. Hot-water bottles should be placed on both sides of his body. Since he is subject to infection, his feeding equipment should be sterile to avoid the danger of his contracting thrush. He should be turned frequently to prevent hypostatic pneumonia, pressure areas on the bony prominences, and skin infections. He requires careful skin care. He should be isolated for his own protection, and nursing personnel who care for him should be free from any kind of infectious condition. Since his resistance is low, he should be kept out of drafts.

The feeding ordered by the physician should be followed carefully and the order checked before each feeding to see whether the feeding has been changed. The infant should be fed slowly and bubbled frequently. During feeding he should be handled gently so that he feels secure in his nurse's care, cuddled and surrounded with emotional as well as physical warmth.

Since collapse is possible in the severely ill infant, he should be watched at all times for the signs of collapse: temperature drop, slow pulse, cyanosis or gray-white color of the skin, and coldness of the extremities.

The nurse will assist with administration of parenteral fluids or blood. Accurate, detailed charting is necessary and includes the amount of feeding taken, refused or vomited, and whether it was taken eagerly or with indifference. It is important for the physician to know the number and type of stools and whether abdominal distention is present. The infant should be weighed at the same time daily to determine the exact gain or loss.

**Prevention.** Prevention of malnutrition is one of the important functions of Child Health Conferences. The amount of the feeding must be adequate and suited to the individual infant. He should be fed with good technique so that he may make full use of the feeding ordered by the physician.

Also important in prevention of malnutrition are early treatment of defects, diseases or infections predisposing to malnutrition and prevention of emotional disturbances.

### Rickets

**Etiology and Incidence.** Rickets is a deficiency disease which occurs in growing children owing to a lack of fat-soluble vitamin D. If the condition occurs after growth has ceased, it is called *osteomalacia.*

Since vitamin D increases absorption of calcium from the gastrointestinal tract and decreases renal excretion of phosphate, lack of this vitamin leads to a disturbance of concentration of calcium and phosphorus in the blood and tissue fluids.

Rickets may occur in any infant, but is most likely in rapidly growing children. It appears to have been a disease common in ancient times. In some early Christian pictures the infant Jesus shows the deformities of rickets.

Factors predisposing to rickets are (1) heredity. Dark-skinned people living away from their natural habitat of hot, sunny climates do not receive an adequate amount of vitamin D from the sun's rays. The dark skin prevents the full effect of the sun's rays upon the body chemistry. (2) Age. Although the age of greatest susceptibility is about eighteen months, rickets may occur at any time from three months to three years (a period of rapid growth). (3) Artificial feeding. A breast-fed infant is less likely to suffer rickets than is the bottle-fed one, provided his mother is receiving an adequate amount of sunshine or vitamin D from some other source. This superiority of breast milk over cow's milk applies only when cow's milk is considered to which vitamin D has *not* been added. Milk produced for sale, as well as evaporated milk, in general contains an ample amount of vitamin D. This has been an important factor in the prevention of rickets in urban low-income homes where children receive little sunshine during the winter months. (4) Prematurity. Prematurity predisposes to rickets because the deposits of calcium and phosphorus at birth are inadequate for the exceptionally rapid growth of the well cared for premature infant. (5) Lack of sunshine. There are many days of cloudy, rainy or foggy weather in some areas. Dirt in the air over cities prevents what sunshine there is from having its full therapeutic effect, and the window glass usually used cuts out a high percentage of the ultraviolet rays in even a sunny room. (6) Season. The incidence of rickets is greatest in the late winter and early spring. In summer the child is likely to be out of doors in the sunlight. During the autumn months he may exhaust the supply of vitamin D stored in his body, with the result that rickets may develop in the winter and spring. Vitamin D is absorbed with fat in the small intestine. The vitamin can be stored in the body, but if a new supply is not available, the amount stored is used up.

**Pathology and Clinical Manifestations.** The manifestations of rickets are most evident in the skeletal system and vary with the age of the child and the amount of stress undergone by the affected bone in performing its function in the child's developing body. Deficiency in the structure of the bone is most pronounced in the lack of calcifi-

**Figure 137.** Deformities in rickets, showing curvature of the limbs, potbelly and Harrison's groove. (Josef Warkany, in Nelson: Textbook of Pediatrics. 7th ed.)

cation of the epiphysis. A detectable enlargement occurs in this area. Besides the bones, the muscles are also affected, lacking normal muscle tone.

The *clinical manifestations* are best described under the various parts of the body affected.

In advanced disease the head appears enlarged, owing to the prominent bossing of the frontal bones. As a result the skull appears to be square when viewed from above, looking down on the top of the head. The anterior fontanel is late in closing, and the cranial bones are soft and make a cracking sound under pressure. This condition is called *craniotabes* and is primarily apparent in the occipital bones. The head is likely to be covered with beads of perspiration.

The thorax shows the rachitic rosary —beading of the costochondral junctions—and Harrison's groove—a bilateral depression at the sites where the diaphragm is attached to the ribs. The chest is funnel-shaped and characterized by an abnormal protrusion or depression of the sternum. When the infant is old enough to sit up, a dorsal kyphosis develops. Lack of muscular tone causes the infant to assume a poor sitting posture which brings pressure upon the weak bones of the spine. Scoliosis with deformities of the pelvis frequently occurs.

The extremities are likely to be deformed. Bowlegs or knock knees accompanied with flat feet are probably the most obvious deformities. There is epiphysial enlargement of the wrists and ankles.

Later the infant, on sitting, assumes a crouching, froglike position. Because of the poor bone growth and muscle tone the infant is retarded in sitting, standing and walking. Eruption of teeth is delayed.

If the pelvis of a female infant is deformed, as often happens in severe rickets, the constricted inlet and outlet will make childbirth difficult.

The so-called potbelly is caused by relaxed abdominal muscles. The loss of strength in the abdominal muscles may cause the child to be constipated.

In less advanced stages of rickets the only obvious signs may be craniotabes and enlargement of the costochondral functions.

Nutritional anemia may be evident. Since the child's general nutritional state is poor, he has a low resistance to respiratory infection and its many complications.

**Diagnosis.** Mild and early cases of rickets are diagnosed by determining the serum calcium, phosphorus and alkaline phosphatase levels. Advanced cases are easily diagnosed by the gross clinical manifestations and the history of a lack of vitamin D. Changes are evident in the radiologic appearance of the bones.

**Treatment and Prevention.** *Treatment* is by oral administration of large doses of vitamin D, generally 2000 to 3000 International units a day for about a month. This usually results in cure of he disease. The physician may order massive doses which will result in more rapid healing. If deformities are present, corrective appliances are used— splints and braces for bowlegs and knock knees. Osteotomy may be necessary.

Although the breast-fed infant is less likely to acquire rickets if his mother has an adequate intake of vitamin D, both he and the bottle-fed infant should receive vitamin D in maintenance amounts to supplement the intake. This is of greatest importance during the winter months. The recommended dose is 400 International units daily for the normal infant. If he lives in the city, he should receive vitamin D throughout the year. The rural infant does not need this protection during the summer months. Since older children grow less slowly, they need less vitamin D and normally receive enough in their diet if it includes irradiated milk and eggs.

**Nursing Care.** Before the newborn leaves the hospital his mother should receive an accurate explanation of the danger of rickets and the need for giving the infant vitamin D and a liberal diet suited to his needs. Such instruction is routine for mothers of infants under the supervision of Child Health Conferences. If the infant already has rickets, the mother should have the treatment explained to her, for it is she who will carry it out unless hospitalization is necessary. Only a child with severe late rickets requires hospitalization, but a rachitic child may be admitted to a hospital for a concurrent infection.

Rachitic children should be handled gently and turned frequently. To prevent deformity they should be kept from sitting without support or from standing (i.e. from putting their weight on the spinal column or legs) during their illness. In lifting the infant undue pressure on the bones of the chest should never be made. The diaper should be applied loosely lest it bring pressure on the long bones of the legs. Proper positioning and frequent change of position lessen the danger of deformity. If the infant lies constantly on

his back or on one side, both his head and chest will be flattened by the pressure of his weight on the soft bones. He should lie on a firm mattress. His back should be supported when he sits up or is carried by his mother or nurse. Great care should be exercised to prevent his falling if he does stand.

Administration of vitamin D presents no problem unless it is in a solution containing oil. Then care must be taken that he does not aspirate even a few drops of the substance, with the possibility of lipoid pneumonia resulting.

It is important to prevent infection. The infant must be kept out of drafts. Frequent changing of his position, required to prevent deformity, will also lessen the danger of lung infection. The physician may order sunbaths for the infant (see p. 277).

**Prognosis.** Rickets is not a direct cause of death, but it is a contributing factor because it predisposes to illnesses. Rachitic deformities may persist, but minor deformities in general disappear during the preschool period. Severe deformities must be corrected either operatively or mechanically.

### Infantile Nutritional Tetany* (Tetany of Vitamin D Deficiency)

**Incidence and Clinical Manifestations.** Infantile nutritional tetany is caused by a deficiency in the intake and absorption of vitamin D. The condition is invariably associated with rickets, but not all rachitic children have tetany. A child may have received sufficient vitamin D to prevent tetany, but not enough to prevent rickets. If a child receiving vitamin D for a rachitic condition acquires tetany, it is probably due to the rapid deposition of serum calcium in rachitic osteoid tissue and depletion of serum calcium in the blood. It may also result from a decrease in parathyroid activity.

This type of tetany has the same seasonal *incidence* as rickets and occurs in the same age group because of the close association of factors causing both conditions.

* For other forms of tetany, see page 379.

*Clinical manifestations* are due to increased neuromuscular irritability. There are two stages in tetany—latent and manifest.

In *latent tetany* the infant or child has a low serum calcium level—less than 7 to 7.5 mg. per 100 milliliters—but no obvious symptoms other than "jitteriness." Muscular irritability may be observed as a result of electrical or mechanical stimulation.

There are four main mechanical or electrical means of producing clinical manifestations of tetany which are used in diagnosis.

1. *Chvostek's Sign.* When the skin in front of the auditory meatus, where the facial nerve is close to the surface, is tapped, unilateral contraction of the facial muscles around the nose, eye and mouth results. Although a newborn infant may have a positive Chvostek's sign normally, a child between three months and three years of age who has a positive Chvostek's sign probably has tetany.

2. *Trousseau's Sign.* If carpal spasm results when the upper arm is constricted for two to three minutes *after the hand has blanched,* the Trousseau sign is positive, showing the presence of tetany.

3. *Erb's Sign.* This test is based on the fact that a patient with tetany has greater muscular irritability than is seen in a normal child. A galvanic current is applied, usually over the peroneal nerve just below the head of the fibula. A positive response consists in dorsiflexion and abduction of the foot as a result of a measured amount of galvanic current.

4. *Peroneal Sign.* This sign is positive when tapping the fibular side of the leg over the peroneal nerve causes abduction and dorsiflexion of the foot.

In *manifest tetany* the serum calcium is often well under 7 mg. per 100 ml. Muscular twitchings and carpopedal spasms occur spontaneously. In *carpal spasm* the thumb is drawn into the cupped palm. The hands are abducted, the wrists flexed. In *pedal spasm* the foot is extended as in talipes equinus or equinovarus. The toes are

*A*

*B*

**Figure 138.** Tetany. *A,* Carpal spasm. *B,* Pedal spasm. (Nelson: Textbook of Pediatrics. 7th ed.)

flexed, and the sole of the foot is cupped. The arms and legs may be adducted and flexed.

There may be spasm of the larynx—laryngospasm—indicated by a high-pitched crowing sound on inspiration, due to spasm of the adductor muscles of the larynx which pull the vocal cords together. If the spasm is severe, respirations may cease and cyanosis may occur. Convulsions—generalized seizures including carpopedal spasm—may occur.

**Diagnosis and Treatment.** The *diagnosis* is made on the basis of the laboratory data and the clinical manifestations of rickets and tetany. The laboratory tests show a low calcium level; low, normal or elevated serum phosphorus level; and increased serum phosphatase.

The objective of *treatment* in hypocalcemic tetany is to raise the serum calcium level above that causing tetany. Calcium may be given in the form of calcium chloride or calcium gluconate. Calcium chloride is given in a 10 per cent solution orally. Calcium gluconate in a 10 per cent solution may be given intravenously if the child cannot take oral medication. Calcium gluconate should not be given intramuscularly or subcutaneously because of the danger of necrosis at the site of injection. The drug may cause cardiac arrest. The antidote for a dose of calcium gluconate which is greater than the child can tolerate is magnesium sulfate given intravenously.

Convulsions may be controlled by oxygen therapy and intravenous administration of calcium gluconate. If these procedures do not give relief, sodium phenobarbital may be administered intramuscularly. Emergency intubation may be necessary if laryngospasm is prolonged and cannot be relieved with sedatives and calcium salt.

After the acute clinical manifestations of tetany have been controlled oral calcium should be continued; in addition, large amounts of vitamin D should be given daily. After rickets has healed the child should receive the usual preventive amount of vitamin D daily.

**Nursing Care.** Nursing care is of the utmost importance. The nurse will give the medications as ordered and will keep magnesium sulfate available when calcium gluconate is to be given.

The nurse should have padded tongue blades, to prevent the child from biting his tongue during a convulsion, and oxygen ready in case of convulsions and laryngospasm. She must be trained to give artificial respiration to infants (see p. 185) and should review the method so that there may be no delay if resuscitation is necessary. Intubation equipment should be in readiness.

**Prognosis and Prevention.** The *prognosis* is good if treatment is given early. Death may occur from laryngospasm or cardiac failure. Further attacks may be prevented by prophylaxis.

Before the infant is sent home the mother, in her conferences with the physician and the nurse, should be told the importance of vitamin D therapy for the infant and also for the other children in the family.

The *preventive measures* for infantile nutritional tetany are the same as those for rickets.

### Scurvy

Scurvy is due to a lack of the water-soluble vitamin C (ascorbic acid). The vitamin is unstable and is destroyed by heat, and also by alkaline solutions or by oxidation when in aqueous solutions. Ascorbic acid withstands heat fairly well in an acid solution and in the absence of oxygen. Vitamin C is generally given to infants in the form of orange juice which should never be boiled, since heat destroys the vitamin.

**Incidence and Etiology.** The newborn has an adequate amount of vitamin C if his mother had a sufficient amount in her diet. Since vitamin C, unlike vitamin D, cannot be synthesized by human beings, the total supply must come from the diet. Although breast milk contains the necessary amount for the infant, if the mother's diet continues to have a sufficient amount for both her own needs and those of her infant, the breast-fed infant should receive a supplementary amount of vitamin C. There is little of this vitamin in commercial cow's milk because much is lost in the pasteurization process. For this reason infants on cow's milk feedings should be given ample vitamin C in some other form.

Scurvy may occur at any age, but is more frequent in infants from six to twelve months of age and in the second year of life. Any infection which increases the infant's temperature may predispose to scurvy, since febrile disease increases the body's need for vitamin C. Scurvy is not seen as often as it formerly was because it is now cus-

*A*

*B*

**Figure 139.** Scurvy. *A,* Scorbutic rosary, depression of sternum and the so-called frog position. (Josef Warkany, in Nelson: Textbook of Pediatrics. 7th ed.) *B,* Hypertrophic bleeding gingivae of scurvy. (Lewis: Practical Dermatology. 2nd ed.)

tomary to include orange juice or some other form of ascorbic acid in the diets of infants.

**Pathology, Diagnosis and Clinical Manifestations.** Pathologically, there is a defect in the formation and maintenance of intercellular substances in supporting tissues, dentin, bone, cartilage and vascular endothelium. Clinical manifestations, including a tendency to hemorrhage, can therefore be seen in the teeth and bones. The tendency to hemorrhage may be the specific result of lack of a maintenance amount of cement substance in the walls of the blood vessels or of collagen around the vessels.

The *diagnosis* is usually based on the history, roentgenographic examination and the symptoms.

X-ray examination shows changes in the distal ends of the long bones. Initially there appears to be atrophy of the bone. In the shaft the bone presents a ground-glass appearance. Subperi-

osteal hemorrhages (hemorrhages beneath the periosteum) of the long bones do not show on the x-ray film *during active scurvy*, but are apparent during the healing process. This is because the periosteum becomes loosened, especially at the ends of the femur and the tibia, and during healing the elevated periosteum becomes calcified.

It is sometimes difficult to distinguish scurvy from arthritis (seldom seen in children), osteomyelitis or poliomyelitis because of the tenderness of the limbs and the pain produced on movement. It may also be difficult to distinguish it from dysentery, hemorrhagic nephritis or blood dyscrasias when the tendency to hemorrhage is the most important clinical manifestation.

Laboratory tests may be done to confirm the diagnosis of scurvy, but the roentgenographic appearance of the long bones is the most significant factor in the diagnosis.

The *clinical manifestations* appear slowly after the body has been deprived of an adequate amount of ascorbic acid. They include fretfulness and irritability. The facial appearance is that of apprehension. The infant fears to be touched because of the pain when he is moved, as in changing his diaper. He may have anorexia.

Subperiosteal hemorrhage causes great pain, chiefly in the legs. The pain causes a pseudoparalysis. The child assumes a frog position; i.e. the hips and knees are semiflexed with the feet rotated outward.

There may be bluish-purple, swollen, bleeding gums and blood in the vomitus and stools. The gums may be so swollen that the teeth are concealed. If the infant is teething, this condition causes him great distress.

Hemorrhages may be seen in the soft tissue around the eyes, and petechiae may appear in the skin. The infant may have the so-called rosary at the costochondral junction. These scorbutic beads are sharper than those of rickets. In rickets they are due to widening of the softened epiphyses; in scurvy they are due to subluxation (partial or complete dislocation) of the sternal plate at the union of the ribs and the sternum.

The infant's temperature may be slightly elevated or even rise to 102° F. Anemia develops, owing to anorexia and hemorrhage. The infant then becomes very pale. The rate of growth, which is rapid in normal infants, is slowed in those with this condition.

**Treatment.** The specific treatment for scurvy is large doses of vitamin C. Orange juice—90 to 120 cc. daily—or ascorbic acid—100 to 300 mg. daily— is given orally or parenterally. After several days of such treatment the normal requirement is all that is needed. An adequate diet is given as a supportive measure. Transfusions may be necessary for severe anemia.

**Nursing Care.** Nursing care centers about the diet and medications and prevention of pain and of infection. The diet is high in vitamin C content. During the acute stage the child should be fed in whatever position appears to be most comfortable for him. His head should be elevated slightly. Later, when he is in less pain, he should be held in a comfortable position and cuddled.

The pseudoparalysis of scurvy is the chief problem in nursing. Great gentleness in handling is necessary. The nurse's movements should be slow and sure. All needless motion and any caress which may cause pain should be avoided. Since the infant fears that he will be moved when a nurse approaches him, it is well not to come too close to the bed unless necessary care must be given. In diapering the infant the buttocks may be elevated and the diaper slid under from the side. The buttocks should never be lifted by elevating the legs as is customary with a well child. A bed cradle may be used to prevent painful pressure of the bed clothes upon the child's body.

Nursing care, medication and treatments should be given at the same time so that the infant may rest without movement between the times when it is necessary to arouse him.

Prevention of infection is of the utmost importance. The infant's position must be changed frequently even though moving causes him pain. Mouth care is also painful, but the mouth should be cleansed with water after each feeding.

**Prognosis and Prevention.** The *prognosis* is excellent if the treatment is adequate. Pain ceases in a few days, and body growth is resumed. But if the condition is untreated, death may occur in a few months from undernutrition or intercurrent disease. Permanent deformity is seldom seen, and orthopedic treatment is required only in unusual cases.

*Prevention* lies in giving the infant an adequate diet containing an ample supply of vitamin C. Starting at 2 to 4 weeks of age, an infant should receive 25 to 50 mg. of ascorbic acid or 1 to 2 ounces of orange juice daily. If tomato juice, fresh or canned, is used instead, 2 to 4 ounces a day are required.

Mothers who breast-feed their babies should take at least 150 mg. a day of ascorbic acid in order to provide enough vitamin C for the infant in the breast milk. An adequate amount of vitamin C is required throughout childhood; older children need 60 to 75 mg. a day, and adolescents 80 to 100 mg. a day, of ascorbic acid.

## GASTROINTESTINAL DISORDERS

### Celiac Syndrome

Celiac syndrome is a state in which the infant or child has chronic nutritional failure. The clinical manifestations are (1) stunting of growth, (2) wasting of the extremities and buttocks accompanied by abdominal distention, (3) pale, foul-smelling, large stools, (4) anorexia, (5) nervous symptoms, and (6) evidence of mineral and vitamin deficiency.

Two relatively common diseases included in the celiac syndrome are true or idiopathic celiac disease (see Chap. 17) and cystic fibrosis of the pancreas.

### Cystic Fibrosis of the Pancreas (Mucoviscidosis)

**Incidence and Etiology.** Cystic fibrosis is a congenital disease inherited as a mendelian recessive trait. For an infant to have this disease, both parents must be carriers. According to the Mendelian Law, the condition may appear in one fourth of all children of such unions. Carriers may be identified by analysis of their sweat.

The disease is uncommon, but not rare, the incidence in the general population being from 1:1000 to 1:10,000, with equal frequency in either sex. The incidence is greatest among Caucasians and rare in Negro infants. More than one child in a family may be affected.

**Pathology and Clinical Manifestations.** There is a widespread change in the mucus-secreting glands of the body, i.e. in the pancreas, lungs and salivary and sweat glands.

The pancreatic changes are due to obstruction by inspissated secretion, beginning in the acini and extending to the ducts. Eventually acinar tissue dilates and atrophies and is replaced by connective tissue, resulting in fibrosis of the entire gland. The islands of Langerhans, which produce insulin, remain normal.

The air passages in the lungs are obstructed by a thick, mucoid secretion which may produce emphysema or atelectasis. Later bronchiolectatic abscesses and areas of bronchopneumonia are found. Eventually pulmonary fibrosis and interstitial pneumonia occur. The acini and ducts of the salivary glands are distended. The saliva contains increased amounts of sodium and chloride. The sweat contains a high concentration of sodium, potassium and chloride.

The *clinical manifestations* may be present at birth if the infant has meconium ileus (see p. 184). Most newborns, however, who have cystic fibrosis may not have meconium ileus because the deficiency of the pancreatic enzymes is seldom complete.

If the infant is normal at birth, between the fourth week and the sixth month there may be a failure to gain weight, indicating the onset of the condition. In the early stage the stools are usually loose, but not fatty or frequent. When the infant receives cereals or fish liver oil, the stools become foul smelling and frothy. Later the stools are light in color and fatty.

There is failure to absorb sufficient food; therefore the child does not gain weight as he should. At last the fat disappears from the main sites of deposit. There is abdominal distention and emaciation.

Behavior disorders result from the child's physical condition. The child is irritable and easily fatigued. In spite of these symptoms there may be a good appetite. There is a change in the physical appearance, growth is stunted, the skin appears loose, the buttocks and thighs are atrophied, and the abdomen is protuberant.

During the early part of the first year the child may have persistent respiratory infections, usually caused by *Staphylococcus aureus*. The infant may have a spasmodic cough which produces vomiting. He may become dyspneic, may wheeze and become cyanotic. Clubbing of fingers and toes may be seen. Because of persistent obstructive lung disease, the right ventricle of the heart becomes strained and hypertrophied.

**Diagnosis.** The diagnosis is made on the basis of the history, physical examination, laboratory tests and roentgenologic studies.

The laboratory examinations show a deficiency of pancreatic enzymes (trypsin, lipase, amylase and carboxypeptidase). These enzymes are reduced in or absent from the duodenal fluid. The tests for the presence of all these enzymes are done on duodenal juices obtained by intubation and aspiration. Usually only a test for trypsin is made, because absence of this enzyme is indicative of cystic fibrosis. The test for tryptic activity can be done on a stool specimen.

The sweat is tested for chloride content, which is higher than normal in patients with cystic fibrosis (note, how-

ever, that this abnormality also occurs among siblings and other relatives who have no clinical manifestations of the disease). In a screening technique the child's hand is placed on agar impregnated with silver nitrate. If the sweat chloride level is high, the hand print is seen on the agar. Later enough sweat may be examined for a more exact accounting of the amount of chloride lost by the patient.

It is possible to test the deficient absorption of fat in the intestines. Microscopic examination of the dilute stool will show excretion of fat in the feces. A low blood cholesterol level may be due in part to poor absorption of fats from the intestines. Since fats are not absorbed, vitamin A given in oily preparations is not absorbed, and some other source of this vitamin must be provided.

Roentgen studies show the changes in the intestinal tract and the lungs. A generalized obstructive emphysema, atelectasis, bronchopneumonia, bronchiectasis and bronchiolectatic abscesses may be apparent. Right ventricular hypertrophy of the heart may be seen in advanced cases.

**Treatment.** Treatment must be planned on a long-term basis, and follow-up care after treatment has been discontinued is extremely important. Good nutrition is essential. The patient should receive a balanced diet which includes a large amount of protein (6 to 8 gm. per kilogram of body weight) and a normal amount of fat. If the child cannot tolerate this, however, the diet should be limited in order to control the bulk and fat content of the stools. In infancy a protein milk formula to which skimmed powdered milk has been added is good. Banana powder and glucose may also be added to the formula. Other foods which are easily digested and are high in protein or low in fat and starches, such as cottage cheese, lean meats, fruits (especially bananas) and vegetables, may also be given.

The caloric intake should be high, from 125 to 200 calories per kilogram of body weight per day, since the child

Figure 140. Cystic fibrosis. This child has a protuberant abdomen and emaciated extremities.

cannot utilize food completely (he loses 50 per cent of the caloric value of his food in the stools). Liberal amounts of salt should be given with the food; in summer and hot weather extra amounts should be provided.

The specific medication in cystic fibrosis is pancreatic extract. The dose varies with the child's age and his need for the extract. One gram of a patent pancreatin preparation may be given for each 6 to 8 ounces of formula. Two or 3 gm. may be given before each meal to replace the pancreatic enzymes which the child's body cannot produce and which are needed in the digestion of foods. In this way the condition of the stools is improved. Vitamins in water-miscible preparations should be given in large amounts.

Prevention of infection, especially respiratory infection, is of the utmost importance. The child should be isolated from other patients and hospital personnel who have respiratory infections. Because of the danger of cross-infection, the period of hospitalization should be as short as possible. This necessitates teaching the mother to care for the child at home.

Antibiotics are given prophylactically as soon as the diagnosis of cystic fibrosis is made, to minimize the danger from a respiratory infection. If, however, the child contracts an infection, appropriate antibiotics such as penicillin, one of the tetracyclines, sulfisoxazole (Gantrisin) or streptomycin may be given.

Digitalis is given if there is evidence of cardiac failure. Oxygen is used for cyanosis due to bronchial secretions or cardiac failure.

Aerosol therapy may be given by mask to an older child, or a tent may be used, with pressure from an oxygen tank or an electric pump, to help remove heavy secretions from the bronchi and to relieve dyspnea. The vapor is given as a fine mist of microparticles at least four times a day. Antibiotics may be added to the aerosol solution. Nebulization under intermittent positive pressure may be used. Since the lungs are inflated by positive pressure during

**Figure 141.** The Bird machine provides nebulization under intermittent positive pressure. It has proved effective when used on children having cystic fibrosis.

inspiration, the aerosols can be administered to every area where ventilation takes place, with the result that bronchial drainage and pulmonary function are improved. Several types of machines may be used for this purpose (see Fig. 141). It is possible to give this treatment to infants if intubation has been done, but it has proved most successful with children eighteen months to two years of age when a mask is used. This treatment is usually given every few hours and continued until the amount of aerosol medication is exhausted. In severe cases aerosol therapy may be given continuously with pressure maintained on both inspiration and expiration.

**Complications.** Rectal prolapse due to emaciation of the buttocks and weak musculature in the rectal area is a possible complication. It occurs most frequently between six months and three years of age.

Heat prostration may result from a high environmental temperature because the child loses electrolytes in perspiration. Osteoporosis may occur because the child cannot utilize fat-soluble vitamin D and therefore cannot make use of calcium in bone growth as the normal child does. Clinical rickets is not often seen, since rickets is a disease of growing children, and these children do not grow. There is vitamin A deficiency due to the child's inability to absorb fats from which the vitamin is obtained. The heart is strained by the exertion required to pump blood through the fibrotic lung. Cor pulmonale, in which the right side of the heart becomes enlarged and dilated, is a frequent cause of death.

**Nursing Care.** The child's nutritional state is important. The nurse must be patient with the child at mealtimes or when giving the infant his bottle. The infant or child is apt to be irritable, coughs and vomits easily and often has difficulty in breathing. Small amounts of food should be offered slowly but frequently so that the child is not tired by his effort to take food. The infant should be bubbled frequently so that abdominal distention is not increased. The diet should be as varied as possible, with consideration for the child's age and ability to digest various foods. The nurse should note and carefully chart her observations of the child's reaction to new foods and the kind of stools which result from additions to the diet.

It is imperative that the nurse accept the personality changes which take place in the child as his illness extends over months. She should give him love and kindness to promote his feeling of security even during the discomfort of his illness.

Skin care is required. The buttocks must be carefully cleansed after each stool, and ointment applied to protect the skin from contact with further stools. If the skin becomes irritated, the buttocks should be exposed to the air or to the warmth of an electric light bulb (see p. 322).

Because of malnutrition the skin may break down over the bony prominences. The patient should therefore be turned frequently, and the entire body must be kept clean to prevent decubiti. More

importantly, changing position lessens the danger of pneumonia. Even if the child is old enough to turn himself, he may be too weak to do so; this is the responsibility of his nurse.

Scrupulous cleanliness of the diaper area will help to reduce the offensive odor from the stools. Soiled diapers should be taken from the unit as soon as they are removed from the infant. An air deodorant is useful, but should never be made a substitute for cleanliness.

The child should not be dressed too warmly, but it is essential that he should not become chilled. If he perspires, his clothes should be changed immediately.

The nurse may be asked to assist in collection of sweat for the sweat test. A small infant may be placed on a plastic sheet in a very warm incubator. A simple method consists of a patch of absorbent material being taped on the child's back. Before the test the child must be bathed to remove dried perspiration from the skin.

The nurse will assist in intermittent positive pressure and aerosol treatments. She must explain to the child, if he is old enough to understand, that he is to take a deep breath under regulated gentle pressure and that a fine mist of medication will reach all areas of his lungs. The child should be positioned correctly and helped to sit up straight. This position allows room for movement of the diaphragm and therefore permits deeper respiration. The child should be encouraged to breathe slowly and deeply at first and to relax during the treatment. Demonstration by the nurse with her own breathing may help him to understand what is wanted of him.

If the child is afraid of the procedure, he should be urged to express his fear. The nurse is then able to give support and encouragement. Eventually most children will cooperate and hold the apparatus themselves (see Fig. 141). The machine must be cleaned thoroughly between treatments because of the danger of respiratory cross-infection between children using the apparatus.

Because of the wasted gluteal muscles, the usual site for intramuscular injections (the buttocks) presents more problems than in the normal child. Injection sites should be examined carefully for hardened areas, and no further medication should be given in the area unless it is normally soft and shows no evidence of trauma. Sites should be rotated whenever injections are given frequently. Massage may help in absorption of the medication and tends to prevent hardness from developing.

Recording of observations should be complete so that the physician may have a clear picture of the child's condition. The stools should be described in detail as to color, odor, consistency and size. The kind and amount of foods taken, as well as those refused, should be charted. Whether the child eats eagerly or indifferently should also be noted. Gain or loss of weight is recorded or shown graphically. The color of the skin has diagnostic value. The nurse should watch for signs of rectal prolapse and report all symptoms of this condition. If the child coughs, the physician wants to know the nature and frequency of the cough. Little children cry readily over trifles, but crying is also a sign of discomfort or pain. The time, kind and frequency of crying are important both in diagnosis and in judging the effect of treatments and therefore should be recorded in detail. A description of the child's crying is helpful in appraising not only his physical condition, but also the personality changes which interact with the physical ones.

Heat prostration may be prevented if the nurse observes and reports to the physician the first symptoms.

Prevention of infection must be a constant aim.

Equally important is education of the parents, who will be responsible when the child leaves the hospital and is under the care of a private physician or of clinic physicians. Conferences with the parents should provide for continuation of the care the child received in the hospital. The mother should be told of the dietary regimen, and time must be taken to be sure that she understands what the diet consists of and also the best ways of making it acceptable to the child. She will also need to know, and emotionally accept, the physician's plan of treatment, including medical follow-up, hygienic measures, prevention of infection, meeting the child's need for adequate rest and the administration of medication. The nurse should not only teach the mother the necessary procedures, but also should explain to her the purpose of each (why it is done and the expected results). She should also explain the necessity for medication which the physician has ordered and the best way to give it to the child.

The loving mother willingly undertakes the time-consuming and difficult task of caring for her child at home. The nurse will help her to use her affection for the child wisely and set limits to his behavior, even though the prognosis is poor and it hurts her to refuse him anything he wants to have or do. It is difficult for her to accept the probable regression in his condition during even mild respiratory infections, and even more difficult if she blames herself for some oversight in his care which she believes caused the infection.

The nurse should help both parents to realize their responsibility in caring for the child and the help they must give him in adjusting to his limitations. The infant under one year of age accepts limitations because he knows no better. The danger for him lies in overprotection by his parents and therefore deprivation of opportunities for normal development. Even at this early age he should be helped to make the best possible adjustment to his handicap.

**Prognosis.** The prognosis is unpredictable, but in severe disease is usually poor. Death may occur in the first year from severe malnutrition or overwhelming respiratory infection. The nurse may be of great support to parents at the time of death, even though they have known the genetic cause of the disease and the prognosis. Spiritual guidance of such parents may be of great value.

## Prolapse and Procidentia of the Rectum and Sigmoid

**Incidence and Etiology.** *Prolapse* of the rectum is an abnormal descent of the mucous membrane of the rectum. The membrane may or may not protrude through the anus. *Procidentia* is an abnormal descent of all the layers of the rectum or sigmoid, or both, which likewise may or may not protrude through the anus.

The *incidence* is greatest during infancy, although the condition occurs in children up to three years of age.

Prolapse is precipitated when the intra-abdominal pressure is suddenly increased. Infants and young children who are malnourished, have diarrhea or are constipated are prone to these conditions. Prolapse or procidentia occurs with straining at defecation if there is a relaxed sphincter and weak muscles of the pelvic floor.

**Clinical Manifestations.** The first manifestation is only protrusion of part of the rectum and sigmoid, which recede spontaneously. Later, manual replacement may be necessary. The color of the protruding mass is bright red to dark purple, depending on the length of time it has been prolapsed and the degree to which circulation has been cut off. The protrusion may be up to 5 to 6 inches in length. The mass may be a flattened, corrugated tumor or just a fold of mucous membrane protruding from the anus.

**Treatment, Nursing Care and Prognosis.** *Treatment* is aimed at the underlying problem, i.e. to correct the child's weight by an adequate diet if he is malnourished, to correct constipation by giving a mild medication (e.g. mineral oil) and instituting proper toilet training, and to correct diarrhea if that is the cause of the difficulty.

During defecation the buttocks should be held together manually or with adhesive tape. If the child is able to indicate when he is about to have a stool, manual pressure is preferable, since it can be adjusted to passage of the stool. The buttocks may be taped together after each bowel movement to prevent repeated prolapse.

*A*                              *B*

**Figure 142.** Rectal prolapse. *A*, Partial prolapse; only rectal mucosa involved. *B*, Complete prolapse of rectum (procidentia); entire thickness of rectal wall involved. (From P. Hanley and M. O. Hines, in Ochsner and DeBakey: Christopher's Minor Surgery. 8th ed.)

For reduction of the protrusion the infant should be placed with his head lower than his body. The protrusion may be replaced with the fingers of the gloved hand. Toilet paper is put over the finger used to insert the bowel and pressed into the opening of the mass as it is pushed back into the rectum. The finger is then quickly withdrawn, leaving the toilet paper in the rectum. The paper will become soft and be expelled later.

Operation may be necessary if other treatment is not successful.

The *prognosis* is usually good with proper treatment.

### Congenital Aganglionic Megacolon (Hirschsprung's Disease) *rare*

**Etiology, Incidence and Pathology.**   In Hirschsprung's disease there is a congenital absence of parasympathetic ganglion nerve cells from the intramural plexus of a part of the intestinal tract, usually in the distal end of the descending colon.

The condition is more common in males than in females. The symptoms may be present at birth or may appear at any time during infancy.

The involved portion of the intestine has a narrow lumen and lacks peristaltic activity. The portion of the colon above this area is greatly dilated and hypertrophied, and feces and gas accumulate in it. The muscular coat of the dilated colon, at first hypertrophied, may become thin; in infants the mucosa may become ulcerated.

**Clinical Manifestations.**   A newborn infant with Hirschsprung's disease may not pass meconium. Lack of meconium, however, does not prove that the infant has Hirschsprung's disease, since a partial or complete obstruction of the bowel due to any cause prevents the passage of meconium. Vomiting, abdominal distention, an overflow type of diarrhea or constipation may appear in the first few weeks of life.

The subsequent course of the disease shows increasingly obstinate constipation with abdominal distention due to the mass of feces and to gas. Abdominal distention may be so great that respiration is embarrassed. Fecal matter may be expelled in pellet-like or ribbon-like form or may be fluid. As the disease progresses spontaneous bowel movements are infrequent. Eventually the abdominal wall becomes thin, and the superficial veins are prominent. The fecal mass may be palpated through the abdominal wall. The more severely affected children may appear malnourished and even stunted in growth. Infants and young children may have periodic attacks of intestinal obstruction due to fecal impaction. As a result there is abdominal pain, vomiting and fever.

**Diagnosis.**   The diagnosis is based on the clinical manifestations. If diarrhea is one of the symptoms, as is often the case in infancy, it is difficult to differentiate this condition from cystic fibrosis of the pancreas. The determining factors are absence of findings positive for cystic fibrosis in the sweat test and the examination of duodenal secretion for trypsin. Roentgen examination after a barium enema in children over six months of age shows the narrowed section of the rectosigmoid. After examination the barium must be removed immediately by colonic irrigation.

Rectal examination shows no fecal matter in the colon lower than the obstruction, in spite of pressure in the bowel above.

**Treatment.**   Treatment will depend on the severity of the condition. Mild cases may respond to dietary control and administration of medications which produce soft stools. Frequent or daily enemas are given to remove fecal matter as it accumulates. Retention enemas of mineral or olive oil may be used, followed by colonic irrigations. Some of the solution given by enema may be retained; therefore only isotonic solution should be used. If tap water were used and absorbed in large quantities, the child might suffer water intoxication.

If surgical intervention is required, the narrowed segment of the bowel in the rectosigmoid area is resected. The normal sigmoid section is pulled through and sutured to the anal opening to reconstruct continuity of the bowel lumen. If the child is not in good condition for operation, a colostomy may be done in preparation for the pull-through operation. The colostomy is made in the distal portion of the colon where normal ganglia are found.

**Nursing Care.**  Good general hygiene is important, since these infants are poorly nourished, apathetic and uncomfortable with distention and nausea. Frequent, small oral feedings are better than three large meals a day. A low residue diet is given to keep the stools soft so that they can be easily evacuated. Mineral oil or mild laxatives may be ordered for the same purpose.

The position of the child is important for his comfort. Because respiration is embarrassed by the abdominal distention, the infant is more comfortable in an upright position. He can be placed in a sitting position and supported with sandbags and pillows. Enemas or colonic irrigations are given as ordered.

The nurse should note and record the child's appetite and the frequency and nature of the stools.

If the child is to be operated upon, *preoperative care* consists in emptying the bowel by repeated enemas and colonic irrigations with physiologic saline solution (never tap water). The physician may order chemotherapeutic agents to reduce the bacterial flora.

The procedure for giving an enema is similar to that for the adult, with

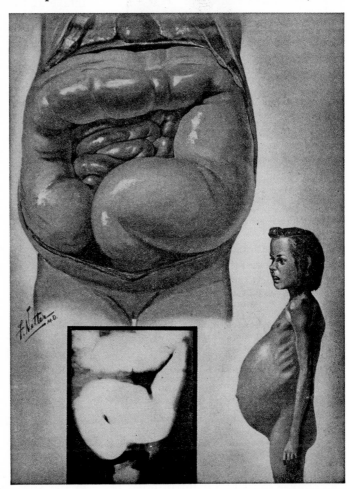

Figure 143.  Megacolon. (Copyright, The Ciba Collection of Medical Illustrations, by Frank H. Netter, M.D.)

**Figure 144.** Positioning the infant for an enema. A pillow is under the infant's head and back. The buttocks are placed upon the bedpan, which has been covered with a folded diaper to protect the infant's back. The legs are restrained in position with a diaper brought under the bedpan and pinned over the legs.

some alterations necessitated by the anatomy and physiology of the child.

1. A no. 10 to 12 French catheter is used. It should be inserted only 2 to 4 inches into the rectum.
2. The temperature of the solution should be 105° F.
3. Physiologic saline solution (never tap water) is used, and is made by dissolving 1 dram of salt in a pint of water.
4. Not more than 300 ml. of solution should be given to an infant unless the physician orders a larger amount.
5. The child is positioned by placing pillows under his head and back. The buttocks are placed upon the pan, which has been covered with a folded diaper to serve as a soft pad under the lower lumbar area. Another diaper is used to restrain the legs in position over the side edges of the bedpan (see Fig. 144).
6. The enema can should not be more than 18 inches above the level of the child's hips so that the solution will run slowly by gravity and without pressure into the bowel.
7. The results of the enema should be fully and carefully charted.

This is one of the procedures which the mother must be taught in order to give the child adequate care when he is discharged from the hospital.

For an oil retention enema a funnel or syringe may be used. From 75 to 150 ml. of oil is usually given at 100° F. Pressure over the anus is necessary after a retention enema so that it will not be expelled. A cleansing enema should be given thirty to forty-five minutes after the oil retention enema.

In *postoperative care* the nurse will probably be asked to assist in the giving of chemotherapeutic agents to reduce the danger of infection.

The infant's temperature after operation is taken by the axillary method rather than by rectum until healing is complete.

There should be careful recording of intake and output of fluids and description of the stools. If a colostomy was performed, the infant must be kept clean and dry to prevent excoriation of the surrounding area. The dressing should be changed frequently. If the area around the colostomy becomes irritated, the abdomen should be exposed to the air and the skin protected with soothing ointment.

**Complications.** The complications to be feared are (1) ulcers in the mucous membrane of the intestine which will cause diarrhea, (2) perforation and peritonitis (unusual but possible), and (3) malnutrition.

**Course and Prognosis.** The child may outgrow the milder forms of megacolon and improve as his body grows. He may have difficulty in controlling flatus. During his early years this creates no serious difficulty, but as he reaches school years it may cause him great embarrassment.

Surgical operation—abdominoperineal resection of the rectosigmoid with suturing of the normal part of the sigmoid to the anal opening—has given excellent results.

## BLOOD DISORDERS

### BLOOD FORMATION

Blood cells begin to form in the fetus in the yolk sac about the fourth week of gestation. They form successively in the liver, spleen, thymus and lymphatic tissues and last in the bone marrow. Although the liver produces the majority of blood cells during the first six months of fetal life, blood formation at term is largely carried on in the bone marrow. During the period of growth nearly all the bone marrow produces blood cells, but after growth has been completed hematopoiesis (blood cell production) is limited to the ends of the long bones, vertebrae and certain flat bones of the body. If, however, in childhood all the marrow is hematopoietic and more demand is made for blood, other organs (liver, spleen) and lymph nodes produce additional cells. At times these organs may enlarge because of the need for extramedullary hematopoiesis in certain disease conditions.

Although erythrocytes, granulocytes and platelets are formed in bone marrow and lymphocytic cells mostly in lymphatic tissue, an examination of peripheral blood may not be adequate for complete understanding of a certain condition. It is therefore necessary to study by direct or indirect means the states of hematopoietic tissue and the spleen, which in the child as in the adult is largely an organ of blood destruction.

*Red Blood Cells (Erythrocytes).* The purpose of red blood cells is to carry hemoglobin. The function of hemoglobin is to take oxygen to the tissues and remove carbon dioxide to be excreted by the lungs. Hemoglobin also acts as a buffer in regulation of the pH of the blood. Production of red cells is stimulated by a reduced oxygen content of the blood as a result of hemorrhage, hemolysis or pulmonary or cardiac disease.

Hemoglobin formation takes place in the reticuloendothelial cells of bone marrow. The red cells are taken from circulation by the reticuloendothelial cells, especially in the spleen. The iron in the hemoglobin is mostly reused; the cell pigment changes into bile pigment and is excreted. When blood is destroyed more rapidly than normal, the liver may not be able to excrete the increased load of bilirubin. Bilirubin accumulates in the plasma, thereby producing clinical jaundice, and may be excreted as urobilinogen in the stools and urine. The spleen and perhaps the liver may enlarge because of increased activity of their reticuloendothelial elements. Rapid formation of new blood cells to replace the old takes place in bone marrow and other tissues.

A mature red cell has no nucleus, but a nucleus is present during the early stage of cell formation. Nucleated red cells are common in fetal blood and may be found in the early days of life, especially in premature infants. Since red cells are constantly being destroyed and created, the presence of some immature cells containing reticulum is to be expected. About 1 to 2 per cent of red blood cells normally are reticulocytes, containing reticulum.

Later in infancy and during childhood the presence of nucleated red cells means that the body is producing them at an abnormally rapid rate in order to meet a demand for them.

The mean number of red blood cells per cubic millimeter of blood is dependent upon the subject's age. In fetal blood the number is 5 to 7 million cells per cubic millimeter. The infant born at term normally has 4.5 to 5.5 million cells. During the first seven to ten days of life the number of red cells decreases rapidly. Because of the immaturity of the liver in early infancy, physiologic jaundice may result (see p. 89).

The destruction of red blood cells then slows down until the lowest point —3.5 to 4.5 million cells—is reached at 8 to 12 weeks of life. By 6 months the infant's blood contains 4 to 5 million red cells per cubic millimeter. The number then gradually increases to 5 million cells and remains at that level.

At birth the amount of hemoglobin is approximately 17.6 gm. to each 100 ml. of blood. By 3 months of age the hemoglobin level has dropped to 11.0 gm. From this level the value rises during childhood to 11.5 to 13.5 gm. per 100 ml., and then by 16 years of age to the adult level.

The useful life of a normal red blood cell is 120 days. Factors such as exposure to hemagglutinins or hemolysins (as in erythroblastosis fetalis or transfusion reactions) or anomalies of structure and shape (sickle cell disease or thalassemia) may shorten the life of a cell to as little as a few days.

### THE ANEMIAS OF INFANCY AND CHILDHOOD

**Etiology, Clinical Manifestations and Prognosis.** Anemia, a deficit of erythrocytes or hemoglobin, is the most frequent disorder of the blood during childhood. It represents a disturbance in the balance between the production and destruction of these substances.

There are many kinds of anemia, but only the fairly common types will be considered here. The major types are due to (1) inadequate production of hemoglobin or red blood cells and (2) excessive loss of blood cells. Causes of underproduction of red blood cells or hemoglobin are (1) lack in the bone marrow of some substance or substances necessary in the formation of cells, (2) depressed functioning of the bone marrow, and (3) specific nutritional deficits in the marrow.

Excessive loss of red blood cells may be due to acute or chronic hemorrhage, e.g. acute hemorrhage in the newborn (see p. 161), chronic ulcerative colitis (see p. 663) or hemolysis of the blood. The most common causes of hemolysis of the blood are (1) a congenital anomaly of the erythrocytes or hemoglobin (e.g. thalassemia—p. 366—and sickle cell anemia—p. 367) and (2) acquired anomalies of the erythrocyte or its environment (e.g. toxic hemolytic anemias due to poisons—p. 454—or drugs, and the hemolytic anemias due to burns—p. 627—and immune reactions such as erythroblastosis fetalis—p. 159).

Although the etiologic factors in anemia are varied, the *clinical manifestations* of the various types are similar. In the early stage the child is easily fatigued, weak and listless; later symptoms are pallor, cardiac palpitation and rapid pulse rate, or tachycardia. Eventually there is mental slowness and physical sluggishness, cardiac enlargement and inability to carry out the usual activities of childhood.

The *prognosis* varies with the type. When anemia is fatal, it is usually because of weakness of the heart and its inability to maintain the normal circulation of the blood.

**Treatment and Nursing Care.** The treatment and nursing care of children with anemia depend upon the severity of the condition, its cause and the age of the child.

Transfusions improve the child's condition, his appetite and his disposition. He becomes more active and like other children. Transfusion is lifesaving when anemia has reached the point at which it interferes with cardiac function. The procedure is like that for intravenous therapy (see p. 317). But the child's reaction is influenced by his anemic condition. The nurse should note any evidence of discomfort such as generalized uneasiness, restlessness, crying or chills, which may indicate the onset of a transfusion reaction. There may also be elevation of temperature and changes in the respiratory and pulse rates and in the color of the skin. Whenever the nurse notes such symptoms, she should stop the transfusion and notify the physician immediately.

One problem with transfusions in infants and small children is blocking of the narrow lumen of the needle by the vein wall. To prevent this the blood may be slowly pumped into a small vein of the infant by using a syringe. The physician must have assistance to do this procedure. When this technique is used, the blood is given very slowly, with care taken to prevent pumping air bubbles through the needle and also to prevent contamination of the plunger of the syringe.

Medication commonly given includes iron, vitamin C and liver extract. Iron is given if the cause of the anemia is an insufficient intake of iron or loss of iron supply through hemorrhage. Iron may be given by mouth in the form of ferrous sulfate, which is absorbed more efficiently than the ferric salt. The child's mother should be told that iron medication causes the stools to become dark green or black. Iron medication should be given between meals when the stomach is empty of milk products and cereals, because these inhibit the absorption of the iron. If the need for it warrants, iron may also be given intravenously or intramuscularly.

Vitamin C is valuable in correction of the anemia caused by scurvy (see p. 349). Liver extract and vitamin B complex may be used in treatment of anemias caused by a megaloblastic bone marrow.

Splenectomy may be performed because of its palliative value or for removal of the pressure of an enlarged spleen upon abdominal viscera.

Preparation of the parents for continued care of the infant or young child having anemia is exceedingly important. In the conference with the mother the physician or nurse will take up the whole problem of the general hygiene of the child. Good hygiene includes an adequate diet, rest, sunshine and fresh air, and will help to build up the child's resistance to intercurrent infections. The child should be dressed according to the weather and kept from other children and from adults who have colds, sore throats or other infections.

As the child grows older—out of the age group considered in this chapter—he should be as self-reliant and as independent of help from his mother as his age and physical condition permit. The mother must further his desire for independence, but keep it within realistic bounds. For instance, when the child is old enough to feed himself, his mother may give him a spoon while she feeds him with another, letting him take turns with her in bringing the food to his mouth. In the hospital the nurse may do the same thing and so accustom him to the procedure before he goes home. In planning play free play activity should be alternated with periods of controlled, quiet play to allow the child to rest. He should never be allowed to exhaust his strength and should be taught gradually as he matures to protect himself against overexertion and emotional strain.

Prolonged hospitalization should be avoided unless it is necessary because of home conditions detrimental to the child's care or because his condition is such that he cannot be cared for at home. Until recently children who had chronic cases of anemia, such as thalassemia or sickle cell disease, were admitted to the hospital for long periods for blood transfusions. These periods of absence from home and their parents and later from school were detrimental to their normal emotional development. The children often developed a fear of the hospital which made each hospitalization more difficult than the last. They felt insecure as to both their health and the normal pleasures of childhood. Much of this was realistic, but they also developed a chronic anxiety which included fears that were completely illogical and unfounded. In the end their whole lives and indeed those of their parents and siblings revolved around their disease. Hospitalization, if paid for at all, was a great drain on the family income, often requiring some sacrifice from every member of the family.

Today children are brought to the hospital for diagnostic examination and initial transfusions. They are then admitted to the hospital on a scheduled basis for a one-day stay for further therapy. Children learn quickly about their diseases and feel less threatened by a brief stay in the hospital unit, during which laboratory studies and transfusions are done, than by prolonged hospitalization. In the pediatric department they are free to talk and play with other children both before the transfusion and afterwards while they are observed for a transfusion reaction. They understand the relation between their receiving blood and their feeling of well-being following the transfusion. Children such as these cooperate best

**Figure 145.** Thalassemia major. Ten-year-old girl who has had frequent blood transfusions for severe anemia. This child understands her illness and the reasons for her periods of hospitalization and visits to the out-patient department. She is a cheerful and well adjusted child.

when they are familiar with the equipment, the procedure and the people who carry it out. They should be permitted to handle the equipment initially and to cleanse the area for injection before the transfusion is given.

If a child must be admitted to the hospital for a longer period for examination, laboratory tests or treatment, the nursing personnel should realize the long-term problem involved and do everything possible to make his stay as pleasant as it can be. Nursing personnel might even keep notes as to his likes and dislikes in food, toys and bed location. Often such children, on a return admission to the hospital unit, greet the nurses warmly as old friends instead of threats to their security.

The education of the anemic child should be as like that of his peers as his condition permits. If he is not able to attend school, he should be taught at home. In many cities and towns the school board sends visiting school teachers to homes or hospitals to teach children who are unable to go to school.

## SPECIFIC TYPES OF ANEMIA

### Hypochromic Anemia Due to Iron Deficiency

**Etiology, Incidence and Pathology.** If hemoglobin is not synthesized, pallor of the erythrocytes results. This hypochromia is accompanied by a variable decrease in size of the cell—microcytosis. If evidence of anemia is also present, as shown by the red cell count, hemoglobin level and hematocrit value below the normal range for the child's age, a hypochromic anemia can be diagnosed.

The cause is a lack of iron in the diet or the child's inability to use the iron he ingests. The infant or young child can produce hemoglobin only if his diet provides a supply of readily available iron. The minimum daily adult requirement is 15 mg. of iron. The infant having iron deficiency anemia may need 100 mg. of elemental iron each day. The iron deficiency anemia of infancy is almost always due to insufficient intake of iron, either because the amount in the child's diet is insufficient to meet his daily requirements or because there is some problem in its absorption or utilization.

Iron deficiency is most apt to occur at periods of rapid growth. The premature infant at three to four months of age grows rapidly and is prone to hypochromic anemia. Infants born at term have a greater reserve of iron than has the premature infant, and the results of a diet low in iron, such as one of milk, potatoes and cereals, are not likely to be severe until the term infant is six months to two years old. At two years the growth rate is slowing down, and children are customarily receiving a varied diet adapted from that prepared for the family.

Behind the poor diet which produces anemia may be social and economic conditions—the low income of the parents or their ignorance of or indifference to the child's dietary needs. They may not know what is an adequate diet for children of different ages or, since the infant will take milk, they do not persist in their efforts at feeding iron-containing foods. This may be because they do not know the technique or lack the time or simply will not take the trouble to accustom the infant to taking into his mouth and swallowing any nourishment which is not in a fluid state.

Only in rare cases is anemia due to abnormal difficulty in swallowing or to prolonged vomiting. Even though an infant ingests an adequate liberal diet suited to his age, there may be insufficient absorption or he may suffer from a chronic disease which diminishes the supply of nourishment, such as celiac disease or a chronic diarrhea.

**Clinical Manifestations.** The onset of hypochromic anemia is insidious and may occur as a complication of an infection or the anemia may itself be complicated by an infection. Infants having hypochromic anemia due to iron deficiency are especially susceptible to infections.

Clinical manifestations of severe anemia include poor muscle tone, slow motor development, weakness and waxy pallor. The heart may be enlarged, and a loud systolic precordial murmur may be heard. The spleen may be palpable. The hemoglobin level is often below 5 gm. The red blood cell count may be below 2,500,000, and stained red cells are pale and microcytic.

**Treatment.** Treatment is aimed at correction of the underlying cause of the condition. An adequate diet includes vegetables and meat. Vitamin supplements are necessary. Vitamin C (ascorbic acid) appears to enhance the absorption of iron. Iron, especially in inorganic form, should be given. Ferrous sulfate is cheap and easily available and has a high iron content. It should not be given in too large amounts, since its absorption is limited and it may produce vomiting. Although other iron preparations may be given, many have a smaller iron content, and

therefore a larger dose must be given. Medications containing iron should not be given with milk or cereals. Iron may be given parenterally, but this method is seldom used if the child can tolerate oral iron therapy. Some types of parenteral iron produce irritation at the site of the intramuscular injection and may cause systemic disturbances in the patient.

Blood transfusions are given if the child's condition is serious, especially if the infant has myocardial insufficiency. Repeated small transfusions of concentrated red blood cells are valuable.

**Nursing Care.** Infants suffering from iron deficiency are usually irritable. Feedings must be given slowly. As the anemia improves, the infant's appetite for food other than milk will increase. The infant should receive no more than one quart of milk daily. Semisolid and solid foods should be introduced into the diet in the same manner as they are for younger children (see p. 281).

The infant must be protected from infection, particularly from nursing personnel who have respiratory infections, and clean technique must be used in his care.

Conferences with the mother are important, since prevention of further difficulties lies in her long-term care of the infant. She should be told that his stools will become dark or black because of iron medication. Parents may become anxious at the color of the stools if they do not know the cause.

Some solutions containing iron should be well diluted and given with a drinking tube or straw to prevent discoloration of the teeth by deposits of iron. The iron solution should be well diluted and for infants given with a medicine dropper. Some newer preparations of iron may be given without a straw because they have no effect on the teeth.

**Prognosis.** The prognosis is, in general, good when iron, given orally, vitamins and an improved diet are given. Recovery usually takes place in four to six weeks, but treatment is continued for eight to twelve weeks longer. The prognosis is variable if the infant has a concurrent infection.

### Thalassemia (Mediterranean Anemia, Cooley's Anemia)

**Incidence, Pathology and Types.** Thalassemia is a chronic, congenital hemolytic anemia in which the chief defect seems to be an inability to produce cells capable of normal incorporation of hemoglobin. It was mistakenly thought that this condition occurred exclusively in children whose parents or ancestors came from countries along the northern shore of the Mediterranean Sea, especially Italy, Sicily or Greece. Cases occur, however, among Negroes, Orientals, Europeans and Jews and their descendants.

The *pathology* is that of chronic microcytic, hypochromic anemia. The specific defect is production of cells of abnormal shape which are deficient in hemoglobin and are destroyed more quickly than normal cells would be. Although these cells are produced, they are not capable of normal incorporation of hemoglobin. The hematopoietic tissue attempts to compensate for this defect by producing more fetal hemoglobin than is normal, but does not produce enough for the effective transportation of oxygen. Large numbers of immature and defective erythrocytes are rapidly destroyed.

There are two types of thalassemia, minor and major. Both are familial conditions.

*Thalassemia minor* occurs when the gene responsible for the defect is a heterozygous trait. The infant or child with the minor form will show mild anemia, moderate hypochromia, and both anisocytosis and poikilocytosis (a condition in which cells are of unequal size and irregular in shape). Sometimes the spleen is enlarged. These children have no incapacitating symptoms, however, and are able to lead normal lives. Their condition is not likely to be recognized unless blood studies are carried out as part of a family survey.

*Thalassemia major* is transmitted when both parents have thalassemia minor. On the average one quarter of their children may be homozygous for the trait of thalassemia major. Such children will have progressive, severe anemia not compatible with long life. This type of anemia responds only temporarily to transfusion therapy. This condition is easily recognized in early infancy because of the onset of a progressive, severe anemia.

**Clinical Manifestations.** *Thalassemia Major.* Since anemia is not present at birth, the newborn never shows signs of the disease. Severe anemia may develop, however, in the first few months of life. The clinical manifestations are, in general, those of any severe anemia, but certain symptoms peculiar to the condition should be noted.

The infant has a decided pallor, especially of the mucous membranes, and a mild jaundice which later becomes a muddy, bronze color. The enlarged spleen of the young infant increases to an enormous size during childhood. This, with an enlarged liver, causes disabling abdominal distention which may lead to cardiorespiratory distress and cardiac enlargement with the danger of cardiac failure. Lymphadenopathy occurs, and skeletal changes are noticeable. Not only the physician but also the mother observes the child's retarded physical development, poor posture, abdominal distention and such skeletal changes as the mongoloid facies—due to the thickened membranous bones of the face and skull, often accompanied with protrusion of the teeth caused by overgrowth of the maxilla—and broad, heavy-appearing hands.

**Diagnosis, Treatment, Course and Prognosis.** The *diagnosis* is made on roentgen examination. By the time the infant is one year old there is widening of the medullary spaces, thinning of the cortices and decrease in the size of the bony trabeculae (connective tissue beams which extend from a capsule into the enclosed substances). In older children roentgenograms of the skull show radiating bony trabeculae traversing the widened space, resulting in a hair-on-end appearance.

The laboratory findings show microcytic anemia in both forms of the condition. In thalassemia major there is a severe anemia, a low erythrocyte count and a low hemoglobin level. There is a rapid turnover of erythrocytes, so that there is an elevated reticulocyte count and an increase in nucleated red blood cell precursors. Even in laboratory examination it is sometimes difficult to distinguish thalassemia from anemia of iron deficiency, other hemolytic anemias of infancy or sickle cell disease. The finding of thalassemia minor in the parents aids in establishing the diagnosis.

There is no *treatment* for thalassemia minor. For thalassemia major frequent transfusions must be given to maintain the hemoglobin level above 40 per cent of normal (6 gm. per 100 ml.). The addition of sedimented cells will increase the efficiency of a transfusion and lessen the danger of cardiac embarrassment due to too much parenteral fluid. These children can live with a relatively low hemoglobin level.

Aspirin with antihistaminic drugs may be effective as prophylaxis against transfusion reactions. If a severe reaction occurs, cortisone may be of some value. Splenectomy may be helpful, since it lessens the discomfort from the enormous spleen; it may also help to prolong the intervals between necessary transfusions and produces more normal growth.

The parents must be encouraged to accept the child's condition with its poor prognosis, and shown how to give the child as normal a life as is possible. As with all children with severe anemias, giving blood transfusions on a brief inpatient or an outpatient basis is preferable to repeated prolonged periods of hospitalization.

Thalassemia minor is a benign condition which does not interfere with normal growth and activity. The *prognosis* is therefore good. Since the trait is genetically transmitted, young people with this condition should be made aware of the danger involved if they marry a person with the same trait.

In thalassemia major the earlier the onset and the more severe the symptoms, the more rapidly is the outcome fatal. From early infancy these children must depend upon transfusion therapy. As they grow older the need for transfusions becomes even greater. The child's growth is stunted, and his activity is limited. There is constant danger of cardiac failure. Today more patients survive to adolescence than in the past. If they do survive, there may be some lessening of the severity of the disease. Death may be due to the severe anemia, to progressive hepatic or cardiac involvement or to intercurrent infection.

### Sickle Cell Disease

**Incidence, Types and Pathology.** Sickle cell disease is associated with an inherited defect in the synthesis of hemoglobin. It is confined almost exclusively to the Negro race and is seldom seen in members of the Caucasian race.

There are two types of the disease— the severe type and an asymptomatic condition. In the *severe* type there is a persistent hemolytic anemia with periodic episodes of painful crises. This severe condition occurs when the abnormality appears in homozygous form (inherited from both parents). When the defect is heterozygous (inherited from only one parent), an *asymptomatic* condition is present—the *sickle cell trait*. This is much more frequent among Negroes in the United States than is the true disease. If both parents are heterozygous, one of their children will have sickle cell disease, on the average, two will have the trait, and one will be hematologically normal.

Pathologically, the hemoglobin in both forms is abnormal (hemoglobin S). Under reduced oxygen tension this hemoglobin is responsible for forming red blood cells into a sickled shape. In sickle cell disease these malformed cells clump together and obstruct capillaries, thereby causing what is known as a crisis in the disease. Capillary obstruction leads to anoxic changes which cause further sickling and thus still further obstruction in the blood vessels. Pain in the area results. Infarcts occur most often in the spleen, but may also occur in bones, kidneys, lungs, gastrointestinal tract, brain and heart. The spleen may be so badly affected through removing blood cells from circulation and by these infarcts that it may become fibrotic and may atrophy and finally disappear.

**Clinical Manifestations.** In children with the sickle cell trait there are no clinical symptoms. In sickle cell disease the onset may be as early as the second or third month of life, when normal fetal hemoglobin is replaced by the abnormal hemoglobin which causes sickling. Approximately half of all children affected by this condition have symptoms by one year of age.

The first clinical manifestation the infant may have is sickle cell crisis. This is an acute disturbance in which the infant has severe pain in the abdomen and legs. The abdominal wall may have a boardlike rigidity. The child may also have extreme pallor, fever, vomiting and severe flank pain with hematuria, convulsions, stiff neck, coma or paralysis. Two to three days after the crisis, jaundice may appear. Between crises the manifestations are pallor and anemia. Icterus may be persistent.

Growth of a child with sickle cell disease is not stunted, but he may have long, thin extremities, a short trunk, barrel-shaped chest and protruding abdomen. If he is under nine years of age, the spleen may be palpable. There is cardiac enlargement, and murmurs are common.

**Laboratory Findings and Diagnosis.** Laboratory examination shows the sickle-shaped cells which are produced under low oxygen tension. This characteristic may be shown on smears of peripheral blood. If it is not seen on a smear, a drop of blood may be placed under a cover slip and sealed off from oxygen by petroleum jelly; if it is kept for one to twenty-four hours at room temperature, sickled forms of blood cells will appear.

Children having a sickle cell trait can be distinguished from those having the disease. In sickle cell trait the red cell count and hemoglobin level are not abnormal. In sickle cell disease the hemoglobin level ranges from 6 to 9 gm. per 100 ml.; in times of crisis it may fall lower. Each child stabilizes at his own level, and any increase in the level as a result of transfusion therapy is only temporary. The reticulocyte count is elevated to 5 or even 25 per cent, and is usually highest up to a week after a crisis as a result of new cell formation. The leukocyte count is elevated, but the platelets are usually normal in times of crisis.

Roentgenograms of the long bones, skull, feet and hands show widened medullary spaces and thinning of the cortices.

The *diagnosis* of sickle cell disease is at times difficult to make, since other diseases may appear similar to it. This is especially true during crises when vascular occlusion occurs. Conditions which might be confused with sickle cell disease are thalassemia, syphilis, tuberculosis, osteomyelitis, rheumatic fever and acute conditions of the abdomen.

**Treatment, Course and Prognosis.** *Treatment* consists of supportive measures such as blood transfusions when necessary, and protection against infections. Treatment during crises includes codeine and aspirin for relief of pain, and maintenance of hydration. Water containing no electrolytes is given by mouth to help reverse sickling and thus to relieve local vascular obstructions. Antibiotic therapy may be necessary if a bacterial infection is present. Transfusion of erythrocytes may be required. Oxygen is given if the hemoglobin level falls rapidly to as low as 4 gm. per 100 ml. and the child has symptoms of hypoxia. Splenectomy usually has no value in sickle cell disease. In older children autosplenectomy may occur as a result of repeated thromboses.

The *course* depends upon the severity of the sickling tendency, the frequency of crises and the age of the child. As the child grows older crises occur less frequently. In the temperate regions, as in the United States, crises occur more commonly in autumn and spring.

The *prognosis* depends on the severity of the disease. The condition may interfere to some extent with the child's growth, nutrition and activity. The life expectancy of the infant or small child is probably less than the average because of the physiologic handicap, but many of these children grow up to adult life and are able to earn a living. Death is usually the result of severe anemia or intercurrent infection.

## ENDOCRINE DISORDERS

### Cretinism (Congenital Hypothyroidism)

**Etiology, Incidence and Onset.** Cretinism is caused by a congenital insufficiency of the secretion of the thyroid gland due to an embryonic defect in which the gland is absent or rudimentary and unable to produce thyroid hormone. The condition occurs sporadically in the United States. The infant appears normal at birth, but clinical manifestations may appear in the first few weeks or months of life. Cretinism is not to be confused with mongolism, which can be recognized at birth (see p. 227).

**Clinical Manifestations and Diagnosis.** Early signs of the condition are prolonged physiologic jaundice and feeding difficulties. The infant is pale because of anemia. He is constipated, and an umbilical hernia develops in the enlarged abdomen, owing to hypotonic abdominal musculature. There is little perspiration, and the skin is dry and scaly. The child is lethargic, cries little, sleeps most of the time and has little appetite. His temperature is subnormal, his pulse slow. The facial appearance is peculiar, for the eyes are far apart, the bridge of the broad nose is flat, the eyelids are swollen, and the tongue protrudes from the open mouth. The anterior fontanel is widely open because of poor bone development. Dentition is delayed, and the teeth decay rapidly.

The general appearance is abnormal: the arms and legs are short, the rela-

A           B

**Figure 146.** Congenitally hypothyroid infant at 6 months of age. Infant fed poorly in neonatal period and was constipated. Had persistent nasal discharge and large tongue. Very lethargic, no social smile and no head control. *A,* Note puffy face, dull expression, hirsute forehead. Serum cholesterol 172 mg. per 100 ml., alkaline phosphatase 4.8 Bodansky units, negligible uptake of radio-iodine. Osseous development that of newborn. *B,* Four months after treatment with U.S.P. thyroid. Note decreased puffiness of face, decreased hirsutism of forehead and alert appearance. (A. M. DiGeorge and J. Warkany, in Nelson: Textbook of Pediatrics. 7th ed.)

**Figure 147.**    Cretin. (Courtesy of Dr. Ralph V. Platou and the American Academy of Pediatrics.)

tively large head is supported on a short, thick neck, and the hands are broad and the fingers short. The hair is coarse, brittle and scanty. The hairline reaches down on the forehead. Bone development is retarded, and both physical and motor development is slow. Mental development also is delayed. These children, then, appear lethargic and are late in sitting, standing and walking. They do not learn to talk at the usual time, and sexual maturation is slower than that of the normal child.

They are dull, placid, good-natured babies. Ignorant mothers are often proud of their crying so little and being no trouble. In areas where routine follow-up of newborn infants is neglected these cases are often missed until much valuable time for early treatment has passed.

Early *diagnosis* may be difficult, for the symptoms appear gradually as the child grows older. Roentgenograms show the retarded bone age in untreated cases; multiple foci of ossification appear in the epiphyses. The basal metabolic rate is decreased. The serum cholesterol level fluctuates, but in general is increased. The normal cholesterol level is 100 to 300 mg. per 100 ml. of serum; in the cretin it is from 250 to 600 mg. The serum phosphatase level is decreased, and the carotene level is many times increased.

A reliable measurement of thyroid function is the protein-bound iodine level of the serum. The values in children with cretinism are usually under 2 gammas per 100 ml. Another test of thyroid function is the degree of uptake of radioactive iodine by the thyroid gland. In infants and children with cretinism a normal concentration in the thyroid is not obtained.

**Treatment.** If treatment is delayed, the infant may become more and more retarded in growth and mental development. The treatment (substitution therapy) is by oral administration of desiccated thyroid. The dose is usually small when the medication is started and is gradually increased to the maximum amount which can be given without producing symptoms of overdosage. This medication must be taken throughout life. The dose may have to be increased at puberty and during the reproductive period.

Besides thyroid therapy, the infant should receive a complete diet with adequate amounts of vitamin D. Since thyroid stimulates bone growth, the child will outgrow his supply of vitamin D if additional amounts are not provided.

The anemia is a problem, since it does not respond readily to hematinics. Constipation, another troublesome symptom, is not easily relieved.

**Nursing Care.** The nurse should observe children being treated with desiccated thyroid for symptoms of overdosage. Such symptoms are rapid pulse, loss in weight, vomiting, cramps, diarrhea, elevation of temperature and personality changes such as increased excitability and irritability.

Because of the tendency for early

decay of the teeth, good dental care should be provided early to preserve the temporary teeth. As soon as the child is able, he should be taught to brush his teeth.

Since one of the major problems in working with these children is their slowness of mental development, neither the child's parents nor his nurses should attempt to push the child beyond his capacity or compare his general development with that of normal children.

**Prognosis.** The prognosis in untreated cases is likely to be poor. Early death may result from an intercurrent infection, or the child may become a mentally retarded dwarf. If treatment is begun early and continued throughout life, the child may be normal physically, but probably somewhat mentally retarded. The earlier and more effective the treatment, the better the prognosis. Even with the best therapy, however, mental development may never be normal.

## DISORDERS OF METABOLISM

### Phenylketonuria

**Incidence, Etiology and Clinical Manifestations.** Phenylketonuria is not a common condition; it occurs in about one in every 20,000 births. Approximately 1 per cent of the patients in institutions for the mentally defective has this syndrome. The condition is equally common in males and females, but the majority of affected infants are blue-eyed blonds.

The condition is due to a congenital defect in phenylalanine metabolism. Phenylalanine is an essential amino acid and is present in all natural protein foods. As the newborn takes in food the phenylalanine accumulates in the blood, and phenylketone bodies are excreted in the urine. The abnormal accumulation of phenylalanine apparently prevents normal brain development.

Phenylketonuria is transmitted by inheritance of the autosomal recessive gene. The majority of affected infants are offspring of two heterozygous carriers of the gene. One fourth of the children from such parents will have the condition, and half will be carriers of the condition.

The *clinical manifestations* begin by about four months of age, when the mother may notice that the infant is not developing normally. Brain development is arrested, and severe mental deficiency results. Since mental deficiency is pronounced, the condition is sometimes called phenylpyruvic oligophrenia. Neurologic symptoms appear; the child may exhibit schizoid-like, disagreeable personality traits. Eczema or convulsions, or both, occur in about one fourth of these children.

**Diagnosis.** The diagnosis is made by a simple urine test for phenylketone bodies and by blood tests for phenylalanine. When the blood phenylalanine level is above approximately 15 mg. per 100 cc. of plasma, phenylketone bodies will usually appear in the urine. These tests should be made as soon as the condition is suspected so as to prevent arrested brain development. The tests are not usually made until the first or second week of life, but are especially necessary on infants born into families with a known history of phenylketonuria or on infants who show signs of mental dullness. The same tests are used for diagnosis and for checking with dietary management.

The *urine test* is made with ferric chloride. One cubic centimeter of urine is placed in a test tube, and 3 drops of a 5 or 10 per cent ferric chloride solution are added. If a green color appears, phenylketone bodies are present. Normal urine, used in the same combination with ferric chloride, remains yellow.

The *diaper test* is done in many Child Health Conferences (see p. 286), hospitals and pediatricians' offices for early detection of the condition. A drop of 5 or 10 per cent ferric chloride solution on a recently wet diaper will turn it green if phenylketone bodies are present. If the urine is normal, it remains yellow. The diaper test should be repeated at intervals, since some children with phenylketonuria do not always give positive results.

**Treatment and Nursing care.** Since the clinical manifestations of phenylketonuria are due to accumulation of unmetabolized phenylalanine, the condition can be controlled by restraining phenylalanine intake from early infancy. Since infants give variable responses to such treatment, management must be individualized on the basis of response to the therapy, as judged by urine and blood levels of phenylalanine, the level of physical and mental development and the relief of physical symptoms. The nutritional status and hemoglobin level should be determined frequently, since the infant is on a limited diet. Intelligence tests and other estimates of mental ability are important for infants who have been treated early to determine the rate of mental growth.

These infants should be observed for evidence of the onset of dermatologic or neurologic symptoms. Nurses should stress in conferences with the parents the importance of health checkups of the newborn and of the diaper test so that the condition, if it exists, can be treated in the earliest stages.

**Prognosis.** The prognosis is at best doubtful, but it is far more favorable if a diet with a low phenylalanine content is begun in the early months of infancy. Once brain development has been retarded, the process cannot be reversed; it can only be arrested. If treatment is not given until the child is three years old, he may show improvement in personality and behavior, but not in mental status. Insufficient research has been done to determine how long the low phenylalanine diet must be continued.

# DEGENERATIVE DISORDERS

## Tay-Sachs Disease (Amaurotic Family Idiocy)

**Incidence and Etiology.** Tay-Sachs disease is one of a group of degenerative disorders which result in functional incapacity. It is the most common of the cerebromacular degenerations. It occurs most frequently among Jewish people originating in eastern Europe and is inherited as a recessive trait.

The *etiology* is not known.

**Pathology, Clinical Manifestations and Diagnosis.** The brain becomes atrophic and firm; the cerebellum is shrunken or smaller than normal. Stores of lipid are found in the neurons.

The infant is apparently normal at birth. At the onset, usually about six months of age, the infant becomes listless, shows regression in motor ability, has muscular weakness and is unable to fix his eyes upon an object. By one year he is flaccid and fat. He has hyperactive reflexes, startles easily at the slightest stimulation and is *blind*. This degenerative disease continues with muscular degeneration, spasticity, seizures, malnutrition, decerebrate posturing, dementia and death.

The *diagnosis* is made when macular cherry-red spots surrounded by a gray-white edematous retina are seen in the fundi of the eyes. Optic atrophy is also noted. No laboratory procedure is performed, since blood and cerebrospinal fluid values usually remain normal.

**Treatment, Nursing Care and Prognosis.** No treatment is known.

The aim of *nursing care* is to give the child as much comfort as is possible during his short life. Stimuli should be reduced to a minimum, for the child startles easily at the slightest stimulation. Nutrition should be maintained by whatever means are possible. Eventually gavage feeding becomes necessary.

The child's emaciated condition necessitates good skin care. He must be kept clean and dry and must be turned frequently to prevent breakdown of the skin and to lessen the danger of pneumonia. Since the child is blind, the nurse should speak before touching him so as not to startle him. She must be careful to prevent his hurting himself in any way.

The gradual deterioration of the child's condition is hard for the parents to bear. They need much sympathy, particularly since they know that his condition is hereditary. Since it is due to a recessive trait, both parents share the feeling of responsibility for the child's disease. The Rabbi will be a source of comfort and emotional support, but the parents will turn to the physician and the nurse to express their grief at the continued degeneration of the child's condition. The nurse should let them express their grief, which is reawakened not only by their pity for his loss of a normal child's life, but also by their comparison of him with other children who are what they had hoped he would be.

The *prognosis* is hopeless. Death usually occurs before the third birthday. By this time the child is in a decerebrate state.

## SKIN CONDITIONS

### Infantile Eczema (Atopic Dermatitis)

**Incidence.** Many different unrelated inflammatory dermatoses may be grouped under the term of "eczema." Here, however, eczema is considered to be an atopic manifestation of a specific allergen, whether ingested or in contact with the skin. Eczema is a common inflammatory skin condition of infants. It is the most frequent evidence of an allergic state seen in the first year of life. Seborrhea or diaper rash may be frequently associated with infantile eczema.

Eczema is most frequent in the first two years of life. It is not uncommon in infants two or three months old, whether bottle-fed or breast-fed, who get some additional solid food. Food proteins which the mother has taken may pass through breast milk into the infant's digestive tract and cause infantile eczema, even though the infant is taking no other food. Eczema is relatively uncommon after the second year.

An infant, even a well cared for infant, may receive antigens through contact or by inhalation.

Eczema occurs in both sexes, in any race and at any time of the year. It is most likely, however, to appear in the winter months and to clear up in the summer. It is most frequent in well nourished, fat infants whose general health is excellent.

**Etiology.** Several factors may be responsible for the condition. There is a decided familial tendency. Anatomically and chemically the skin of an infant differs from that of an adult. The infant is likely to show greater response to scratching and to other irritants. His skin is more irritable and has a higher water and sodium chloride content than that of the adult. These attributes are exaggerated in the skin of an infant with eczema. His skin may be abnormally sensitive to irritation from clothes, wool garments, soaps, cold, strong sunlight or mild skin infections. Some physicians believe that overfeeding, especially of carbohydrates or fat, may have an adverse effect on infants prone to eczema. It is difficult to prove this, although eczema in obese infants has improved when they lost weight as a result of dietary restriction of fat and carbohydrate.

Although there is general agreement that infantile eczema is due largely to allergy, it is difficult to show specific causes for the sensitivity. The most common allergies are due to various foods, e.g. egg white, cow's milk, wheat cereal and oranges.

Some investigators believe that there is a disturbance in the mother-child relations among infants and children

**Figure 148.** Seborrheic eczema in overweight infant. (Pillsbury, Shelley and Kligman: Dermatology.)

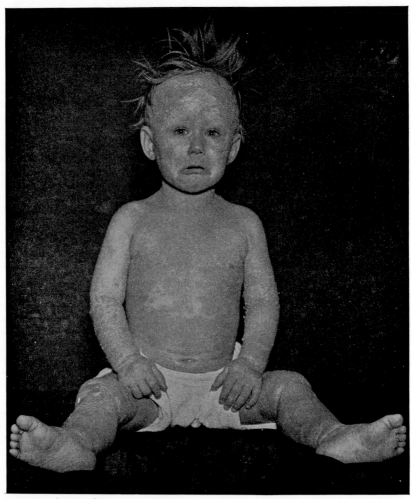

**Figure 149.** Atopic dermatitis. The considerable unhappiness of infants with extensive forms of this disease is well shown. (Children's Hospital of Philadelphia.) (Pillsbury, Shelley and Kligman: Dermatology.)

who have eczema. Such children are smothered with love by their parents.

**Pathology, Clinical Manifestations and Diagnosis.** *Pathologically,* the capillaries of the skin dilate, thereby producing erythema and edema. Fluid escapes from the capillaries into the tissues. Papules and then vesicles form. These rupture and exude yellow, sticky material which dries and forms crusts on the skin. The infant scratches, and excoriation of the skin results. Mild and severe lesions may exist at the same time on different parts of the body. The skin becomes thickened, and

fissures form. Secondary infection results from scratching the lesions. The itching is usually intense. The regional lymph nodes swell in the area. The cervical lymph nodes may swell if there is an infection of the scalp.

The eczema has periods of exacerbation and remission which are discouraging to the mother, who hopes for steady improvement. The areas where eczema most commonly occurs are the cheeks, forehead and scalp. It occurs also, but less frequently, behind the ears, on the neck and on the flexor surfaces of the arms and legs. There may be lesions on the trunk, abdomen and back, but these are usually drier and more scaly than elsewhere. The palms of the hands and the soles of the feet are not involved, though the rest of the body may be.

Because of the constant and intense itching the infant may not be able to sleep and may be highly irritable. If the lesions become infected, he may have a low-grade fever. Although most infants with eczema are overweight, malnutrition may be present if an infant has anorexia, dietary restrictions, a chronic infection, or diarrhea.

Eczematous lesions may flare up after prophylactic immunizations. These infants should not be given smallpox vaccination because of the possibility of generalized vaccinia developing. This condition might also occur if the infant were to come in contact with a sibling or another child who was recently vaccinated. Such contacts should be carefully avoided.

The *diagnosis* is made on the characteristics and distribution of the eruption, the family history, symptoms of severe itching, demonstration of protein sensitivity and a tendency to improve in summer.

**Treatment and Nursing Care.** Even the most intensive *treatment* may not produce a cure, but most infants can be helped by therapy.

The mother should be instructed as to the course to be expected, the treatment and the nursing care. She should understand that these infants are prone to infections of the skin and the respiratory tract and that they should be treated at home if at all possible because of the danger of infection in the hospital. Hospitalization may be necessary if the infant already has a secondary infection or if he requires more intensive care and local treatment than the mother can provide. Sometimes there is less external irritation in the hospital environment, and the infant can be kept on a stricter dietary regimen. If the mother is exhausted because of caring for the infant, he should be hospitalized for her sake as well as his own.

If hospitalization is necessary, the infant should be isolated for his own protection, not only from recently vaccinated children, but also from all persons with herpesvirus infections or pneumococcal or streptococcal infections. These infants are uncomfortable and need mothering. If possible, the mothers should visit frequently, and the nurses should give these infants extra attention.

In local treatment, restraints are important, though they should be applied only when necessary to prevent scratching. These infants scratch their irritated skin instead of crying when they are angry or frustrated. The nurse should help the infant to express his feelings outwardly by encouraging active play or physical movement. Restraints are necessary, of course, when the mother or nurse cannot be with him constantly.

There are many types of restraints, and their use depends on the specific type needed. The following are self-explanatory: elbow cuff, abdominal, jacket, face mask, and ankle and wrist restraints.* Cotton socks may be put over the hands and feet after the fingernails and toenails have been cut as short as possible to prevent the infant from digging his skin. Any needed combination of restraints may be used, but they must be checked frequently to

**Figure 150.** Eczema vaccinatum. (T. F. McNair Scott, in Nelson: Textbook of Pediatrics. 7th ed.)

* An effective elbow-cuff restraint for an infant may be made with tongue blades inserted into a stitched muslin restraint. This restraint may be secured in place by turning the end of a long-sleeved shirt back over the restraint and pinning it securely (see Fig. 69).

determine whether they are constricting the circulation.

When the infant is restrained, care must be taken to apply the restraints securely but gently. The restraints should be removed every few hours to allow free movement. If the infant is extremely uncomfortable because of itching, restraints should be removed from only one extremity at a time so that the nurse or mother can easily prevent him from scratching uncontrollably. If he has a paroxysm of scratching, the improvement of several weeks may be undone, and the skin may be opened to infection.

The infant should be picked up frequently and his position changed as often as possible to prevent respiratory infections, especially pneumonia. He should have supervised periods of play out of his crib to minimize his anger at being restrained and to give him opportunity to learn about his surroundings if he is old enough to walk.

To prevent irritation of the skin from rubbing against the sheet, heavy plastic or cellophane sheeting should be placed over the cotton sheet so that the infant can be turned from side to side and lie upon his back without increasing the severity of the lesions. This will also prevent absorption of ointment by the bedclothes. If the parents cannot afford new plastic sheeting, an old pliable plastic table cover can be used. In the hospital large pieces of exposed and washed x-ray film—the sharp edges covered with adhesive tape—may be used beneath the infant's head.

The infant may be bathed in water if it does not irritate his skin. In general it is better not to use soap; a substitute containing hexachlorophene may be used. Oil baths may be ordered if both soap and this substitute are irritating to the skin. Oil should be applied with a piece of cotton and patted rather than rubbed on. The crusted areas may be soaked with mild antiseptic solution compresses. Saline soaks kept continuously wet for one or two days may be helpful in removing crusts. If large areas are covered with papulovesicles, a soluble starch and sodium bicarbonate

bath may be ordered. The water for the bath should have a temperature of 95° F., and the soak should be continued for 15 to 20 minutes. Floating toys may be used to divert the infant's attention. During the bath only one extremity should be removed from restraint at a time. Although the bath is comforting to the irritated skin, the infant may attempt to scratch his body; if both his arms were free, his nurse or mother would be unable to control him.

It is not advisable to take the infant outdoors if the weather is cold or if there is a strong wind. His clothing indoors should be such that he is sufficiently warm, but not overheated. He should be dressed in as little clothing as possible to avoid overheating and skin irritation. No woolen garments should be used, since he may be sensitive to wool. The diapers should be changed promptly to avoid irritation of the buttocks.

The infant should be held for his feedings in the same way that healthy infants are held. He needs love for his emotional growth. Holding him for his feedings also ensures periods in the nurse's or mother's arms which will tend to change his position and prevent respiratory difficulties. Allowing him to suck on a nipple or pacifier provides relaxation and reduces tension during the first year of life.

Local medication applied to the irritated skin is important. Since different types of lesions may be present on different areas of the body at the same time, different kinds of medication and treatments may be ordered for the various areas. Ointments are not used for weeping areas. On indurated areas the ointment should be thoroughly rubbed into the skin. Whatever ointment or lotion the physician has ordered should be kept on the skin constantly and applied with long, soothing strokes.

Many kinds of ointments and lotions have been used in the treatment of eczema. It is difficult to apply ointment to the skin of the face so as to be effective because crusts are usually present, and it is difficult to keep ointment on this area. Crusts may be removed by wiping with gauze soaked with liquid petrolatum or by applying saline compresses constantly for one or two days. If an ointment is to be applied to the face, a mask made of gauze or stockinet may be used to keep the medication in close contact with the skin.

Holes are cut in the material for a face mask to correspond in shape and location to the eyes, nose and mouth. The holes are stitched so that the edges cannot fray. The mask is secured in place on the infant's head by draw strings. In applying it care must be taken to avoid binding or friction which would irritate the lesions.

If infection has occurred in the acute inflammatory phase of the eczema, various types of lotions or ointments may be used which contain bacitracin, bacitracin with neomycin or other antibiotics.

If the skin surface is dry, red and papular, an ointment containing crude coal tar may be ordered. The ointment should be applied as often as necessary to keep the area covered. Before its application a small area should be treated with it to determine the infant's sensitivity to it. All areas treated with tar ointment should be constantly bandaged, and uncovered only when new ointment is to be applied. Every day all the ointment should be removed with liquid petrolatum, and fresh ointment should be applied. A starch bath

**Figure 151.** Face mask which can be used on a child with eczema to keep medication in close contact with the skin.

may be used to remove ointment from large areas of the body covered with papulovesicles.

In teaching a mother to use tar ointments the nurse should emphasize that the ointment must be kept in tightly covered jars to prevent evaporation of volatile ingredients. Stains on linen can be removed by rubbing both sides of the soiled area with lard and washing with soap and water. The mother should also be told not to expose the infant to sunlight, since tar ointment contains a photosensitizing fraction that will produce further skin irritation. After the papules and the intense itching have disappeared the tar ointment is often discontinued, and a milder medication such as petrolatum or zinc oxide is used.

Many infants improve under these local applications, but if there is no improvement, further specific measures must be taken. Specific treatment involves a search for the specific allergens which cause the condition. Whether these are foods, wool or inhalants such as dust, they should be removed.

Wool should be removed from the child's environment. Neither his clothing nor his blankets should be of wool, and adults caring for him should not wear wool. The area about the crib should be kept free from dust. Carpets and drapes harbor dust and should not be used in his room.

A careful history or an elimination diet can be used to determine allergenic foods. If the infant is on an elimination diet, his mother should be given a list of foods he may have rather than a list of foods to be avoided. She should adhere strictly to the diet ordered. Synthetic vitamins may be given to supplement the diet. The diet should be increased so as to be as complete as possible. When a new food is added, the mother or nurse should watch for an allergic reaction to it. Such foods and reactions should be noted for the physician's consideration.

Skin testing as a means of finding allergenic substances is not very helpful in young infants or in children who have eczematous lesions covering their bodies. It is used with older children.

Many infants with eczema are allergic to cow's milk. Substitutes for cow's milk must therefore be provided in their formulas. Some infants can tolerate cow's milk if it has been exposed to a high temperature, thereby altering its protein so that it is less allergenic. For this reason evaporated or dried milk is of great value in the treatment of such children.

Infants sensitive to cow's milk in any form may be given goat's milk, vegetable protein substitutes, formulas made from meat or products made from hydrolyzed casein. Vegetable protein substitutes, largely made of soybeans, are available commercially in liquid or powdered form. With any substitute formula vitamins C and D, as well as other essentials, must be included in the diet.

Various nonspecific treatments may be ordered. In evaluating their use, however, it must be remembered that fluctuations in clinical manifestations of eczema may occur in the natural course of the condition. Measures which produce mild dehydration are helpful in the treatment of eczema, but dehydration is difficult, since by reducing fluid intake the intake of other nutritional elements in the formula may also be reduced. If a lowered sodium intake is ordered, water retention may be decreased.

Corticosteroids may be given systemically as well as locally to produce relief in severe cases, and are useful in controlling inflammatory skin reactions. Antibiotic therapy by oral or parenteral administration is essential if infection of the skin or other parts of the body is present. Mild sedation may be necessary if the infant is unable to sleep.

Charting is important and should include the condition of the skin (changes in the appearance and location of the rash and the general appearance of the infected areas), reaction to food (both the articles added to the diet and the formula), treatments given, additional allergic manifesta-

tions such as asthma and rhinitis, the amount of discomfort caused by itching of the skin, and alteration in personality characteristics.

The psychologic aspect of nursing is as important as the physical aspect. These infants should receive as much attention and affection as normal infants, if not more. Although their appearance may not encourage the nurse to handle, fondle and play with them, they need loving care to prevent emotional deprivation.

Toys suited to the child's age should be provided. The toys must be washable, safe and soft (if possible) and have a smooth surface. Stuffed toys which contain substances such as wool, feathers or kapok, to which children may be allergic, should not be used.

The nurse should understand the needs of the parents. Some mothers feel that they have failed to fulfil their maternal role, some are overprotective toward the infant, and others are afraid that their infants have a chronic condition which will result in disfiguring scars and retarded development. The nurse should help the mother to verbalize her feelings about the infant and the care he will need. Helping the mother to overcome her fears about her child while he is in the hospital will ensure better care for him at home.

The nurse must instruct the parents in the methods of local therapy and the diet to be given the infant. She must demonstrate to the mother the ways of applying restraints and providing exercise and diversion for the infant or small child. The nurse must help the mother find ways of giving adequate compensation for the kissing and skin-to-skin contact which other infants enjoy and of providing a happy environment in which the infant can lead as normal a life as is compatible with the necessary restraint of his hands and with local applications of ointments. The infant or small child should be permitted to move around his crib, play pen or room and feel that he is part of the family group. Normal activity and satisfactions are necessary so that he will not feel frustrated by the discomfort of his itching skin. The mother should have an opportunity to care for him in the hospital with the help of the nurses. This will reduce her fears about caring for him after his discharge.

**Prognosis.** The prognosis is good, but the course is long-drawn out, and there are remissions and exacerbations. Parents are likely to become discouraged, especially if they have tried their best to care for the child. The nurse must help them to see the situation realistically and without unwarranted anxiety over the child's evident discomfort. Infantile eczema usually clears up spontaneously toward the end of the second year of life. The condition can be controlled earlier if the causative allergens are eliminated. After two years the child may exhibit other allergic manifestations such as asthma and hay fever.

If infection develops during hospitalization of the infant, the prognosis may be poor, but will depend upon the severity of the condition. To prevent this danger these infants should spend as little time as possible in the hospital.

# DISORDERS OF THE CENTRAL NERVOUS SYSTEM

## Tetany

Tetany is extreme irritability of the neuromuscular system. It may be caused by any one of a number of conditions. These may be divided into groups: those characterized by a decrease in serum calcium (hypocalcemic tetany) and those in which a state of alkalosis exists (tetany of alkalosis).

Symptoms of *hypocalcemic tetany* occur when the total serum calcium concentration falls below 7 or 7.5 mg. per 100 ml. (normal serum calcium is from 9 to 11.5 mg.). In tetany of the newborn—i.e. in the first week of life —there is hypocalcemia due to hypofunction of the parathyroid glands. Hypocalcemia also occurs in vitamin D deficiency associated with rickets and is termed infantile nutritional tetany (see p. 347). In celiac disease, tetany results because of deficient absorption of vitamin D and calcium (see p. 465).

*Tetany of alkalosis* occurs when the acid-base balance is shifted to an alkaline level. It is not associated with changes in the serum level of calcium and phosphorus. It occurs with hyperventilation (excessive breathing) and in gastric tetany due to excessive vomiting and the concomitant loss of chloride. It may be observed in pyloric stenosis or in high intestinal obstruction which causes vomiting.

## Convulsions

**Incidence and Etiology.** A convulsion may be termed a symptom of a disease rather than a disease entity. Convulsive disorders are far more common during infancy and the second year of life than in any other age period.

Convulsions during early childhood are due to a variety of conditions, any of which may affect the nervous system.

In the newborn, birth injury, a congenital defect of the brain, and the effects of anoxia and intracranial hemorrhage are the most frequent causes of convulsions. During later infancy and early childhood acute infections of the central nervous system or other parts of the body, with accompanying elevation of temperature, are the most common causes. Less frequent causes are tetany (see p. 347), pertussis immunization (see p. 291), spontaneous hypoglycemia, poisoning by a convulsive drug or by lead (see p. 473), asphyxia, fluid and electrolyte imbalance, progressive degenerative diseases, neoplasms and postnatal intracranial trauma (see p. 381).

**Nursing Care.** Though children rarely die in convulsions, few other conditions frighten parents to the same extent. The nurse must be understanding of their fear and help them to a realistic attitude toward the child's condition. They should be told that though seven infants in every hundred have a convulsion, few of them suffer permanent damage. In the other cases the condition is indicative of some deep-seated pathologic state.

The nurse should place the child who

has had a convulsion or in whom a convulsion may occur where continuous observation is possible. In most pediatric units this would be near the head nurse's desk or in a unit for acutely ill children. It is essential that the child have no convulsion when the nurse is not there to give him care and to observe and report accurately to the physician.

A young child may show changes in behavior indicating the onset of a convulsion, such as irritability, restlessness or the reverse, listlessness. Such changes should be charted with the report of the convulsion. The nurse should note the types of movement and whether they are clonic (i.e. twitching, jerking movements) or tonic convulsions (those in which the child becomes stiff and the muscles are in a state of constant contraction), the time the convulsion begins and ends, the areas of the body involved, the amount of perspiration, movements of the eyes and change in the size of the pupils, incontinence (this will be influenced not only by the severity of the seizure, but also by the distention of the bladder at the time of the convulsion), the rate of respiration, color, bodily posture, foaming at the mouth or vomiting, the apparent degree of consciousness during the seizure, and the infant's behavior after his return to consciousness.

*Seizure Precautions.* The patient must be protected from injury. All hard toys should be removed from the bed, since he might be injured if he fell upon them. A padded tongue depressor should be kept on the bedside stand or taped to the bed to put between the teeth to prevent his biting his tongue. The sides of the crib should be padded if he has had a convulsion recently or is likely to have one. If the child has repeated convulsions, there should be in readiness an aspirating machine with which to remove accumulated secretions from the nasopharynx, and an emergency oxygen setup in case he has sudden respiratory difficulty.

If the child's temperature is elevated, tepid sponge baths may be ordered. The procedure is as follows.

The water should be tepid. Alcohol is added only if it is ordered. Long, soothing strokes with a wash cloth should follow the course of the large blood vessels of the trunk and extremities. In sponging the extremities the stroke is from the neck to the axilla and down to the palms of the hands, and from the groin to the feet. Gentle friction is used to bring the blood to the surface. Moist cloths should be placed over the superficial blood vessels in the axillae and the groins. A warm water bottle should be put to the feet to prevent a feeling of chilliness. This may not be practical with an active infant, but is generally used with an older child. An ice bag is applied to the head for greater comfort.

### Febrile Convulsions

**Incidence and Diagnosis.** About 7 per cent of all infants and children have febrile convulsions between 6 months and 2 or 3 years of age. After seven years of age convulsions due to elevation of temperature are usually rare. Males are more affected than females, and there appears to be an increased incidence of febrile convulsions in some families.

*Diagnosis* of the cause of the febrile convulsions involves diagnosis of the disease of which fever is a symptom. Most convulsions occurring between six and twelve months of age and in early childhood are initial symptoms of an acute febrile disease. A convulsion in this situation is equivalent to a chill experienced by an adult under the same conditions. Any young child who has a febrile convulsion, however, should be examined to eliminate the possibility of other etiologic factors.

In order to rule out other factors and to be certain of the cause, a careful history of previous convulsive episodes and illnesses and a complete physical examination, including a neurologic appraisal, should be obtained. Laboratory examination for calcium, inorganic phosphorus and electrolytes in the blood serum and for sugar and urea nitrogen in the whole blood will aid in the diagnosis. If the convulsion is due to fever, the physician will determine whether the infection is intracranial or extracranial and what the specific problem is.

**Treatment, Prognosis and Nursing Care.** *Treatment* is aimed at (1) direct control of the seizures by sedatives such as phenobarbital sodium, the dose depending on the age and size of the patient—and (2) control of the systemic conditions causing the convulsion. Therapy includes antipyretic drugs and measures to reduce the body temperature, such as aspirin and tepid sponge baths; anti-infectious therapy, depending on the organism responsible for the illness; aspiration if the nasopharyngeal secretions are excessive; and oxygen inhalation if the infant is cyanotic.

The *prognosis* depends upon the cause of the convulsion. A single febrile seizure is not indicative of a later chronic epilepsy, but repeated febrile convulsions increase the probability of subsequent nonfebrile convulsions (see p. 574).

The *nursing care* is the same as that for convulsions in general (see p. 379).

### Subdural Hematoma

**Etiology and Incidence.** A subdural hematoma is a collection of blood and fluid within the potential subdural space between the tough dura mater, which lines the inner surface of the skull, and the arachnoid. It may be acute, subacute or chronic. The chronic form is generally seen during infancy. The cause is trauma to the head, either extensive molding at birth or injury after birth. The condition is most frequent in infants who have not received adequate care or have been more often exposed to trauma; it may also be seen in infants who have bleeding tendencies such as in purpuric states. If the infant has scurvy, the possibility of subdural hematoma following injury is increased. Meningitis may also cause subdural collections.

Subdural hematomas are not rare. They are more common in males than in females and generally appear between the second and fourth months. The incidence decreases thereafter to fourteen to sixteen months, after which time the condition is less common. In about 80 per cent of cases it occurs bilaterally.

**Pathology, Clinical Manifestations and**

**Diagnosis.** At the time of the injury the delicate subdural veins are torn, and small hemorrhages occur in the subdural space. As a result fluid collects, and a sac forms in the subdural space between the dura and the arachnoid layers of the meninges. The sac enlarges with further accumulation of fluid and contains a mixture of old and fresh blood and xanthochromic fluid. The brain beneath the sac becomes compressed, and brain atrophy and clinical signs develop. In the longstanding subdural hematoma the fluid may disappear, leaving a constricting membrane that prevents normal brain growth.

*Clinical manifestations* of subdural hematoma are varied.

In the *acute* subdural hematoma, usually following trauma, there may be a rapid onset of signs of increased intracranial pressure previously described. In the *chronic* form clinical manifestations may have an insidious onset. The mother states that the child had anorexia, irritability, restlessness, vomiting or convulsions. The child who fails to thrive and attain normal developmental milestones may also have a chronic subdural hematoma.

Other signs such as recurrent fever, changes in reflexes, bulging and tense fontanels, enlarged head and possibly abnormal eyegrounds may be present at the time the mother is interviewed, or she may tell of them. The sutures may be separated. The infant may have anemia due to loss of blood. The cerebrospinal fluid pressure is increased, and the fluid may contain increased numbers of blood cells and an increased amount of protein. On subdural puncture a greater than normal amount of fluid can be obtained.

The *diagnosis* is frequently difficult because of the insidious onset of the signs and symptoms and is best made by bilateral subdural taps. In infants this procedure is easily done by inserting the needle in the lateral corner of the fontanel or farther out through the suture line. In older children burr holes must be made through the skull before the needle can be inserted.

**Treatment and Prognosis.** Subdural

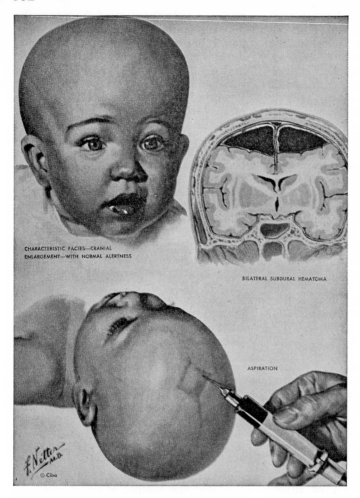

CHARACTERISTIC FACIES—CRANIAL
ENLARGEMENT—WITH NORMAL ALERTNESS

BILATERAL SUBDURAL HEMATOMA

ASPIRATION

**Figure 152.** Subdural hematoma. (Copyright, The Ciba Collection of Medical Illustrations, by Frank H. Netter, M.D.)

hematoma is usually treated by a neurosurgeon. The aim of *treatment* is to remove abnormal fluid and the membrane which forms the sac. Subdural fluid is removed before a craniotomy is done. Frequent aspirations of fluid are performed. Sometimes all the fluid can be removed in this way. Trephine holes may be made to determine whether a membrane is present, and also the estimated degree of cortical atrophy. After confirmation of the membrane a craniotomy is performed to remove as much of the adherent membrane and clot as possible. If the hematoma is bilateral, craniotomies are performed at intervals of several days. In some instances aspiration of fluid must be continued even after craniotomy.

Transfusions are given to correct the anemia. If scurvy is the cause of the condition, vitamin C is administered. Infection is treated with appropriate antibiotics.

The *prognosis* may be determined by the appearance of the brain when craniotomy is done. If the brain is severely atrophied, the prognosis is poor. After removal there is often a remarkable clinical improvement. The mortality rate varies in the acute and chronic forms because of underlying brain damage.

**Nursing Care.** One of the most important nursing responsibilities is that of early recognition and prompt treatment of the infant or young child suffering from subdural hematoma, so that the brain will be able to grow normally. If the infant does not receive treatment early, the brain will be damaged, and mental deficiency will result.

The infant should be placed on a sponge rubber mattress and turned frequently to prevent pressure areas on the skin. The nurse who assists the physician in withdrawal of subdural fluid should shave the anterior portion of the child's scalp and cleanse it thoroughly. She should hold the infant securely to avoid injury caused by a sudden movement. After the procedure she should observe the dressings for drainage. If drainage seeps through, the dressing should be reinforced to prevent organisms from gaining entrance to the wound, and the physician should be notified at once. The nurse should differentiate between serous drainage and frank hemorrhage. She should also observe the infant for signs of increased intracranial pressure.

Someone must stay with the infant to prevent his attempting to pull the head dressings off, or else his hands must be restrained with elbow cuffs (see Fig. 69) or the clove hitch restraint (see Fig. 51). Before applying restraints, every effort should be made to quiet him, since restraints make him more restless and increase intracranial pressure. For more detailed care of the postoperative patient see page 656.

## SKELETAL DEFECTS

### Craniosynostosis

**Etiology and Pathology.** Craniosynostosis is a premature closure of one or more sutures of the skull. Since other defects of the skeleton may be found with craniosynostosis, it is thought that the skeleton is adversely affected early in embryonic life.

In the normal newborn infant the bones of the skull are separated. The sutures, which can be located soon after birth, are separated by a layer of fibrous tissue. The bones of the skull grow in this fibrous strip.

In craniosynostosis one or more of the sutures are closed before or shortly after birth. Growth of adjoining bones is stopped, and there is a reduction in the diameter of the skull in this direction. Where open sutures remain, a compensatory growth or enlargement is found. The result is various deformities of the skull, depending on which sutures are closed.

**Clinical Manifestations.** Since most of the brain growth is completed in early childhood, any pressure which interferes with normal expansion may cause brain damage and resulting mental retardation.

In *scaphocephaly* the sagittal suture is closed prematurely. The head develops in a long, narrow shape. Symptoms of intracranial pressure may be evident.

*Oxycephaly* is a condition in which the coronal suture closes prematurely, either completely or partially.

Other sutures may also close and various deformities result. Complications arise since the brain may be severely compressed, with resultant headache, loss of vision, and convulsions. Exophthalmos may occur. Examination

**Figure 153.** Craniosynostosis in a child 5 years of age who also had mental deficiency and paralysis of the ocular muscles. (Josef Warkany, in Nelson: Textbook of Pediatrics. 7th ed.)

is likely to reveal strabismus, nystagmus and papilledema. Mental retardation is common. Syndactylism may be associated with this deformity.

Roentgenograms reveal the abnormal shape of the skull and absence of one or more sutures.

**Diagnosis and Treatment.** Craniosynostosis must be differentiated from microcephaly, which results in a small head because the brain fails to grow. Increased intracranial pressure does not occur in microcephaly.

Surgical intervention may prevent mental and visual defects if it is done before compression of the brain occurs. Early repair of the skull also produces a better cosmetic effect. Operation is therefore done as soon as a definite diagnosis is made during infancy. The surgical procedure includes linear craniotomy along the prematurely closed suture and lining of the edge of the suture with polyethylene film to slow its reunion.

**Nursing Care.** The nurse has an important role in early finding of these cases. Often the public health nurse who visits in the home may be the first person to observe the condition in a supposedly normal infant. Although she cannot diagnose this condition, she should refer such a child to a physician.

The nursing care of a patient after operation is similar to that after a craniotomy for brain tumor (see p. 656).

**Prognosis.** The prognosis is excellent if treatment is instituted before permanent brain damage occurs. Because of rapid bone growth resulting in closure of the sutures, revision of the craniotomy may be necessary.

## EMOTIONAL DISTURBANCES

**Causes of Anxiety in Infancy.** Every infant experiences inevitable frustrations because, basically, "he wants what he wants when he wants it." He may want to eat when his mother is busy; he may desire to suckle when he is supposed to eat solid foods; he may want his mother to carry him around instead of learning to walk.

These frustrations bring him pain, discomfort and anxiety. Gradually he learns that he can rid himself of these uncomfortable states by adopting new methods of behavior—e.g. by learning to eat solid foods and learning to walk. Infants learn new skills, therefore, because initially they were frustrated and uncomfortable as a result of depending only upon old skills. Learning new skills eventually brings new pleasures and fewer frustrations.

An infant will desire to learn new skills only if he has an optimum period of satisfaction with the old mode of behavior before the period of frustration begins. Infants should be allowed to experience the inevitable frustrations of life slowly and in small doses. Sudden, overwhelming frustrations, such as weaning within a few days, have an adverse effect on the immature personality.

**Behavior of the Infant Who Is Anxious.** The anxious infant may react in one of three ways: he may resent or fight against the cause of his discomfort; he may turn away or move from it, without fighting; or he may remain immobile and do nothing.

*Anxiety Due to Frustration in Feeding.* Young infants frustrated in the feeding process will react in the only way they know, i.e. by kicking, crying and by constant bodily movement. If the breast-fed infant cannot get adequate amounts of milk because of inverted nipples, he may regurgitate what he has already taken, he may turn away and refuse to suck, or he may fall asleep. Likewise the infant weaned too abruptly may show the same problem behavior.

The infant may react similarly to complementary foods if the food is too hot, if it contains lumps or if it requires excessive chewing. In such a situation he may vomit repeatedly, may turn his head away from his mother or may become immobile and refuse to participate in the feeding process.

Any of these reactions affects the

eating process directly. If the infant blames, as it were, his mother for the discomfort in feeding, he may turn away from her when she approaches him, refuse to eat, cry when she touches him or, when he is a little older, do exactly the opposite of what she requests.

*Anxiety Due to Frustration of Sucking.* If the desire to suck is frustrated, as when the breast produces milk too freely or when the hole in the nipple is too large, the infant will not receive adequate sucking pleasure. He will then suck on non-nutritive objects such as fingers, the blanket or toys for long periods of time and will continue this activity past the second or third year, when such activity is usually given up.

If the parents permit such sucking on non-nutritive objects, the infant will gain his needed satisfaction. But if the parents disapprove of such activity because they fear that it will deform the child's mouth, the infant may reject food or will stop the sucking activity completely and learn to find pleasure in frustration.

*Anxiety Due to Lack of Parental Love.* The newborn cannot distinguish between himself and his environment. Soon, however, he distinguishes between himself and his mother, who is the source of all pleasure. If his mother loves him and introduces frustrations slowly, he will respond in a way to please her. If his mother does not love him, he senses this and feels overwhelming frustration. In such a situation he will refuse food or go into a condition of semistupor and pay no attention to her. This is especially liable to happen if the mother gives the child minimal attention because of her own mental illness, depression or psychosis. Such infants may become emotionally deprived and later may become autistic (see p. 581).

*Overwhelming Frustration Which the Infant Cannot Handle.* When the infant lives in a situation in which there is persistent tension, noise and disturbance, he may not eat or may vomit after eating. He may respond as does the adult who is extremely depressed. He

may appear to wish death through starvation. The infant seems to decide that living with overwhelming frustration is not worth the effort.

A brief case history may illustrate such a situation.

Timmy, a two-year-old boy, was admitted to the children's unit. He weighed 7 pounds 5 ounces. He had multiple skin infections and suffered from malnutrition and dehydration.

His birth weight was not known. He was the illegitimate child of a fifteen-year-old girl. Shortly after his birth his mother left him with a sister and disappeared. His aunt subsequently married and gave him to a neighbor. During the two years of his life he had about eight substitute mothers, neighbors who passed him around at their convenience. Eventually he was given to a woman who really cared for him, but by that time he was so physically retarded and emotionally underdeveloped that her efforts were in vain. He would not suck on a nipple or respond to anyone. She brought him to the hospital, but in spite of gavage feedings, intravenous therapy, antibiotics and the best of nursing care, Timmy died.

The infant equates food with love. Timmy, who received rejection and no love, refused his food and literally died of starvation.

**Symptoms.** *Anxiety symptoms* include excessive crying, inability to sleep, restlessness or rhythmic rocking movements and possibly vomiting. In overwhelming anxiety the infant may experience depression with weeping, screaming when strangers approach, withdrawal, and arrest of physical and emotional development.

*Feeding disorders,* ranging from refusal of food to air swallowing and repeated vomiting, are common. Eventually marasmus may develop, and the infant may die of starvation.

*Antagonistic behavior* consists in a lack of enjoyment in the companionship of his parents, in a refusal to enjoy interaction with them or in doing the opposite of what they request of him.

**Treatment and Nursing Care.** Prevention of emotional disturbance is much to be preferred to treatment of the disturbed infant. Many mothers want to be loving and warm to their infants and yet seemingly reject them in greater or less degree because of disapproval by their husbands, relatives or neighbors of a truly maternal attitude toward the infant. Some mothers, for instance, want to care for their infants constantly during the first year of life, but because their husbands want them to leave the infant at home during vacation, they go away without him, leaving him with someone who gives good physical care, but no maternal love. Other mothers want to provide warm loving care for their babies, but are separated from them because of their own illness or that of other members of the family.

Such mothers could be helped to a great degree by education in the emotional needs of infants. Such education, given during the prenatal period, could make them more sure of their own judgment and less sensitive to external disapproval of others. Although intellectual understanding is not a cure-all for such problems, the support of an outside authority is reassuring. The physician or nurse can help such women to trust their own maternal feelings as guides in their behavior. Those women who have a conflict between their love for the child and their selfish desire to do the things that give them pleasure cannot be good mothers regardless of the guidance they receive. Their immature wish for pleasure causes them to be unaware of the infant's need for love and to be unable to give love even when they comprehend the necessity of a warm mother-child relation in the emotional life of the child.

In treating an infant for an emotional disturbance, the cause must first be found. The infant's need which is being frustrated must be clearly understood. It is important, then, for both the mother and the physician to treat the child as though he were a little younger than he was when the traumatic experience occurred. For example, if the infant reacts violently to supplementary solid foods, his mother should cease offering them for a while. Then the foods should be introduced gradually *without force* or even undue urging.

Sometimes the feeding difficulty, vomiting or refusal to eat may become so severe that the infant may need to be removed from his mother for a time. He may be cared for at home by a warm, loving person or may be placed in a hospital. Often such infants may begin to eat well after a brief period of adjustment to the new situation. During the period of separation the parents should receive guidance so that they may create a more loving environment for the infant when he returns to them.

If the infant is hospitalized, it is the nurse's responsibility to provide the love and tender care such an infant needs. She must hold him closely and show the warmth of her affection, cuddle him and be kind and patient in her feeding methods. Often the nurse can demonstrate to the mother how to hold the infant close to her body to feed him and to give him the loving care he needs.

## TEACHING AIDS AND OTHER INFORMATION

*Mead Johnson and Company*
   Phenylketonuria: Low Phenylalanine Dietary Management with Lofenalac.

*The Children's Medical Center, Boston, Mass.*
   Pancreatic Fibrosis.
   Eczema.

## CLINICAL SITUATIONS

Michael O'Brien, a four-month-old infant, was brought to the Child Health Conference by his mother. He appeared to be well nourished and well developed for his age, although he had had no previous medical supervision. During Mrs. O'Brien's conference with the nurse the mother asked several questions.

1. "Michael has been breast fed since birth, but I have been thinking about weaning him to a cup. When should I do this?"
   a. "As soon as you can after he is five months old, because continued sucking may cause his teeth to protrude."
   b. "As soon as Michael shows a desire to give up sucking and to drink from a cup."
   c. "Before summer comes regardless of his age, because it is difficult to wean an infant in warm weather."
   d. "Before he is a year old, because he will have several teeth and will not be able to suck properly."

2. "The doctor said that Michael should eat solid food, but he refuses it after he is breast fed. What should I do?"
   a. "Force him to eat, because he will lose weight and develop anemia if he continues to take only milk."
   b. "Give him only breast milk as long as he refuses solid food."
   c. "Mix the puréed food with some cow's milk and feed it through a large-holed nipple."
   d. "Offer small amounts of puréed food before each breast feeding when he is hungry."

3. Michael at four months of age has the following abilities. Select the one that is *not* typical for a child of his age.
   a. Enjoys sitting alone.
   b. Lifts his head and shoulders at a 90-degree angle when on his abdomen and looks around.
   c. Attempts to roll over.
   d. Moves his arms rapidly at the sight of a toy.

4. The nurse understands that Michael should be immunized against certain diseases during infancy. These diseases include
   a. Measles, pertussis, scarlet fever, chickenpox and diphtheria.
   b. Smallpox, pertussis, diphtheria, poliomyelitis and tetanus.
   c. Chickenpox, poliomyelitis, measles, diphtheria and typhoid fever.
   d. Smallpox, tetanus, diphtheria, pertussis and measles.

5. The important point about Michael's immediate safety to stress to Mrs. O'Brien at this time would be
   a. "Do not give Michael dry toast to chew, because he may aspirate it."
   b. "Do not permit Michael to chew paint from the window ledge, because he might absorb too much lead."
   c. "When Michael learns to roll over, you must supervise him whenever he is on a surface from which he might fall."
   d. "Lock the crib sides securely because he may stand and lean against them and fall out of bed."

Mrs. O'Brien brought Michael back to the Child Health Conference when he was six months old and said that he had been ill for about three days. The physician observed that Michael's anterior fontanel was sunken, his skin turgor was poor, and his skin was warm. Mrs. O'Brien said that he had had about six stools which were watery and foul-smelling each day and that he had vomited all his feedings. He was referred to the local hospital and was admitted promptly with a diagnosis of diarrhea and vomiting.

6. On admission a blood specimen was drawn from his jugular vein. The nurse restrained the infant by using a
   a. Clovehitch restraint.

   b. Mummy restraint.
   c. Abdominal restraint.
   d. Elbow restraint.

7. Intravenous therapy was started promptly. The most important responsibility of the nurse when caring for such an infant is to
   a. Check the number of drops of solution running into the vein frequently and regulate the flow of solution as ordered.
   b. Remove the needle as soon as the fluid which has been ordered has run into the vein.
   c. Change the bed linen promptly if it becomes moistened from the intravenous solution.
   d. Add a new bottle of solution when the present one is empty, with or without a physician's order.

Mrs. Smith brought her first infant, a five-week-old son, Bruce, to the pediatric clinic because he had been "spitting up" since he was three weeks of age. Bruce had been breast fed for the first four weeks of his life, and then had been put on a formula.

8. The physician made a diagnosis of pyloric stenosis on the basis of the infant's history and clinical manifestations which included
   a. Projectile vomiting beginning abruptly, normal stools, and malnutrition.
   b. Rumination of feedings, normal stools, and a sausage-like abdominal mass.
   c. Constant abdominal pain with crying, frequent liquid stools, and an olive-shaped abdominal mass.
   d. Gradual increase in vomiting, finally becoming projectile in nature, constipation and weight loss.

9. The vomitus of an infant having pyloric stenosis is the color of his formula and does not contain bile because
   a. The obstruction is above the opening of the common bile duct.
   b. The liver does not secrete bile, since its functioning is impaired.
   c. The obstruction at the cardiac sphincter prevents the flow of bile to the stomach.
   d. The stenosis of the common bile duct prevents bile from flowing properly.

10. A Fredet-Ramstedt operation was done. Mrs. Smith asks how Bruce will be fed after the operation. In order to answer her question you should know that the feeding regimen after a pyloromyotomy is based on the principle that
   a. Thickened feedings aid mechanically in helping food pass through the pylorus because its weight stretches the hypertrophied muscle.
   b. Clear liquids are tolerated well because they contain no curds which would have difficulty passing through the pylorus.
   c. Easily assimilated fluids are given in increasing amounts so that the newly

incised muscle can accommodate gradually.

d. Easily digested fluids are given in large amounts in order to combat dehydration.

11. Bruce's mother asks you to recommend a book which she could read on child care. You would suggest
   a. Hurlock, E.: Child Development.
   b. Spock, B.: Baby and Child Care.
   c. Gesell, A.: The First Five Years of Life.
   d. Erikson, E.: Childhood and Society.

When Bruce was seven months old, he was readmitted to the hospital with a diagnosis of eczema. He was irritable and restless, and scratched his skin whenever he could. The skin on his face and scalp was secondarily infected. Mrs. Smith said that Bruce had received a wide variety of foods in his diet and that his appetite had been excellent.

12. Eczema is a skin condition caused by
   a. Bacterial invasion primarily by the streptococcus.
   b. Excessive secretion of the sebaceous glands.
   c. Inflammation around the sweat glands due to excessive heat.
   d. Allergy to internal and external irritants.

13. When dressing Bruce after his bath, it is important to dress him
   a. In as few cotton clothes as possible according to the temperature of his environment
   b. In warm woolen clothing, because these infants frequently contract respiratory infections.
   c. In only a diaper, because clothing increases the infant's discomfort.
   d. In cotton clothing, but wrap him in a woolen blanket for warmth.

14. When using restraints they must be
   a. Kept on constantly to prevent Bruce from scratching.
   b. Removed once a day to allow active motion of his extremities under supervision.
   c. Kept securely in position so that Bruce remains on his back at all times.
   d. Checked frequently to determine whether the restraints are constricting his circulation.

15. Even though Bruce has not yet received his smallpox immunization, it will not be given until he is completely recovered because of the danger of development of
   a. Acrodynia.
   b. Aganglionic megacolon.
   c. Generalized vaccinia.
   d. Hypocalcemic tetany.

16. Bruce was hospitalized for several weeks. Mrs. Smith was not able to visit him more frequently than twice a month. In order to prevent emotional deprivation during this time, the most important measure the head nurse could take would be to
   a. Place him each day in a play pen near another seven-month-old infant so they could interact with each other.
   b. Place his crib near the entrance to the unit so that he would not become lonely.
   c. Give him many toys to keep him occupied.
   d. Assign the same staff nurse to provide care for him each day.

Mr. and Mrs. Jones had had three children. The first child died at one week of age after an operation for intestinal obstruction due to meconium ileus. The second child is normal. June, their third child, seemed normal at birth and had a good appetite, but she gained weight slowly. At five months bronchopneumonia developed, which responded well to chemotherapy. At eight months she again had bronchopneumonia and continued to have a chronic cough after discharge from the hospital. Upon readmission to the hospital at eleven months because of weight loss, a diagnosis of cystic fibrosis was made.

17. Before the collection of sweat for diagnostic testing an immediate important responsibility of the nurse is to
   a. Encourage a large amount of fluids.
   b. Give a bath.
   c. Give an enema.
   d. Give the child her medication.

18. During an evacuation June's rectum prolapsed. After it had been replaced by the physician the nurse prevented the recurrence of the prolapse by
   a. Giving a daily colonic irrigation to prevent constipation.
   b. Giving a mild laxative each night to prevent constipation.
   c. Restraining the child in bed with her head lower than her body.
   d. Taping the buttocks together after each defecation.

## GUIDES FOR FURTHER STUDY

1. During your experience at the Child Health Conference observe several infants under one year of age with their mothers. Note the apparent differences of maternal attitudes toward the infants when their mothers feed them, comfort them or give them physical care. What immediate effects do these various attitudes have on their individual infants?

2. A mother of an apparently normal two-month-old infant at the Child Health Conference has complained to you that in spite of all her efforts to teach him to sit alone, he shows no progress toward accomplishing this ability. What would your response be on the basis of your knowledge of the principles of motor development and your understanding of the interrelatedness of maturation and learning?

3. The women's group of a local church has offered to donate toys for the infants hospitalized at Christmas. List the specific toys you would request for infants of various ages and give the reasons for your choices.

4. Visit a foundling home in or near your community. Observe the infants to determine whether their behavior shows any evidence of maternal deprivation. In terms of your knowledge of the care the infants receive, evaluate your findings and make suggestions in seminar as to how the emotional needs of the infants could be more adequately met.

5. Trace the steps in motor development through which an infant must go before he finally is able to stand alone.

6. During your experience at the Child Health Conference or the pediatric clinic list several questions asked by mothers of infants of various ages. Discuss your answers to these questions in seminar. Evaluate your own progress in being able to establish rapport with these mothers and in being able to answer their questions to their satisfaction.

7. Plan a daily menu for infants of three months, six months and one year. Check each of these diets with the recommended dietary allowances given for infants on page 280.

8. What are the most recent statistics in your state on infant mortality? What are the most frequent causes of death? After investigating provisions made for the health supervision and care of infants, give suggestions as to how the infant mortality rate in your state could be reduced.

## REFERENCES

Andersen, D. H.: Cystic Fibrosis and Family Stress. Children, 7:9, 1960.

Berry, H. K., and others: Chemical and Clinical Observations during Treatment of Children with Phenylketonuria. Pediatrics, 21:929, 1958.

Berry, H. K., Sutherland, B., Guest, G. M., and Warkany, J.: Simple Method for Detection of Phenylketonuria. J.A.M.A., 167:2189, 1958.

Bowlby, J.: Maternal Care and Mental Health. Geneva, World Health Organization, 1952.

Dodd, S. G., and Shannon, V.: Care of Children with Nephrosis and Cystic Fibrosis of the Pancreas in a Crippled Children Program. Am. J. Pub. Health, 48:15, 1958.

Fakkema, La Verne: How to Help the Child with Cystic Fibrosis. Am. J. Nursing, 59: 1269, 1959.

Gross, R. E.: The Surgery of Infancy and Childhood. Philadelphia, W. B. Saunders Company, 1953.

Harvie, F. H.: Pediatric Methods and Standards. 3rd ed. Philadelphia, Lea & Febiger, 1958.

Kiesewetter, W. B.: Pre and Postoperative Care in the Pediatric Surgical Patient. Chicago, Year Book Publishers, Inc., 1956.

Lewis, G. M.: Practical Dermatology. 2nd ed. Philadelphia, W. B. Saunders Company, 1959.

Liebman, S.: Emotional Problems of Childhood. Philadelphia, J. B. Lippincott Company, 1958.

Nelson, W. E. (editor): Textbook of Pediatrics. 7th ed. Philadelphia, W. B. Saunders Company, 1959.

Ochsner, A., and DeBakey, M. E. (editors): Christopher's Minor Surgery. 8th ed. Philadelphia, W. B. Saunders Company, 1959.

Perlman, H. H., and Falk, A. B.: Pediatric Dermatology. Pediatrics, 21:502, 1958.

Pillsbury, D. M., Shelley, W. B., and Kligman, A. M.: Dermatology. Philadelphia, W. B. Saunders Company, 1956.

Reed, S. C.: Counseling in Medical Genetics. Philadelphia, W. B. Saunders Company, 1955.

Reynolds, A. H., and Joos, H. A.: Eczema Vaccinatum. Pediatrics, 22:259, 1958.

Robertson, J.: Young Children in Hospitals. New York, Basic Books, Inc., 1958.

Spitz, E. B.: Neurosurgery in The Prevention of Exogenous Mental Retardation. Pediat. Clin. North America, 6:1215, 1959.

Stephan, P. J.: Nebulization under Intermittent Positive Pressure. Am. J. Nursing, 57:1158, 1957.

Stevenson, S. S., and Bonine, G.: Mucoviscidosis. Am. J. Nursing, 56:866, 1956.

Wolman, I. J.: Laboratory Applications in Clinical Pediatrics. New York, McGraw-Hill Book Company, Inc., 1957.

Wortis, J., and Giancotti, A. M.: A New Simple Test Paper for Mass Detection of Phenylketonuria. Am. J. Pub. Health, 49:463, 1959.

# The Toddler

# Chapter 15

# The Normal Toddler: His

# Growth, Development and Care

THE PERIOD of infancy covers the first year of life. During this time the basis is laid for subsequent stages of development. The infant by his first birthday has learned to *trust* or *distrust* the adults who care for him. This attitude is modified by experiences throughout childhood and adolescence, but its direct influence on the way he perceives experience during the toddler stage is evident to all who know him.

During the first year the infant has developed from the complete dependency characteristic of the newborn to the satisfaction of many of his wants without help from others. He experiences pleasure in practicing newly acquired motor skills. He can pull himself up by holding onto furniture, can stand alone and may take a few steps without help. He can understand what others say to him if they use simple words which he has learned and use short sentences. He may even be able to respond with a few words of his own.

As he moves from passive dependency to active interaction with those about him, society or that small section of it which he knows—his family—guides him in conformity with social norms. The most important demand made upon him during the toddler period is that of toilet training.

## OVERVIEW OF THE TODDLER'S EMOTIONAL DEVELOPMENT

### Sense of Autonomy

As the infant passes from infancy into the toddler stage (one to three years) he uses his increasing ability to help himself and to develop his *sense of autonomy*. He makes his wants known to those about him to get what he wants. He shows that he has a mind and a will of his own. If he has learned to trust others, he accepts their gentle, considerate guidance in learning new

**393**

skills. But when they deny him what he wants, he is angry and hates the very people whom he has learned to love—mother, father, siblings and nurse. Their response to his anger is important in forming his personality. If they show him love while refusing him what he wants, he quickly returns to the loving relations which he has learned bring pleasure. He has learned that an angry attitude does not get him what he wants, but that a pleasant response, even when he is denied what he wants, brings him happiness. He becomes conditioned to being happy.

Understanding love for the child of this age is shown by giving him all the freedom he can safely use, by giving him all the love and help he needs to keep him safe in an environment which he is unable to control and in which he is dependent upon others for the satisfaction of bodily drives, and by giving him guidance in avoiding the hazards in the changing social situations in which he feels himself to be the focal point.

If he has learned by the end of the toddler period to accept and utilize guidance, he has gained a new level of self-control without losing his self-esteem. If he has not learned to be self-helpful, within the limits of his ability and in the way that those about him want, and, equally important, to accept adult direction in situations in which he cannot carry on alone, he is likely to feel insecure in his ability to meet the physical and social problems in his environment. He appears withdrawn and may have a *sense of doubt* about himself and others and a sense of what an adult would feel as shame. He avoids new experiences and thus has fewer opportunities to acquire new skills than has the child with an outgoing personality.

## NEEDS OF THE TODDLER

The basic needs of the toddler are the same as those of the infant. The toddler needs security and love, but he also needs graded independence.

**Figure 154.** The toddler needs security, but she also needs a degree of independence so she can explore her world. (H. Armstrong Roberts.)

### Love and Security

Love enables the toddler to grow up and reach out for more mature goals because he feels secure in his parents' affectionate care of him. Since he feels secure, he can endure the frustrations which come to every child in the process of maturation.

Both boys and girls give their first love to their mothers because mothers give them tender, loving care. As the needs of children become more diversified—less for physical care and more for social pleasures—their attachment to a loving father increases. In a family in which the father gives the infant the same care the mother does—bathes and feeds him, changes his diaper and takes him out in the stroller or in the family car—the infant generally feels as secure with one parent as with the other. But many infants hardly know their fathers until they reach the toddler stage. Then the father plays with them and takes them about with him. These toddlers still turn to their mothers when they want physical care or feel sick and wish to be petted. The more an infant is with his father, the more affection is he likely to show toward him, and the more secure he feels in his father's company.

## Graded Independence

Independence is learned gradually and is given the child only in situations in which he can guard himself from physical and emotional trauma. Independence must be denied him while he is too young to use it successfully. He might be seriously injured, or a painful experience might make him afraid to try out new skills.

### FULFILLMENT OF NEEDS

The toddler whose parents give him graded independence which brings pleasurable results develops a sense of self-reliance and adequacy, of autonomy. He finds that he is an individual who may make choices under the guidance of his parents. He may decide to play on the floor or on the chair, to eat the food offered him or reject it, to welcome a visitor or cling to his mother's skirt. Sooner or later he learns that there are many things he would like to do, but *can* not or *may* not. He easily learns that he cannot touch all the objects he wants because some are out of his reach, and that he may not cross the street whenever he wants to because cars are coming and he may be frightened by a narrow escape or hurt if he runs in front of them. It will take him a little longer to learn that there are some things he *can* do without being hurt, but *may* not do because his parents say "No."

The child wants to do many things he is not physically able to do. He will try and try again even if he sits down hard or rolls over in his attempts. Climbing upstairs is an example of his persistence. If he is constantly with a sibling only a few years older than he, he will attempt many activities which he is unable to do successfully.

As the child's muscular system matures he develops simple muscular skills, but finds that he cannot coordinate these diverse patterns into a purposeful activity such as he sees older children do so easily. Although he has learned to walk, to hold on and let go, to grasp and manipulate objects in various ways, he is often frustrated in his efforts to make his hands and feet do what he wants them to do. The toddler age is a frustrating age.

Regulating the toddler's activities is an important part of his training and is a challenge to the most mature and resourceful adult. The toddler cannot realize the consequences of what he does. Even if there is no danger of his being hurt, he may make himself ridiculous so that people laugh at him. This hurts his self-esteem if he cannot also join in the laughter. The adult must be loving, considerate and firm in setting limits and forbidding conduct which is harmful to him or brings too heavy a strain on other members of the household or his playmates or the neighbors. If he causes too much trouble to others, they will consciously or unconsciously dislike him.

A gradually expanding area of growth in a safe environment must be provided for him. Since one reason for adult control is that failure may injure his self-esteem, it is evident that an adult should never use shame or ridicule as a means of punishment or of prevention of forbidden activities. Shaming makes the toddler feel even smaller than he is; if it is used to excess, the child may comply when he is watched, but do as he pleases when he is not observed. This has been the cause of many serious accidents.

A certain amount of defiance is normal and may be more apparent than real. "No, no" does not always mean that he will not do what he is asked to do. It may mean, "Don't look so cross, Mama," or "I don't know what you mean." "No" is an easy sound to make, and he may use it for personal pleasure rather than for expressing a negative feeling. Even with the two- or three-year-old it may not mean refusal, but rather a bewildered response to injunctions he does not understand. All too often, however, it means that he will not do what the adult asks of him. His defiance is likely to be increased by anger on the part of the adult. This is because the child is likely to become confused and also because he follows the adult's lead with expressions of anger. He lacks words to convey his meaning and strikes the adult, has a temper tantrum, cries or becomes sullen.

Although a certain amount of defiance is part of his growing independence, excessive defiance becomes a habit and, unless wisely corrected, may be a factor in poor adjustment in kindergarten and school, in the Scouts, at summer camp or even in the contacts with his playmates in his yard or theirs. The repercussion upon himself of the irritation he arouses in others is likely to make him withdraw into himself or become more defiant. A disliked child is an unhappy child who has little pleasure in group activities. If his defiant attitude is not corrected before adolescence, he may find others like himself who are defiant of adult restraint. If he can get along with them, he may become one of the gang whose delinquent acts fill our newspapers. If he cannot fit into the gang because he will not accept the restraint the gang exercises over its members, he may become a solitary delinquent. He may learn to dislike the real world, in which he is disliked, and turn to daydreaming. Then he envisions an image of himself which he admires, and situations in which he not only does what he wants to do, but also controls others. Outwardly he may appear to be a quiet, obedient child in whom defiance is not suspected. He seems to be meek and dispirited, causing no one any trouble; neither does he contribute to group activity or any form of social interaction. This child is likely to have poorer mental hygiene than the delinquent.

Parents or their substitutes should have a deep sense of the value of preserving their own dignity as the child sees it, as well as the child's self-respect.

By building on the sense of trust in others which he developed during his first year of life the child normally gains a sense of autonomy during the toddler stage. He must be respected as an individual and helped to internalize the social norms of his group so that he *wants* to do what is *right* and, conversely, hurts his image of himself if he does what is *wrong*.

This developmental task takes two full years to make even a good beginning on which further guidance can be given as the child grows older. Some adults make the mistake of pushing him and forget that he is just out of babyhood and must learn slowly as he matures.

Three specific areas in which the toddler must be given guidance are (1) control of bodily functions of urination and defecation, (2) learning to talk, and (3) learning social norms.

### Control of Bodily Functions

Control of the bodily functions of defecation and urination is important, for it is the most personal phase of the young child's learning, closely related to his sensations. The child would like to continue emptying his bladder and bowels whenever he is conscious of discomfort from tension in these organs. Society does not sanction such behavior, and so gradually the toddler must learn to face the frustration of retention, and gain control of defecation and urination with the help of those he loves. Toilet training is at best difficult for the young child, especially if his family places an extreme value on cleanliness. If cleanliness has for his mother a moral aspect (if he dirties himself he is naughty, and if he keeps clean he is good), the child who is not able to keep clean and dry begins to develop feelings of guilt and anxiety because he cannot live up to the expectations of adults who care for him.

The infant, who for the first year received all care, love and attention, is now asked to assume the responsibility of giving up his comfort and to contribute to the comfort of others. He must learn to excrete urine and feces only at the appropriate time and place, although he cannot understand the necessity for this. He is motivated to try only because he wants to please his mother.

In more technical terms, the infant lives according to the *pleasure principle* (wanting what he wants when he wants it). Toilet training is foreign to the desire of the infant who is living according to this principle. The toddler must begin to accept the *reality principle* (giving up an immediate pleasure in order to gain another pleasure later). In this instance the toddler must give up the pleasure of excreting where and when he wishes in order to gain his mother's approval. If he does not have a trusting relationship with his mother, he will not be strongly motivated to succeed in toilet training.

Other factors, of course, influence him. If he sees an older brother or sister using the toilet and pulling the handle, he may want to do the same. As he becomes more active his wet clothing is more uncomfortable. If other children point at the puddles he makes and laugh at him, he may laugh too and put his finger in the puddle, but he does begin to connect keeping himself dry with part of the life pattern of the older child whom he imitates and who can do many pleasant things which the toddler attempts, but fails to accomplish.

Learning a new skill is difficult before the stage of maturation at which the child is motivated to learn and is physically able without too great an effort. If he is urged to learn before this stage, unfavorable attitudes may develop. To wait beyond the optimum stage when he is ready to learn a new skill is a mistake, because the happiness of using this skill is kept from him. Then, too, skills normal for his age evoke a favorable response from other people, and his self-image, taken from their attitude toward him, is more satisfying.

**Age for Beginning Toilet Training.** Toilet training should be started about the end of the first year when the child is psychologically and physiologically ready. By that age he is usually able to stand alone; this indicates that the tracts of the spinal cord are myelinated down to the level of the anus. It is useless and too frustrating to the child to attempt toilet training before the neurologic pathways are formed which enable him to control the anal sphincter and the urethra under tension and to excrete when his mother tells him to do so. Toilet training should be considered in relation to the general pattern of life which little children lead in our society. It is a great mistake to make an issue of this single phase of his training. He is learning at the same time to drink from a cup and is shortening his periods of enjoyment from sucking. He is learning to be away from his mother for longer periods.

Most pediatricians advocate that toilet training may be attempted at the end of the first year, but if the child does not understand what is wanted of him, it should be postponed until later. If training is started before the child is a year old, it is probable that the child is neither controlling nor expelling excreta at will, but rather that his mother has put him upon the toilet chair at the time when tension causes release of the anal or urethral sphincter, or both. As long as the child's diet and fluid intake are about the same each day this procedure may be successful, but any change in routine is likely to change the time of excretion, and he will soil his diaper or training pants. The mother is then apt to feel that the child has retrogressed and may show her disapproval by a scowling face or severe tone of voice.

Bowel training should be started before bladder training, since the number of stools in a day is less than the number of times the child urinates. Bladder training may be started one or more months after bowel control has been

**Figure 155.** The toddler should feel secure when placed on the training chair. She should be able to touch the floor with her feet and should be supported adequately by the back and arms of the chair.

fairly well established. Extraneous factors such as moving to a new house or the birth of a sibling may make the process of toilet training more difficult than it would usually be.

**Method of Toilet Training.** The first step is to observe the child's usual time of defecation. A little before this time he should be placed on a comfortable infant toilet seat or training chair on which he feels secure. There should be a rest for his arms and feet. He should not be given food or toys at this time, for these distract his attention from the purpose for which he is put on the chair. He may be kept upon the chair for ten to fifteen minutes. The mother or nurse should indicate to him by gestures and tone of voice that he is

expected to pass his eliminations in this place and at this time. A specific word indicating the act should be selected, a word easily understood by everyone. This is important, for many a child at nursery school or visiting with friendly adults has not been able to tell the adults that he wants to relieve himself, because he does not understand the words they use and they do not know what he is saying. The word used by the child's mother and taught to him often reflects the social class of the parents. Nurses should never show disgust at any word a child may use, though he can be taught a more appropriate one.

Much patience is required of the mother, for the child learns only as the result of repeated attempts over a period of time. Training should not be made a tense issue for either the mother or the child. The mother will find it easier for herself as well as better for the child if she assumes a casual, matter-of-fact attitude. Toilet training generally covers one or two years, so that there is no need to hurry the process. When the child defecates or urinates in the toilet or training chair, he should be praised and cuddled. But when he fails to do so, the mother should never show disappointment or disapproval, for a child of this age has difficulty in releasing the contents of the bowel or bladder at will.

When the child is old enough to go to the toilet by himself, he should have clothing which he can manage without help so that he can develop increasing independence. His pants should be such that he can slip them down or open them with a zipper. A girl's training pants should have elastic at the waist so that they may be easily pushed down below the knees. Steps which the toddler can climb to reach the adult toilet (with or without the child's toilet seat) are helpful. Boys learn to stand for urination by watching older boys urinate. A step may be necessary for him to urinate into the toilet bowl without wetting the floor.

Enemas, cathartics or suppositories should not be used unless ordered by the physician. The mother should understand that not all children have a daily bowel movement.

**Age at Which Toilet Training Is Accomplished.** The average healthy, intelligent child usually accomplishes bowel control by the end of the eighteenth month. Daytime bladder control may be fairly well established by two years of age, and night control by three years. Night control should not be hurried. It is not a good plan to wake the child and take him to the toilet, for he may stay awake for a long time after he has been put to bed again. Withholding fluids in the late afternoon and evening may be tried, but if the child is not physiologically ready, this will not help him to retain urine during the night. Also, he may be thirsty and cry for water during the night.

**Training during Illness.** If the child is not already trained when he enters the pediatric unit, he should not be taught to use a bedpan or urinal or little toilet chair while he is hospitalized. He would not be motivated to learn because there would be no one person whom he loves and attempts to please by doing what she asks of him. Then, too, a sick child should not be subjected to the strain of breaking old habits and acquiring new ones.

If the mother on admission of the child says that he is toilet trained, this should be noted in the habit history on the admission chart. The technique used by the mother and the words the child associates with the acts of elimination should be recorded. If the child is old enough to understand, he should be shown the hospital equipment, such as the bedpan, urinal and training chair, if the physician permits him to be out of bed. The nurse should try to keep him on the same schedule as that used by his mother, but should not be worried if he wets or soils himself and certainly should not show disapproval. The sick child in a strange environment generally regresses to infantile toilet habits. When he is well again, his mother can help him to resume his former habits of elimination.

**Meaning of Toilet Training to the Child.** The child is now asked to do what his mother wants him to do, whereas when he was a baby, she gave him loving care without asking any other response from him than his loving dependence upon her. Instead of being irresponsible, he is now asked to assume some responsibility for himself.

*Fecal Smearing.* The child has not yet acquired the adult's distaste for bodily excretions. He appears to enjoy the odor. He likes to manipulate fecal material and smear it upon the floor, wall or furniture. This sort of behavior occurs between the ages of fifteen and twenty-one months. The toddler thinks of his feces as coming from him and in this sense regards it as a gift, just as he offers his mother his toy or a piece of bread to get a pleasant response from her. He does not understand why fecal material is thrown away after he has been urged to expel it into the toilet chair. (This is one advantage of a toilet. He can help pull the handle and see the feces disappear with the swirling water. This is to him a satisfying accomplishment.) The parent or nurse should accept the child's feeling about his excretion and never express strong disapproval of his smearing it upon himself or any object.

Figure 156. Toddlers enjoy playing in sand. This is a more socially acceptable activity than smearing feces. (H. Armstrong Roberts.)

His desire to smear should be gratified in a socially acceptable way by giving him clay, damp sand or mud pies to manipulate. Later he may enjoy smearing in finger painting, using bright, light, cheerful colors on large sheets of paper.

Smearing with feces can be reduced if the child is cleaned immediately after a bowel movement. If this is not possible, diapers should be applied securely, using four pins, so that the child cannot put his hands upon the excrement. After he has learned to use the training chair or toilet, smearing is no longer a major problem.

**Influence of Toilet Training on the Child's Personality.** *Ambivalence* toward his mother is common during the training period. He loves her, but now she asks him to give up the comfort of relieving himself when and where he feels the desire to do so. He therefore feels antagonistic toward her. His ambivalent attitude is composed of love and hate at the same time. He may strike at her and pull away and a moment later turn to her for comfort. If she maintains an attitude of friendliness and understanding, love will predominate over hostility in him. It is important to minimize his antagonism so that he does not grow out of the training period with feelings of hostility, rebellion and resentment. In addition to having difficulty with bowel and bladder regulation, a hostile child will have more temper tantrums and show more disobedience and destructiveness than is normal in little children.

**Summary.** If a mother gives love to her child during his first year, he is normally conditioned to please her and will respond to toilet training without too much difficulty. She will not be discouraged if she has confidence in his intelligence and his desire to do what she asks, and she will give him a reasonable length of time in which to learn.

On the other hand, if the mother shows disgust about the whole process of excretion, the child will feel ashamed of his body. He may feel that he is not lovable. He may even feel that he is a naughty child if he fails in toilet training. Eventually he may acquire the attitude that all physical functions should be brought under rigid control. He may extend this feeling to all his activities and be constantly afraid of doing something which will displease his mother or other adults. He takes over and adapts her attitude toward toilet training into his concept of what she wants of him at all times when he plays or eats his meals. He is apt to be a child afraid to soil his hands or dirty his clothes when playing. When other children make mud pies, he stands back. Such a child may develop a persistent attitude of anxiously trying to please anyone in authority over him for fear he will lose their approval.

If a mother forces a child to give up soiling himself before he is psychologically ready to control himself, he will become extremely nervous. For fear of displeasing her he may become overanxious to keep clean. In his mind he equates overcleanliness with being good. Unfortunately his desire to keep clean usually inhibits normal active play. Such a child lacks spontaneity and creativity. Not only must he be perfect himself, but also he expects his friends to be likewise. He becomes rigid and inflexible and bound by compulsive rituals which to his mind will minimize the danger of his displeasing someone and thus will lessen his anxiety.

### Learning Language

Learning to talk takes a long time. From the newborn's cry to the first spoken word is the change from a reflex utterance to speaking words which have a meaning for both the child and others. The infant uses motions, particularly movement of the hands, to indicate his wants. Motions are his substitute for speech.

The little infant coos and later babbles, using a wide variety of sounds. If his mother smiles and talks to him when he makes these sounds, he will continue. Babbling reaches a peak by about eight or nine months.

Between the ages of one and three

years the child is increasingly able to understand others and to express his feelings and ideas in words. Infants and little children may continue to use gestures, however, such as holding out their arms and smiling when they want to be picked up, even when they are able to say what they want.

Long before a child can use words in sentences he understands the meaning of many words. The mother's facial expression, gestures and tone of voice help the child to understand the meaning of her words. She may teach him a new word by pointing to an object while she says the word. Or when he is interested in an object, such as a doll, he may say the word as she gives it to him.

**Incentives to Speech.** In order to speak a child must have satisfying relations with his mother. Unless he feels that she will respond to his words, he is not motivated to speak. He must find it rewarding to talk or he will not be interested in trying. He speaks to express his needs. His need may be only for a pleasant response or to call attention to his discomfort. When he says, "Ma-ma," he is expressing a need for all the pleasant things she does for him. If he says, "Ma-ma," and points to something, he means, "Please give me that." When he learns the names for objects, he will use the names, e.g. cup, dog. If all his needs are supplied without his asking, he is poorly motivated to speak until he feels the need for words to express attitudes, ideas and emotions.

Normally a child's first speech is an expression of his wants. This is followed by words or phrases which indicate ideas or what he thinks the function of objects to be. His idea of animals is expressed in terms of what they do; e.g. a dog barks. He early learns the value of speech in pleasant social relations. He takes great pleasure in talking and talks to anyone, his toys, pets or himself. Even when he can say only a few words, he uses these words to obtain information about himself, other people and things. "Go bye-bye" is not only a request; he is also asking whether he is going outdoors. When he says, "Dog," he may be asking where the household pet is.

**Methods of Learning.** A young child must have a good model or he will not learn to speak correctly. He will imitate poor speech as readily as correct speech, perhaps more easily because it is often more simple and direct and apt to be accompanied with gestures. If an adult uses baby talk in speaking to him, the child has no model for learning the correct words for objects, experiences and attitudes. He needs not only a model talking *to him,* but also the opportunity to use the word immediately in his answer. Talking to toys, to animals and to himself gives him practice in using words, but since he hears only himself, he may be confirmed in his baby mispronunciation and misuse of words.

There is a plateau stage in learning to talk at which a child makes little progress. The plateau occurs when the child has learned to walk and is so interested in walking that he pays little attention to acquiring new words. Although he makes little progress in learning to speak, he appears to be increasing the number of words he understands.

The child with his limited vocabulary may cry because he is frustrated in his efforts to express his wants or feelings and because he does not get what he wants. He still hits out when he is angry and cries when he is hurt. He has not yet acquired the ability, physically or psychologically, to control his actions and to use words to express antagonism and unhappiness. Later on instead of hitting his mother or a playmate, he may express his feeling by saying, "I hate you!" or "I wish you'd go away," and instead of crying because he may not go out and play he may say, "Why does it rain? I want to play," or simply wail, "I want to go out and play." In either case he is asking for the comfort which crying brought him when he was a baby. Even when he is able to speak, if his emotions are too great for him to control, putting them into words is not a sufficient outlet, and

**Figure 157.** The toddler cries because she cannot express her needs in words. (H. Armstrong Roberts.)

he resorts to the immature outlets of anger and disappointment. Whenever he speaks or cries, the child needs acceptance of himself and his feelings, however unreasonable they appear from the adult's point of view. Crying is a distress signal with him as with an infant.

Examples of this sort of situation are often found in the hospital. When a child thinks that he will be hurt because he will get a needle and is reassured by what we say to him, we see the value of his understanding verbal communication and of his ability to put his fear into words. He needs a simple explanation as a preparation for the procedure and both verbal and physical demonstrations of affection so that he does not feel that these strange adults want to hurt him (technically speaking, that he is being attacked). The nurse in such a situation must not say, "Don't cry." To do so would indicate a lack of understanding of how the child perceives the situation and of his stage of development. He is still too young not to be afraid of pain. The nurse or mother should explain the

need for his being hurt and what is to be done, so far as he can understand the reason or the procedure. If possible, his mother should be there to hold him; if not, one of the nurses whom he knows or at least has made friends with should take her place. The nurse should tell him that she knows he is frightened, saying, "All children feel that way. It will be over soon."

**Vocabulary Building.** The child builds up a vocabulary in the following ways. The first words he learns are nouns of one syllable, nouns like the sounds he has babbled ("Ma-ma, da-da"). He attempts more difficult words until eventually he can give the names of objects and people in his daily environment. He next learns verbs that mean some form of action which he sees about him and whose meaning he understands (e.g. give, take, run). Adjectives he learns from eighteen months on. The first adjectives he learns are usually "good" and "bad," because he hears them frequently. The first adverbs he uses are usually "here" and "where." These are words used by his mother in speaking to him. Last he learns the meaning of the different pronouns. These are confusing to him because they vary with the person using the word. Johnny is "me" and "I" to himself, but "you" to his mother when she speaks to him, and "he" when she tells his father about him. The same confusion exists with other pronouns.

The size of a child's vocabulary depends on whether he has been helped to learn new words, on whether he has had an incentive to learn and on his intelligence. At nine months he can say "Ma-ma" and "Da-da," and at one year two or three more words. From eighteen months to three or four years his vocabulary increases rapidly. At 2 years he can say approximately 300 words, and at 3 years approximately 900. During school age his general vocabulary increases rapidly as the result of being taught new words and of his pleasure in reading.

**Sentence Formation.** The child's first attempt at making sentences consists in combining two or more words into a phrase and supplementing these words with gestures. Early sentences contain nouns, verbs and, at times, adjectives and adverbs, e.g. "Baby go bye-bye."

**Delayed Speech.** The normal child will begin to speak by about fifteen months of age. If he does not speak by the time he is two years old, the cause for delayed speech should be investigated. Some of the common causes are as follows.

*Intelligence.* Speech is delayed in children of low intelligence. The size of the vocabulary depends to a great extent upon the child's intelligence.

*Social and Cultural Environment.* Children of poorer social environments are delayed in speech development because they often have poor models to imitate, see few books and have little constructive play material. Children in an orphanage or a similar institution may have extreme language retardation because adults seldom speak to them individually, and when they do, the subject is likely to be merely what the child is to do or not to do.

*Illness.* Children who are ill in an institution for a long time have slower speech development than well children because they have fewer contacts with other children and also because their needs are answered before they have to ask for what they want. A child who receives a great deal of adult attention at home when he is sick may increase his vocabulary rapidly. It is the hospitalized child who is likely to be retarded.

*Poor Models.* Not only does a poor model make for poor speech, but also if the child does not love his model, or have much contact with the adult, his speech may be both incorrect and retarded. This occurs in institutionalized children, in those cared for by nurses who speak a language foreign to them and in children separated from other children, such as those in wealthy families.

*Negativism.* The child may decide not to talk because he was forced to talk when he had not matured to the point at which he wanted to imitate his mother's words. He may have been laughed at for his babyish pronunciation and had his self-image lowered.

*Deafness.* If the child cannot hear what others say, he cannot imitate them and therefore will not speak unless he has had special training. Even then he will have a smaller vocabulary, poor pronunciation and a peculiar, flat tone of voice.

*Sex.* Boys are usually slower than girls in learning to talk. They also have a smaller vocabulary than girls have and make more grammatical errors.

*Learning two languages* at the same time for the child under five years of age is likely to delay his learning to speak and also causes confusion as to both vocabulary and grammatical forms.

### Cultural Development

The toddler must begin to learn many other patterns of behavior besides toilet training and language. He learns how to make the simple basic movements in washing and bathing himself and brushing his teeth. He understands what his mother means when she wants him to keep clean, to put his toys away when he has finished playing with them, and to keep his play space neat.

The child is attempting an over-all mastery of his world. When he learns to do something by himself, he has a real sense of mastery, independence, and adequacy in meeting his needs. His parents should help him to learn and should approve his success. If parents do not show their approval in ways he can understand, the child experiences a conflict between enjoying what he can do himself (even if this is to get an ashtray and empty it on the floor) and the disapproval of his parents. Since he knows that they will disapprove, he must make a choice between the two pleasures (the pleasure of doing what he wants and the pleasure of having his parents' approval). Through such decisions the child eventually learns how to make appropriate judgments, choosing what is considered right in the culture of the group he belongs to.

His basic motivation is love for his parents, a love acquired in infancy and strengthened during early childhood.

### PERSONALITY TRAITS OF THE TODDLER

#### Negativism

In his desire for independence or autonomy the child wants to do many things he should not do. From infancy through the toddler period he has heard his mother say "No" to his many efforts at self-assertion. Gradually he learns to use the words "No, no" to mean "Don't" and a rather stubborn "I won't." In this way he is substantiating his power as an individual in controlling those who love him. The developmental task of this period is to curb his negative responses and adjust his conduct to the social norms of those in authority.

Each child goes through this period of negativism during his growth toward maturity. Two years is said to be the "No, no" age and has been called "the terrible twos." He wants to act as an individual and appears to want power —to have his own way—more than the pleasure of the forbidden activity. Yet when he is frustrated in achieving what he wants independently of the help of others, or when their reaction toward him leads him to believe that they do not love him, he is likely to turn to the adults against whom his aggression was aimed, for comfort in the unpleasant situation which he has created for himself.

Sometimes he seems to want to be dependent and independent at the same time. For example, when he is offered ice cream, he may say, "No," and yet eat it quickly in spite of his answer.

A child acts in a negative fashion because he is unable to tolerate the frustration of a desire. He cannot accept parental restrictions and at the same time cannot find an acceptable way to gain the results he wants. When he says, "No," he feels as strong as his parents.

Sometimes a child appears to be negativistic when he really is not. He may not object to doing what his parents want, but he does not want to stop what he is doing, e.g. if he is playing happily and is asked to put away his toys and go to bed. If parents put too much pressure upon a child, he may become extremely negativistic about going to bed.

The period of negativism is usually a short one if the child's needs are understood. He needs the support of his parents' love in order to learn how to satisfy his new powers of independence in socially acceptable ways.

**Handling Negativistic Behavior.** An adult should not use opposition to overcome opposition in a child. Opposition increases the child's desire to show his independence.

An adult should not give the toddler too many commands or interrupt his activities too frequently.

The adult should help the child to participate in what is expected of him by giving physical help—for instance by putting the toys away when it is bedtime. This allows the toddler to feel that he and the adult are working toward a common goal and not that he is forced to do what the adult wishes. When the mother places food in front of a two-year-old, she may feed him a few spoonfuls, speaking gently to him as she does so. The child may then take the spoon in his hand and feed himself.

The mother must recognize indications of independence in the child. Such recognition increases the child's self-esteem and makes him want to cooperate even more. It helps him to feel self-important. All children learn to know themselves through the attitude of others (particularly members of their own families) toward them. If the mother has a wholesome concept of the child, he has a wholesome concept of himself. If he accepts himself at this age, he can later accept others.

#### Ritualistic Behavior

The toddler engages in much ritualistic behavior. He makes rituals of simple tasks because he knows that he can master himself in this way by doing these rituals. Ritualistic behavior is most common between the ages of two and four years; it reaches its height at approximately two and a half years. As the child leaves the toddler period he has less and less need of a strict routine because he is more sure of himself and can adapt to changes better than he could when he was younger. Adults should recognize these rituals in such phases as bathing (hanging the wash cloth in a certain way), eating (having his bib on always in the same way) and sleeping (always taking his favorite blanket to bed with him), because the adult saves time and energy by doing so and also gives the child a feeling of security and mastery of himself.

### Slowness in Carrying Out Requests

The toddler is gradually learning the difference between right and wrong. He cannot decide which of two actions to take. He is therefore likely to carry out both actions. For example, when his mother calls him from play to use the training chair, he is likely to finish carrying out his play activity first and urinate on the way to the training chair, partly because of his nervousness and haste to do what his mother has asked. This slowness in carrying out an adult's request is typical of children in this age group. When the child learns through experience which action he should take, he will be able to make decisions more wisely and more quickly.

### Temper Tantrums

Temper tantrums occur when the child cannot integrate his own internal impulses and the demands of reality. He is frustrated and reacts in the only way he knows—by violent bodily activity and crying. When no substitute solution is available, temper tantrums result. Such situations are most common during the toddler and early preschool periods; hence occasional tantrums of variable intensity occur in these years. If the tantrums are abnormally frequent or continue into school age, the child should be taken to a

child guidance center so that he may have professional help with his problems or with a deep-seated emotional maladjustment.

In the hospital children may have tantrums because they fear the unknown and are away from those they love. Such children need help in understanding their environment and their care. They also need the security resulting from their mothers' frequent visiting.

In a temper tantrum the child is completely oblivious of the reality of the situation. He does not hear or react to what is said to him unless it shocks him so severely that it penetrates his consciousness.

His release of emotion through muscular activity is either aimless or is directed against himself. He is likely to bang his head against the floor or otherwise inflict pain upon himself. Only rarely does he attack the adult who has provoked the tantrum.

**Handling the Child.** The child should not be given extra attention, but he should be observed and restrained from self-injury or from something in the physical environment which may be a source of injury to himself. Restraint increases the severity of a temper tantrum because it prevents the one outlet which the child knows for his angry emotion. If he hurts another child or an adult or breaks a cherished possession, he may feel guilty when the tantrum is over.

The tension in the child will be reduced if he can be removed from the immediate cause of the tantrum and be with only one adult who he knows loves him. This adult, usually his mother, should be calm and patient with him, but should not force attention upon him until he indicates that he is ready for the comfort of knowing that he is loved and that his unhappiness can be changed to happiness. A child often fears his own aggression and the disagreeable state into which it throws him. He can be helped to release his tension in a socially approved way—one in which he may acquire skill in a game or in making something he can give to his mother or enjoy playing with himself. The sick child may hammer rubber balls through holes in a board or toss bean bags into a can placed on the floor. In the home there is a wide range of activities which can be used as an outlet for his tension. If he may go outdoors, digging in the garden and helping rake the leaves or shovel snow are tension-releasing activities. In the house he may use a hammer and pegs or build a block tower which he can then knock down.

If the tantrum is caused by an adult's refusal to grant a request the child has made, the adult should be firm and not yield to the child. Only by consistency in adult behavior can a child learn to adjust his own behavior to his expectation of the adult's reaction to what he intends to do. Unfortunately, perfect adults can no more be expected than can perfect children. The child does not and never will live in a world of perfect people, and his own imperfections are less likely to arouse guilt feelings in him if he sees imperfections in those nearest him. One value of a large family is that the children talk over imperfections in their parents—whether real or imaginary—and develop a healthy, realistic love of others even while recognizing their faults. It is a comfort to a two-year-old to know that the four-year-old thinks that mother is sometimes mean. The modern mother knows that she is sometimes mean and that the child knows it, but loves her just the same as she loves him with all his naughtiness.

Sometimes when a child feels anger and tensions rising, he isolates himself. This is all right as a temporary measure, but if he always withdraws, he will need help in learning to face problems more directly.

**Care after Tantrums.** It is advisable to make as few comments as possible upon the child's behavior during a tantrum. He should not be punished in any way. If he will cooperate, it is soothing to wash his face and hands. He may be given a toy to divert his attention from the experience he has undergone. He has been so emotionally upset that he needs to quiet down before he is given food.

The mother, knowing the child, may see that a tantrum is imminent. She should try to show him better ways of solving his problem and provide more socially acceptable outlets for his anger and frustration. To allow him to have his own way so as to prevent a tantrum only leads to further difficulties in the future. He learns to feign a tantrum in order to have his own way and from force of habit tends to use a tantrum as the most effective way of getting what he wants.

## DISCIPLINE

The toddler experiences a conflict between wanting to express his impulses and at the same time keeping the approval of his loving mother. He strives for increased independence, but the expression of it must be guided, for he is a human being who must learn to live and work with others. Children do not live solitary lives; rather, they are members of families and the community.

Discipline has as its goal *self-control*. It is not merely a way of forcing the child's obedience to adult authority. To be most effective, discipline must be carried out through guidance, helping the child to learn how to live comfortably with others. Discipline, if it is to be constructive, must help the child to direct unacceptable, unrealistic and often futile ways of reaching the goal toward which his impulses are directed into socially approved channels that are effective. This socialization process is begun by the parents and should function without demanding too great sacrifice of the child's individuality and creativity.

As the child learns to control himself in his relations with others, he feels more secure and less anxious. To achieve self-control he needs the help of adults in accepting his feelings and handling them in a constructive way. He needs a positive rather than a forbidding, negativistic parent-child relationship.

Discipline is a broad term which includes much of the interaction between the mother or some other adult and the child. A parent uses discipline to establish limits, grant permission, help the child to understand social standards and guide him to direct his impulses into socially acceptable ways of behaving. Much of this is not recognized as discipline by either the parent or the child. It is part of family life or the expression of happy parent-child relations. The way in which a parent approaches the problem of discipline is perhaps the best indication of his feelings toward the child.

**Setting of Limits.** Limits must be set to the child's behavior if he is to feel secure; otherwise he will constantly be suffering the consequences of his mistakes in situations in which he is not old enough to function without guidance. Small children do not know the difference between right and wrong; they must learn the difference from their parents. When limits are imposed, the child will probably be angry momentarily, but he is likely to feel more secure because he knows that his parents can create happier situations for him than he can for himself. This is an extension of the sense of trust in adults the infant learned in the first year of life.

It is essential for a child's happiness in relations with other people that he form habits of behavior limited by social approval. If he does not, he will not have the approval of the adults about him and later will find it difficult to make successful, lasting friendships with other children. He will be an unhappy child whose personality repels rather than attracts others. Parents who establish habits of behavior which win the toddler friends and give him an acceptable self-image reflected from what others think of him are fulfilling an important part of their function in the training of their child.

The way in which a toddler accepts discipline from his parents or other adults depends upon his love relationship with those adults. Parents who won the trust of their child during his infancy established a relationship in which he was passively cooperative. Passive cooperation lays the foundation for his active cooperation.

**Constructive Discipline.** Parents should be reasonable in their requests and tolerate some delay in the child's response. They should not be overanxious about small details of the child's behavior or say "No" too often. They should never expect from the toddler behavior which is beyond his ability.

The child who has learned the pleasure of cooperating with his parents will carry over the same attitude toward other adults and reap the reward of being liked and included in many pleasant situations in which he strengthens his habit of accepting discipline and lays the foundation for self-discipline. Such a child is free to grow, but is given the help he needs with his problems. He is given graded independence, but is not forced to accept more than he can utilize constructively. The adult should do things *with* the child, whenever possible, and not *to* or *for* him, thereby making desirable behavior easy and satisfying to the child.

The child should be shielded from unnecessary fear, but should learn to meet fearful situations courageously. "Courageously" means retaining the ability to use clear thinking, and maintaining full use of all the resources of his body to meet the emergency. This is just what the child loses when he is paralyzed with fear.

If the mother is not consistent in her discipline or if the adults about the child do not make consistent demands upon him, he becomes confused and cannot use his developing power of reasoning to determine what will happen if he responds in this way or that. Even if he is motivated to do what the adult says because he loves the adult, he will often disobey because the other parent, whom he also loves, has asked just the opposite behavior from him.

**Punishment.** Some form of punishment should be given the child who breaks rules which he understands and which are enforced by all adults responsible for his discipline. The child should be allowed to maintain his self-respect when punished, and never be made to feel that his parents do not love him because he has done wrong.

Love should not be used as currency with which to buy good behavior. Love should call forth love, and the central element in love is furtherance of the welfare, the happiness, of the one loved. Such love is not developed in the child under two years.

Some parents make the mistake of blaming themselves if any time they feel antagonistic to or angry with (hostile toward) their child. Nurses may also have similar feelings. They never punish a child, because they believe that punishment is an expression of anger. This is a mistake. Punishment is a useful tool in discipline if it is used with discretion. It often clears the atmosphere for further interaction. The child will not resent it if he feels that he "had it coming to him." He should be punished knowing that the adult still loves him. Punishment should never appear to him as an angry retaliation by the adult. Fear of punishment should be reduced to the minimum which serves to reinforce in the child the habits established during infancy of accepting adult decisions to please the adult. Then the child learns the necessity of obedience as he matures and has decisions to make as to what he will and will not do.

If possible, the child should be shown that punishment is the logical consequence of his wrong decision. When a child burns his hand because he disobeys his mother and touches a hot stove, he sees the result of his disobedience, but he also knows that his mother did not inflict the pain. He remembers not to touch the stove again, for he sees the connection between the pain and his act. The connection is not clear to him when his mother punishes him for disobedience. Only if he has learned to trust his parents' judgment and knows that they do not punish him without good reason does he accept the connection between punishment and what he has done in the same spirit with which he accepted the burnt fin-

ger when he touched the stove.

It is even harder for him to learn what is morally right and wrong. Burning his finger had no moral implications (unless his mother had told him not to go near the stove); it was a matter of poor judgment on his part. By being hurt he learned about the physical environment in a painful way. If he has learned that "mother knows best," he believes her when she says that he might get hurt or sick, lose his penny, break his toy or tear his new shirt. But when she forbids behavior which interferes with the rights of other members of the family or of the people he meets when she takes him out with her, the reason for her decision is not clear to him. Nevertheless a child who loves his parents does accept their decisions about what is morally right and wrong as he accepts their decisions on the physical results of behavior. He learns to accept punishment as just when it follows his wrong actions. He learns to fear his own extreme impulses which are followed by unpleasant results in his relations with other people and learns to try to do right.

If a child feels guilty over something he has done which his mother did not find out and for which he was not punished, he may purposely do something naughty in order to be punished and so reduce his feeling of guilt over the first offense. Some children who are ignored and rejected by their parents may actually seek to be punished so as to gain some response from their parents. Although this is not a loving response, it is better than being ignored.

Parents should not show emotion which they would not wish to have the child imitate. An angry parent increases the anger of an angry child.

Although the child must be guided in unfamiliar situations, his natural curiosity should be neither overstimulated nor repressed. Directed activity must be provided for him so that his curiosity about his physical and social environments may be satisfied.

Before condemning what a child does, his reasoning, motive and experience must be considered. The child should never be made to feel that the adult condemns him. He must be helped to understand that it is what he has done that is condemned and that he is still loved as before. Punishment should relate to the wrong act and follow directly upon the act so that wrong doing and punishment are brought together in the child's mind. Punishment should not be cruel, and corporal punishment should not be used if it can be avoided and never given so as to embarrass the child before other children or adults.

It never helps to nag a child. His accomplishments should be praised and his success in self-control noticed.

### Summary of Emotional Development

The problems of this period center mostly around the child's need to develop a *sense of autonomy*. He needs to learn to hold on and let go, as in toilet training. He needs help with the conflict between carrying out his new-found abilities and his continuing need for security and parental love.

Parents should remember that the child has many years in which to complete the developmental tasks begun in the toddler stage of development. They should not try to force him too rapidly into more mature behavior. If they do, the child, instead of submitting, may rebel and defeat the parents' attempts to use compulsion. He may become negativistic.

Two kinds of parents fail in guiding a child during this period. The first is the overdemanding parent, the second is the parent whose policy is *laissez-faire*. With such parents the child has no help in his striving for maturity.

The adult must define reality for the child. If adults do not set limits to his behavior, he cannot learn to live satisfactorily in his society.

## OVERVIEW OF PHYSICAL GROWTH AND DEVELOPMENT

Physical growth and motor development are slower in the period between one and three years than during infancy. This is a period marked primarily by increasing strength and skill in performance. By the end of the second year the major types of muscular activities have appeared. Skilled performance in new areas is simply a utilization of old skills in new ways. Old skills become more and more perfected. The result is fewer errors and more speed with smoother, graceful movements. After the basic motor skills have been acquired the repertoire of added skills varies widely, depending upon the child's interest in new activities, his environment and his ability to learn.

**Significance of Delayed Motor Development.** Although most children progress through the stages of infantile development at approximately the ages given in Chapter 12, some do not. These are not only late in reaching the stage of independent action characteristic of the toddler period, but also are prevented from interacting with other children and from achieving normal social development. The young child whose motor development is retarded cannot join in play with other children who can run and climb as he cannot. He refrains or is excluded from their play and may develop feelings of inferiority which later are the bases for antisocial behavior.

**Schedule of Growth and Development.** The developmental schedules for toddlers (Table 5) are only representative of averages. They are not typical of any one child. There are individual differences among toddlers just as there were among infants. The ages given are *approximate* for the various activities and learnings listed. These developmental schedules provide only a general outline of the growth of a child between one and three years.

*Table 5.    Developmental Schedules, 15 Months to 2½ Years*

---

### 15 Months

*Motor Control* (See also Figure 158.)

At this age the toddler has reached a plateau of motor development

Walks alone at 13 to 15 months, but with a wide-based gait to steady himself. After he has learned to walk it is to him a form of play

Creeps upstairs

Builds a tower of 2 blocks

Throws objects repeatedly and picks them up again. Throwing is evidence of his new ability to release an object in his grasp

Opens boxes

Pokes finger in holes

Holds a cup with fingers grasped about it. He is apt to tip it too quickly and spill the contents

Grasps a spoon and inserts it into a dish. He cannot fill the spoon well. If he brings the spoon to his mouth, it is likely to be turned upside down, and the contents spilled into his lap

*Vocalization and Socialization*

Uses jargon

Names familiar pictures or objects

Responds to familiar comments

Vocalizes his wants and points to the desired object

Pats pictures in a book and turns pages

Indicates when his diaper is wet

---

### 18 Months

*Physical Development*

Anterior fontanel is usually closed (may be closed as early as 12 months)

Abdomen protrudes

*Motor control* (See Figure 159.)

Walks and runs with a somewhat wide stance, but increasingly more like the adult gait. He seldom falls

Pulls a toy behind him

Can walk sideways and backward (16.7 months)

Climbs stairs or upon furniture

Seats himself on a small chair

Throws ball into a box, puts block in a hole

Scribbles vigorously. Attempts straight lines. Differentiates between straight and circular strokes

May build tower of 3 blocks

Holds cup to lips and drinks well with little spilling. Hands cup to his mother or drops it on the floor

Can fill his spoon, but has difficulty inserting spoon into his mouth. Is apt to turn the spoon in his mouth. Spills frequently

*Vocalization and Socialization*

Knows 10 words

Uses phrases composed of adjectives and nouns

Shifts attention rapidly from one thing to another. Moves quickly from place to place. Explores drawers and closets. Gets into everything

Has a new awareness of strangers

Begins to have temper tantrums if things go wrong

May resist sleep for some time after he has been put to bed. Calls for his mother

May control bowel movements

May smear stool

Thumb-sucking may reach a peak. It usually occurs just before sleep or goes on all night

Enjoys solitary play or watching others' activities

Hugs his teddy bear or doll

Begins to select a favorite toy or object such as a blanket

**Figure 158.** The 15-month-old (A) walks alone, (B) creeps upstairs, (C) builds a tower of 2 blocks, (D) holds a cup with fingers around it, (E) grasps spoon, but spills contents, (F) pats picture in book.

## PLAY

**Purposes.** The main function of play during infancy was physical development and early association. As the child grows older the importance of play increases. (1) Physical development continues through play. Muscles are developed, and exercise is given to all parts of the body. Surplus energy can be worked off during active play. (2) Social development occurs when the toddler participates in group activity with other children. Although at this age social interaction is limited, he enjoys parallel play (playing *beside* another child, but not *with* him). (3) The therapeutic value of play is psychological as well as physical, for it sublimates drives so that they are released in an approved way, and helps the child to release emotional tensions. For instance, an angry child or one irritated by having to stay in the house all day may find relief by pounding boards, tossing bean bags or even in the quiet activity of playing with mud or clay or in finger painting. (4) Play is a means of education. The toddler who plays with toys of all sorts learns to know colors, shapes, sizes, and textures of play materials. He also develops muscular skill in handling his toys. (5) Play develops a beginning understanding of moral values. The toddler begins to learn right from wrong. He begins to learn not to hurt other children by rough play.

Figure 159.    The 18-month-old (A) has a protruding abdomen, (B) climbs upon high toy box, (C) hands cup to mother, (D) moves rapidly from place to place and enjoys pulling toy behind her, (E) begins to have temper tantrums. This toddler shows increasing frustration because she wants to get out of her high chair. A temper tantrum occurred shortly after this picture had been taken.

Table 5.    Developmental Schedules, 15 Months to 2½ Years (Continued)

2 Years

*Physical Development*
Weight: 26–28 pounds
Height: approximately 32–33 inches tall (gain of 3–4 inches in second year)
Pulse: 90–120 per minute
Respirations: 20–35 per minute
Teeth: approximately 16 temporary teeth
Abdomen protrudes less than at 18 months

*Motor Control* (See Figure 160.)
More grown up, steady gait
Can run in more controlled way, has fewer falls and may run away
Can jump crudely. In initial attempts he usually falls, since his body is propelled forward
Walks up and down stairs, both feet on one step at a time, and holding onto a railing or the wall
Builds a tower of 5 or more blocks. Can make cubes into a train
Can open doors by turning door knob
Scribbles in more controlled way than at 18 months. Imitates vertical stroke
Drinks well from a small glass held in one hand
Can put a spoon in his mouth without turning it

*Vocalization and Socialization*
Has a vocabulary of approximately 300 words. Can use pronouns and names familiar objects. Can
    tell about his experiences. No longer uses jargon
Makes short sentences of 3 or 4 words
Shifts attention less rapidly than child of 18 months
Behaves as though other children were physical objects. He may hug them or push them out of the
    way. Would like to make friends, but does not know how
Does not readily ask for help
Obeys simple commands
Helps to undress himself. Can pull on simple garments
Is toilet-trained in daytime. Verbalizes toilet needs
May still smear with stool
Thumb-sucking decreased
Does not know right from wrong
Number of relatively violent temper tantrums is decreasing
Is proud of accomplishment of motor skills
May fear parents' leaving
Shows increasing signs of sense of individuality
Enjoys parallel play—no interaction with other children even though their activity is the same.
    Interaction that does occur may consist in snatching toys from one another, kicking or pulling hair
Manipulates play materials. Dawdles frequently
Enjoys playing with dolls, placing beads in box and dumping them out, pulling blocks piled in wagon
Cannot share possessions. Has great sense of "mine," little of "yours"
Learns to replace toys in their proper place
Enjoys hearing stories illustrated with pictures
Begins play which mimics activities of parents
Takes favorite toy to bed with him, which helps to quiet him. Has many demands before going to bed.

**Figure 160.** The 2-year-old (A) runs in a more controlled way than she did at 18 months and seldom falls, (B) walks up and down stairs, both feet on one step at a time and holding on to the wall or railing. (H. Armstrong Roberts.)

**Table 5.   Developmental Schedules, 15 Months to 2½ Years (Continued)**

30 Months (2½ Years)

*Physical Development*
   Has full set of 20 temporary (deciduous) teeth
*Motor Control*
   Walks on tiptoe
   Rides a Kiddy Kar
   Stands on one foot alone
   Can throw a large ball 4 to 5 feet
   Piles 7 or 8 blocks one on top of the other
   Copies horizontal or vertical line
*Vocalization and Socialization*
   Temper tantrums may continue
   During the whole toddler period the child has begun to develop a self-concept from reflected appraisal
      of significant people—his parents and other adults who care for him. He is beginning to know him-
      self as a separate person, and to have a conscience when he can control some areas of his behavior
      to conform to social demands

The toddler has strong feelings about his toys, clutching at them and saying, "Mine, mine." But he slowly learns the importance of sharing even though it may be difficult for him to do so. He should not be forced to give up his toys until he is older and can understand that play with others involves giving up some pleasures on his part in order to have the greater satisfaction of participation in common projects in which he receives as well as gives pleasure.

**Characteristics of Play.** Each age group enjoys its own type of play. Play during childhood follows a pattern of development based on the maturity of the group. Certain play activities are popular at each age no matter what the socio-economic status, the environment or the ethnic culture is in which the child is brought up. In general, play

with toys is popular until the eighth year. After this children enjoy games which encourage large muscular activity such as running. After this stage, games or sports for which there are strict rules become all-important.

During the toddler period, play is active and is based on the motor and emotional development of the child. Walking in the early toddler period is a delightful game. He has acquired greater skill in the use of his arms. The fifteen-month-old toddler enjoys throwing objects and picking them up again, putting them into receptacles and taking them out again.

At eighteen months the toddler is exceedingly active. Since his attention span is short, he moves freely from place to place and gets into everything. It is difficult to keep him out of bu-

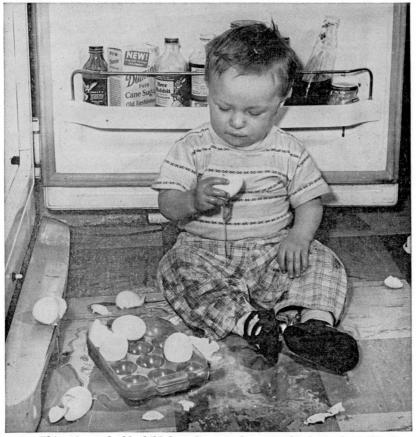

**Figure 161.** This 18-month-old child has discovered a new kind of play. (H. Armstrong Roberts.)

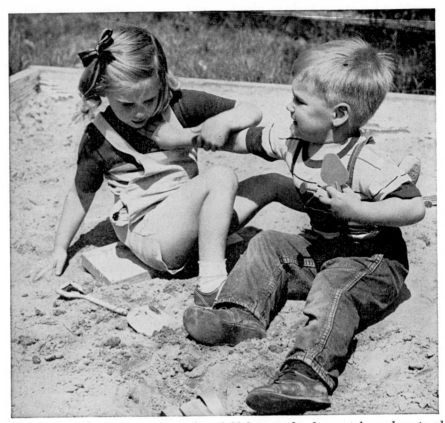

**Figure 162.**  A toddler may attack another child because he does not know how to play cooperatively with her. (H. Armstrong Roberts.)

reau and kitchen table drawers. By this age his balance has improved so that he can pull toys behind him or carry a doll or stuffed animal about with him. He enjoys playing alone or watching other children play, but has not learned to play with them in any game requiring group consensus. He notices the activities of his parents and may imitate them.

The two-year-old has less rapid shifts in attention than the younger child. He may dawdle in his play activities. He enjoys manipulating play materials, pounding, patting and feeling mud, sand or clay in his hands. He plays with dolls, strings large beads and puts his blocks into his wagon.

In parallel play the toddler plays beside another child in such activities as making mud pies. He wants to be friendly with other children, but does not know how. He may attack another child in his attempt. For this reason adult supervision of toddlers' play is necessary.

The two-and-a-half-year-old toddler has developed finer use of his muscles than the two-year-old. He enjoys handling smaller blocks and balls in a sensory way, but he still needs larger blocks and balls for play. He also has enough coordination to ride a Kiddy Kar fairly well.

Play in the early toddler period is mostly free and *spontaneous*. There are no rules and regulations to follow. The child explores as he desires and stops when he pleases. Since he has poor motor coordination, he is apt to be destructive. His toys must be carefully examined to determine whether he might injure himself on broken parts. He does not intentionally break his toys, but his exploration of them—shaking, pushing, rattling—is sometimes more than the toys can stand.

By the end of the second year most children begin to impersonate adults whom they are with and who do what the child considers interesting, e.g. setting the dinner table. If they play with older children, make-believe use of materials leads to make-believe situations such as playing house. Usually when toddlers play house with preschool children, the toddlers are the children in the family.

Even in the early toddler period *constructive* play is seen, such as making mud pies, making holes in sand and playing with clay. Toddlers also enjoy crayons and use them in drawing and scribbling on paper. The product usually has no practical use, but its educational value is great. Toddlers enjoy moving their arms in time to music and singing simple songs, but they are unable to coordinate complex movements of their bodies with the music.

Toddlers, because of their short attention span, require a variety of activities and playthings to keep them busy. They spend most of their waking time in play. Since the average span of attention of a two-year-old child is approximately seven minutes, they may leave an activity to do something else, but return later to their original play.

Play is informal. The toddler plays when and where he wishes. He does not need special clothes, toys or play space.

**Selection of Play Materials.** A few of the toddler's likes and dislikes should be remembered when selecting his toys. He is active and curious. He explores his environment, using his large muscles rather than small ones. He likes to pull and push toys and enjoys pedal-propelled toys, a Kiddy Kar (tip-proof) and low rocking horses. He likes to pour from a pitcher into another pitcher or a cup. He enjoys toys that open and close. Since he is imaginative, he likes to play with dolls and stuffed animals. His constructive and manipulative ac-

tivities include playing with sand box toys, water toys, clay, finger paints, blocks, peg boards (large), pounding sets and thick, large crayons. He enjoys being read to while he looks at the pictures in his book.

**Safety Factors in Selection of Toys.** The toddler needs toys which are safe for him to play with. He should not be given toys that are sharp, have rough edges or small removable parts, nor should he have flammable toys, or beads, marbles and coins that he can put in his mouth to swallow or aspirate. Toys painted with lead paint are dangerous, since he ingests a little of the paint if he sucks them.

## CARE OF THE TODDLER

In caring for the toddler the mother or nurse should adjust adult procedures to the difference in size between the adult and the child. For instance, when

Figure 163. A toddler should not be permitted to play with toys that have small removable parts which could be aspirated or swallowed. (Courtesy of the Metropolitan Life Insurance Company.)

talking to him, the nurse should squat down so that she is on his eye level. If she merely bends over, her image will still be overpowering for the small child. The toddler lacks the adult's resistance to force and loud sounds; he responds best to a light touch and a quiet voice.

Procedures should also be adapted to his level of understanding and endurance of frustration. Although he should be allowed to make decisions on the level of his understanding, he responds best to simple statements of what he should do or to directions indicating what his mother or nurse wants him to do. Too many choices confuse him, since he does not understand the implications of each choice. He may not ask for what will give him the most pleasure.

The toddler who has learned to trust others knows that the limits they set to his behavior are for his safety and happiness.

Adults often forget that during his daily care the toddler is developing his concept of self and that his self-image is formed from the attitude of others toward him and his behavior. Toddlers are susceptible to the facial expression of those about them, reading into it their response to him, to what he does and to his efforts at verbal communication. Because of his ambivalent attitude of love for and aversion to the adults about him, he has difficulty in building his self-image from their behavior toward him. At one time he wants to accept their image of him, at another time repudiate it. It is during the daily routine contacts with him that loving adults help him build his ego and conscience, or super-ego. He internalizes the wishes and demands of others, particularly of those he loves the most. The beginning of a conscience is seen when even to a slight extent he is able to control his behavior in those areas in which he is most mature in order to conform to social norms.

## Bathing

The toddler's bath need not be as detailed a procedure as that of the infant. It is part of his daily program, but the time when it is given makes little difference. He should have a reasonable schedule which fits in with that of his mother and the rest of the family, but it should be fairly regular and consistent in order to establish good habits. Many mothers believe that bathing the child before the evening meal is relaxing and induces a quiet mood for the hour before bedtime. He may be bathed in the adult tub, but care should be taken to clean and dry it thoroughly before the water is run for his bath. His face and hands should be washed before meals.

## Care of the Teeth

Brushing the teeth should be commenced as soon as the temporary or deciduous teeth have erupted. Even the child of three or four should be taught to brush his teeth after eating and especially before bedtime. Doing it himself establishes interest in keeping his teeth clean and helps to establish a routine which is useful as he grows into later childhood and has so many interests that he is likely to forget the care of his teeth. At first he will not be able to use the brush with perfect technique, but he will improve with practice. His mother should supervise his efforts as long as necessary.

## Clothing

Clothing should be light or bright in color, because children like bright colors, and adults delight in seeing them dressed in delicate shades. Light colors show the dirt readily, but they look fresher and cleaner after being laundered than do the darker hues. Bright colors also have value in accident prevention in that the child is easily seen and is therefore less likely to be injured by bicycles on the pavement or by cars if he runs into the street.

Clothing should have large, easily managed buttons and snaps which should be placed where the child can reach them. Girls should wear panties which can be readily slipped down, and boys may have zippered flies which they can manage themselves. All clothing should be easy to put on and remove so that the child can help himself in dressing and undressing.

The average toddler is learning control of urination and defecation and, when two or three years old, may go to the toilet alone. When the mother has decided that the child is old enough to be trained, training panties should be used instead of diapers. A change of panties whenever they are even slightly wet will accustom him to being dry. He feels more grown up and like his siblings when he no longer wears diapers and can be changed while standing. If possible, after he has become accustomed to panties, diapers should not be put on him except at night and at nap time. Children find attractive panties a great incentive to keeping dry.

Outdoor clothing should be warm, but not bulky, since the toddler enjoys active play and is irritated when his movements are restricted. He should have rubber boots for rain and snow and some sort of waterproof coat and hood or cap.

## Shoes

When the toddler begins to walk, his shoes should be selected with reference to the free development of his feet and his posture. Shoes should have firm soles and should conform to the shape of the foot; i.e. they will be straight along the inside and have broad toes and relatively narrow heels. The soles should not have even a low heel and should be rough to prevent the child from slipping; they should be ½ inch longer and ¼ inch wider than the foot. The heels should fit snugly.

A little child outgrows his shoes rapidly. It is well to buy inexpensive ones, for they will last until they are too small and should be replaced with the next larger size. If expensive shoes are bought, the mother is tempted to have them used until they are worn out. In so doing she is likely to force the child's feet into shoes which are too small for him. He is then not only uncomfortable, but also in danger of having the shape of his feet distorted by the pressure of tight shoes.

### Fresh Air, Sunshine and Exercise

Toddlers enjoy activities in which they use their large muscles. They are active, curious and fond of outdoor play. Although the child of eighteen months or two years may be suspicious of strangers, as long as he is with his mother he likes to watch other children play. He enjoys playing beside children whom he knows, but not with them; i.e. he likes parallel play, but is not yet ready for cooperative play. As he approaches his third birthday he has matured to the stage at which he makes motions of friendliness to other toddlers and some attempt to join in cooperative play. He welcomes a sunshiny day when he may play outdoors, making mud pies, digging in the sand pile or, on a hot day, splashing in water. In winter he likes to play in the snow for a while, but cannot manipulate it as he can mud and sand.

Toddlers need freedom to play in a safe area where they can wander without danger of being harmed. An adult should be near, however, for it is impossible to foresee what a child is likely to do. Although he wants to run about freely and does not want anyone to be constantly saying "No, no," he feels more secure when he knows that an adult is with him.

### Sleep

The amount of sleep the toddler needs depends upon his age, health, emotional tension, activity during the day and depth of sleep. From one to three years the amount of sleep needed gradually decreases. The child may resist sleep for some time after being put to bed, crying for his mother or demanding a drink of water or some other form of attention—anything so that he may have company.

At two years the toddler is likely to

have a set ritual which he insists on following when he goes to bed. From one and a half to three or four years he likes to take a favorite toy to bed with him. Since this helps him to relax, he should be allowed to have the toy. As he grows older he will voluntarily give up the habit. Other methods he may use to relieve his tension before going to sleep are head-rolling, singing or talking to himself. He should not be restrained or told to be still, for that only increases his tension and delays his going to sleep. The typical child will outgrow these habits by the time he is three years old or shortly after, but may resume them when he is under a strain and anxious, as he is likely to be in the hospital.

Toddlers spend, on the average, twelve to fourteen hours in sleep out of the twenty-four, including a daytime nap of one to two hours. Naps may become a source of rebellion in the two-year-old. Few mothers escape the nap time battles, and mothers should not place too much importance on a child's refusal to go to sleep when put to bed for his nap. His outer clothing should be removed, he should be given a drink of water and taken to the toilet, and then he should be placed comfortably in bed. The shades should be drawn and the room door closed. He may have one toy in bed with him, but a variety of toys tends to keep him awake, for he handles first one and then another. A cuddly toy is the best kind to take to bed. The mother should be firm in keeping to the daily scheduled time for his nap even if he does not sleep.

Dreams and nightmares or night terrors are not uncommon, beginning in a mild form at two to three years of age.

### Safety Measures

**Importance of Accident Prevention.** Prevention of accidents is an important aspect of the care of children of all ages. Accidents are the principal cause of death among toddlers and account for many permanent handicaps and disfiguring scars. The majority of accidents occur in or near the home. In approximate order of frequency are deaths due to motor vehicles, burns, drowning, miscellaneous causes, falls and poisons.

Although there has been some advance in the prevention of accidents in early childhood, their incidence has not been reduced as rapidly as has that of serious illnesses which formerly were the main causes of death or permanent disability.

The interests of boys and girls of any age lead them into hazardous situations. When we know the hazards, we are better able to protect the children. In our society there are many hazards which cannot be done away with. Children should be taught what is safe and unsafe for them to do and, until they are old enough to use good judgment, should be under adult supervision.

Nurses as well as physicians must help parents to understand this approach to accident prevention. Then the parents will be able to judge more accurately how much freedom each child should be allowed as he gradually takes over more and more responsibility for his own safety. This applies to the kind of toys given him and to his experimentation in climbing, opening and shutting doors—including slamming the door of the family car—and running ahead of his mother or lingering behind her on the street. If he hurts himself, while sympathizing with him she should point out in simple terms he can understand the reason why he hurt himself—give him his first lesson in cause and effect of activities which are dangerous for him and cause him pain. In this way his knowledge of what he can safely do will be increased.

Nurses must assume the responsibility of teaching parents the importance of accident prevention. Not only the parents, however, but also the children must be taught, and the most effective way for them to learn is through carefully safeguarded, graded experiences in self-protection. There should be a reciprocal relation between protection of the child and the education appropriate to the child's stage of maturation.

**Specific Hazards of Toddler Years.** Toddlers naturally fall frequently. In general they sit down suddenly or fall flat without hurting themselves, but if they fall down steps or from some height, they may injure themselves severely. They not only fall, but they also tug at the end of table covers and pull objects over on themselves because they cannot see the top of the table. The modern formica-topped table for the family meals is far safer and more convenient to use than the polished wooden dining table covered with a table cloth. Covers which extend far over the tops of dressers and tables are out of date, and with them has disappeared one source of danger for little children.

To satisfy a child's curiosity about what is on top of a table and what mother is doing there, he may be lifted up or placed beside her in his high chair. The average child of two years is tall enough to see over the table edge if he stands on tiptoes, holding on to the table, but this is an uncomfortable position and does not give a complete view of what is there. Also he is so unsteady that if he reaches for something, he is likely to sit down suddenly. This is frustrating and may produce a temper tantrum or tears.

When exploring objects, children poke and probe with their fingers, which may be hurt in one way or another.

The two-year-old's curiosity leads him into danger. He searches in lower closets and climbs to reach the higher ones. Falls are frequent. His curiosity prompts him to taste anything he finds in a can or bottle and to break off and swallow bits of dried paint or plaster from the walls. In this way toddlers often ingest poisonous substances. They are proud of their new ability to turn door knobs and may open a door, while mother is in another part of the house, and wander away from home. If the weather is cold or if it is raining, they suffer from exposure, for they seldom stop to put on outdoor clothing. They may be injured in traffic or, if they are

**Figure 164.** The toddler's curiosity may lead him into danger. *A,* He may taste or swallow anything he finds in this cabinet containing cleaning products. *B,* The toddler may climb to high places and possibly fall. (H. Armstrong Roberts.)

**Figure 165.** A toddler may climb on a chair to see what is on top of the table and possibly burn himself. (Courtesy of the Metropolitan Life Insurance Company.)

in the vicinity of a body of water—even artificial pools in well kept gardens—may be drowned.

The child from two and a half to three likes to climb, to run and to jump. He is, in fact, no longer a toddler except in name. He is much quicker in his movements than he was six months before. He is very much interested in cars and is likely to be injured while playing about motor vehicles. Three-year-olds enjoy running simple errands, but should not be asked to do anything potentially dangerous such as crossing the street alone or carrying glass containers which might break in their hands if they fell, cutting some part of their bodies. The greater use of unbreakable substances for kitchen equipment and play toys has decreased this sort of accident.

Toddlers should be taught the reason for safety measures such as keeping the floor clear of toys so that no one will stumble over them.

**Specific Safety Measures: Shared Parent-Nurse Learning.** Safety measures should be designed to prevent accidents which

are likely to occur in the daily life of the child. The nurse should help the mother with her individual problems of accident prevention. Both the mother and the nurse will find it helpful to keep in mind the common sources of accidents among toddlers and the preventive measures which can be taken for their safety.

*Motor Vehicle Accidents.* Little children are taught to cross the street holding an adult's hand. Their attention is directed to the custom of crossing at the corner rather than in the middle of the block. If there are traffic lights, they are taught that green means "Go" and red means "Stop." They are too immature to gauge the speed of an oncoming automobile with reference to the time it takes them to cross the street, but they will slowly learn while crossing with adults who do not hurry them across while a light is changing

Children should be supervised when playing outdoors on a Kiddy Kar, tricycle or sled to prevent their darting into the street between parked cars or coasting down a driveway into street traffic. Parents should be careful when backing a car into or out of the garage for it is difficult to see a small child who is directly behind the car.

The incidence of children injured while riding with their parents is increasing as more family cars are on the road. Children share the adult's danger from collision or overturning of the car. Modern door catches prevent falls from an open door of a moving car. When a child stands upon the seat beside the driver, a sudden stop in city traffic or on the road is likely to throw him forward.

*Burns.* Matches should be kept away from young children, even though few of them in this age group can strike a safety match. Little children should be watched closely in the kitchen so that they do not touch or fall against a hot stove or investigate the top with its fascinating open flames and pots and pans. Pans with handles extending from side to side or toward the back of the stove are less likely to attract the toddler's attention and are harder for him to reach than are pans with handles extending at a right angle to the front of the stove. Hot radiators are a source of minor burns, particularly if the child falls against one. Modern recessed radiators protected by a built-in screen eliminate this danger. Toddlers are interested in electrical outlets and are likely to poke a pin or other bit of metal into them. Safety plugs may be used to prevent this activity.

*Drowning.* Children like to play in water, but if they fall, they may be unable to get out of even a shallow pool; if they fall into a swimming pool, they are completely helpless. There is also danger of their drowning in the home. Children should not be left alone in the bathroom after the water for the bath has been drawn. The bath tub is slippery, and in climbing over the side the child may fall into the water. Should he hit his head or fall into very hot water, he might collapse and drown before his mother returns to bathe him. The old-fashioned wash tub is seldom used except in rural areas. Serious accidents have occurred when such a tub was filled with hot water and the child's

Figure 167. Children like to look out the window, but their curiosity may result in their falling if the window is not closed or properly screened. (Courtesy of the Metropolitan Life Insurance Company.)

mother went for a pail of cold water. The child investigated the tub in her absence. If he fell in, he was burned even if he was rescued before drowning. Pails of hot water used for mopping floors are also a danger to small children.

*Falls.* Children like to climb, and climbing is a normal activity useful in their development. Until their muscular coordination and judgment have developed to the stage at which they can climb with safety, special equipment should be provided (e.g. small wooden crates), and all climbing should be under adult supervision.

Children like to look out of windows, but they are so short that they often climb on a chair to see what is going on outside. While standing on a chair and leaning forward or balancing on a sill they are likely to lose their balance and fall head foremost. Hence all windows should have screens.

Falls on stairs are dangerous. In in-

Figure 166. The toddler may be injured when attempting to climb into a bath tub alone. (H. Armstrong Roberts.)

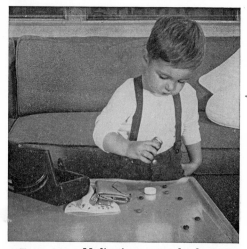

**Figure 168.** Medications must be kept out of the child's reach. (Courtesy of the Metropolitan Life Insurance Company.)

stitutions for children gates should be placed at the top and bottom of stairways. This would be ideal in the home, but is seldom practical. The modern ranch type of house or one-floor home has obviated the hazard of falls on stairs. If the house has a basement, the door leading to the stairs should be locked. A child who fell down the basement stairs and was too stunned to cry might lie at the bottom for some time before being discovered.

Falls from open porches were formerly a common source of injury to small children. In modern buildings, however, especially in urban housing developments, porches are likely to be screened and so present no danger for the little child.

The side gate of a toddler's crib should be kept up at all times and fastened securely so that it will not go down if the child leans against the top of the gate.

*Poisoning.* The incidence of poisoning in children is greatest between the ages of one and four years. Children are curious about the taste of substances and often ingest poisonous liquids, powders and even solids which they find in the house. The main source of danger to the little child is the house-

hold supply of washing powders, and substances for cleaning sinks, toilets, and the like.

Medicines which are beneficial in small amounts are often poisonous when taken in quantities. If a medicine has little or no taste or if the unpleasant flavor has been camouflaged with some sweet syrup or sugar coating, the child may finish the bottle. All harmful substances should be kept out of the toddler's reach, and common household poisons and medicines should be kept in locked storage places or on high shelves inaccessible to children. Harmful substances should never be kept in containers intended for food.

Mothers should be taught what to do if a child does take any of these harmful substances. She should telephone the physician or clinic at once or, if she lives close to a hospital, take the child to the receiving ward. If she cannot get medical attention for the child and she lives in a city having a Poison Information Center, she should telephone there for advice. If she knows what substance the child took and the approximate amount, she should give this information clearly and concisely. If the child has taken the contents of a bottle or can whose ingredients are listed, she should give this information. The Center will tell her the emergency treatment and may furnish emergency transportation for the child to the hospital. In most cities the police car is always available. The container from which the poison was taken should be given to the physician who treats the child. If the child vomits spontaneously or after being given an emergency emetic, the vomitus should be examined chemically. This is particularly important if the mother does not know what the child has taken or the ingredients of some commercial product which she knows the child has swallowed.

In some cities the public health nurse is responsible for visiting the home after the child's return from the hospital. She helps the parents to correct the situation in the home which led to the accident and gives them a better understanding of the child's level of growth and development so that further accidents may be prevented.

### Health Supervision

Visits to the physician or the Child Health Conference, at intervals suggested by the physician, are important during the toddler period. During the second year these visits may be scheduled every two to four months and thereafter twice a year for continued health supervision. During these years defects may be determined in an early stage. If they yield readily to treatment, they may be prevented from developing into serious handicaps. The physician also records growth progress and gives advice about safety measures, nutrition, the establishment of desirable habits and the prevention or correction of objectionable habits in the child. He will give booster doses at twelve to eighteen months to continue the immunization program against diphtheria, pertussis, tetanus and other diseases, particularly poliomyelitis, as needed.

The toddler period is one in which the physician can establish and develop a rapport with the child that will be valuable when the child is sick, particularly if he must be hospitalized.

Dental care and supervision of daily mouth hygiene are important after the child has his full set of temporary teeth, i.e. by about two to two and a half years. Visits to the dentist should be made about every four to six months. The modern dentist, like the physician, builds up a rapport with the child which is valuable later on when painful dental work must be done. Cleaning the child's teeth and work on superficial cavities in the temporary teeth are seldom painful. The dentist should have a kindly approach to children, explain procedures to them and allow them to handle his instruments.

## NUTRITION

Nutrition is an important factor in the maintenance of the toddler's health and normal growth and development. Diets for young children should include food which supplies the essential nutrients in the amounts necessary for maintenance, replacement and increase of tissue and for energy.

Food should be offered in three well spaced meals. The child will then be hungry and ready to eat the well balanced, varied yet simple diet offered him.

**Influence of Growth and Development on Eating Behavior.** During his second year of life the child needs less food than during infancy, because he is no longer growing at so rapid a rate. He also has greater interest in the social and physical environment. Many children at this age have anorexia. The mother should remember that the child needs less food per unit of body weight and that this is the primary reason for his anorexia (*physiologic anorexia*). He may have developed food preferences through imitation of his parents or siblings. He may even refuse food for a short time. Food should not be forced upon him. Unless he has some organic disease, he will develop serious feeding problems only because adults have tried to impose upon him their ideas of what and how much he must eat. If food is forced upon him when he refuses his meals, he is likely to rebel and a real feeding problem will develop.

Children should be allowed a reasonable freedom of choice in both the amount and the kind of food they wish to eat. Strong likes and dislikes should be respected. The child who dislikes essential food substances should be gradually taught to eat them, or they may be included in the diet in some disguised form, e.g. putting mashed carrots in mashed potatoes. The child may take additional milk if it is used in custards.

At times the toddler may be demanding not only in what he wants to eat, but also in the dishes he uses and the way his food is served. His behavior may be bizarre. He enjoys feeding himself even though he may be slow and clumsy. The mother should be flexible and humor him when the matter is not

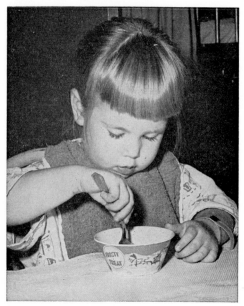

Figure 169.  A two-year-old child can put a spoon in her mouth without spilling its contents. She can feed herself most foods fairly well, provided she has had earlier experience in doing this.

too essential, since this makes him feel important and reinforces good mother-child relations.

Many children are negativistic at this age, especially in the matter of eating. A toddler may test his parents to see how far they will let him have his way. Although eating is basically his responsibility, limits to his behavior must be set within which he is allowed to explore, feeling secure in his parents' decision of what he may and may not do. He feels uncomfortable and often fearful if he is allowed to attempt anything his fancy suggests. A child may refuse his food only to be hungry soon after the meal is over. He may feel sick after eating too much or too rapidly. What an affectionate mother asks her child to do is likely to be what makes him feel good physically and emotionally.

The amount of his activity influences a child's appetite. A reasonable amount of running about increases his appetite, but if his curious searching of the environment is too long continued, he

becomes overfatigued. A rest period before meals serves to lessen fatigue and his resistance to adult suggestion. Furthermore, mealtime may appear to him as an interruption of his play, and so, even though he is hungry, he may resist being called to the table. His mother must work out a schedule which is best for him by experimenting with a schedule of meals, snacks, naps and indoor and outdoor play.

The toddler has such a short attention span that he appears to be even more restless than his biologic need for activity demands. He may wander away from the table before he has finished eating. Forcing him to remain in his place may precipitate a temper tantrum. Often his newly discovered interests may be used to bring him back to the table. If he has gone to get his teddy bear, his mother may say, "Here, let's make a place for Teddy at the table."

The toddler is ritualistic in his eating habits; he may have strong preferences for certain utensils and dishes. He may insist on eating foods in certain sequences. Adults should not impose their own eating habits upon the child, whose ritualistic behavior is a normal part of development at this age. His ritual will tend to coincide with family habits if he is made to feel that he is one of the group and not a baby set apart from the group. His meals should be served at regular intervals and with a fixed routine, but whether he eats with the family or is served alone depends on what is convenient for his mother. There are many reasons, however, why a toddler in his third year should eat with his siblings; he is much less likely to acquire eating whims and fancies if they have none than if he eats alone.

Handedness becomes evident during this period. The child should be permitted to use either hand in feeding himself. The spoon should be placed in front of him so that he can pick it up with the favored hand.

It is well to give a variety of foods so that the child learns to like various tastes. It may be difficult during the toddler period to add new foods because the child is likely to have become discriminating in his tastes and detects and appraises new consistencies and flavors in the foods offered him.

**Development of Eating Skills.** Children differ in their ability and willingness to feed themselves, but the following represents the typical advances in skill.

12–15 months—Drinks from a cup which he himself holds
15–18 months—Holds his own spoon. The mother should spread newspaper on the floor, and he should wear a coverall bib. Help should not be forced upon him, but should be offered if he needs it. The dishes should be unbreakable
24 months—Feeds himself fairly well, provided he has had the requisite early experience in helping his mother feed him. The mother should not make the mistake of feeding him in order that he may not spill his food

**Dietary Allowances.** Table 6 gives the recommended daily dietary allowances for children between one and three years of age.

**Table 6. Recommended Daily Dietary Allowances for Children between 1 and 3 Years of Age**

| | |
|---|---|
| Calories | 1300 |
| Protein | 40 gm. |
| Calcium | 1 gm. |
| Iron | 7 mg. |
| Vitamin A | 2000 I.U. |
| Thiamine | 0.7 mg. |
| Riboflavin | 1 mg. |
| Niacin equivalents | 8 mg. |
| Ascorbic acid | 35 mg. |
| Vitamin D | 400 I.U. |

From the Food and Nutrition Board, National Research Council: Recommended Daily Dietary Allowances (1958).

**Specific Suggestions for Feeding.** By the time the child is eighteen months or two years old he should be eating table food and three meals a day. Nurses and mothers should remember the following helpful points.

1. Serve food in small portions. The child likes plain food and eats one food at a time.
2. Chop or cut the food into small pieces.
3. The diet for each day should include the following (the particular diet may depend upon the cultural preferences of the family):
   a. Meat or fish, one serving; one egg daily, or cheese
   b. Liver, one or more servings a week
   c. Green and yellow vegetables, two or more servings a day
   d. Citrus fruit, raw or cooked fruit, two or more servings a day (one could be in citrus or tomato juice)
   e. Cereal and bread, enough to meet his caloric needs
   f. Butter or margarine
   g. Milk—maximum of 1 quart, part of which may be used in cooking or on cereals.
4. Satisfy the child's appetite with nutritious foods and avoid offering him candy, cake, ice cream, and the like. Nutritious snacks may be given between meals.
5. Give vitamins as suggested by the physician.
6. Since the child is growing less rapidly, he may eat less at this age than he did at the end of the first year. Do not force him to eat.

**Food to Avoid.** Parents should realize that the small child does not miss what he has never had and does not need. Foods to be avoided include chocolate, sugar, large amounts of fat (this is difficult to digest), nuts and seeds (there is danger of inadequate chewing and also of aspiration into the lungs), foods which are highly seasoned and stimulants such as tea and coffee.

**Importance of Good Eating Habits.** During the toddler and preschool years eating habits and attitudes toward foods are developed which tend to persist through life. Meals should be served at regular intervals and in a physical and social situation in which the child feels secure. He should have three or four simple meals a day. Some children with small appetites may need a midmorning, midafternoon or evening snack. Snacks should not be given at a time or in an amount which will interfere with normal appetite at mealtime.

Toward the end of the toddler period most children eat with the family. If his siblings and parents have good or poor eating habits, a toddler will imitate them. Parents who have not already experienced this difficulty with the older children must be told of this problem. They should be advised how to handle problems which may arise and be reminded that the basic factor in

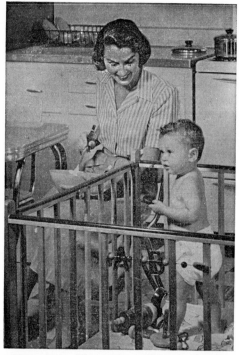

**Figure 170.** The young toddler is protected from harm while mother cooks. (Courtesy of the Metropolitan Life Insurance Company.)

forming good eating habits is that eating time be made a happy time. Toddlers are too young to learn good table manners. Eating is an enjoyable experience; it is the culmination of the mother's planning and work, in which the toddler may have had a small but to him important part. Mealtime is a family gathering to share this important and pleasurable activity.

## SEPARATION

**Meaning of Separation to the Toddler.** During the toddler period, although his security depends upon both his parents, the child is much closer to his mother than to any other adult or to his siblings. He knows his mother as a very special person. His need for her love is as great as his need for food. His attachment to her is possessive and selfish. She can, he believes, protect him from

all harm. His parents, especially his mother, make the toddler's world secure and stable.

By the end of his first year the child realizes that it is his mother who gives him love, protects him from harm and provides pleasurable experiences for him. He believes that he cannot survive without her. Because of this feeling he is fearful when his mother is out of his sight. The infantile game of peek-a-boo is one way by which the child can master his fear of separation from his mother. Since he can bring her back easily, he finds that he can master his separation anxiety more easily. He discovers later, in the game of hide-and-seek, that his mother will search to find him. In these ways he gradually learns that he can bring his mother back to him through his own activity.

We know from his behavior that a child needs his mother, almost an ever-present companion, until about his third birthday. During the toddler period he gains increasing mastery over his fear of separation, and he learns to share his love-object, his mother, with others.

**Reasons for Separation.** The young child cannot understand why he should ever be separated from his mother. As he matures, however, he becomes increasingly aware that there are others (siblings) whom his mother also loves. He may become resentful of them, and yet his mother expects them to love him and him to love them. At this stage the toddler must be helped to accept his siblings, but he must be shown that he is loved even if he shows hostile feelings toward them. He must have all his needs fulfilled, because this means love, even though he cannot understand the words which adults say to him while caring for him. Since his mother expects the toddler, who is secure in her love for him, to be like his siblings, he learns one of the first lessons in socialization: to like to be with other people. In this way he gradually matures socially as well as physically. He wins his mother's approval and strengthens her love for him.

As he matures, his mother may work away from home, may continue her studies in a college or university, and may not be with him constantly. She may become ill or go to a hospital for delivery of another child. The toddler himself may become sick or be injured and be placed in the children's unit of a hospital. His specific response to hospitalization will be discussed in the next chapter.

## TEACHING AIDS AND OTHER INFORMATION*

*American Dental Association*
Tommy's First Visit to the Dentist, 1954.
Your Child's Teeth.

*Bureau of Publications, Teachers College, Columbia University*
Baruch, D. W.: Understanding Young Children.

*Child Study Association of America*
Auerbach, A. B.: The Why and How of Discipline, 1957.
Wolf, K. M.: The Controversial Problem of Discipline, 1953.

*John Hancock Mutual Life Insurance Company*
Between One and Five.
Safe at Home . . . and in the Community, 1955.

*Public Affairs Pamphlets*
Baruch, D. W.: How to Discipline Your Children.
Dietrich, H. F., and Gruenberg, S. M.: Keeping Your Child Safe.
Idem: Your Child's Safety.
Hymes, J. L.: Enjoy Your Child—Ages 1, 2 and 3.
Yahraes, H.: Your teeth—How To Save Them.

*Ross Laboratories*
The First and Second Years of Life.
Your Children and Discipline.

*Science Research Associates*
Krug, O., and Beck, H. L.: A Guide to Better Discipline.
Ridenour, N.: Building Self-Confidence in Children.

*U.S. Department of Health, Education, and Welfare*
Accidents and Children, 1959.
A Healthy Personality for Your Child, 1952.
Foods Your Children Need, 1958.
Into Childhood, Help Your Baby to Grow Up, 1949.
* Complete addresses are given in the Appendix.

Nutrition and Healthy Growth, 1955.
Your Child from One to Six, 1956.
Your Children's Feet and Footwear, 1957.

## REFERENCES

American Public Health Association: Health Supervision of Young Children. New York, American Public Health Association, 1955.

Breckenridge, M. E., and Murphy, M. N.: Rand, Sweeney and Vincent's Growth and Development of the Young Child. 6th ed. Philadelphia, W. B. Saunders Company, 1958.

Cooper, L. F., Barber, E. M., Mitchell, H. S., and Rynbergen, H. J.: Nutrition in Health and Disease. 13th ed. Philadelphia, J. B. Lippincott Company, 1958.

Erikson, E. H.: Childhood and Society. New York, W. W. Norton and Co., 1950.

Foster, C. J., and English, O. S.: What Kind of Discipline? Parents' Magazine, 33:48, Jan., 1958.

Fraiberg, S. H.: The Magic Years. New York, Charles Scribner's Sons, 1959.

Gesell, A., and others: The First Five Years of Life. New York, Harper and Brothers, 1940.

Gilbert, B. M.: Mothers in Hospital. Nursing Outlook, 7:690, 1959.

Hurlock, E. B.: Child Development. 3rd ed. New York, McGraw-Hill Book Company, Inc., 1956.

Josselyn, I. M.: The Happy Child. New York, Random House, 1955.

Krause, M. V.: Food, Nutrition and Diet Therapy. 2nd ed. Philadelphia, W. B. Saunders Company, 1957.

Mackintosh, J. M.: Accidents Are Not Accidental. World Health Organization, World Health, 13:17, May-June, 1960.

Nelson, W. E. (editor): Textbook of Pediatrics. 7th ed. Philadelphia, W. B. Saunders Company, 1959.

Recommended Dietary Allowances. Revised 1958. Washington, D.C., National Academy of Sciences, National Research Council.

Spock, B.: Baby and Child Care. 3rd ed. New York, Duell, Sloan and Pearce, Inc., 1957.

Spock, B., and Lowenberg, M. E.: Feeding Your Baby and Child. New York, Duell, Sloan and Pearce, Inc., 1955.

Stuart, H. C., and Prugh, D. G. (editors): The Healthy Child. Cambridge, Harvard University Press, 1960.

Watson, E. H., and Lowery, G. H.: Growth and Development of Children. 3rd ed. Chicago, Year Book Publishers, Inc., 1958.

Witmer, H. L., and Kotinsky, R.: Personality in the Making: The Fact-Finding Report of the Midcentury White House Conference on Children and Youth. New York, Harper and Brothers, 1952.

# Chapter 16

# Conditions of Toddlers Requiring

# Immediate or Short-Term Care

## HOSPITALIZATION OF THE TODDLER

To THE young child hospitalization appears as something dreadful that his parents have inflicted upon him. His emotional insecurity is often harder for him to bear than his physical pain and general discomfort. This may be his first separation from his home.

**Personality of the Sick Toddler.** The personality of the child remains basically unchanged when he becomes sick, but he is more irritable, and his basic traits are exaggerated, while the acquired habits are submerged. He may regress to infant behavior, and is liable to be apprehensive and insecure. He is too young to understand the necessity for treatments and accepts them only if he has a sense of trust in adults and has experienced love and kindness at their hands. He will build up good relations with his nurses as he learns to know them. The importance of his experience during admission and the

first hours after his mother has left him with the nurses is obvious.

### Specific Responses of the Toddler

When a child is admitted to the hospital and is separated from his mother, he experiences a feeling of intense loneliness and suffers from the lack of security in his new environment. Love provided by parents and siblings is necessary to his development of a sense of trust. But trust in others may easily be changed to distrust by unpleasant experiences with strangers. Trust is strengthened or impaired during the toddler period.

On being hospitalized the toddler experiences basic fears: loss of love, fear of the unknown and fear of punishment. He is too young to be reasoned with; he knows only that his mother, for whom he is calling, does not respond. His distress, whether vocally expressed or repressed, is potentially

430

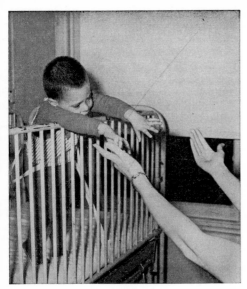

Figure 171. The toddler is extremely disturbed when mother begins to leave him. He is restrained with a jacket restraint which will prevent his trying to climb over the sidegate to follow her. The tapes of the restraint are tied to the springs of the bed.

harmful to his developing personality and may be dangerous to his physical condition. On separation from his mother he suffers from acute anxiety. He may manifest behavior difficulties, sleep poorly, regress in toilet habits and exhibit excessive anger and grief. Such reactions have the highest incidence when the child is two or three years of age.

## Adjustment to Hospitalization

The child shows his initial distress by screaming, crying, calling for his mother, shaking the crib and throwing himself about. This is a normal reaction. The nurse, however, may not realize that the fundamental difficulty is not hospitalization itself, but separation from the mother. Instead of ignoring his cries, the nurse should try to give the child all the reassurance and affection which are possible in the midst of her other duties.

After a few hours, days or weeks the child apparently becomes accustomed to hospital life. He becomes quieter and

less demanding. Nurses at this time may think that he has adjusted to the hospital situation. Upon discharge, however, it may become evident that his apparent contentment was a mere façade, since he may display signs of regression and emotional disturbances which are indicative of the emotional strain under which he suffered during his absence from home.

The stages in the child's apparent adjustment to the hospital are generally as follows:

1. The child is grief-stricken. He calls for his mother almost constantly. He may reject the nurse when she gives him attention.

2. The child sinks into apparent depression. He is quieter, withdrawn and apathetic. He mourns deeply for his mother. At this point he may be greatly upset when his mother visits him, because a short visit does not satisfy his need for her.

3. If the child stays in the hospital long enough, he will eventually reach the stage in which he is no longer depressed. He takes greater interest in his surroundings and seems to be happy. At this stage he can no longer tolerate the poignancy of his distress

Figure 172. The toddler is depressed between mother's visits and makes no attempts to play with a toy offered to him.

and represses all feeling for his mother. When she visits him, he barely notices her and does not cry when she leaves.

There are, after all, many pleasures in hospital life. He begins to know the nurses and the other children. He likes his bed, the toys, the radio and the television, and the refreshments between meals. He scarcely notices his mother unless she brings an attractive toy, and then it is the toy, not her presence, to which he responds. On discharge he may not want to go home and clings to the nurse to whom he is accustomed. At home it may be some time before the mother-child tie becomes re-established, as strong as it was before his hospitalization.

If the child's stay in the hospital is prolonged, he will eventually settle down to hospital life and apparently require neither his mother nor mothering from the nurses. Yet such a child may be severely emotionally disturbed. He may have developed a "hospital" personality with no deep attachment for anyone. He is likely to become a pet of the entire staff. Yet no one has the time or sufficient interest in him to form the loving relation which is needed to stimulate him to learn self-control in order to please his love-object. Nurses find it easier to give him superficial attention or some little gift and pass him on to the next person. If he is naughty, correction is left to someone else. He becomes accustomed to hospital routine, but is not guided in the development of habits of self-control and obedience through tutelage and discipline. He is not motivated by love for anyone to do what he does not want to do at the moment.

### Problems in Care of the Toddler

**Rotation of Personnel.** Many different nurses offer the child daily care, with the result that no single one loves and cherishes him. Eventually he becomes accustomed to nurses being with him for a short time only and accepts the constant change of nurses. He gradually loses the ability to form deep relations with others. He interests himself in material satisfactions and in superficial relations with any adult who notices him. On his return home he may provoke great stress and family friction. He may suffer from varying degrees of the emotional disturbance induced by hospitalization.

**Visiting by the Mother.** The toddler, when separated from his mother, has great difficulty in mastering his fear of the loss of her presence. He cannot understand why the separation is necessary, nor can he understand that it is a hospital rule that his mother is not permitted to visit him at all times. Consequently he feels that his mother does not want to be with him. He does not realize that his mother has to obey rules, for he has previously known her as the decision-maker in the home. Since he feels that his mother has deserted him, he becomes angry and frightened or, if he is very sick, accepts the situation with what in an adult might be called resignation. Such a reaction within him has no reasoned basis as it does with the adult and may represent a bewildered, hopeless loneliness. These feelings, whether of anger, fright, resignation or hopeless loneliness, are psychologically devastating and, through the psychosomatic interaction, physiologically harmful.

When his mother does visit the child, he will express strong emotion. This is good, because then his feelings will not be suppressed, to be expressed later. If his mother understands the reasons for his strong reaction, she will not feel that it would be better if she did not come to visit him. His emotional reaction to her presence may occur on first seeing her, during the visit or when she is ready to leave. If, in spite of his anger, he clings to her and cries, she may be so distressed that she may dread visiting again. Yet at the same time she will be gratified by his evident dependency upon her.

The nurse must not only be able to understand and interpret to the mother the meaning of the child's behavior, but must also anticipate that he will have the same feelings toward her when he has become attached to her as a substitute for his mother. In fact, the toddler may show more clinging behavior and anxiety toward his new love-object, the nurse, than he did toward his mother at home, because he has already had one experience of separation from the adult he loves most dearly and fears to be hurt again in the same way.

**Toilet Training.** The child who is separated from his mother will be hindered in the process of achieving control of both his bodily and his socially acquired drives. He thus is likely to lose what ability he has acquired for the control of urination and defecation. He may regress to the infantile lack of sphincter control and wet and soil himself. After his return home he will again feel pride in pleasing his mother by keeping himself clean and dry.

The nurse should know and record on the admission sheet the child's stage of development before his admission to the hospital. She should learn from the mother what methods of training (the equipment, words used and the frequency with which he was placed on the toilet seat or potty) were used at home so that as far as is possible the same methods can be continued in the hospital. The nurse must not be too rigid and demanding of success, since the child is under an emotional strain due to his feeling of abandonment by his mother. The nurse should sympathetically accept the child's inability to cooperate. He needs to learn about the bedpan and the urinal in his mother's presence. Her approval will motivate him to use the new equipment.

If a young toddler has not yet started toilet training, the nurse should not feel it necessary to initiate training immediately. If he has a prolonged convalescence, training may be begun when he feels stronger. In order for it to succeed, the mother who visits the child frequently and one nurse for whom the child feels affection should carry out the training process. He should get the pleasure he needs from regulating the excretory process; normally this is through his mother's praise.

The nurse herself may have feelings of repugnancy toward soiling by urine and feces on the diaper and the child's clothing (possibly also a soiled bed). She should understand her own feelings and gain control over them. She also needs to understand the toddler's instinctual pleasure and his feelings about his own excretory products.

The nurse should be prepared to forgive accidents, which are bound to happen. Young children who have achieved control of urination and defecation tend to be upset when an accident occurs. The child needs acceptance. The nurse should reassure him by telling him that his mother will help him to develop his former control when he is well again. If he knows that the nurse understands and is willing to help, he will more readily cooperate as far as he is able.

Some children use soiling themselves as a means of gaining attention or getting even with the parents who left them in the hospital or as a retaliative measure against the nurses who manifest a lack of understanding of children's needs. They may refuse to ask for a bedpan or urinal and then have an accident before or even after it is brought to them. If the nurse makes the child an object of censure because of an accident, he may repeat the performance to gain her attention or annoy her.

The nurse must endeavor to find the reason for his soiling and should plan ways to help him to cooperate. The child who resorts to such techniques is in a state of emotional turmoil. The nurse, on whom he depends for guidance, must meet his needs and also help him to work out his problem in a more satisfactory way. She must accept his behavior and yet help him to gain love and attention in a more appropriate fashion.

### Hospitalization of the Toddler with His Mother

It is a truism that the most effective way to prevent trauma to a child from hospitalization is to provide the care at home when he is ill so that there will be no need for removal to the hospital. But if it is essential that he receive hospital care, every effort should be made to have his mother remain with him. This is not always possible, however, and then ways must be devised to reduce the problem of maternal deprivation.

The child and his mother should be taken to his crib. The nurse should exhibit an unhurried, friendly, sympathetic attitude. The mother should be provided with a chair and helped to relax. Although the nurse should show an affectionate interest in the child, she should not assume the role of a mother-substitute, but rather that of "mother's kind friend."

The admission procedure discussed in Chapter 4 should be carefully explained to the mother. The nurse should accept the verbalization of the mother's anxiety and provide emotional support. She should then explain how the mother can help the child in the hospital milieu.

Since the child gains much of his own attitudes from his mother, she should be as calm as possible and in every way provide emotional support for him. By her courteous attitude toward the nurse she can increase the child's faith in his nurse. The mother can explain to the child the hospital procedures and the use of equipment which is new to him. If he is not to use the potty, but rather the bedpan and the urinal, she can explain this in familiar terms he understands. She can undress him and put on his hospital garments.

The nurse should ask the mother about her methods of dealing with the child at home so that the hospital personnel may follow them as closely as possible. If the child's condition permits, the nurse should introduce the mother and her child to other parents and children. She should further orient the mother to the physical facilities of the hospital unit so that the mother can participate conveniently in the child's care. The mother should explain to the child that she will remain with him so that he need not fear abandonment when he sees other children who have been left alone.

A collapsible bed or one of the newer chair-beds can be placed in the unit for the mother. She can then be with her child day and night and provide not only the comfort of being with his mother, but also physical care under the supervision of the nurse.

Hospital personnel do not always realize the advantages of having the mother stay with the child. They fear that she will be difficult to work with and that they will have to spend much time in bolstering her morale—time which should be reserved for caring for the patient. They are mistaken. The more her maternal feelings are satisfied, the less anxious she will be, and much of her emotion can be expended in doing something for her child and seeing to his comforts as no one else can. Then, too, if she is permitted to feed and bathe him, she will feel it less necessary to bring expensive gifts and complain when they are broken. She will also help her child to stay on a diet if one is necessary instead of feeding him candy to compensate for lack of mothering. If his physical condition permits, the mother may continue his toilet training regimen during the hospital stay.

The nurse in a unit where mothers give care to their children must be able to determine how much each mother can safely be trusted to do for her child and how much guidance she will require. Mothers are generally able to give routine care, but the nurse should instruct them in new skills or in any adaptation of methods which the child's condition makes necessary. A mother should never be urged to attempt procedures she does not feel equal to, for she, like the child, is under a heavy strain which may make her less capable than she is at home. Most mothers will help their children through these difficult experiences if they feel that they themselves have the support of the physicians and nurses. There are times, however, when it would be unwise to permit the mother to be with the child, for if she is unable to control herself, the effect upon the child would be disastrous. Whether she stays or not depends upon the individual situation and upon the reaction of the mother, the physician and the nurse.

When the mother stays with the sick toddler, her place at home will have to be filled by the father or the older children in the family. Friends and relatives may have to help keep the home functioning smoothly. This will require ample planning. At all events, the child should be protected from maternal deprivation and also from its effects upon his emotional development in years to come.

### Hospitalization of the Toddler without the Mother

Children in private accommodations and in some ward units may have their mothers stay with them during hospitalization. Most sick children, however, are not so fortunate. The reasons for this are that (1) the physical setup of most pediatric units is not adequate for a visiting parent; (2) some emotionally disturbed children seem to be more upset when mother is present than when they are left alone, and (3) some mothers are too anxious and bewildered and are unable to provide care for their sick children.

**Unrestricted Visiting.** An increasing number of hospitals are permitting unrestricted visiting. Although this arrangement is not as comforting to the child as having his mother with him continually, it is far better than restricted visiting. If unrestricted visiting is permitted, the child is able to vent his feelings of distress and anger frequently instead of suppressing them until he has returned home. Parents, in spite of the tears of their children, are often less anxious than they would be if they could see their children only at restricted intervals.

Hospital personnel often feel that unrestricted visiting hours produce confusion on the unit because of the number of parents present. This does not usually happen if parents are shown how to care for their children and if the unit routine is changed to include their services. In general, unrestricted visiting hours have improved the relations between parents and hospital personnel.

If the mother cannot visit her child frequently, the nurse must exhibit a sympathetic understanding of his feelings of loneliness and anxiety. She must tell him that she knows that he wants his mother and wants to go home with her. She should not try to make him forget his mother. Instead she should help him to understand that the close tie with his mother is not broken, even though she is not with him. The nurse, of course, will make life in the hospital as pleasant as possible for him. When he becomes accustomed to his new environment, he will be happy there if he is sure that his mother and father and siblings are waiting for him.

Measures to help the child feel secure in the intervals between visiting hours include permission to have a favorite toy or blanket with him, allowing him to keep a handkerchief, glove or other object belonging to his mother, and providing cards for him to send to his mother and having her send him cards, which the nurse can read to him. If it is practical, he may speak with his mother over the telephone.

At the close of visiting hours the mother must be firm and truthful in telling the child that she must leave and when she will return. She should never sneak out of the unit because she is afraid he will cry if she tells him the truth. The nurse should stay with the child after visiting hours until his initial grief at her departure has passed.

**The Nurse as a Mother-Substitute.** If the mother cannot stay with the child constantly or visit him frequently, he should be assigned to a small group of children whom one nurse regularly attends. The nurse functions as a substitute mother for the children. She should be relieved during her time off by a nurse who is also familiar with the children.

Those who care for toddlers who must stay in the hospital for a long time should be permanent members of the staff—graduate nurses, practical nurses, aides or foster mothers. Students should not be assigned to the care of these children, since students must be rotated in order to acquire a varied learning experience. Nurses who are given a long-term assignment to a small group of children or who function on a nursing team caring for a somewhat larger group are able to give the kind of care that toddlers need during a prolonged stay. Such individual care prevents much of the emotional trauma seen in hospitalized children who are cared for by a constantly changing series of attendants.

### Preparation for Hospitalization

Preparation for hospitalization is minimal, because children of this age cannot grasp the idea that their mothers will really leave them. Emphasis should be placed on how the mother and her child can be kept together.

## ACUTE CONDITIONS IN THE TODDLER

### Retropharyngeal Abscess

**Etiology and Incidence.** A retropharyngeal abscess is a suppurative lesion involving one or several of the retropharyngeal lymph nodes. It is generally secondary to a nasopharyngeal infection caused by bacteria or due to a penetrating foreign body, e.g. a sliver of a chicken bone or a small fish bone. It is most common in the first three years of life and is rare in children over three years of age because of the normal atrophy of these nodes (the nodes are present in the normal newborn). The incidence even in the toddler period has decreased in recent years, owing to better medical supervision of children and more effective therapy.

**Clinical Manifestations, Diagnosis and Differential Diagnosis.** Abscess formation is rapid after an acute respiratory infection. The abscess makes it difficult and painful for the child to swallow, and therefore drooling of saliva is prominent. To relieve the pain and facilitate swallowing he tends to keep his mouth open. The muscles of his neck are stiff, and he cries when his head is moved. If the lesion is in the upper portion of the pharynx, a bulging of the posterior pharyngeal wall may be visible. Respirations are noisy and are accompanied with a gurgling sound. If the swelling is excessive, obstruction to breathing may occur with stridor and possibly dyspnea. The child's temperature is variable, but tends to be high. Prostration is often severe.

The *diagnosis* is made by inspection if the abscess is in the upper part of the pharynx. Palpation generally discloses a soft midline mass, although the swelling may be greater on one side than on the other. When the mass is sufficiently low in the throat, it may be seen in a lateral roentgenogram. Decision as to when drainage should be established depends on detection of fluctuation within the mass by digital examination. The physician may use a laryngoscope through which he can inspect the abscess.

*Differential diagnosis* must consider peritonsillar abscess (quinsy) and tuberculosis of the cervical vertebrae (cold abscess).

**Treatment.** If antibiotic therapy is started immediately upon the early symptoms, regression of the infection often occurs without abscess formation. When the abscess is ready for incision, this is done by puncture; the opening is then spread apart with a hemostat. To remove the drainage, frequent aspiration of the pharynx is performed. If hemorrhage occurs, owing to erosion of one of the branches of the carotid artery, ligation of the vessel may be necessary despite the danger of cerebral sequelae.

A general anesthesia is not given, for these reasons: (1) it would abolish the cough reflex, and the child might aspirate the purulent discharge; (2) it would prevent the use of the accessory muscles of respiration; and (3) the child might not be able to breathe after relaxation induced by the anesthetic and before relief of the respiratory obstruction by drainage and decompression of the abscess.

**Nursing Care.** Nursing care includes assisting the physician in his examination of the throat and incising the abscess, and in postoperative care of the child. When the physician examines the child's throat, the child should be restrained with a mummy restraint (see p. 149). The nurse holds the child's head still with one hand on each side of his head. The child must be securely restrained so that the examination may be done gently and quickly without damage to the wall of the pharynx and with a minimum of pain and fright to the child.

During incision of the abscess the child is restrained as for examination of the throat. The nurse holds the child's head lower than his body to prevent aspiration of purulent material into the larynx.

When the child is put back to bed after the incision has been made, a position suitable for drainage from the mouth must be maintained. The foot of the bed is elevated, and the child is placed on his abdomen. A pillow may be placed under his chest and abdomen so that the discharge from the abscess will drain through the mouth rather than down the throat.

The child should be encouraged to take fluids as soon as he can swallow. He must be closely observed for symptoms of respiratory distress and hemorrhage. Frequent swallowing may be an indication of bleeding and should be reported so that an examination can be done.

**Prognosis.** The prognosis is good if the abscess is incised as soon as the mass is fluctuant and if proper antibacterial therapy is instituted in the early stage of abscess formation. An untreated abscess may rupture spontaneously, externally through the side of the neck or internally into the esophagus, mediastinum or the auditory canal.

Death from retropharyngeal abscess may occur in untreated cases or in cases in which the child is not brought to a physician until death from anoxia is imminent. Death may occur suddenly because of edema of the glottis, pressure upon the larynx, rupture of the abscess into the larynx or erosion of blood vessels in the area with severe hemorrhage. Less immediate and less frequent causes of death are pneumonia and pulmonary abscess caused by infection carried to the lungs from the draining abscess.

## ACUTE INFECTIONS OF THE LARYNX

Acute infection of the larynx is more frequent in toddlers than among older children and is more serious because their narrow airway is more readily obstructed.

Usually other parts of the respiratory tract besides the larynx are involved. Laryngeal obstruction produces clinical manifestations which are the same even though produced by various types of organisms. The clinical manifestations are aphonia, hoarseness, inspiratory dyspnea, stridor and retraction of various respiratory muscle groups (intercostal, substernal, subcostal, suprasternal) on inspiration.

A specific diagnosis can be made by laryngoscopic and bacteriologic examinations.

### Croup (Acute Spasmodic Laryngitis)

**Etiology and Incidence.** Croup is a mild catarrhal inflammation of the larynx. The predominating clinical manifestation is a reactive spasm of the muscles of the larynx which produces a partial respiratory obstruction.

Spasmodic croup is relatively common between the ages of two and four years, but may occur in any child under five. There appears to be a familial and individual predisposition to the condition. The child who is hyperactive and nervous seems to be affected more often than the quiet one. Susceptible children are likely to have more than one attack, and the attacks invariably occur at night. A susceptible child is more likely to have an attack of croup if he has had an upper respiratory tract infection than when he is in good health.

Cold air may precipitate an attack at any time in susceptible children, particularly if an upper respiratory tract infection is present. Even moving the child from a warm room where he has spent the day to the cooler bedroom for the night may induce an attack of croup.

Croup has a low order of communicability, and mothers should be told this. If they have other children close to the same age, they are likely to fear that these siblings will acquire the condition. Although children seldom, if ever, die of uncomplicated croup, because the child appears to be strangling, croup frightens parents as do few other conditions of like severity.

**Clinical Manifestations and Diagnosis.**
*Clinical manifestations* may appear in a child who has shown no symptoms of an upper respiratory tract infection or other illness. The onset is dramatic, all the more so since it often occurs during sleep.

In a typical attack early in the night the child wakens with dyspnea and coughing. The cough is tight, the sound barking and metallic. Respirations are noisy. The cough wakes the parents, who find the child sitting up in bed, extremely frightened and struggling for breath. He may grasp at his throat because of his feeling of suffocation. With each inspiration a high-pitched rasp, or a sharp stridor, occurs. The child's face is red, and his lips and nails may be cyanotic. The alae nasi may flare with each inspiration. There may be substernal, suprasternal and supraclavicular retractions. The voice is harsh, the pulse rapid, and the child perspires freely. His temperature is seldom over 101° F. After one to three hours the severity of the spasm diminishes, and all clinical manifestations abate. Sometimes more than one attack will occur in a night, or attacks may occur on subsequent nights. The morning after an attack the child may have a loose cough. In a mild attack he may have a croupy cough, but only moderate laryngospasm and dyspnea.

The *diagnosis* is made on the basis of the history, the type of respiratory difficulty and lack of other clinical manifestations. The physician must differentiate croup from diphtheritic laryngitis, the laryngospasm of tetany (see p. 348) and acute streptococcal laryngitis.

**Treatment.**    Treatment is directed toward reduction of the spasm of the laryngeal muscles. The child should be placed in an atmosphere of high humidity, for this tends to liquefy the secretions in the throat and also reduces the spasm. The physician may order an emetic such as syrup of ipecac to induce vomiting. Vomiting tends to reduce the laryngeal spasm. The dose of the emetic may be repeated once or twice if necessary. A sedative such as phenobarbital may be given after the child has vomited. Chemotherapy may be ordered if the infection is severe, but as a rule this is not necessary. Only in rare cases is intubation or tracheotomy needed.

**Nursing Care.**    The nurse carries out the treatment outlined by the physician. In the hospital, as in the home, the provision of moist air is a primary consideration. The equipment to be used should be shown to the child, and the procedure, if he is old enough to understand, should be explained to him. The water vapor serves to liquefy secretions, and the warmth, if ordered, tends to reduce the spasm of the muscles and to relieve the inflammation of the mucous membrane of the throat. A drug such as benzoin may be added to the water, but actually it is steam vapor that is therapeutic. The child is put in a croup tent to concentrate the warm moist air about him.

*The Croup Tent.*    The tent is made in the following way.

Over the upper half or two thirds of the child's crib (top and sides) are draped a blanket, a mackintosh and a sheet (the blanket forms the inside layer and absorbs moisture). The mackintosh is placed between the blanket and the sheet. The sheet and the blanket should be pinned neatly and firmly in place. An electric vaporizer is used to provide steam and should be large enough for an adequate and continuous flow for several hours. The spout of the vaporizer should be pointed forward inside the top of the tent. To prevent burning the child, a piece of wood or protective wire should be placed or tied to the crib rails between the spout and the child. A thermometer should be fastened to the roof of the tent on the crib rail so that the temperature within the tent can be ascertained. Unless the nurse or the mother can stay with the child, a restraining jacket may have to be applied to keep him in the tent. If the child fights the restraining jacket and thereby causes himself further respiratory embarrassment, the jacket should be removed. During acute respiratory distress the mother or nurse should stay with him to comfort him and support him in a sitting position if he finds that position most comfortable.

Since the tent is not closed, most children are not frightened by it, but a toddler who is afraid may be told that it is his own little house or tent.

HOME MODIFICATION OF THE HOSPITAL PROCEDURE. The quickest and easiest way to provide warm moist air for the child with an attack of croup is to run hot water in the bath tub or shower, take the child into the bathroom and close the door. This arrangement cannot be continued for long, however, for the steam might damage the paper or plaster on the walls and the supply of hot water might give out. It does give emergency relief, however, while a croup tent is being prepared.

The child's crib may be covered as is done in the hospital. A plastic table cover may be substituted for the mackintosh. If the mother does not have a vaporizer, a kettle of hot water may be used. A gas or electric plate can be used to heat the water. Every precaution must be taken to prevent burning the child.

If the child does not sleep in a crib, a sheet or blanket may be draped over a baby carriage, or a card table or an adult-size straight-back chair—tilted—may be placed on an adult's bed, and the child laid under the table or chair. An umbrella may be used instead of the chair, but it does not give a firm support for the tent.

POINTS IN THE USE OF THE CROUP TENT. (1) The child must be protected from burning any part of his body by a protective device (a piece of wood or wire netting) placed in front of the outlet nozzle. The nurse must check frequently to make sure that it has not slipped out of position.

2. If it is necessary to remove the child from the tent for some time, as when he is given a bedpan or urinal in the hospital or the potty in the home or his bath or morning care, a warm blanket should be thrown around him so that he is not chilled by exposure to air at room temperature.

3. When his condition improves and he is

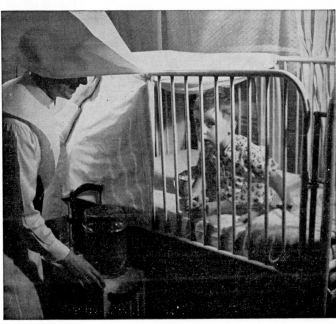

**Figure 173.** Warm moist air can be provided for the child when a vaporizer and a croup tent are used. (William M. Rittase.)

removed from the tent, chilling should be prevented by wrapping him in a blanket.

4. The child must be kept dry. Steam condenses on the clothing and bed covers. These should be changed when damp.

5. The covers forming the tent must be securely fastened in place so that they do not fall upon the child. Such an accident would frighten him and would impede his respiration until they were removed. They should be pinned on the outside of the tent so that he cannot reach the pins.

6. Leaving the lower half or third of the crib uncovered is important, for it permits free circulation of air and also enables the nurse or mother to watch the child without constantly sitting beside him.

7. The temperature within the tent should be checked frequently and kept below 90° F. If the temperature goes up much above this, the child's body temperature will also be elevated.

8. The child should be kept as contented as possible. He should have his favorite toy with him. An adult should be with him as much as is practical.

The physician may order that the child in the hospital be given cool moist air, rather than steam, to liquefy the secretions in the larynx. This cannot be given in the home, for it requires special equipment such as a Croupette. With the Croupette cool mist can be provided, using the pressure of oxygen or, if the child does not need oxygen, compressed air. (For setting up the Croupette, see p. 304.) One reason why cool moist air is ordered rather than hot steam is that cool air may lower the child's body temperature, while the warmth of the steam-heated croup tent may raise it. Some hospitals use devices which mechanically vaporize water and fill the cubicle or room with mist. In such units the toddler need have no fear of being enclosed in a tent, and the nurse can work in the humidified environment around him rather than outside his closed-in "house."

*Other Points in Nursing Care.* Since syrup of ipecac causes vomiting, the nurse or mother should stay near the child until after he has vomited. He is already anxious because of his respiratory distress, and vomiting increases his anxiety. Soiling his clothing and bed with vomitus may frighten him even if he knows that he will not be blamed for the accident. After he has vomited, a sedative, usually phenobarbital, ordered by the physician may be given.

When the child is resting quietly, the nurse should help the mother relieve her anxiety by expressing it in words and extend sympathetic emotional support. The nurse can explain to the mother the child's condition, why treatments and medications are given and the progress of his illness. The mother will then be less frightened if a second attack occurs on the following night.

The nurse is responsible for the administration of any chemotherapeutic agents the physician may order.

In order that the physician may have information essential to the diagnosis and treatment of the condition, the nurse must observe and record all signs and symptoms, not only those which are objective, but also those which are subjective, so far as the child is able to communicate. So far as possible the nurse should teach the mother the importance and meaning of these observations.

The most important symptoms to be observed during an attack are the color of the child, the rate and nature of the respirations, the degree of restlessness, the level of anxiety, the presence of cyanosis and the degree of prostration.

If at any time the child's respiratory embarrassment increases, intubation or tracheotomy may be necessary. The nurse must promptly report to the physician this change in the child's condition.

**Prognosis and Prevention.** The *prognosis* is invariably good, although both parents and child are thoroughly frightened.

There are no specific *preventive measures*, but conditions which increase the probability of an attack of spasmodic croup should be avoided in the care of children known to be susceptible. If there is evidence of an impending attack, such as coughing or hoarseness, particularly on the night after an attack, general preventive measures which may be taken include keeping the bedroom warm (temperature approximately 70° F.), humidifying the air of the room and giving the child subemetic doses of syrup of ipecac, and phenobarbital for sedation.

## Laryngotracheobronchitis

**Incidence and Etiology.** Laryngotracheobronchitis is an acute inflammation of the larynx, trachea and bronchi. The *incidence* is greatest during the first three or four years of life.

Several viral and bacterial agents may cause the infection. The bacteria usually responsible include *Hemophilus influenzae,* hemolytic streptococci, pneumococci and staphylococci.

**Pathology, Clinical Manifestations and Diagnosis.** The *pathology* is manifested in the inflammation and edema of the mucosa and submucosa of the larynx, trachea and bronchi. Such infections may produce little or no exudate. Rarely a purulent exudate which produces crusts is present. If these accumulate, they may obstruct the air passages.

*Clinical manifestations* include a preceding acute respiratory infection for one or more days before laryngotracheobronchitis ensued. Often, however, the onset is sudden and accompanied by prostration, elevation of temperature and severe dyspnea. During the onset respiratory difficulty is usually in the inspiratory phase, since the larynx is involved. Later there may also be expiratory difficulty because of involvement of the bronchi and bronchioles.

The child may become restless, owing to lack of oxygen. Hoarseness or aphonia may be present. The chest shows both substernal and suprasternal retractions. His color may be ashen gray or cyanotic. His temperature may be as high as 104 to 105° F., and febrile convulsions may occur as the result of the fever. His cough is likely to be persistent. If there is an exudate, the cough is loose, croupy and noisy, but if the exudate is too thick to move, the child may not cough at all. When obstruction due to exudate is nearly complete, breath sounds may be barely audible, and dyspnea may be severe.

The *diagnosis* is confirmed and the causative organism is found by laboratory examination of a culture of exudate. Sensitivity tests are performed to determine which antibiotic agent is most effective. The material for laboratory examination should include a direct smear and culture to rule out diphtheria. Blood cultures should also be obtained. Fluoroscopic and bronchoscopic examinations may be done to rule out the possibility of an aspirated foreign body.

**Treatment.** The basis of treatment of laryngotracheobronchitis is the provision of (*a*) sufficient oxygen. This should be given whenever the accessory muscles of respiration are used for breathing. (*b*) Sufficient humidity to liquefy secretions and so to prevent crusts from forming. Either hot steam or cool vapor may be used for this purpose. Cool vapor is preferred, however, because it does not tend to raise the child's body temperature. (*c*) Drugs to control the infection. Antibiotics are always given; if the infection is of bacterial origin, they are effective, but if it is caused by a virus, no striking response will be observed. Cultures of the nasopharyngeal secretions are made to determine the causative organism. Broad-spectrum antibiotics are generally started before the results of these laboratory examinations are available. These antibiotics include oxytetracycline (Terramycin), chloramphenicol (Chloromycetin), tetracycline (Achromycin) and penicillin.

During the foregoing treatment a patent airway must be maintained. When there is severe obstruction, relief must be provided by an emergency tracheotomy. *Tracheotomy* consists in an incision into the trachea. It is made in order to open up a passage for air to enter the trachea proximal to the site of laryngeal obstruction. The incision also aids in the draining of secretions. Indications for a tracheotomy with insertion of a tracheostomy tube are restricted expansion of the lungs (this shows that only a minimal amount of air can enter the lungs), signs of cardiac failure and prostration with severe pallor or cyanosis. The incision is made just below the first tracheal ring (see Fig. 175).

mm.   4   5   5.5   6   7   8   9

size   00   0   1   2   3   4   5

| New-born | No. 00-0 | 3 to 6 years | No 3 |
| Up to 1 year | No. 1 | 6 to 12 years | No. 4 |
| 1 to 3 years | No 2 | 12 to 20 years | No. 5 |

**Figure 174.** Tracheotomy set. *A,* Outer cannula. *B,* Inner cannula. *C,* Obturator. Diagram below shows sizes of tubes (with the diameters in millimeters) usually used for children of various ages.

Drugs such as atropine and opiates are contraindicated because atropine tends to dry up secretions in the respiratory tract, and opiates dull the cough reflex. Digitalization is necessary if clinical signs of cardiac failure appear.

Parenteral fluids may be required to maintain the necessary state of hydration.

**Nursing Care.**   After performance of a tracheotomy maintenance of this artificial airway is of fundamental importance. It is also the outlet for pulmonary drainage. Accidents arise in maintenance of this airway which endanger the child's life. Most of them can be prevented by intelligent nursing care and observation of the child's condition. The nurse must be prepared to care for emergencies as they arise. Sometimes she will be able to handle the situation herself, and it will not be necessary to call the physician. If he is needed and she puts in a call for him, she will have to give emergency care until he arrives.

Since the situation is frightening, the nurse must use all possible means to reduce the anxiety of the situation. Confidence in her own ability to give the child optimum nursing care is essential to inspiring confidence in him and his parents.

After a tracheotomy the nurse must provide constant care and observe indications of respiratory difficulty and the child's general reaction to treatment. She must observe such danger signals as restlessness, extreme fatigue, dyspnea, cyanosis or pallor, fever, rapid pulse, retractions and noisy respirations. She must also watch for bleeding or indications of infection around the incision.

Control of the environment is im-

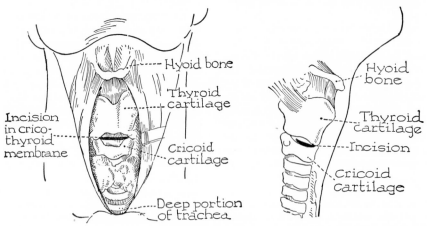

**Figure 175.**   Diagram showing landmarks and horizontal incision for emergency tracheotomy. (M. G. Lynch, in Ochsner and DeBakey: Christopher's Minor Surgery. 8th ed.)

portant in preventing emergency situations from arising. Since inspired air is normally filtered, warmed and moistened in the upper respiratory tract, the environment of the child must be such that the air he breathes is to some extent moistened and not too cool before it enters the tracheotomy tube. The room should be warm, the temperature of the air he breathes about 80°

F. (this temperature will also keep the child warm and prevent his being chilled). To moisten the air, a humidifier or croup tent is used. Oxygen may also be necessary. If continuous oxygen is not necessary, an emergency setup should be kept in readiness.

An aspirating machine with good negative pressure must be kept at the bedside.

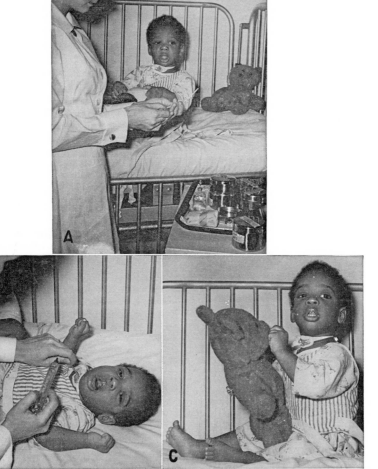

**Figure 176.**  Tracheotomy care. *A,* The nurse cleans the inner cannula with a pipe cleaner. Containers are labeled on their tops and sides to prevent accidental interchange of lids. Note the favorite toy of this little boy in the corner of his crib. *B,* Aspiration is done after sterile saline solution from the syringe has been instilled into the tracheotomy tube. *C,* The toddler with his tracheotomy tube in place. After his own aspiration he enjoys aspirating his teddy bear.

A tray should also be kept at the bedside on which is sterile equipment for the routine care of the tracheostomy and for emergency use.

Such equipment includes duplicate tracheotomy tubes with tapes attached, two curved clamps, scissors, obturator, pipe cleaners or tonsil wire, gauze bandage, gauze dressings, a medicine dropper or syringe and needle, applicators, tongue depressors, an extra catheter (no. 8 to 10 French which has additional holes near the tip to facilitate the process of aspiration of the nasopharynx) and an open-tip catheter, preferably of the whistle tip type (this is used in tracheal aspiration, i.e. clearing the tracheal tube of secretions). In addition, there should also be on the tray a covered jar of hydrogen peroxide or other solution to cleanse the tracheotomy tube, a covered jar of physiologic saline solution and a covered jar of sterile petrolatum or petrolatum gauze. The jars should be labeled on both the sides and the lids so that the nurse cannot confuse their contents.

The hydrogen peroxide or some other solution is used to soak the inner cannula, which is removed during aspiration of the outer, larger tube. Hydrogen peroxide may also be used to cleanse the area around the incision. Sterile physiologic saline solution is used to liquefy secretions in the lower respiratory tract (a few drops are inserted into the tube) and so facilitate aspiration of mucus. The sterile petrolatum may be used to lubricate the end of the tracheostomy tube when the physician changes it, and also to coat the area around the tube. The petrolatum may be applied with a tongue depressor.

*Care of the Tracheostomy Tube and Incision.* The nurse should wash her hands thoroughly before touching the tracheostomy tube and equipment. She *removes the inner cannula* and cleans it by soaking it in hydrogen peroxide or another solution and then passing the pipe cleaners or tonsil wire and gauze through the tube. She aspirates the outer cannula and tracheobronchial tree. If the obstruction persists or if the physician has ordered it with each aspiration, a few drops of sterile saline solution may be instilled into the cannula before aspiration. To do this she uses the medicine dropper or syringe.

The aspirating catheter should be pinched so that the lumen is closed while it is inserted into the opening of the outer tube. It should be slowly and gently inserted. After withdrawal for rinsing with sterile physiologic saline solution the catheter should be rotated 180 degrees between the fingers so that its normal curve will carry it down to another bronchus when aspiration is repeated. The catheter should be reinserted and aspiration continued until all drainage has been removed. The inner cannula, throughly cleansed, is reinserted and locked in place after the aspiration procedure has been completed.

If the nurse is unable to aspirate the tracheobronchial tree successfully, and if respiratory difficulty or noises on respiration persist, the physician should be notified so that the lower airway can be investigated.

The frequency of aspiration depends upon the need of the individual child. Immediately after tracheotomy aspiration is usually performed every fifteen minutes, later every thirty minutes or every hour. The need for aspiration gradually decreases with improvement in the child's condition.

If the nurse is to change the dressing around the tracheostomy tube, as is ordered in some hospitals, she cleanses the area around the tube with hydrogen peroxide and then coats the area with sterile petrolatum, using a tongue depressor. A gauze square cut to the center should be slid behind the tube and under the tapes to hold it in position.

The prevention of accidents is an important part of the nursing care of these children. The toddler is too young to understand the importance of leaving the tube in place, and so his hands must be restrained. For this purpose elbow restraints may be used. The older child who is restless and has nothing to occupy his mind may attempt to put bits of food or debris into the tube. The nurse should explain the importance of the tube to such a child. She must be certain that the inner cannula is securely fastened in place so that it will not fall out, and that the tapes are applied to the tube properly and securely tied so that the tube is held firmly in the correct position and the child cannot dislodge it.

If by accident the outer cannula is removed from the trachea, the physician should insert the extra tracheostomy tube. The incision in the trachea must be held open with a hemostat by the nurse while another nurse summons the physician.

If the child stops breathing, it may be because of some obstruction of the airway. The inner tube should be withdrawn and the outer tube thoroughly aspirated. The child should be given oxygen through the tracheal tube. If the outer tube has become dislodged, oxygen should be given through the incision. Artificial respiration may be given; the method, if the tracheostomy tube is or is not in place, is that ordinarily given children (see p. 185), with the fundamental difference that the nurse places her mouth to the opening in the neck rather than over the child's mouth. Other methods of artificial respiration may also be used. When the physician arrives, he will attempt to relieve the obstruction by bronchoscopic examination, if need be.

When the child no longer needs the tracheostomy tube, the lumen is partially obstructed by a cork. This compels the child to breathe through his nose, but still permits entrance of supplementary air through the tube. When he can tolerate complete occlusion of the tube, a cork filling the entire opening is placed in position. If this does not cause him distress, the tube can be removed, and a sterile dressing can be placed over the incision. In *decannulation* there is danger of puddling of secretions in the lungs with a subsequent rise in temperature and with restlessness. The child should be under close observation for several days.

There are few conditions in which the nurse's record of observations and the care given the child are more important than in the nursing of a child with a tracheostomy. Whenever the tube is aspirated, the time should be charted, as well as the amount, consistency and nature of the return (whether it contains blood, mucus or crusts), and whether the child breathed more easily after the aspiration. The time when the tracheostomy tube is changed should be charted, together with the child's reaction to the procedure.

Psychologic care is extremely important. The child needs his nurse because he is in physical danger without her, but he also needs her for emotional stability. The nurse must be in constant attendance to give him physical and emotional support. He has a physical basis for his fear of being alone, and his respiration is further embarrassed when he becomes anxious and excited. In his condition he cannot cry or call for his nurse, and he is in danger of respiratory obstruction at any time. He must learn to get used to breathing through the tube, which is at first difficult. He needs the love and reassurance of both his mother and his nurse. He is afraid, and the nurse increases his fear when she aspirates the tube, so that he feels insecure and unhappy when she is near him. When he becomes accustomed to aspiration of the tube and finds that it makes him more comfortable, he will learn to depend upon his nurse for relief as he does upon his mother for love. He may even play at aspirating his favorite toy (see Fig. 176, C). The importance of the tube can be explained to an older child, but the toddler is too young to comprehend its function until he learns from experience that he feels better after it has been cleared.

Until the toddler becomes accustomed to the tracheostomy tube, he is afraid to try to swallow. By placing small quantities of fluid or food in his mouth he will learn that swallowing will cause him little or no pain.

Excitement should be avoided, but the child should be amused with toys and stories, particularly if his hands are restrained and he is unable to play with toys.

*Other Points in Care of the Child.* The vital signs should be taken as ordered by the physician. If the child cannot change his position, the nurse should move him frequently to prevent puddling of secretions. Older children seem to find a semi-Fowler's position most comfortable; it may be tried with the older toddler to see whether he also finds it comfortable. It may be necessary to give mouth care if the child is not taking an adequate amount of fluid to keep his mouth moist. He should be helped to get as much rest as possible and never be disturbed for unnecessary examinations. His care should be scheduled so that his rest is not broken. It is desirable to give enough fluids—preferably warm fluids —orally to prevent dehydration. If he will not take the required amount, parenteral fluids should be given. His oral intake may be increased by offering small amounts of any fluid which he likes at frequent intervals.

Drugs and antibiotics will be given as ordered by the physician.

The physician may discharge the child from the hospital before the tracheostomy tube has been removed. In that case the mother must be taught the care of the child before he leaves the hospital. He will probably be referred to a public health nurse if he is not under the care of a private physician, and his mother will be instructed to take him for periodic return visits to the outpatient department of the hospital. Not all mothers are sufficiently intelligent and resourceful to undertake the responsibility of such a child's care, but if his mother can be taught to care for him, he is better off at home than in the hospital after he has learned to live with the tube in place and to cooperate in the care it necessitates. The mother should be taught not only the procedures she must carry out, but also what observations she should make of his condition, and what she should report to the physician. She should also be told where she can obtain the required equipment and oxygen for emergency use.

If the mother was with the child during his stay in the hospital, the nurses will have had an opportunity to teach her what she should know in order to be successful in the child's care. If she has not remained with the child or visited him daily, it will be difficult for her to learn. The nurses will have to spend some hours in demonstration and explanation before it will be safe to discharge the child in her custody.

The mother must take great care when bathing the child or when he is near a wading pool with other children that he is not momentarily submerged in the water, for liquid will be drawn through the tracheostomy tube directly into his lungs, and he will drown.

**Prognosis.** The prognosis depends upon the age of the child, the severity of the infection, the length of illness before treatment was instituted and the kind of treatment the child receives. Death may occur from the primary infection, from a secondary pneumonia or from respiratory obstruction. Septicemia may cause death, but is an uncommon cause.

Occasionally chronic bronchitis and bronchiectasis may follow laryngotracheobronchitis.

### PNEUMONIA

Pneumonias may be classified in several ways on the following bases: anatomic distribution, causative organism, pathologic changes in tissue and response to antimicrobial therapy. None of these methods of classification is completely satisfactory.

In any type of pneumonia the portions of the lung which are affected are not aerated because the alveoli or air spaces are filled with inflammatory exudate. Because of this fact and also because the child breathes in a shallow manner, often owing to pain on breathing, the blood is not oxygenated as it should be. The oxygen saturation of the blood is invariably reduced when the child has pneumonia.

Since there are many varieties of pneumonia and since some kinds occur principally in one or more age groups, only selected types of pneumonia are discussed in this text. Pneumonia of the newborn and aspiration pneumonia were discussed in Chapter 10. Interstitial pneumonitis or bronchiolitis and lipoid pneumonia were discussed in Chapter 13. Pneumonias caused by pneumococci and staphylococci are discussed here, since the nursing care of any other type is essentially the same in the toddler period.

## Pneumococcal Pneumonia

**Etiology, Incidence and Predisposing Factors.** Pneumococcal pneumonia is a disease involving lung tissue and causing more or less consolidation of the affected areas. It is caused by the pneumococcus organism, of which there are about seventy-five types. Certain types are more prevalent among different age groups. Serums were formerly used against many of these types of pneumococci, but are no longer necessary, owing to the effectiveness of antibiotic therapy.

In the past the pneumococcus was the chief cause of pneumonia in infants and young children. More recently the incidence of this type of pneumonia has decreased because of the response of most pneumococcal infections to antibiotic or sulfonamide medications, which are usually given early in the infection before a fully developed pneumonia exists. Pneumococcal pneumonia is generally a primary infection. Lobar pneumonia, in which one or more lobes of the lung may be affected, is more common after the period of infancy. The disseminated type, such as bronchiolitis (see p. 302), is seen more often in infancy.

The peak *incidence* of pneumonia is in the late winter and early spring months. In the temperate zone pneumonia is endemic in the general population. Although pneumonia may occur in more than one member of a family, this is seldom the case. Family members may, however, harbor the pneumococci without showing clinical symptoms of pneumonia; they are carriers of infection. As a result of constant exposure to the infection, most persons have antibodies in their blood against many types of pneumococci.

*Predisposing factors* are age (the highest incidence of the disease is during the second year of life, the toddler period), and lowered resistance due to malnutrition or severe chilling of the body.

**Pathology and Clinical Manifestations.** Pneumococci reach the lungs by way of the respiratory passages. The first stage in the attack is termed *engorgement*. During the period of only a few hours the lung becomes dark, bluish-red and heavy. In the next stage, that of *red hepatization,* the infected lobe becomes solid with red cells and fibrin, and air is displaced. In the third stage, *gray hepatization,* the pleural surface lacks luster and is dull in color. The alveoli are filled with leukocytes and fibrin. In contrast to the two previous stages, the third stage is prolonged. In the final stage, that of *resolution,* a creamy purulent material forms and is evacuated via sputum or resorption. At autopsy this material can be expressed from the cut surface of the lung.

The typical *clinical manifestations* differ with the age of the child and are more variable in children than in adults. The onset is abrupt, although it may be preceded by a mild upper respiratory tract infection. In older children and in adults the onset is characteristically preceded by a chill, but in younger children the first symptom may be a convulsion. Symptoms referable to the nervous system are more common in children than in adults. Children also have more gastrointestinal symptoms—vomiting and possibly diarrhea —than do adults.

In the early stages the cough is dry and may cause pain. In the stage of resolution the cough is loose and productive. Fever is a characteristic of the early stage as well as of the course of the disease. The temperature rapidly reaches 103 to 104° F. and may or may not show extreme fluctuation within the 24 hours of the day. Among untreated older children the temperature drops abruptly, usually on the sixth or seventh day. This marks the crisis of the disease.

The respiratory and pulse rates are characteristic of pneumonia. The rate of respiration may be increased to 40 to 80 per minute in infants and to 30 to 50 per minute in older children. Respirations tend to be increased out of proportion to the increase in the pulse rate. They are shallow in order to reduce the pleural pain. The accessory muscles of respiration may be used, with resulting retractions. In children the alae nasi usually expand and contract with respiration.

The pulse rate is increased. The strength and rate of the pulse beat are indicative of the prognosis of the disease. If the pulse becomes weak and the rate extremely rapid or slow, the prognosis is guarded. Chest pain is due to pleural involvement and is felt especially on coughing or respiratory movement. The pain may be referred to the abdomen.

Gastrointestinal symptoms are common in the toddler. At the onset of the disease he may vomit or have diarrhea. Anorexia is common during the course of the disease. The older child may complain of a headache. Rigidity of the neck may be present.

**Diagnosis, Differential Diagnosis and Complications.** Examination of the chest is paramount in the *diagnosis* of pneumonia. The physician determines the number and extent of the pneumonic areas by the presence of rales, nature of breath sounds and evidence of consolidation. A roentgenogram is taken to corroborate the foci of consolidation found on examination and the presence of any complications such as atelectasis or empyema.

Laboratory tests may show a slight reduction in the red blood cell count and hemoglobin level and an increased white blood cell count—commonly from 16,000 to 40,000 per cubic millimeter. The urine has a high specific gravity, is dark amber in color and scanty in amount. There is usually an acetonuria and a mild to moderate albuminuria. The pneumococcus can usually be isolated from the nasopharyngeal and pharyngeal cultures. Bacteria may or may not be seen in the blood cultures.

Lobar pneumonia must be differentiated from atelectasis and pleural effusion and, if there is severe abdominal pain, from gastroenteritis and appendicitis. If nervous symptoms predominate, meningitis may be suspected.

A common *complication* of pneumonia is plastic pleurisy. It exists to some degree in nearly all cases. The incidence of other complications has been reduced since sulfonamides and antibiotics have been used in the treatment of pneumonia. Abdominal distention or tympanites is a serious complication; if it persists, it may be a reflection of toxic paralytic ileus. Other complications such as empyema or meningitis are extremely rare.

**Treatment and Nursing Care.** Today more cases of pneumonia in children are treated in the home than were treated in past years. The modern treatment with sulfonamide or antibiotic therapy, or both, is successful and easily carried out by the mother. When these drugs are given early in the course of the disease, administration of oxygen (difficult and dangerous for the mother to give in the home) is seldom needed. If severe complications arise, the child is hospitalized.

The child with pneumonia can be cared for at home if the physical environment is satisfactory and the mother or some other adult in the family can nurse him. This imposes on the physician or nurse the responsibility of teaching the mother how to nurse the child.

Much of the nursing care of the pneumonia patient is symptomatic and geared to the needs of the individual child. He should have adequate rest both physical and psychological. He should be disturbed as little as possible. At the first indication of pneumonia the physician orders administration of a sulfonamide or antibiotics, or both. The pneumococcus is susceptible to practically all such medications except those which are poorly absorbed. Penicillin in full dosage seems to be the drug of choice.

An increased fluid intake is necessary to supply the body's increased demand for fluid due to the infection. If the child vomits, fluids must be administered parenterally. Fluids should be given in sufficient quantities to maintain the normal specific gravity of the urine. This is important for excretion of toxic products and for avoidance of kidney complications when sulfonamides are given. As the child feels better, anorexia becomes less of a nursing problem. He should not be encouraged to eat more than he desires, however.

The child tends to lie on the affected side to lessen the pain. His position should be changed frequently. Although changing position causes pain at the time, it ultimately reduces his discomfort and facilitates drainage from the tracheobronchial tree.

Drug therapy is important throughout the course of the disease. The antibacterial agent should be given for four or five days after the temperature has returned to normal. For fever, aspirin is given, and cooling sponges (see p. 380) may be ordered. Oxygen is administered for restlessness or severe dyspnea, even though the child is not cyanotic. A Croupette or an oxygen tent may be used to give oxygen. If oxygen is given early, the need for analgesics and sedatives will be reduced. In severe cases aspirin and phenobarbital may be given.

Modern drug therapy prevents many of the complications which formerly occurred. Abdominal distention is a serious complication which still occurs in some cases. Prophylaxis includes early antibacterial treatment of the infection, oxygen therapy before the appearance of cyanosis, and the avoidance of constipation. If distention occurs, an enema may be given and the rectal tube left in place. Prostigmin is the most effective treatment and should be given for even mild distention. It may be repeated if the distention is not relieved.

An adequate convalescent period is essential even though the child seems well after antibacterial therapy. Recovery from uncomplicated pneumonia is usually rapid, but adequate convalescence is essential. Before the child is permitted to return to his daily activities he should have gained the weight lost during his illness and not be fatigued by normal exercise. Complete recovery usually takes two weeks.

**Prognosis and Prevention.** Sulfonamides and antibiotics have dramatically changed the course of pneumococcal pneumonia and reduced the mortality from it. After therapy has been begun the temperature usually returns to normal in twenty-four hours, the child's clinical condition improves, and complications are extremely rare. With early treatment the mortality rate is usually less than 1 per cent in both infants and children.

*Prevention* consists in isolating the child from contact with patients with pneumonia. This is important in the children's unit of a hospital and in the home if any member of the family has pneumonia. Often, however, the infection is spread before the sick person calls a physician and his condition is diagnosed as pneumonia. The importance of isolating children and adults with respiratory conditions is evident. Conditions predisposing to contracting pneumonia include excessive fatigue, chilling and upper respiratory tract infections.

### Staphylococcal Pneumonia

**Etiology, Incidence, Clinical Manifestations, Pathology and Diagnosis.** The causative organism is *Staphylococcus aureus*. Recently staphylococcal pneumonia has become the most important type of pneumonia in childhood. This is due to the emergence of a virulent strain of staphylococci resistant to the common antibiotics. Most other types of bacterial pneumonia are effectively controlled by antibacterial agents.

Staphylococcal infection may be acquired in the newborn nursery, in the hospital unit, in the home or in the community. It may begin as a skin infection, and the child may then become a carrier of virulent staphylococci in his nasopharynx. Later either he or another member of his family may suffer from staphylococcal pneumonia.

The onset of the disease is rapid. Multiple lesions occur in the lungs, pulmonary tissue is destroyed, and abscesses are formed. Lesions on the periphery of the lungs may erode into the pleural space and cause tension pneumothorax or empyema. Other *clinical manifestations* are similar to those of pneumococcal pneumonia.

Roentgenograms of the chest often

show multiple lesions and confirm the *diagnosis.* Nasopharyngeal and sputum cultures are examined and are found to be positive for the organism. Blood cultures are taken and may also prove positive.

**Treatment and Nursing Care.** Two essential points in the *treatment* of staphylococcal pneumonia are strict isolation and constant nursing care. Antimicrobial therapy consists in full dosage of two of the broad-spectrum antibiotics effective against a wide range of strains of staphylococci. Such antibiotics are novobiocin, erythromycin, oleandomycin, chloramphenicol, kanamycin and Staphcillin. Sensitivity tests should be done for the particular organism involved, and drugs should be chosen accordingly.

Oxygen therapy and maintenance of the fluid and electrolyte balance are important. The nurse must observe the child for any symptom suggesting the development of tension pneumothorax, such as the abrupt onset of pain, dyspnea or cyanosis.

**Prognosis.** When sulfonamides and antibiotic therapy were first used, recovery occurred in a number of cases, but now virulent, resistant strains of staphylococci have appeared, and the prognosis is guarded. Even with adequate treatment the mortality rate may be as high as 25 per cent.

Empyema and pneumothorax are unfavorable complications requiring decompression or surgical drainage.

### INTESTINAL PARASITES

Children who have intestinal parasites have few if any symptoms. Symptoms attributed in the past to such infestations included picking the nose, restlessness in sleep and possibly convulsions. These are more likely to be due to emotional disturbances, however.

There are several varieties of intestinal parasites which infest human beings, and toddlers are frequently infested by them. The two most common in the United States are pinworms and roundworms.

### Oxyuriasis (Enterobiasis; Pinworm, Threadworm or Seatworm Infection)

**Etiology.** Oxyuriasis is a parasitic infection produced by the pinworm, *Enterobius vermicularis,* which invades the cecum and the appendix. The worm is white and threadlike in appearance. The adult male is 2 to 5 mm. in length, the female 8 to 13 mm. The worms attach themselves to the mucous membrane of the cecum and the appendix by means of their "lips." Gravid worms become detached, migrate down the bowel and crawl out onto the perianal and perineal skin, where they lay thousands of eggs and provoke itching. A few hours after deposition the eggs become infective.

**Epidemiology and Pathology.** Oxyuriasis is the most common variety of parasitic infestation. It is spread by person-to-person contact. Children are especially susceptible. The condition is frequent where large groups of children are in close contact, as in an institution. The individual child reinfects himself by contaminating his hands when he scratches the itching skin around the anus where the eggs are lodged, or by handling soiled bedclothes, sleeping garments or contaminated objects. He then puts his fingers in his mouth, and the infested eggs repeat the life cycle upon maturing in the intestinal canal. The child may also become infective by breathing air-borne ova. Fertile eggs stay infective for about nine days in the average environment.

In short, the route by which reinfestation is accomplished is anus to fingers to mouth or anus to clothing to fingers to mouth.

Pathologically, eggs which are swallowed hatch in the duodenum and migrate directly to the cecum and appendix. Adult worms develop from eggs in forty-five days or less. Generally there is no damage noticeable at the site of attachment, though the worms may cause small hemorrhages from the appendiceal wall or provide an opening for pathogenic bacteria which may cause an abscess of the submucous tis sue. Gravid worms entering the vagina may cause vaginitis or a salpingitis and encapsulate in the tubules or migrate to the peritoneal cavity and encapsulate there. The gravid worms usually come out of the anus at night. The worms cause a severe pruritus, and secondary infection and scarification may occur from scratching.

Infestation usually cannot go on without reintroduction of the eggs by mouth.

**Clinical Manifestations.** Clinical manifestations are variable. Sometimes there are no symptoms other than itching about the anus at night which causes the child to be irritable and restless. There may, however, be symptoms of acute or subacute appendicitis from appendiceal lesions. Bacterial infection of the skin may develop from the pruritus ani, which produces weeping eczematous areas. Vaginitis often occurs, and little girls are frequently irritable, have a poor appetite, lose weight and suffer insomnia. These difficulties may cause a chronic emotional disturbance. Eosinophilia is present in some cases. On inspection worms may be seen on the surface of the child's stools or around the anus after he has been in bed for some hours.

**Diagnosis.** A conclusive diagnosis can be made if, on examination, worms are seen to emerge from the anus. The most practical and effective method of diagnosing the condition is by placing a tongue blade covered with cellophane tape, sticky side out, against the anal or perineal area, where it picks up the eggs. The sticky side of the tape is then placed downward on a slide, which can be microscopically examined at any time by allowing a drop of toluene to filter between the tape and the slide. Anal swabbing is best done in the early morning before arising or just before dressing, bathing or defecation. Eggs are not found readily in the stool.

**Treatment.** The aims of treatment are to destroy the ova and the worms in the intestine and to prevent reinfection from other persons in the environment.

One specific drug used is gentian violet in enteric-coated Seal-Ins or Enseal tablets which permit the drug to travel to the lower ileum before it is released. No cathartics are given before or after treatment. The tablets are given orally with the child's meals. Defective tablets may cause gastrointestinal irritation; hence the tablets should be tested by running water over them to see whether they will crack. Gentian violet may cause nausea and mild abdominal pain, and the nurse or mother should watch the child for these symptoms. It must be used for ten days to be effective.

Oxytetracycline (Terramycin) is as effective as gentian violet if the child is given the full course of treatment. The most harmless and effective drug is piperazine citrate (Antepar), a pleasant-tasting fruit-flavored syrup. It produces no side effects. Pyrvinium pamoate (Povan) has recently been introduced and promises to be an effective single-dose, nontoxic oxyuricide. Enemas may also be prescribed.

All infected persons in the household or group must be treated together. After eradication of parasites from the family or group new parasites can be acquired only from outside contacts.

**Nursing Care.** The nurse has an important part in the cure of children with oxyuriasis. Anthelmintics are dan-

**Figure 177.** Scotch tape test is usually done early in the morning for the purpose of locating the eggs of the pinworm.

gerous drugs. Mothers should be warned of the danger of overdosage. Some mothers are so anxious to rid the child of intestinal parasites that they may give more of the medication than is ordered.

The mother should learn how to give the medication and to carry out any procedures ordered by the physician. If the mother does not know how to give the child an enema, she should be shown the procedure (see p. 360).

The mother needs to know how to prevent reinfestation. The child should wear mitts or socks over his hands so that he cannot pick up the eggs under his fingernails when he scratches about the anus. His nails should be cut as short as possible. Hand hygiene should be carried out carefully, especially before meals and in the morning. The child should wear a tight diaper or panties so that he will be unable to reach the infested area. The anus should be cleansed carefully with soap and water after each defecation, and a soothing ointment should be applied to allay the itching. The toilet seat should be scrubbed daily. Underclothing, bed linen, night clothing, and towels used to dry the child should be boiled to destroy the eggs which are likely to be on the cloth. In the hospital the child should be prevented from coming in contact with others. His bedpan should be cleansed and sterilized after use.

The worms are removed from the bowel if necessary by enema, cathartics or other drugs prescribed by the physician. This phase of therapy is not often necessary.

**Prognosis and Prevention.**   The *prognosis* is generally good.

*Prevention* lies in scrupulous personal and group hygiene.

### Ascariasis (Roundworm Infection)

**Etiology and Epidemiology.**   This condition is a parasitic infestation by the giant roundworm, *Ascaris lumbricoides,* found most commonly in the lumen of the small intestine. The mature worm is similar in both shape and size to a white or pink earthworm and is 6 to 15 inches in length. The circumference of the mature female worm is that of a common pencil; it is slightly less in the male.

These parasites are found in warm climates and in the temperate zones up to latitude 40 degrees north or south. The fertile egg is capable of withstanding almost all external conditions except heat. The egg is contained within the feces of an infected person. Where hygienic toilets are not used, eggs may be deposited upon the ground, in cracks between stones or on the flooring. The egg embryonates and contains a motile first-stage larva in nine days in a warm environment. A week later the larva moults, and the egg becomes infective, but does not hatch in the soil. It hatches only after having been swallowed by the infected person.

Where little children defecate upon the ground, those who harbor the worms in their intestines seed the soil with the ova. Even if toilet facilities are available, little children may defecate where they are playing rather than take the time to go to the toilet. They spread the eggs where other children are likely to be contaminated. The eggs develop in the top soil, and the children take them into their mouths on toys, contaminated fingers or food, or by eating dirt. A large proportion of children from ages one through ten years have ascariasis where these unsanitary conditions prevail. They are the main source of infestation of older children and adults.

**Pathology, Clinical Manifestations and Diagnosis.**   In the infective stage the Ascaris is swallowed and enters the duodenum, where it hatches. The larvae penetrate the intestinal wall, mesenteric lymphatics or venules, commonly migrate to the liver and then proceed to the lungs through the right side of the heart.

The larvae invade the air sacs of the lungs by way of the pulmonary capillaries and cause the discharge of minute pools of blood at the sites. This results in an acute cellular infiltration which blocks passage of the larvae into the respiratory tree. The larvae moult a second time while in the lungs, ascend to the glottis and are swallowed, becoming established in the small intestine.

If the worms become irritated with their environment, they may proceed down the intestinal tract and be excreted, or they may migrate into the stomach and be vomited or be regurgitated through the nares. Worms may block the appendiceal lumen, perforate the intestinal wall, enter the pleural cavity, block the common bile duct or migrate to the liver and into its parenchyma.

The *clinical manifestations* are those which would be assumed from the pathology. An atypical pneumonia may occur when many larvae are in the lungs. Migrating larvae may cause an allergy; manifestations of such allergies include asthma, urticaria and eosinophilia. Intestinal symptoms may not be present or may include nausea and vomiting, anorexia and loss of weight. Other symptoms are insomnia, mild fever, nervousness, irritability and physical and mental lethargy. The most frequent symptom in small children is intestinal colic. Large masses of clumped worms may cause intestinal obstruction, perforation of the intestinal wall, intussusception or paralytic ileus.

The *diagnosis* is usually made by recovery of fertile or infertile eggs in microscopic fecal films. Occasionally the diagnosis is made by examination of the worms which have been passed in the stools, or have been vomited or have emerged from the nares.

**Treatment, Prognosis and Prevention.** Older methods of *treatment*, usually with hexylresorcinol crystoids, required elaborate preparation, fasting and post-treatment purgation. The modern drug of choice is piperazine citrate (diethylene diamine), which comes in a pleasant-tasting fruit-flavored syrup (Antepar). It requires none of the auxiliary preparation which other anthelmintics require and has no side effects when given in the recommended dosages.

The *prognosis* is excellent when an appropriate anthelmintic is administered. It is good to fair when secondary complications arise, such as lobar pneumonia, intestinal obstruction or intestinal perforation.

*Preventive measures* are essential in areas where the condition is common. Reinfestation occurs every three months in endemic areas. Children and adults must be provided with comfortable, clean toilets and must be taught to use them for every defecation. The infested top soil, 2 inches down, should be turned under. All infected persons must receive treatment; otherwise preventive measures are not likely to be successful.

## ACCIDENTS

Although not all the varieties of possible accidents can be discussed here, the care of the child who has suffered one of the more common accidents can be considered. These include the insertion of foreign objects into the nose or ears, poisoning, and fracture of the femur.

### Foreign Bodies in the Nose

**Incidence and Types.** This kind of accident usually occurs in early childhood. The infant does not appear interested in so small an orifice as his nostril, and the older child knows that he should not put anything in it. A toddler puts small objects into his nose, such as beads, pebbles, cherry stones, peas and watermelon seeds. He is likely to insert any small object of this sort if he happens to get hold of it.

**Clinical Manifestations, Diagnosis and Treatment.** The child rarely pushes the object far into the nostril because it hurts him to do so. Inexpert attempts to remove it may push it farther in, however. If the mother does not know that the child has put something up his nose, the first symptom which calls her attention to the accident is his complaint of pain when his nose is touched, obvious obstruction to respiration, and possibly wheezing. If the object is capable of absorbing fluid, it will swell and cause discomfort soon after insertion. If the object is hard and smooth and is not capable of absorbing fluid, it may not produce symptoms for weeks or months. On the other hand, it may irritate the mucous membrane and cause swelling and obstruction. A unilateral bloody, purulent discharge, which drips from the nostril in which the object has been lodged for some time, may result.

The *diagnosis* is made by examination with a speculum or nasoscope.

*Treatment* depends on the individual case. Sometimes forcible blowing of the nose with the other nostril compressed may dislodge the object. If the foreign body is not easily removed, the physician should spray the nasal cavity with a local anesthetic and attempt removal under direct vision.

### Foreign Bodies in the Ear

**Incidence, Types and Treatment.** This kind of accident usually occurs only in early childhood. The child may put any small object, hard or soft, into his ear.

If the object is visible and within easy reach and the child cooperates, it can be gently removed; otherwise it should be removed under general anesthesia.

Ear irrigation should not be done if the material is organic, since the object will swell from absorption of water. A postauricular incision may have to be made in some rare cases. A small mass of tightly packed cerumen may be removed by careful extraction with a curet or hook. If the mass is large, it should be softened with oil or detergent soap solution and removed by irrigation with warm water.

### Poisoning

Poisoning is a morbid condition caused by a poison. Poisons refer to a multitude of toxic substances accessible to the inquisitive, untutored or inexperienced child within his environment. Approximately 500 children under 5 years of age succumb annually in the United States from the ingestion of poisonous substances commonly found in the medicine chest or kitchen cabinet.

We shall limit this discussion to those poisons which children take into their mouths. A child may spit a distasteful poison out, but is also likely to swallow minute particles. He may even swallow repeated mouthfuls. For our purpose we speak of poisons as any substances which, when ingested, even in relatively small amounts, by their chemical action are capable of damaging tissues and disturbing bodily functions.

Poisons may include (1) those which a child is likely to find in the medicine cabinet or kitchen cabinet, such as carelessly stored insecticides or potent exterminators for insects, mice and rats; (2) those which have an immediate corrosive effect, such as lye or phenol; and (3) others in which the growth of bacteria produces toxins, as in various foodstuffs.

Food poisoning due to bacterial toxins requires the same kind of nursing care as digestive disturbances (see p. 316) and is spoken of here only in connection with teaching mothers the importance of discarding all spoiled food promptly. Bacterial poisoning from spoiled food is far more common in the low-income groups of large cities than in other social classes or in rural areas. Custards and salads do not keep well without good refrigeration and are a common source of food poisoning.

For our purpose poisons must also be divided into those which have an immediate action, as an overdose of sleeping pills or rat poison, and those which have a slow but cumulative effect, as chronic ingestion of small quantities of paint or plaster which contains lead.

The student should keep these divisions in mind as she reads this section, since each cannot be discussed separately.

**Incidence, Diagnosis, Clinical Manifestations and Treatment: General Principles.** In the United States poisoning accounts for many cases of accidents, and accidents are the leading cause of death among children over one year of age. Poisoning in children is always an accident due to lack of supervision of the child or to carelessness in leaving poisonous substances within his reach.

Many children die of poisoning each year, and more have permanent disabilities such as hepatic damage, esophageal stricture or damaged glomeruli. There are a few cases on record of children being given poison accidentally by mothers or nurses, but these accidents are so unusual that they need no discussion here.

There are more than 500 toxic substances used in the home. These include cleaning agents, detergents, bleaches, insecticides, heavy metals, paint solvents, polishing agents, kerosene, cosmetic preparations and drugs such as hypnotics, sedatives and tranquilizers. The Federal Food and Drug Administration requires that poisonous substances be so labeled. Some commercial preparations have the chemical composition stated on the label, but this is not always so.

Poisoning is more frequent in boys than in girls in the age group under five years. This is probably because boys are more active and venturesome than girls. The poison which children are likely to take varies with the part of the country and with rural or urban status. There is also a class differential. In tenement areas rat and roach poisons are a leading cause of quick poisoning among the toddlers. In old sections of many cities poisoning from outmoded lead paint used generations ago on walls is frequent (see p. 473).

In all cases of ingestion of rapidly acting poisons the *diagnosis* must be made promptly so that the antidote can be administered before the poison is absorbed. For this reason the mother or nurse should endeavor to give the physician a complete history of what has happened. Often, however, she does not know what the child has taken or whether, in fact, he has taken any poison at all. She may think that he has suddenly become sick and take him to the physician for treatment some time after ingestion of the poison. It is essential that anyone who cares for children should know the first indications of poisoning and not make the mistake of believing the child's symptoms to be due to sickness and thereby delay treatment.

Mothers and nurses cannot know the sources, actions and therapy of all known poisons. It is important, however, to know the general principles of management, for in many cases treatment must be instituted before the child can be seen by the physician.

The first step is to identify the poison if this can be done quickly. If it is not known, immediate measures described later should be taken. The mother may see the container from which the child took the poison, or relatives, bystanders or friends may give the information. The physician needs this information when he institutes treatment. If the child vomits spontaneously or if the mother has made him vomit by causing him to gag (see below), the vomitus should be saved for the physician's inspection. If the child voids, the urine should also be kept for examination. The physician, nurse or the mother may be able to identify the poison by its characteristic odor on the child's breath.

If time and facilities are available, laboratory studies should be made. Unfortunately the immediate treatment (induction of emesis or administration of gastric lavage by the physician or nurse) does not always remove all traces of poison from the child's stomach before a certain amount has been absorbed into the system. It is therefore advisable to give a specific antidote if one is available. Spectroscopic examination of the blood will show the presence or absence of methemoglobin, sulfhemoglobin and carboxyhemoglobin. The photoelectric colorimeter is used to reveal traces of lead, thymol and many other toxic substances. Later x-ray studies of the bones can be made to show evidence of lead and bismuth poisoning.

The clinical manifestations and treatment of the different poisons may be found in handbooks on the subject or obtained from the Poison Control Centers. But these symptoms are seldom peculiar to poisoning; they occur in many common diseases of childhood. Poisoning should be thought of if a child suddenly becomes sick, even though there is no reason to believe that he has taken any harmful substance.

Common clinical *symptoms* of poisoning include (1) gastrointestinal disturbances: (*a*) abdominal pain, (*b*) vomiting, (*c*) anorexia, (*d*) diarrhea; (2) respiratory and circulatory symptoms: (*a*) shock, (*b*) collapse, (*c*) unexplained cyanosis; (3) central nervous system manifestations: (*a*) sudden loss of consciousness, (*b*) convulsions.

These clinical manifestations in a little child are not specific and may indicate acute illness rather than poisoning. The physician must keep in mind the possibility of poisoning; this is essential because he cannot wait for time-consuming laboratory tests to confirm a diagnosis. In most cases of poisoning the effectiveness of the antidote depends upon the time which has elapsed between ingestion of the poison and administration of the antidote. If the physician does not know the exact nature of the poison or whether the child has actually taken poison, but wishes to rule out that possibility, he may consult the Poison Control Center.

If the poison which the child is believed to have taken is a patent preparation, the ingredients are commonly marked on the container, but if the mother has carelessly put the poison in an old glass jar, its composition may not be known to the mother or physician. The Poison Control Center can usually establish its identity and advise about treatment if there is a clue.

The general principles of *treatment* for ingested poisons may be summed up as follows:

1. Excessive manipulation of the child and overtreatment should be avoided. He should not be treated with large doses of sedatives, stimulants or antidotes. These may cause more damage than the poison itself.

2. In acute poisoning the mother or nurse should remain calm and collected so that she can institute treatment and carry out the physician's orders.

3. Prompt treatment is necessary. Time is of great importance in treatment because the amount of absorption of the poison depends on the interval between ingestion of the poison and its removal.

The immediate procedure is to induce vomiting. This may be done by giving the child a glass of milk and then, while holding his head downward, placing a finger, tongue blade or handle of a spoon in his mouth, far back upon the base of the tongue, and depressing it until emesis ensues. Vomiting should be induced in all cases except those in which the child is comatose or in which the poison he has taken is a petroleum distillate or a corrosive.

After this the child should be taken immediately to a physician in the hospital or clinic. If the mother or nurse knows from what bottle or other container the child got the poison, she should take it with her for the physician's inspection. She should also take any stomach contents which the child has vomited.

If it is not possible to induce vomiting or if there is reason to believe that not all the poison has been vomited, lavage is advisable. Few mothers have the equipment or know how to lavage the child. This is therefore done by the physician or nurse and is often a lifesaving measure.

Apomorphine given subcutaneously usually causes vomiting at once, and the physician may give this instead of lavaging the child, or he may follow up the vomiting with lavage as a precaution against any poison being retained in the stomach. Apomorphine is a respiratory depressant and should not be given if the child is in a coma, if poisoning is due to a respiratory depressant or if the respirations are slow or labored.

The antidote, if one exists, for the poison is then given. The label on the container may state the antidote; if not, the Poison Control Center should be called to obtain the information. The antidote is given even if the child's stomach has been emptied by lavage, for some absorption of poison has taken place.

Symptomatic and supportive treatment for shock or metabolic disturbances is given if necessary. The physician may order oxygen therapy and parenteral administration of fluids and electrolytes. Exchange transfusions may be given in certain types of poisoning.

*Universal Antidote.* If the poison the child has taken is not known, a universal antidote may be given to render the poison inert or prevent its absorption by changing its physical nature. Such an antidote may be made from the following common household ingredients:

Pulverized charcoal (made from
    burned toast) .............. 2 parts
Magnesium oxide (milk of magnesia) .................... 1 part
Tannic acid (*strong* tea) ...... 1 part

This solution should be given as soon after ingestion of the poison as possible. The carbon will absorb phenol and strychnine; magnesium oxide neutralizes acids; and tannic acid precipitates alkaloids, certain glucosides and many metals.

*Treatment for Poisoning from Corrosive Chemicals.* If the child has swallowed a corrosive chemical such as lye, tissues with which the chemical comes in contact are destroyed. Lye is one of the most common causes of poisoning in children. Sources of lye are washing powders, paint removers and drainpipe cleansers.

The manifestations of corrosive esophagitis may be seen in the tissue of the alimentary tract from the lips to the stomach. The symptoms are pain, inability to swallow, and prostration. The mucous membranes of the area are white immediately after the accident, but later become brown, ulcerated and edematous. The edema may be sufficient to obstruct respiration, and tracheotomy may be necessary. The pulse is feeble and rapid, and the child may collapse.

If the child survives, acute symptoms subside, and for a time he may appear well. But esophageal obstruction invariably appears within four to eight weeks, as a result of contraction of scar tissue. In severe obstruction the child may be unable to swallow either food or fluids.

The immediate treatment is neutralization of the chemical which was swallowed. This may be done with dilute vinegar or lemon juice. Pain may be relieved with sedatives. Olive oil taken by mouth may also relieve the pain by its demulcent action. Emetics or lavage should not be utilized for fear of traumatic perforation through the necrotic mucosa.

If the child cannot swallow, food and fluids must be given parenterally. To prevent stricture of the esophagus, the physician may pass a rubber eyeless catheter of appropriate size and filled with small shot at intervals determined by the child's condition. The first treatment is given about four days after the accident. Dilatation by bougie is continued for at least a year. The size of the catheter used is gradually increased. The child may be fed by gastrostomy if obstruction has been complete until the lumen is adequately dilated.

**Nursing Care.** The nurse should prevent the anxious parents from overstimulating or handling and caressing the child too much.

When the child is brought to the clinic, the nurse will save all vomitus and urine specimens for laboratory examination. She assists the physician with lavage or carries out his order for the procedure (see p. 329).

The child in a mummy restraint is positioned with his face to one side. A well lubricated large-bore catheter is passed. Size 28 French may be used; the actual size depends upon the child's age and the stomach contents. An Ewald aspirating bulb is attached. A small amount of the lavage solution (150 to 200 ml.) should be injected into the stomach and aspirated as necessary. The procedure is continued until all traces of the poison are removed. In all, 2 to 4 liters of solution should be used.

For immediate emptying of the stomach, water or weak salt and sodium bicarbonate solution may be used until a more suitable solution can be obtained. Later activated charcoal, tannic acid, magnesium oxide or other solution may be used, depending on the poison the child has taken.

Routine lavage procedure is used with the following exceptions.

If the child has taken a corrosive poison, there is danger of perforating the esophagus. In strychnine poisoning the stimulation of passing a lavage tube may induce a fatal convulsion. If the child has been poisoned by kerosene, lavage may provoke aspiration of the fluid, and pneumonia may ensue.

Good general supportive therapy increases the effectiveness of removing the poison and giving a specific antidote. Supportive therapy will depend, of course, upon the action of the particular poison ingested.

The nurse must watch for evidence of stimulation or depression of the nervous system. Stimulation results in convulsions, restlessness and delirium. Depression results in stupor and coma.

There may be symptoms of respiratory depression, of pulmonary edema or pneumonia. To relieve pulmonary distress, the patient may be given artificial respiration (see p. 185) or oxygen, or establishment of a patent airway may be necessary.

The nurse must watch for peripheral circulatory collapse or cardiac failure. Intravenous administration of fluids or digitalis may be necessary.

Some poisons cause intense vomiting and diarrhea. Water and electrolyte loss must be replaced by parenteral fluids.

The nurse must observe the frequency of voiding and collect samples of urine as ordered by the physician. The extent of renal damage varies in different cases. The most important aspect of therapy in relation to the influence of poison on the kidneys is administration of the correct amounts of electrolytes and fluids.

The child's temperature must be taken at frequent intervals, since the physician should be notified if hypothermia or hyperthermia occurs.

The child who is poisoned is prone to infection. He must be isolated from other children, and no nurse who has even a slight infection should care for him. The nurse will give antibiotic therapy as ordered by the physician.

Both the child and his parents are in need of emotional support from the nurse, particularly if the child is in pain. The mother may feel guilty, blaming herself for the accident. She should be counseled to avoid such sentiments of recrimination. Competent, comprehensive nursing care is essential.

**Prevention.** Most cases of accidental poisoning in young children are due to the carelessness of the adults responsible for the care of the children. The immediate responsibility lies with the child's parents. It is also the responsibility, however, of all members of the health team who teach parents the hygiene and care of little children to stress the danger to these active, curious toddlers of leaving poisonous substances in any receptacle within easy reach.

All dangerous substances should be kept out of the toddler's reach, on a high shelf or, better still, in a locked cupboard. All drugs, household chemicals and poisons should be kept in the containers in which they were sold, for these are plainly marked, and no adult is likely to carelessly leave them in easy reach of the child. If poisonous substances are stored in containers used for food, there is danger that someone will leave them where the child can sample the contents.* Children should also be protected from poisoning by spoiled food, thus preventing bacterial poisoning.

### Fracture of the Femur

**Incidence, Etiology, Types and Diagnosis.** Many injuries occurring among toddlers are the result of falls. The toddler is learning to climb. He goes up and down stairs and climbs on and off chairs and benches for the sheer joy of it. Although a fracture of the femur is not the only injury he may receive, it is one of the most common serious fractures caused by his many falls. The nurse should stress this danger in her conferences with the mother.

The stairs should have handrails so that the child may hold on to the rail as he goes up or down one step at a time. Ideally there should be gates at the top and the bottom of the stairs. The one-story house is safer than the two-story house for the toddler in this

* This same precaution applies to inflammable materials.

respect. Generally there is a door to the cellar steps which can be kept shut.

Fracture of the femur, sometimes accompanied by other serious injuries, also results when the child is struck by a passing car when he chases into the street after a ball or is struck by a car being backed out of a driveway or garage. If the driver is the child's parent, that fact adds to the emotional impact of the accident upon the parents. Climbing over the side of the crib or springing on the bed mattress frequently results in severe falls and skeletal injury.

A *greenstick fracture* is one in which one side of the bone is broken, the other side being bent. This type of fracture is common in children because their bones are soft and not fully mineralized. A severe injury, however, will result in a complete break. In young children

healing may occur with some deformity, though this usually disappears during the process of growth.

The *diagnosis* is made by his history of inability to bear weight, pain on movement and local tenderness. X-ray examination confirms the findings and the position of the broken fragments.

**Treatment and Nursing Care.** The child's clothes should be removed gently, first from the uninjured side of the body and then from the injured side. The injured limb should be moved as little as possible. It is sometimes necessary to cut off the clothing.

The physician may order cold applications or ice caps for the first twenty-four to thirty-six hours to prevent swelling and edema. Aspirin or some form of salicylate is effective for relief of pain.

The method of fixation of the legs is

**Figure 178.** Bryant traction is used for the young child who has a fractured femur. Sufficient weights are used to elevate the child's pelvis from the bed. (Courtesy of the Gilbert Hyde Chick Co., Oakland, California.)

by traction. It is developed by a system of weights and pulleys and is applied to both legs by means of skin traction. Traction is applied to reduce the fracture, to maintain the bones in the corrected position and to immobilize both legs. The type of traction apparatus commonly used for children having a fractured femur is *Bryant traction,* and the method is by vertical suspension.

The fundamental principle of the Bryant traction system is a bilateral *Buck's extension* applied to the child's legs. The procedure is as follows:

1. Shave the child's legs if any hair is present, and paint the skin with tincture of benzoin so that the adhesive will grasp to the skin more firmly. Benzoin also serves as a disinfectant for the skin and allays itching and excorciation beneath the tape.
2. A strip of moleskin should be cut for each leg, long enough to extend above the knee on each side and under the foot. In the center of each strip, at the level of the sole of the foot, place a thin flat board 3 inches long and an inch broader than the widest distance between the malleoli. There should be a hole in the center of the block through which the traction rope is to be passed. In order to hold the piece of board in place, a second piece of moleskin must be placed on the side facing the child's foot. This piece of moleskin must be as wide as the other and long enough to reach from above the malleoli on one side under the foot to above the malleoli on the other side. This is done to protect the malleoli from pressure from the adhesive. Metal attachments may be used instead of the pieces of wood.
3. Two overhead bars placed longitudinally, or one longitudinal bar with a crossbar, are fastened securely over the crib. One or two pulleys are attached to the bar, in position to apply traction at the desired angle.
4. The moleskin is applied and held in place by gauze or Ace bandages. A rope is threaded over the pulleys. Sufficient weights are applied *to elevate the child's hips from the bed.* The legs should be at right angles to the body and the buttocks elevated and clear of the bed. A jacket restraint should be used to keep the child flat in bed and unable to turn from side to side. The child may lie upon the mattress of the bed or be placed upon a Bradford frame within the bed. The nurse should never remove the weights once they have been applied, for the traction should be kept constant. In moving the bed the weights should not be supported, but neither should they be permitted to swing against the bed.

*Care of the Child in Traction.* The nurse should observe the traction ropes to see whether the child's body is in correct alignment. She should feel his toes frequently to note any sign of impaired circulation. The toes should be pink and warm. Any cyanosis, tingling or loss of sensation is an indication that the bandage is too tight. The nurse should be sure that the weights hang free and that the ropes are in the wheel grooves of the pulleys. Little children in Bryant apparatus are tempted to turn from side to side when they are interested in what is going on about them. This interferes with the even traction exerted by the weights. Movement of the body is an indication that the restraining jacket is not fastened correctly.

Lying constantly on his back with the friction which the slight movement of the restraining jacket permits is likely to chafe the child's back. Hence he needs good back care. The nurse should reach under his body and rub his back and buttocks. The bed must be kept dry and free from wrinkles and crumbs or other particles of food.

Lack of exercise often results in the child's becoming constipated. His abdomen may become distended. The physician may order a mild cathartic to relieve the distention. Roughage in the diet and the fluid intake should be increased. Enemas may be needed, but continued use of cathartics is avoided.

These are children who need their mothers with them. Application of the Bryant traction is frightening to toddlers, and later, when they are accustomed to it, the restraint makes time pass slowly. Unless amusement is provided for them and their mothers visit them daily, they will find hospitalization a traumatic experience.

**Prognosis.**   Femoral shaft fractures in little children heal quickly. There is usually solid union within three to four weeks after the injury.

### TEACHING AIDS AND OTHER INFORMATION*

*Community Service Society of New York*
Some Parasitic Infections Affecting Man, 1957.
* Complete addresses are given in the Appendix.

*State of Illinois, Department of Public Welfare*
  Going to the Hospital.
  You and Your Child—Getting Sick.

*U.S. Department of Health, Education, and Welfare*
  Accidents and Children, 1959.

# REFERENCES

American Academy of Pediatrics, Committee on Accident Prevention: Accidental Poisoning in Childhood. Evanston, Illinois, American Academy of Pediatrics, 1956.

American Medical Association, Committee on Toxicology: First Aid Measures for Poisoning. Am. J. Nursing, 58:98, 1958.

Arena, J. M.: Diagnosis and Treatment of Poisoning. Clinical Symposia. Summit, New Jersey, Ciba Pharmaceutical Products, Inc., 12:3, 1960.

Batson, R., and Young, W. C.: The Administration of Oxygen to Infants and Small Children (An Evaluation of Methods). Pediatrics, 22:436, 1958.

Cann, H. M., and others: Survey of Poison Control Centers. Pediatrics, 23:359, 1959.

Citizens' Committee on Children of New York City, Inc.: Liberal Visiting Policies for Children in Hospitals. J. Pediat., 46:710, 1955.

Cooper, M. L., and Keller, H. M.: Severe Staphylococcal Infections in Young Children. A.M.A. J. Dis. Child., 95:245, 1958.

Dietrich, H. F.: The Role of Education in Accident Prevention. Pediatrics, 17:297, 1956.

Dimock, H. G.: The Child in Hospital. Philadelphia, F. A. Davis Company, 1960.

Goddard, J. L.: Childhood Accidents. Children, 6:83, 1959.

Harvie, F. H.: Pediatric Methods and Standards. 3rd ed. Philadelphia, Lea & Febiger, 1958.

Hemmendinger, M.: ℞: 'Admit Parents at All Times.' Child Study, 34:No. 1, 3, 1956.

Hohle, B. M.: We Admit Parents Too. Am. J. Nursing, 57:865, 1957.

Holthaus, L. S.: Cooperation to Prevent Home Accidents. Am. J. Nursing, 56:1160, 1956.

Hunt, A. D.: An Experiment in Teamwork. Child Study, 34:No. 1, 10, 1956.

Hunt, A. D., and Trussell, R. E.: They Let Parents Help in Children's Care. The Modern Hospital, 85:89, Sept., 1955.

Illingworth, R. S.: Young Children in Hospital. Nursing Times, 52:112, 1956.

Larson, C. B., and Gould M.: Calderwood's Orthopedic Nursing. 4th ed. St. Louis, C. V. Mosby Company, 1957.

Livingstone, H. M.: Nursing Care in Oxygen Therapy. Am. J. Nursing, 57:65, 1957.

Loeb, D. G.: Problems of Children in Hospitals. Understanding the Child, 24:7, Jan., 1955.

Macpherson, C. R.: Oxygen Therapy—An Unsuspected Source of Hospital Infections? J.A.M.A., 167:1083, 1958.

Moore, B. R.: When Johnny Must Go to the Hospital. Am. J. Nursing, 57:178, 1957.

Nelson, W. E. (editor): Textbook of Pediatrics. 7th ed. Philadelphia, W. B. Saunders Company, 1959.

Ochsner, A., and DeBakey, M. E. (editors): Christopher's Minor Surgery. 8th ed. Philadelphia, W. B. Saunders Company, 1959.

O'Connell, E. A., and Brandt, P.: Liberal Visiting Hours for Parents. Am. J. Nursing, 60:812, 1960.

Paterson, D., and McCreary, J. F.: Pediatrics. Philadelphia, J. B. Lippincott Company, 1956.

Press, E.: Poison Control Centers. Nursing Outlook, 5:29, 1957.

Pryles, C. V.: Staphylococcal Pneumonia in Infancy and Childhood. Pediatrics, 21:609, 1958.

Robertson, J.: Young Children in Hospitals. New York, Basic Books, Inc., 1958.

Rodman, M. J.: A Survey of Potentially Harmful Household Products. J. Pediat., 46:171, 1955.

Slotkowski, E. L., and Voorsanger, E. L.: Pneumonia in Infants and Small Children. Am. J. Nursing, 59:1720, 1959.

Starbuck, G. W.: Recent Trends in Accident Prevention. Pediatrics, 22:761, 1958.

Thomas, J. M., and Ulpis, E. B.: A Seasonal Hazard—Laryngotracheobronchitis. Am. J. Nursing, 61:52, March, 1961.

Tonyan, A., and Jensen, J. S.: The Nurse's Part in Poison Control. Am. J. Nursing, 58:96, 1958.

Williams, F. J.: Nurses Have Much to Do about Poison Control. Nursing Outlook, 6:93, 1958.

World Health Organization: Technical Report Series No. 118, Geneva, Switzerland. Accidents in Childhood. W.H.O. Palais des Nations, 1957.

# Chapter 17

# Conditions of Toddlers Requiring

# Long-Term Care

## LONG-TERM HOSPITALIZATION

LONG-TERM hospitalization of the toddler or young child presents a more serious problem of maternal deprivation than does short-term hospitalization. This is partly because many hospitals do not permit too frequent visiting by parents on units for children with a long-term illness. Such visiting is supposed to be upsetting to the routine, and the personnel find it difficult to have the parents on the unit as often as is permitted on an active service. Then, too, working parents have neither the time nor the money for transportation required for daily visiting. There may be other children at home for whom some arrangement must be made if the mother leaves them to visit the sick child.

Student nurses are usually not assigned to the care of children for long periods, since that would interfere with gaining wide clinical experience. None of the permanent personnel may be assigned to the care of a child long enough for him to become attached to them and feel secure in their love.

**Prevention of Maternal Deprivation.** The personnel of the children's hospital or pediatric unit in a general hospital should be educated to understand the child's emotional need for his parents so that they appreciate the importance of frequent visiting. If the expense of transportation or loss of time from work is the reason given by parents for not visiting the child, the social service worker may find ways of assisting them. Every effort should be made to keep young children at home, with care given on an outpatient basis. If this is not possible, children should be hospitalized near their homes and, if possible, sent home on weekends and holidays. Arrangements might be made for other young children in the family to go to nursery school so that the mother may be free to visit the sick child. The child's older brothers and sisters should be permitted to visit him.

If the mother is unable or unwilling to visit the sick child frequently, the hospital should compensate for his loss of maternal love by supplementing her visits with a mother-substitute.

1. The case-assignment system should be used exclusively in long-term care of little children.

2. The same personnel should be assigned to a small group of children throughout their period of hospitalization. This is possible only if nursing care is given by a permanent staff and students are supernumeraries assigned to the care of patients solely for the learning experience involved.

3. Children needing long-term hospitalization may be placed in hospital units resembling a children's home where medical attention is provided. The main part of the care would be given by women skilled in meeting the needs of little children; they would not be nurses, but would be nonprofessional foster-mothers. Each would act as "Mother" to a small group of children. Physicians and nurses would come in only when necessary. In such small family groups a child could form stable relations and lead an emotionally satisfying life.

4. These children confined to the hospital should have as many of the pleasurable activities available to normal children as would be possible to give them. For instance, they would play with sand and water and do finger painting. In the typical children's hospital unit such play is difficult to provide. In the model hospitals planned solely for the care of chronic and orthopedic cases and in convalescent hospitals a variety of play materials are provided for the children.

## LONG-TERM CONDITIONS

### Cleft Palate

The incidence, etiology, pathology and clinical manifestations of cleft palate were discussed in Chapter 11 (p. 201). Only the long-term program of care, including surgical correction, will be taken up here.

**Total Program of Care or Habilitation.** The care and habilitation of the child with cleft palate may require many years of medical, dental, surgical and speech treatment. The personnel involved act as a team in the care of the child, functioning better as a group than if care were given by them individually. The *cleft palate team* includes the pediatrician, plastic surgeon, dentist, prosthetic dentist, orthodontist, otolaryngologist, medical social worker, nurse in the hospital, speech pathologist, psychologist or psychiatrist or both, and the public health nurse. The child's physician may act as coordinator of the group so that the mother is not confused by the apparent complexity of the treatment. The mother may need guidance from each of the team members at various times as treatment progresses. Cleft palate teams such as these are usually located in the clinics of the large medical centers.

If the parents cannot afford to pay for this expensive care, the child is treated at one of the large medical centers connected with the state program for crippled children or at a children's hospital under private auspices. In either case he is treated without cost to his parents or for whatever fee they are able to pay.

Dealing with the anxieties of the parents is one of the main functions of the cleft palate team, and specifically of the nurses in the newborn nursery, the public health nurses in the home or clinic, and the nurses in the hospital when the child is admitted for surgery. The parents should be reassured that all possible therapy will be given the child. They must also be told that improvement will take time and will require their full cooperation. The parents must not only accept the child with his disfigurement, but also must help him to adjust to his deformity. The physical defect can be corrected more successfully than can hampering personality traits which may develop if he believes that others turn away from him because of his cleft palate.

**Surgical Correction.** The child should be placed under the care of the cleft palate team as early as possible in order that changes occurring with growth can be observed and plans can be made for long-term needs.

The time for operation is delayed until the child is between one and five years of age because the surgeon wants to take advantage of changes in the palate which occur with growth. The time for operation varies with the individual child because of differences in the size, degree and shape of the deformity. The surgeon tries to correct the defect so that there is optimum union of the cleft in the palate, without injury to the developing maxilla, and so that intelligible speech will be possible.

If operation is postponed until the child is learning to speak—about the third year—a dental speech appliance can be fitted so that the child can speak clearly enough for others to understand him. If the deformity is too severe and surgical repair is not possible, a prosthetic speech appliance is used as an important means of speech habilitation. Such appliances must be replaced periodically as the child grows.

**Surgical Management and Nursing Care.** *Preoperative care* is minimal. Any infection is a contraindication to operation. The nurse must watch the child closely and report any evidence of infection. The clotting and bleeding times should be determined preoperatively. Feedings are given until six to eight hours before operation if the child is in good nutritional condition, with good fluid and electrolyte balance.

*Postoperative care* is extremely important. Special nursing care is essential immediately after operation to keep the mouth clean and free from irritation. Antibiotics are ordered only if infection is suspected. Directly after the operation the child is placed on his abdomen to prevent aspiration of drainage material. His head is turned to one side. The nurse should watch closely for signs of an occluded airway and for hemorrhage. If necessary, the child is placed in a position favorable to postural drainage.

The physician may order aspiration of the nasopharynx to reduce the possibility of development of pneumonitis or atelectasis. Many physicians, however, prefer that no suction be used. If it is ordered, it must be done very gently.

The suture line must be kept clean. Restraint is necessary to keep the child from putting his fingers or even toys in his mouth. His arms must be securely restrained with elbow restraints. The restraint should be placed over the shirt, with the shirt sleeves turned back and pinned in position. The restraints should be removed periodically and passive exercise given.

The diet is limited to clear sterile or other fluids as ordered by the physician. Milk is usually not permitted immediately after the operation because of the danger of curds forming along the suture line. The child's mouth should be rinsed or cleansed with sterile water after each feeding. If the child is uncooperative, a mouth gag or tongue blade is used to hold the mouth open. The nurse should tell the child not to rub the site with his tongue, in words he can understand, such as, "Don't put your tongue on the part of your mouth which feels sore."

As far as possible all strain on the sutures must be prevented. The first postoperative feeding is given with a rubber-tipped medicine dropper or from the side of a spoon. After the first day a cup may be used if the child prefers it. A straw is not used, for he should not suck.

If possible, crying should be prevented. The child should be kept warm, dry and as comfortable as possible. Quiet diversion such as showing him pictures in his favorite picture book and reading the accompanying story will help to keep him from crying. The physician may order sedatives to be given.

The diet is fluid or semifluid for ten days to two weeks after operation. For the following two weeks a soft diet is given, and after that a regular diet.

The nurse may be asked to assist the physician in giving parenteral fluids.

This procedure is not always necessary, however.

**Instructions to the Mother on Discharge of the Child.** The mother must be cautioned to prevent injury to the palate. Since the area may be without sensation, the child may show no sign of pain if the healing area is scraped with some hard object such as the spoon with which he is being fed. The child must wear arm cuffs constantly except when he is bathed or when his mother gives him passive exercise and allows him to move his arms freely. At such times she must guard against his putting his hand into his mouth.* Sucking and blowing movements bring a strain upon the wound. If the mother sees that he is amusing himself in this way, she should play with him and divert his attention with a toy.

Upper respiratory tract infection increases his discomfort, and he should be kept from infection by isolating him from anyone who has a sore throat or a cold.

**Complications.** These children have recurring attacks of otitis media with resulting loss of hearing. The mother should report any indications of otitis media to the physician. Excessive dental decay may accompany cleft palate. The mother should be taught the correct method of brushing the child's teeth so that she can keep them clean when the physician says that it is safe for her to use a brush. Later she will teach the child the correct technique. The mother should also be told of the need for dental supervision of the child. If displacement of the maxillary arches and malposition of the teeth occur, orthodontic correction may be necessary.

**Prognosis.** The prognosis is fair, but depends upon the extent of the deformity at birth. A speech defect may still exist after good surgical correction of the palatal defect or after insertion of a speech appliance. Speech therapy should be given if the speech defect persists.

---

* The mother can make arm cuffs out of rolled cardboard and tie them in place with string. Care must be taken that the restraints do not rub the skin in the axilla.

## True or Idiopathic Celiac Disease (Chronic Idiopathic Steatorrhea or Chronic Intestinal Indigestion)

**Incidence and Etiology.** True celiac disease is characterized by chronic intestinal malabsorption as evidenced by steatorrhea with varying degrees of losses of other nutrients, resulting in malnutrition and deficiency diseases. [handwritten: fatty stools]

The disease is a chronic condition of infants and children which may begin insidiously with digestive disturbances when the child is six to twelve months old. The disease appears in both a mild and a severe form. It occurs in both sexes and has its highest *incidence* in the white race.

Celiac disease in children seems to be related to sprue in adults and may occur among different members of the same family. The *etiology* is not known, but because of the familial incidence, there may be a constitutional peculiarity, possibly of genetic origin. In most patients glutens, or protein, of rye, wheat and oats produce a gradual or acute increase in the characteristic symptoms. Parenteral infections and emotional disturbances may lead to exacerbations.

**Pathology and Clinical Manifestations.** The *pathology* is evident in severe malnutrition and secondary deficiency diseases, of which rickets is the most common, but scurvy or hypoproteinemia may also occur.

Typical *clinical manifestations* appear in the second year and may last to the fifth year of life; they are most severe in the second year. Episodes of diarrhea occur, and the child is prone to respiratory infections. At intervals the clinical picture is complicated by constipation. Anorexia, if it occurs, results in failure of growth and normal gain in weight. Severe abdominal distention may be caused by collections of gas and fluid and by relaxed abdominal musculature. There are fluctuations in weight. Slow gain and loss in weight are most noticeable in the limbs, buttocks and groin. The skin over the flattened buttocks may be wrinkled and hang in folds. The face usually remains plump,

**Figure 179.** Celiac disease. This child has abdominal distention and growth failure. (Courtesy of Dr. Ralph V. Platou and the American Academy of Pediatrics.)

and the rounded cheeks may be flushed even if the child is anemic. This gives a deceptive appearance of health. Dentition is often delayed. The child may show increasing irritability and other changes in behavior.

A celiac crisis may be precipitated by even a mild respiratory or gastrointestinal infection. The child has diarrhea and vomiting with resulting dehydration and acidosis. This condition may result in death if the child is not promptly and adequately treated.

In this severe form of the disease his sleep is restless, and the child cries out frequently; sweating is excessive, and his extremities are cold. His restricted diet and his anorexia are likely to result in dietary deficiencies, including deficiencies of vitamins.

The nature of the stools varies with the diet and the severity of the disease. The typical celiac stools are bulky, heavy, fatty and of more than normal frequency (particularly during a crisis), mushy, foul-smelling, pale and frothy. The excessive fat in the stools is largely split fat, i.e. free fatty acids and soaps. With improvement in the child's condition the stools become formed and normal in color, but may still contain fat. There is no actual impairment in the digestion of fat, since pancreatic lipase and bile acids are present. The impairment is in the *absorption of fat.* There is also impaired carbohydrate absorption. Nevertheless the carbohydrate which is absorbed in the intestinal tract performs its natural function in the body.

In a fully developed case of celiac disease there is a mild hypoproteinemia or protein deficiency. Minerals—calcium and iron—are lost in the stools in amounts depending on the severity of the disease.

The relation between the mild and the severe forms of celiac disease is not established. In the mild uncomplicated form of the disease (*starch intolerance*) the clinical symptoms are (1) excessive extracellular starch granules in the feces after feeding of starch, (2) chronic diarrhea, (3) growth failure, and (4) the transitory complication of steatorrhea. There is some question whether this mild uncomplicated form is to be considered celiac disease or is a different condition.

**Treatment.** Treatment consists in supervision of the diet by the physician on the basis of the child's improved behavior, his growth, and the anxiety of his parents over his condition and the dietary restriction. Specifically, the diet depends on the child's condition and age. If the child is very ill, he is given skimmed or protein milk sweetened with glucose, sucrose or banana powder. Gradually other foods are added, one at a time, at intervals of two or more days until at the end of two or three weeks a full but gluten-free diet is given. Foods which can be added are eggs, cottage cheese, meat, fruits and vegetables.

The diet must meet the child's caloric needs. It should contain an optimal amount of protein for growth and repair of tissue. Two forms of carbohydrate, both monosaccharides and disaccharides, may be given. If polysaccharides (starches) contain no gluten, they can be given without difficulty. Gluten-containing grains such as rye, wheat and possibly barley and oats should be eliminated from the diet. Other starches such as rice, potato and corn may be given. Normal amounts of fat may be given in a gluten-free diet. During a celiac crisis, however, fat is withheld, as it would be with any child having a gastroenteritis. Generous amounts of vitamin and mineral supplements should be given to every celiac patient to prevent deficiencies. The parents should be given a list of food products which contain wheat or rye gluten, such as gravies, meat loaf, puddings and processed meats, and should be told why these foods are contraindicated for the child.

Treatment during a celiac crisis involves fluid and electrolyte replacement and maintenance therapy. If symptoms of tetany occur, calcium is given until the serum calcium level returns to normal. Antibiotics are given for any infections which may develop. Adrenal steroid therapy produces remissions in celiac disease, but a relapse occurs as soon as the medication is discontinued.

**Nursing Care.** Nursing care involves helping the parents to accept not only the child's physical condition, but also his behavior problems. Typically, the child is irritable, moody, negativistic and difficult to manage. The nurse must have a sympathetic understanding of their problem. Parents may feel guilty or ambivalent toward the child. They may overprotect him or communicate to him their great concern about the nature of his stools.

During hospitalization for diagnosis and treatment the child may need emotional support from the nurses. He is confused and unhappy because of the initial food deprivation. His parents should visit him frequently or, if possible, stay with him. When he is hungry, he becomes frustrated and angry and may have temper tantrums or be withdrawn. The hungry child should feel free to complain either by crying or, if he can talk, with words. The understanding nurse will help him to express his feelings in words and will show her sympathy if he cries.

Feeding the child is a problem. Although hunger may be the fundamental cause of his irritability, his appetite is capricious. He should be fed slowly and given small amounts at a time. He should not be forced to eat; when he feels better, he will eat more. New foods should be introduced gradually, one at a time, and may be masked in foods he likes. If he will not take a particular food, this fact should be reported to the physician, and the food should be eliminated from the diet and tried again at some future time.

Recording of the child's food intake is important. The nurse should observe and chart the kind and amount of food taken, the child's appetite and his reaction to different foods. With each new addition to the diet the nurse should note the nature of the stools, the child's behavior and the degree of abdominal distention.

It is imperative to prevent infection. Good hygiene must be maintained, since the child is anemic and malnourished. He perspires freely and must be kept dry. If he is confined to bed and tends to lie in one position, he should be turned frequently.

As the child recovers, every effort should be made to provide him with special treats when he cannot have the food which other children in the pediatric unit are enjoying or, after his return home, which the family members are eating.

Children with celiac disease are often withdrawn and do not enter into play with other children. Their play is likely to be passive, since they find active play exhausting. The toddler may retain infantile habits of self-comfort such as sucking his thumb, or he may carry his favorite toy or object wherever he goes to give him a feeling of security. The nurse must be patient and try to provide security for the child in companionship with other children and the unit personnel. As his physical condition improves, his emotional behavior will also change; he will give up infantile habits and seek the companionship of others.

**Instructions to the Mother.** The parents should learn the underlying concepts of the child's illness and his treatment so that they can give him adequate care after his discharge from the hospital. In her conferences with the mother the nurse stresses (1) the necessity of preventing infection and emotional disturbances from any cause, (2) the importance of strict adherence to the dietary regimen, and (3) the need for follow-up supervision. This instruction should be given slowly without frightening the mother, for if she becomes too anxious, she will overprotect the child and restrict his activities beyond the limits set by the physician. Overprotection is harmful to positive mental health, particularly in the toddler, who has no relations with a teacher or other professional workers to counteract his mother's attentions.

**Prognosis.** The incidence of death from celiac disease is low, owing to the better understanding and more common use of parenteral fluid therapy, dietary management and control of infection by antibiotics. Recovery takes several months. The course of the condition is an intermittent process of exacerbations and remissions. Since celiac disease is a constitutional defect, actual cure does not occur, but clinical manifestations decrease in later life.

## Nephrotic Syndrome (Nephrosis)

**Etiology, Types and Incidence.** The *etiology* is unknown. It is seldom possible to relate the onset of nephrosis to another condition or disturbance. Exacerbations of the condition often follow acute infections.

The nephrotic syndrome can be divided into two groups: lipoid nephrosis and a nephrotic phase of subacute or chronic glomerulonephritis. It is not known whether these are, in fact, separate entities. Nephrosis is a disease of

childhood, the average age at its onset being two and a half years. It is seldom seen in children under one year of age and for an unknown reason is more common in boys than in girls.

**Pathology and Clinical Manifestations.** Pathologically, the kidneys are yellowish and enlarged. The cortices are thickened and the tubules dilated.

The *clinical manifestations* may be produced by glomerular lesions which permit excessive loss of plasma protein in the urine. Reduction in serum albumin is due principally to loss in the urine.

The onset is insidious. Edema is usually the first symptom noted. In the beginning of the sickness the child rarely appears ill. The edema, apparent around his eyes and at his ankles, becomes severe and later is generalized. As the fluid accumulates the child gains weight rapidly. In some cases he may double his normal weight. This state may last from several weeks to months. The common sites of collection of fluid are the peritoneal cavity (*ascites*), the thorax (*hydrothorax*) and the scrotum. In some cases the swelling is so great that it seems as if the skin would break. Striae may appear from overstretching of the skin. The edema in the peripheral tissue shifts with postural change. The urinary output varies inversely with the edema.

Pallor may be out of proportion to the degree of anemia.

Anorexia is a nursing problem. Malnutrition may be severe, but the loss of body tissue is obscured by the edema. Vomiting, diarrhea and abdominal distention may occur. During periods of edema other clinical manifestations seen in some cases include inguinal and umbilical hernias (see pp. 333, 337), respiratory distress, rectal prolapse (see p. 357) and decreased motor activity. The blood pressure usually remains normal, but if the child has advanced renal insufficiency, hypertension is seen. The child is generally afebrile. Behavioral concomitants of his condition are irritability and lassitude.

Nephrotic children are susceptible to infection. Formerly pneumococci or streptococci caused the majority of concurrent infections, but today other infections are also common. It is interesting to note that if the child contracts measles, a remission of the nephrotic condition may result.

A nephrotic crisis during the course of the illness may produce such signs and symptoms as fever, abdominal pain and at times erysipeloid skin eruptions. These subside in a few days, and diuresis may occur.

In the final stage of the disease cardiac failure may occur. The child may have hypertension, azotemia and hematuria.

The laboratory findings on the urine and blood are important in fitting the treatment to the needs of the individual child. Typical findings include proteinuria (the presence of protein in the urine), with an albumin-globulin ratio between 5:1 and 1:1. There is heavy loss of albumin in the urine, up to 10 to 15 gm. or more of protein daily. Diuresis of large amounts of urine results in disappearance of the edema. Persistent hematuria (red blood cells in the urine) may indicate a serious prognosis. Blood changes involve protein and lipids. Sufficient lowering of the serum albumin level takes place to produce a reversal in the normal albumin-globulin ratio. There is an increase in the blood lipids, especially the cholesterol fraction, with levels of 300 to 1800 mg. per 100 ml. A secondary anemia may be present. The erythrocyte sedimentation rate is rapid.

**Complications and Treatment.** *Complications* are infrequent today, since infections are controlled with antibiotics.

The objectives of *treatment* are control of infections, normal adjustment of the disturbed processes, control of edema and promotion of good nutrition and, of equal importance, good mental hygiene.

Control of acute infection is achieved through administration of sulfadiazine or penicillin between exacerbations of the disease, and prompt antibacterial therapy if an acute infection develops.

The diet should be well balanced, complete, and high in protein to compensate for the constant loss of protein in the urine. It may be advisable to limit the salt intake for short periods during the course of the disease. Children do not accept salt-poor diets, however, and their nutrition is likely to suffer if such a diet is all that is given them.

Reduction of the edema through diuresis is induced in the following way. Corticotropin or one of the corticosteroids is about the only practical, effective way to do this. Hormonal therapy is widely used in the treatment of nephrosis. Short-term therapy stimulates diuresis, but today more prolonged therapy is being used. Corticotropin is given parenterally, and prednisone is commonly given orally. This therapy is started when the condition is first recognized. Steroid is given daily for about four weeks. Then there is a clinical remission with disappearance of the proteinuria. Diuresis usually occurs in seven to fourteen days.

Intermittent hormonal therapy may be given between exacerbations. Smaller doses are ordered than when the child is on intensive therapy during an exacerbation. If the blood pressure is elevated, hormonal therapy is withdrawn. Since hormonal therapy masks the signs of infection, antibiotic therapy should be given with it.

Attempts to elevate the serum protein levels by giving blood plasma have not been very successful in inducing diuresis. Plasma, concentrated salt-poor albumin or other plasma substitutes may be tried only temporarily. Diuretics are usually ineffective in reducing edema. Nitrogen mustard may induce diuresis, however.

Peritoneal drainage may be necessary if a large ascitic collection of fluid is causing respiratory or cardiac distress. If advanced renal failure is evident, fluid intake should vary with the urine volume and the child's capacity to concentrate urine.

Complete bed rest is necessary only during severe edema and when other symptoms are present. The child is allowed out of bed for supervised activity as often as his condition permits, but he must be protected from infectious contacts.

Reduction of anxiety in parents and

child is important. The physician should give the parents support and encouragement during the course of the illness. He should discuss the nature of the disease with them and the therapy he is using. Whenever possible, children should be treated at home and brought to the hospital only for special therapy or expert care.

**Nursing Care.** Nursing care is the most important element in treatment. The parents should be allowed unlimited or frequent visiting and permitted to help in the care of the child. Thereby the harmful effects of maternal deprivation will be avoided, and the parents may express their love for the child in a normal way which brings relief from their frustrating feeling of helplessness, and a sense of security to the child.

Careful attention must be given to protect the edematous skin from injury or infection. The child should be bathed frequently, with special attention to the moist parts of the body. A boy's genitals should be bathed several times a day and dusted with soothing powder; they may be supported with a soft pad held in place by a T binder. Adhesive should never be used on edematous skin. A pillow should be placed between the knees when the child is lying on his side.

All skin surfaces that are in contact should be separated and cotton placed between them, in order to prevent intertrigo (see p. 110).

The edematous area about the eyes and lids requires attention. The eyes should be irrigated with warm saline solution to prevent a collection of exudate. The child's head should be elevated during the day to reduce discomfort from the edema.

In order to prevent respiratory infection the child should be kept warm and dry and turned frequently. He should not be exposed to infection through contact with other children in the unit or with personnel who have a cold, sore throat or other infection.

Nutrition is important, but difficult to maintain, since the child is not hungry during periods of severe edema. A well balanced diet should be given, high in protein to compensate for that lost in the urine. The food should be attractively served on colored dishes, with colored straws provided for the taking of liquids. Small amounts of easily digested foods should be offered, and the child may be permitted to help himself to "seconds."

The child should be weighed as ordered by the physician—usually daily or two or three times a week. The gain or loss in weight is evidence of the amount of edema present.

An accurate record of intake and output is always valuable. This is difficult, if not impossible, with little children who are only partially toilet-trained and may have regressed during their sickness. If the urine cannot be measured, the amount voided can be estimated by noting the size of the moist area. The color of the urine should also be charted.

If the child has ascites which interferes with respiration, he may be placed in a semi-upright position until a paracentesis can be done. When abdominal paracentesis is to be performed, the nurse should explain the procedure to the child in order to gain his cooperation. The child should void just before paracentesis so that there will be less danger of puncturing the bladder. The equipment and the exact procedure used vary in different hospitals.

In general, the responsibilities of the nurse are as follows:

Nurse No. 1: Sets up the equipment and prepares the area, collects samples of ascitic fluid for culture, and checks the child's color during the procedure.

Nurse No. 2: Explains the procedure step by step to the child. She places him in a sitting position on the edge of the table and supports his back with her body. She clasps the child's hands in hers. No further restraint is necessary if the child cooperates. The nurse should talk to him, have him close his eyes and turn his head away from the site of the puncture.

Ascitic fluid is not permitted to run

too quickly or in too large amounts from the abdomen because too rapid reduction of intra-abdominal pressure causes the blood to distend the deep abdominal veins and reduce the normal supply to the heart. This may cause shock.

When the procedure is over, an abdominal binder is applied rather snugly, and the child is put to bed. The nurse must observe and carefully chart the amount of drainage and the child's condition.

During the long course of the disease, when his condition permits, the child should be allowed play activities appropriate to his age, interests and state of health. The Play Lady may visit his bed, or he may be taken to the play room if there is no danger of his contracting an infection from the other children.

**Instructions to the Mother on Discharge of the Child.** The physician explains the nature of the illness and its therapy to the parents. The nurse may further discuss the child's specific diet, the administration of medications, prevention of infection, skin care and the need for continued medical supervision.

Discipline is a serious problem in any long-term condition in the toddler. Parents should be consistent in their discipline of the child and in setting limits to his freedom. A happy home atmosphere is probably the most important factor in establishing discipline. In a happy situation a child is conditioned to cooperate.

**Prognosis.** The course is variable, and is usually characterized by recurrent episodes of edema which may be of short duration or may last for some time. Since antibacterial therapy has been successfully used to control intercurrent infections, a large number of children survive until nephrosis spontaneously disappears.

Corticotropin or one of the corticosteroids has had favorable results in many nephrotic children. It has been used in both short- and long-term therapy.

If the child does not die from concurrent infection, he has a chance of complete cure, or chronic nephritis or renal failure with a fatal outcome may ensue.

## Acrodynia (Pink Disease, Erythredema)

**Etiology, Incidence and Diagnosis.** The *etiology* is not proved. The disease is believed to be caused by poisoning or unusual sensitivity or idiosyncrasy to mercury. Mercury is excreted in the urine. The sources of mercury poisoning include accidental poisoning, calomel, mercurial ointment and diaper rinses. Other less probable causes are chronic infections, poisoning by chemicals and viral infections.

The condition occurs most frequently during late infancy and early childhood (the toddler period). Acrodynia is disappearing from most parts of the United States, owing to the declining use of mercurial teething lotions and powders, local ointments, and anthelmintics. Children must still be protected from accidental ingestion of substances containing mercury.

The *diagnosis* is based on the distinctive clinical appearance and the course of the disease.

**Clinical Manifestations, Laboratory Findings and Pathology.** The *clinical manifestations* are unusual and form a characteristic pattern. The onset is insidious. The child becomes increasingly miserable, irritable, restless and at times apathetic. The palms of the hands and soles of the feet are red and slightly swollen. This *pinkness* is accompanied by painful itching which causes the child to rub and scratch the affected areas constantly. Later the red skin desquamates. The redness of the hands fades into pink at the wrists and gradually turns to the normal color of the flesh. The child experiences perverted sensations, and older children complain of burning. The body presents a diffuse erythema and profuse perspiration. The cheeks and nose are a pronounced pink. In severe cases the gums are red and swollen. The deciduous teeth are lost, and there is increased salivation. The nails loosen and fall out, and there is loss of hair. The blood pressure is high,

Figure 180.   Extreme hypotonia and photophobia in a child with acrodynia. This bizarre position may be maintained for hours. (J. B. Bilderback, in Nelson: Textbook of Pediatrics. 7th ed.)

the pulse rate elevated. Fever is not usually present unless there is a concurrent respiratory infection or pyuria. Acute upper respiratory tract infection with moderate fever is associated with acrodynia.

The child's personality changes. The hyperesthesia of the skin and muscles results in dislike of and resentment at being handled. Fretfulness and irritability are frequent characteristics of the condition. There is a decrease in muscular activity (sitting, standing and walking), and the child is hypotonic. He may assume bizarre positions. The knee-chest position is characteristic. Because of photophobia he hides his face.

Anorexia results in malnutrition. Since the child may have moderate fever and perspires freely, he drinks large quantities of water. He has difficulty in sleeping, owing to severe pain. He is thoroughly miserable and constantly dejected and does not smile or play. He is unlike his normal self, and this change in personality causes his mother as much anxiety as does his physical condition.

The main *laboratory finding* is mercury in the urine.

No characteristic *pathologic changes* have been observed.

**Treatment.**   BAL (British anti-lewisite) is effective against some heavy metal poisons such as mercury. Treatment should be started early. The drug is administered intramuscularly in a 10 per cent solution. It often causes undesirable side effects such as lacrimation, nausea and vomiting, salivation, headache, burning sensation, pain in the teeth, sweating, a feeling of tightness in the chest, fever and restlessness.

Opiates are not given except in temporary emergencies for discomfort; there is too much danger of addiction. Paraldehyde in olive oil may be given rectally to reduce discomfort. Priscoline may also be given to produce symptomatic relief.

The diet should be high in proteins, minerals and vitamins. If anorexia is extreme, gavage feedings may be given. Copious amounts of fluids are needed to replace those lost through profuse sweating. If a child will not drink fluids in sufficient amounts, parenteral fluid therapy may be necessary.

If the acrodynia is believed to be due to a focus of infection, this should be removed; if respiratory infection occurs, it should be treated with antibiotics.

**Nursing Care.**   Nursing care must be adapted to the personality changes in the individual toddler. The child may be active, restless and irritable, but is usually negativistic or apathetic. The nurse must be firm but kind, and react to his behavior with insight into the cause. These children cannot respond in the usual way to kindness from the nurse. She must understand this and accept the child's reaction, knowing that it is conditioned by his sickness. She must attempt to alleviate his discomfort and anxiety. When he feels more comfortable, his reaction to the nurse will be more normal.

To keep the child from injuring himself, the sides of the crib should be covered on the inside with soft pads or blankets. When he is placed in his high chair, he must wear a restraining jacket because he is likely to fall. Elbow restraints are required to prevent his chewing his fingers or pulling his hair.

Because of his profuse perspiration and to minimize the chances of a secondary pyogenic infection, the child should have frequent baths. Tub baths rather than sponge baths should be given, since a sponge bath increases the painful itching. The clothing should be light and preferably of cotton; it must be changed frequently because of the perspiration.

Mouth care should be given to prevent infection when the gums are inflamed. Gentleness is necessary so that trauma does not occur to the mucosa. Because of photophobia, the child should be protected from bright lights.

The child should be offered high vitamin fluids at frequent intervals. The nurse should feed him if his palms are sore or if the exertion of feeding himself causes fatigue. He should not be forced to eat, since vomiting may result. If necessary, he may be fed by gavage (see p. 150).

Every precaution should be taken to prevent cross-infection from contact with other children, and he should not be nursed by personnel who have upper respiratory tract infections. He must be kept warm, for chilling predisposes to contracting infection. Sedation may be needed for insomnia and is given as ordered to prevent exhaustion. If BAL is given, the nurse should watch for indications of undesirable effects. The child should be weighed routinely to determine weight loss.

Recreation suited to his condition should be provided. During the acute stage of the disease these children are seldom eager to play. But a child who feels secure in his nurse's care will enjoy having her read aloud to him or play his favorite pieces on a record player. Recreation helps the child, and also his parents, to adjust to his condition.

**Complications, Course, Prognosis and Prevention.** *Complications* which may arise are pneumonia, pyuria, diarrhea and prolapse of the rectum.

The *course* of the disease may extend from several months to a year. Mortality rates are low, but are higher among hospitalized children than among those treated at home, owing to the greater probability of contracting respiratory infections, particularly pneumonia.

Home is the best place for the acrodyniac toddler. The parents should be made familiar with the nature and the course of the disease. They must be taught how to give the child adequate care.

*Prevention* lies in avoidance of medications containing mercury and in keeping the child safe from the accidental ingestion of mercury preparations.

### Lead Poisoning

**Etiology, Incidence and Clinical Manifestations.** Lead poisoning is most common during later infancy and the toddler period. Lead can enter the body through the gastrointestinal tract, skin or lungs. The usual route of entrance in children is through the mouth. Infants may suck lead nipple shields. Little children suck, or chew when teething, painted or lead toys, crib rails, window sills and furniture. (Revarnished or repainted wood is apt to come off in flakes.) Toddlers put colored crayons into their mouths and may swallow bits scraped off by their teeth. Outdoors, toddlers may chew upon painted stair railings, swings or fences, but are more likely to break off and swallow bits of dried paint from painted wood surfaces.

Water carried in lead pipes may contain a trace of lead. Lead may be inhaled with the fumes caused by burning storage batteries, though this is seldom the cause of poisoning in the toddler group.

The *incidence* of lead poisoning appears to be increasing in the tenement areas of large cities. The walls in old tenement buildings are likely to have layer upon layer of paint. Paints used years ago had a higher percentage of lead than house paints used today. Paint made for outdoor use today has more lead than that for indoor use, which has less than 1 per cent. In old buildings layers of paint come off in thick flakes which the child may put into his mouth, chew and swallow. This increase in the incidence of lead poisoning may be more apparent than real, however. Today there are fewer missed cases, because children of the lower-income group receive better health supervision than in the past.

The residual effects of lead toxicity on the nervous system may be permanent and progressive.

The *clinical manifestations* and severity depend upon the degree of cerebral irritation. The onset is insidious except in the rare cases of acute poisoning. Progressive poisoning usually occurs as the result of slow absorption or accumulation of lead in the blood and soft tissues. Vascular changes occur in the brain, with destruction of brain cells, intense edema and neuroglial disintegration. Lead is transferred slowly from the soft tissues to the bone. The symptoms depend upon the amount of lead in the soft tissues and the blood. Lead is excreted in the urine.

*Acute lead poisoning* is rare and occurs only after accidental ingestion of lead salts or inhalation of lead fumes. The child has nausea, vomiting, abdominal pain, convulsions and finally coma. Renal damage is common. Shock may cause death in two or three days. If the child recovers from the acute stage, symptoms of chronic poisoning may follow.

The clinical manifestations of *chronic lead poisoning* depend on the degree and rate of transport of lead from the intestine or bone (lead is stored in

bones) to the blood or soft tissues. In mild cases the child has weakness, loss of weight, irritability and vomiting. He is pale and suffers from headache, abdominal pain, anorexia and insomnia.

In severe cases there are lesions in various systems of the body. Encephalitis occurs after a short period of exposure, owing to the extreme vulnerability of the child's central nervous system. Children suffering from lead poisoning are anemic, and have colic, peripheral neuritis, muscular incoordination, joint pains and a labile pulse rate. Convulsions may occur, followed by stupor and death in coma.

**Diagnosis and Treatment.** The *diagnosis* is suspected from the history of exposure to lead and the clinical manifestations of poisoning: the so-called lead line (a bluish line) on the gums, roentgenographic evidence of increased density at the ends of the long bones, basophilic stippling of red blood cells seen on a smear, excessive concentration of lead in the urine or blood, excretion of coproporphyrin in the urine, a mild degree of glycosuria and, when lead encephalopathy is present, findings of cerebrospinal fluid under pressure and possibly containing large amounts of protein and a few cells.

The immediate *treatment* of acute lead poisoning is by gastric lavage, if poisoning has resulted from the ingestion of lead, followed by catharsis with magnesium sulfate and, if necessary, specific measures to counteract shock. The child should be given milk to form insoluble salts in the intestines. To increase the excretion of lead which may have been absorbed, and thereby decrease its concentration in the blood as rapidly as possible, EDTA (calcium disodium versenate) may be given. This forms a nonionized chelate with lead which is excreted in the urine. EDTA is usually given by intravenous infusion; it may be administered orally, but its action is delayed when it is given by this route. BAL also causes an increase in the urinary excretion of lead, but since it does not combine with lead in the tissues, it is of little value and is not used.

Chronic lead poisoning may follow

acute poisoning if all traces of lead have not been removed before absorption takes place. For this reason, after emergency care, if there is any reason to believe that absorption of lead has taken place, the treatment outlined below is given.

Chronic lead poisoning is commonly the result of taking into the body (with children almost always by ingestion) small amounts of lead over a period of time. When a child is brought to the hospital for chronic lead poisoning, it is not probable that he has ingested lead recently. Lead may be in the intestines, but is not likely to be in the stomach. For this reason lavage is not given routinely. The other measures outlined for the treatment of acute lead poisoning may be ordered.

The objective of further treatment is to reduce the concentration of lead in the blood and tissues, and to promote its deposition in the bones. Treatment to prevent absorption from the intestinal tract has been outlined. Further ingestion of lead must be prevented by removing from the environment all sources from which the child might ingest lead.

To promote and hasten the deposition of lead in the bones, large amounts of calcium, phosphorus and vitamin D are given. Since both electrolyte imbalance (acidosis) and infections inhibit deposition of lead in the bones, such conditions must be corrected.

Lead colic is treated with antispasmodics such as atropine or opiates. Convulsions due to encephalopathy are controlled with phenobarbital. Increased intracranial pressure may be reduced by repeated lumbar punctures, removing a small amount of fluid at a time to prevent brain-stem herniation. In some children surgical decompression by craniectomy may be necessary. Oxygen may be given for respiratory depression. Parenteral fluids may be administered for fluid and electrolyte imbalance. Urinary retention may be relieved by catheterization.

Treatment to delead the tissues completely takes months, but is essential to prevent recurrence of the symptoms of lead poisoning.

**Nursing Care.** Nursing care is symptomatic, meeting the needs of the individual child. If the child has convulsions, all unnecessary handling should be avoided, since it may stimulate the central nervous system. Nursing care should be planned around periods when medications are to be given.

If the child is in coma, he is fed by gavage. He must be turned frequently from side to side, and good skin care is essential. For collection of urine specimens the receptacle must be very clean and free from lead, because the amount of lead found in the urine is exceedingly small.

**Prognosis and Prevention.** The *prognosis* is generally poor. About half of the affected small children have manifestations of encephalitis. The mortality rate is about 25 per cent in these cases. Many of the children who recover have permanent mental or neurologic sequelae, such as mental retardation. Close observation is necessary after treatment for a long time in order to prevent further damage to the central nervous system. The incidence of permanent damage to the central nervous system increases with the duration of exposure to lead.

Children who have pica or perverted appetite may continue to ingest lead over long periods. All possible sources of lead should be removed from their environment, and they should be closely supervised to keep them from obtaining lead from those sources which it is not feasible to remove.

*Prevention* is doubly important because treatment is not highly successful. Manufacturers in the United States are required to use lead-free paint on all children's toys and furniture. Amateur painters in the home, however, may repaint furniture with paint containing lead. The public is being educated constantly about the danger involved in the ingestion of paint. The public health nurse also does this in part while visiting in a home where potential sources of lead poisoning exist.

In many areas the incidence of lead poisoning must be reported to the public health department. The public health nurse then makes a visit to the home to guide the parents in removing any source of lead from the child's environment.

### Cerebral Palsy

The diagnosis and treatment of cerebral palsy are particularly important during the toddler period if parental attitudes are to be properly formed and the child is to have the foundation of experience necessary for normal emotional development in the years to follow. Although for many years such children have been treated during infancy for the physical manifestations of the condition, it is only recently that the intellectual and emotional aspects have been studied.

Diagnosis may not be possible during the first year of life, but can usually be made during the toddler period, at which time the question of the child's normal mentality arises. Proper handling of his intellectual and emotional development is as important as his physical care.

**Incidence and Etiology.** Cerebral palsy is the term commonly used for difficulty in controlling the voluntary muscles due to damage to some portion of the brain. There is no common etiology, pattern of clinical manifestations, treatment or prognosis for such children. The problem ranges from very mild to severe. The damage is fixed, however, and does not become progressively greater. For this reason it is possible to map out a long-term program of development of those capacities which the child possesses.

The *incidence* of the condition is from 100 to 600 cases per 100,000 population.

The specific *etiology* is obscure. There are many causes of brain damage which result in this condition; some of these causes are clear, others are not. Damage occurring prenatally, at birth or during infancy has already been discussed. Examples of such causes of cerebral palsy are developmental malformation of the cerebrum, anoxia (see p. 184), narcosis at birth

with anoxia, erythroblastosis fetalis (see p. 159) with resulting kernicterus, and intracranial hemorrhage (see p. 166). Damage which may occur in infancy or the toddler period includes lead poisoning (see p. 473), head injury with subdural hematoma (see p. 381), brain damage due to febrile illness, encephalitis (see p. 542), meningitis (see p. 544) and hydrocephalus (see p. 218). In many children no single etiologic factor can be established.

**Diagnosis, Types and Clinical Manifestations.** In some children the *diagnosis* can be made soon after birth. It is based on the following symptoms: feeding problems, afebrile convulsions and failure to follow the normal pattern of motor development (see Chap. 12). In other children the diagnosis is not made until the toddler period.

Two *types* of cerebral palsy account for about 75 per cent of all cases. They are those cases marked by either spasticity or athetosis. *Spasticity* is characterized by tension in certain muscle groups (see Fig. 181, *A*). The stretch reflex is present in the involved muscles. This is the most common type of cerebral palsy. *Athetosis* is characterized by involuntary or excess motion (fine wandering movements) which interferes with normal precision of movement (see Fig. 181, *B*). Various degrees of muscle tension are present.

A third type of cerebral palsy is *ataxia*, which is characterized by a disturbance of the sense of balance and posture. Children with this condition walk as though they were inebriated. A fourth type, marked by *rigidity*, is characterized by resistance in the extensor and flexor muscles. A fifth type is characterized by *tremor*, in which there are fine muscular movements with a rhythmic pattern.

The *clinical manifestations* vary with the type of cerebral palsy.

Spasticity is the most common evidence of motor disability. The child is unable to control the voluntary muscles, nor can the examiner control them. Certain muscle groups have abnormally strong tonus which keeps portions of the body, mostly the extremities, in characteristic positions. In severe cases deformity of position may occur. The child's voluntary efforts to move such muscles result in jerky motions, making walking, eating and other co-ordinated movements difficult. The parts of the body commonly affected are the lower extremities (the child crosses his legs and points his toes), the arms (the fist is clenched, the fore-arm flexed, the upper arm pressed against the wall of the chest) and the trunk (the head is extended and the back arched).

The spasticity varies from very mild to a severe involvement which produces a helpless child. In very severe cases swallowing may be difficult because of involvement of the muscles of the face, jaw, tongue and pharynx.

In some cases of spasticity groups of muscles are weakened. Weakness may be present without spasticity, however.

Disturbances other than these physi-cal problems may be due to brain dam-age, but they may be caused or accen-tuated by the parents' reaction to the total problem. Psychologic and emo-tional problems may be more hamper-ing to the child's development than his motor difficulties. There may be vary-ing degrees of mental retardation, but this is not always an accompaniment of cerebral palsy. Speech, sight and hear-ing defects may complicate the case and influence the child's interaction with other members of his family and, later, with his social life in the com-munity. Convulsions further compli-cate the problem.

The child with cerebral palsy appears to be emotionally unstable. Emotional instability is due primarily to his physi-cal condition, but also to the psycho-logic treatment he has received. His basic human needs for acceptance, for love from his parents, his peers and others, for exploration of his environ-ment, for play, for learning as other children do and for the feeling of status which comes through gradually increas-ing independence are seldom satisfied. He is therefore likely to be chronically emotionally depressed.

If the child has speech problems, he is unable to communicate verbally in a normal manner, if at all, with others. If he cannot see well, he is unable to have vicarious experiences through reading or motion pictures—experi-ences which would enrich the limited use he is able to make of his physical

**Figure 181.** Cerebral palsy. A, Spasticity. B, Athetosis. (From Courville: Cerebral Palsy, San Lucas Press; in Cardwell: Cere-bral Palsy—Advances in Understanding and Care. New York, Association for the Aid of Crippled Children.)

A          B

and social environments. If he cannot write, he has further difficulty in establishing satisfactory relations with others. It is in the toddler period that the basis for development of what capacities he has must be laid.

Although the mentality of these children is likely to be affected, many have normal levels of intelligence. With education and special training they may become useful citizens. Even those with intelligence below normal may be trained to earn their living or at least to provide self-care.

**Treatment and Nursing Care.** If children with cerebral palsy are to develop to the fullest extent their capacity to lead normal lives, they should be under the supervision of the cerebral palsy team. This team includes the pediatrician, social worker, surgeon, orthopedist, psychologist or psychiatrist, physiotherapist, speech therapist, teachers, nurses and the child's parents.

It is difficult to identify all children with cerebral palsy during infancy and the toddler period. Missed cases are found at school age, since attendance at school is compulsory. The missed cases are usually in the low-income group, particularly in families living in isolated rural areas. Middle-class parents seek help if they see that their child is not normal; also their children are under the care of a private physician from infancy throughout childhood. Follow-up by public health nurses of newborn infants and continued health supervision through clinics and Child Health Conferences have decreased the number of cases in which professional help has been delayed until school age.

Before treatment can be begun it is necessary to evaluate not only the child's physical condition, but also his intellectual capacity, since his treatment will be determined by his individual needs. It is difficult to evaluate the mental capacity of a child until he is old enough to cooperate on performance tests which use motor abilities. On the best available information realistic short- and long-term programs are planned and re-evaluated as treatment progresses.

The goal of therapy differs with each child. No treatment can restore a damaged brain to a normal functioning level. The aim is *habilitation,* because new habits have to be established rather than lost functions replaced. The goal is to appraise individual assets and potentialities and to capitalize on these in order to create as useful and well adjusted a person as possible. Muscles must be used for new functions, and this training must be made a satisfying, rather than a frustrating, process for the child.

Parents must be helped to accept the child with his assets and liabilities while he is still an infant or as soon as the team is able to evaluate his potentialities. They need help in learning how to care for the child and to feel secure in their ability to fulfill the parental role which they have learned to adapt to his needs.

Care includes planning for special problems connected with respiration, feeding, relaxation, play and education.

*Problems of respiration* in early life are due to cerebral lesions or to mucus in the infant's throat, or to both. Mucus can be removed by aspiration. The infant's position should be changed frequently to reduce his discomfort.

*Feeding problems* may be caused by his difficulty in sucking and swallowing. The child may vomit easily. To help him take his feeding, he should be fed slowly. The nurse must be patient when giving him solid food, since often he cannot control the muscles of the throat. Feeding these children requires skill, acquired only by experience, and the student nurse should not be discouraged if at first she is not successful. Helping the child to learn to feed himself is even more difficult. He needs a spoon and a fork (if he is able to control his hand adequately) with special handles so that he can grasp them readily (see Fig. 182). The plate should be attached to the table so that he does not push it about when he attempts to get food on his spoon or fork.

*Problems of relaxation* have a special meaning for these children, who are under a constant strain even when at

Figure 182.    Independent eating is facilitated by practice with special equipment. (Courtesy of Children's Division, Institute of Rehabilitation and Physical Medicine, New York University–Bellevue Medical Center; in Cardwell: Cerebral Palsy—Advances in Understanding and Care. New York, Association for the Aid of Crippled Children.)

empting to perform the simple acts which others carry out unconsciously

without giving attention to their movements. Although palsied children tire easily, they find it difficult to relax. They need frequent rest periods in a quiet room with few stimuli of any sort. They should not be excited before rest time or bedtime.

These children must be disciplined with understanding. If they feel secure and relaxed, they have far better control over their movements than if they are nervous, angry or afraid. The adult who can be firm, but not rejecting, in her manner and words not only wins their cooperation, but also provides the social environment in which they are physically able to cooperate. The child's success in muscular control, whether of the muscles of the legs and arms or of those involved in speech and swallowing, reduces his frustration. The palsied child is happier with adults who set limits within which he can function successfully and is thereby less likely to arouse irritation in others. Relaxation is for him a skill which must be learned; it is not a natural capacity as it is with other children. After he has learned to relax he can learn purposeful motions which enable him to get the results he desires.

*Play problems* are many, but can be

Figure 183.    Parallel play. (Courtesy of National Society for Crippled Children and Adults; in Cardwell: Cerebral Palsy—Advances in Understanding and Care. New York, Association for the Aid of Crippled Children.)

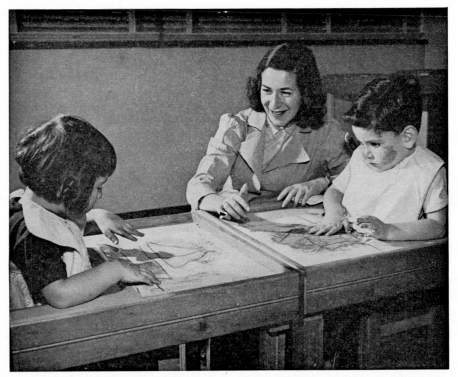

**Figure 184.**  The occupational therapist helps these children to have fun as they learn to finger paint. (From Mary Stewart: Role of the Nurse in Pediatric Rehabilitation. Health News, Vol. 33.)

met successfully (see Fig. 183). No child leads a normal life if he does not play. But play with these children must be gentle, without excitement, and involving only slow changes in stimulation. Mothers and nurses must show creativity and ingenuity in finding toys which will be safe for him and also have educational value. He needs toys for enjoyment, but he also needs others which foster learning, encourage self-expression or help in social interaction with other children. When he reaches school age, it is important for him to play in groups so that he will make friends and learn to interact successfully with his peers. He should feel that other children are his peers, that he is their equal, even if he cannot do all that they do and makes uncouth blunders which interfere with play.

The child's *education* includes training in self-care and social relations as well as formal education. It should begin in nursery school, if not earlier and must be adjusted to his capacity so that he has joy in achieving what is expected of him. When he enters grade school, his work must be adjusted to his mental capacity as well as to his physical limitations. In most cities there are special schools, or special classes in the regular schools, for handicapped children. In these classes or schools, teachers plan the educational programs to meet the needs of small groups of children who have somewhat similar abilities. These schools provide for muscle re-education and physical therapy and often psychologic help for the child who has emotional problems.

The cerebral palsy team may give other forms of therapy either at the school or in conjunction with the school program. Children whose handicap is not so great may attend the regular school classes, or be in special classes for some subjects and in the regular classes for other subjects in which they can be taught with normal children. When education is adapted to the palsied child's individual potential, the child can gain security from being able to be with normal children. Possibly he may excel in some area of study. Working with other children will help to eliminate feelings of inferiority and self-pity. If the child has difficulty in articulation, speech training will be necessary.

One advantage of the special school or classes for these children is that the furniture is designed so that the cerebral palsied child can work in comfort.

*Hospitalization.* Parents may need help in meeting the problems connected with hospitalization of the child. Long-term hospitalization is a financial drain upon the income of the average family. When hospitalization is necessary, the parents, even if they carry hospitalization insurance, may be unable to pay the full hospital and medical bills and still maintain the family level of living which is essential for the other children in the family, as well as for the sick child when he returns home. Such cases are referred to the social worker, who will arrange for financial assistance from a state or community agency.

Parents may not understand why the child must be hospitalized, the treatment he will need or how long he must be away from home. They may be unwilling to leave him in the hospital because they think that he, more than a normal child, will suffer from maternal deprivation. The nurse can do a great deal to help the parents view the child's condition realistically.

Life in the pediatric unit of a general hospital or in a children's hospital should be planned for the emotional growth as well as the physical improvement of the children. Absence from home may be made a maturing experience for these children, particularly if they have been overprotected at home.

The physical care of children with cerebral palsy includes the prevention of contractures. This is difficult for the parents to understand. They have tried

**Figure 185.** Group play helps the child to achieve satisfactory relations with others and prepares him for daily life after his return home. (From Mary Stewart: Role of the Nurse in Pediatric Rehabilitation. Health News, Volume 33.)

**Figure 186.** The modern concept of total habilitation is to help the child attain the highest degree of independence of which he is capable. This child shows obvious delight in walking for the first time without braces. (From Mary Stewart: Role of the Nurse in Pediatric Rehabilitation. Health News, Volume 33.)

to make the child as comfortable as possible by allowing him to assume any position and maintain it for as long as he wanted. Corrective splints may be ordered. Usually these are applied only at night, but leg splints may be used during the day also to enable the child to stand. Programs of remedial exercise depend upon the specific needs of the child.

Surgical treatment for orthopedic deformities may be necessary. This may involve the severing of nerves leading to the spastic extremities, lengthening of the tendon of Achilles or other surgical procedure to improve the child's muscular control.

If the child has had a cast applied, the nursing care is that of other patients in casts (see p. 237). If he has not achieved control of bladder and bowel, he may be placed on a Bradford frame (see p. 215). Medical treatment may include drugs to decrease nervous tension or a tendency to convulsions.

Braces may be used to enable the spastic child to control his motions or to correct his deformity. Physiotherapy is important to prevent contractures and stimulate control of movement.

Public health nurses and hospital nurses are members of the health team caring for children with cerebral palsy. The team serves the children in their homes, in hospitals, schools and summer camps. Nurses help mothers learn how to give the daily care the child needs and to interpret his needs to other members of the family, and to his school teachers. As the child grows older his contacts outside the home increase. Even the toddler is admitted to some nursery schools for handicapped children, and older children go to camp in the summer and join play groups planned particularly for them. Nurses contact professional workers in these areas of the child's life and help them to coordinate these special services with the general plan of treatment made by the cerebral palsy team for the individual child.

In large cities there are organizations which offer guidance to the parents of children with cerebral palsy. The nurse works closely with the staff of such an organization. Many of these organizations provide group play for the children and vocational training for the adolescents. Each year more such groups are supporting research on the etiology and treatment of cerebral palsy and providing funds for the application of research findings to the habilitation and education of these children.

**Prognosis.** The prognosis depends upon the severity of the physical condition, the child's mental capacity and the treatment which is available. The child of wealthy parents can be taken to one of the leading centers for treatment, and the low-income family is eligible for assistance under state and community programs. These programs vary in quality and the extent of service given, and the prognosis in any case must take into consideration the treatment the child will receive. In general the child with normal intelligence who receives adequate care improves to the extent that he can care for himself and can possibly succeed in a vocation or profession suited to his limitations.

**Summary.** The objective in the care of cerebral palsied children is that each develop his potential capacity. In a physically and socially favorable environment many children develop a healthy personality. The foundation is laid during the toddler period. These children must be helped to face reality, to accept themselves objectively, if they are to make a successful adjustment to the problems caused by their handicaps. A child's attitude toward himself and his relations with other people are formed in early childhood, and successful adjustment in adolescence and adulthood is conditioned by his experiences while still a little child. Adults are tempted to make life easy for him rather than helping him face his problems, solve them and go on to the more complex experiences which come with maturation. He needs help with the developmental tasks which come with growing up. Finally he must face the responsibilities of adulthood. If it is possible, he will want to support himself; if he cannot be self-supporting, he must accept support from others. To assume total self-care gives him a feeling of security and of self-respect. He must adjust to his sexual role in life and to the degree of emancipation from his family which is advisable in his condition.

## Deafness

**Importance of the Problem.** Care of the deaf child is a comprehensive problem which requires teamwork for its solution. There are degrees of deafness. Complete bilateral deafness is an extreme handicap. The deaf miss all the pleasure which sound brings to people with normal hearing and are without the natural means of communicating with others.

Deafness may not be recognized until the child fails to develop speech or is unable to relate himself to others in the family. If the infant or young child fails to respond to loud noises, the acuity of his hearing should be investigated. A child of twelve months who has ceased to vocalize or one of eighteen months who neither speaks nor recognizes words should be examined for deafness.

Unilateral deafness is a different handicap from bilateral deafness and may not be suspected until some accidental occurrence calls the mother's attention to the child's inability to hear in the affected ear. Unilateral deafness, whether partial or complete, should be treated with the same care that is given in bilateral deafness. The child is, of course, not so seriously hampered in his social relations as is the totally deaf child.

Deafness, whether partial or complete, may cause behavior problems and poor adjustment in group relations. Children who are deaf and have no means of communication may become physically aggressive and unmanageable. They may be alert children with normal or above average intelligence and may be remarkably dextrous.

**Etiology and Diagnosis.** Deafness may be congenital, owing to anomalies of the ear, or acquired as the result of disease or injury to the auditory nerve or auditory center in the brain. Diseases causing deafness include congenital syphilis (see p. 164), meningococcal meningitis (see p. 544), encephalitis (see p. 542) and serious chronic otitis media (see p. 296).

Early *diagnosis* is essential. Congenital deafness, if complete, is generally recognized in infancy. Unilateral or partial bilateral deafness may not be recognized until the toddler period, when it may be discovered during a routine check up (see Fig. 187). In

**Figure 187.** The child's speech and hearing are evaluated. Gross hearing tests are followed by audiometric testing if hearing loss is suspected. (From Mary Stewart: Role of the Nurse in Pediatric Rehabilitation. Health News, Volume 33.)

children who are not under health supervision it may not be found until a health examination in nursery or grade school is done. Detection of impaired hearing by routine audiometric tests should be part of the school health examination and repeated every three years. The school nurse or public health nurse may give these tests. When the child has 70 per cent or less of normal hearing, he cannot hear all that the teacher or his classmates say. He needs special help in order to cover the same amount of material as other children.

**Treatment.** Members of the health team necessary for successful treatment of the deaf or partially deaf child are the physician, otologist, audiologist, speech therapist, possibly psychologist or psychiatrist, social worker, nurse, the child's family and the child himself.

Early detection of deafness is necessary for proper speech development and for emotional growth. Training is nec-

essary in understanding the facial expression which goes with words of approval or disapproval, of permission or denial, and in lip reading. Lip reading may start as early as two and a half or three years of age, the period when a child normally learns to talk in sentences. A specialist in work with the deaf, in training children in lip reading and in speaking, seldom begins her work until the child is of nursery school age. The mother should learn to move her lips correctly when speaking in order to supplement the work of the specialist in lip reading. If deafness is partial, a hearing aid is provided for the child at an early age.

Parents are given instruction in the care of their deaf children, and individual conferences are held in which they can receive help with particular problems.

If deafness is due to recurrent otitis media or blockage of the eustachian ube, the services of the otologist should be procured.

If there is a serious hearing loss, special education may be necessary. Nursery schools have been organized for deaf children in many communities, and speech training is often given in connection with them. In some communities instruction in lip reading must be postponed until school age, since there are no facilities for younger children. The sign language or finger language may be taught to supplement lip reading. Training to communicate with others lays the foundation for vocational or professional training or for manual labor, skilled or unskilled, in industry.

Deaf children should be treated as normal children in all respects except their one great handicap; they are normal children who have a hearing loss. Adults who work with them must be patient. Until the child learns to communicate by speech, signs must be used or, if the child has learned to write, signs supplemented with written words.

**Role of the Nurse.**   The nurse helps in discovering deafness or impaired hearing in the infants and little children brought to the clinic or Child Health Conference. The school nurse often gives the routine tests for impaired hearing. If a child who has been ill appears to have difficulty in understanding what is said in class, the teacher may send him to the nurse for testing. The school nurse routinely sees children who are known to have impaired hearing so that she may supervise the physician's program of treatment. Nurses work closely with the personnel of special classes and special schools for the deaf. In clinics for deaf children and those who are hard of hearing nurses have direct contact with not only the child, but also his mother.

**Prognosis.**   The prognosis for the improvement or cure of deafness depends on the degree and nature of the pathologic state or structural defect and on whether the child receives optimal treatment. How well a hearing aid suited to his need and training in lip reading may overcome his physical handicap depends on the availability of such devices and the services of a specialist in teaching deaf children to communicate through speech. If the community does not furnish such help to the child, he may attend a state school for the deaf or a privately supported institution.

If the prognosis is defined in terms of ability to lead a normal life, then for most deaf children it is excellent. This assumes that deafness is their only handicap. If the child is blind as well as deaf or has low mentality, the prognosis is poorer for social adjustment.

**Prevention.**   The prevention of acquired deafness consists in the prevention of infectious disease which is likely to involve the ear. Respiratory infections are a common example. It is difficult, if not impossible, to prevent all infections, but prompt treatment can be given in all cases of upper respiratory tract infections and otitis media.

Impacted wax impairs hearing and may lead to a lesion of the ear. The wax should be removed by the physician. Sinus infection and infected lymphoid tissue in the nasopharynx should be treated promptly. Drugs which endanger the eighth nerve should not be used indiscriminately.

Relatively few cases of deafness in children are caused by injury. Nevertheless the possibility should be considered. The ear drum can be injured when a child puts something sharp into his ear. Injury to the external ear has little effect on hearing. Injury to the brain can affect the centers of hearing and speech.

### Blindness

**Etiology and Importance of the Problem.** The child may be born blind or may acquire blindness from retrolental fibroplasia (see p. 153), trauma, infection during delivery (ophthalmia neonatorum—see p. 162) or congenital syphilis (see p. 164). Other conditions causing blindness in childhood are numerically of relatively little importance.

Children who are blind or have extremely poor vision require special edu-

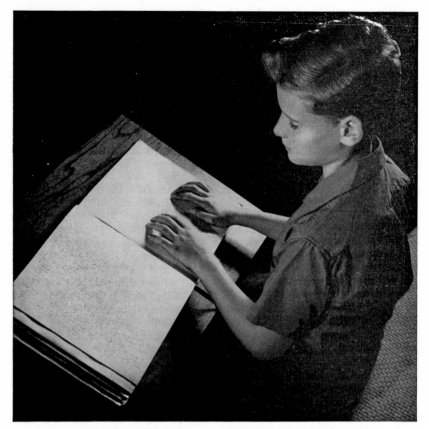

**Figure 188.**   A blind child learns to read Braille. (H. Armstrong Roberts.)

cation and training for daily life activities. Their condition may be improved by medical or surgical procedures and the use of glasses. They may need help in acquiring the everyday skills needed in self-care. Instruction must be given through the sense of hearing or touch. If the child has normal mentality, he is able to take the same subjects in school as normal children do, although his progress may be slower than theirs. Without the same education that normal children receive, the blind child does not grow up with the same interests, attitudes and abilities that the sighted possess.

**Treatment.**   The physical condition is treated, if that is possible, in order to restore or improve sight or to prevent further impairment of vision.

The totally blind child of school age should be enrolled in a school for the blind or, in a school for normal children, in a special class for children with visual problems. Special classes have been established in public and private schools for children whose vision is so poor that they cannot profit from the regular school system of instruction. These schools emphasize the use of auditory instruction and the development of reading skills through touch perception by the Braille system (see Fig. 188). For children who are not totally blind books are printed with extraordinarily large type so that eye fatigue is minimized. Good lighting and correct posture are emphasized.

Children who have some vision may attend regular classes if a teacher skilled in working with blind children gives them help when it is needed. This contact with normal children tends to develop skill in making friends and joining in the activities of the sighted. Being one of the normal group promotes normal social and emotional development.

Parents of blind children must be instructed in the needs of the child. Blindness at birth or developing early in childhood prevents the child from knowing what others mean by colors he cannot see and objects he cannot handle (e.g. the sun, a river or a baby robin). The mother should use such words in their context so that the child gets some idea of the meaning. Blind children need to handle as much of their environment as is practical and build up concepts which other children acquire by sight. If these children have been protected from hurting themselves while exploring the world about them, meeting their own needs and doing what gives them pleasure, they acquire a skill in self-help which children blinded later in life seldom acquire.

Parents must be instructed in the special care required by the blind or partially sighted child. The tendency is to overprotect the child. They find it hard to give him the freedom he must have to build up skills and experience which are necessary when he reaches adolesence and must prepare himself for adult life. Vocational training is given the blind, and for those who are capable and desire it a higher education and preparation for the professions which are open to them. Scholarships and maintenance are provided from private or public sources if the student is in need of financial assistance.

**Role of the Nurse.**   Early detection of impaired vision and blindness is essential for the treatment and education of the child. Infants who do not reach for their bottle or toys and who do not smile when the mother smiles should be examined for blindness. A toddler who walks into the furniture, has no interest in even large pictures and does not respond to the motions of other people should be seen by a physician and have his eyesight tested. Undetected cases of blindness are rare since

facilities for health supervision of children in all economic classes have improved, and since physicians and nurses test for vision as part of the routine physical examinations given in Child Health Conferences and children's clinics.

The blind child needs happiness as all children do and is more dependent than normal children upon the moods of the adults about him. The nurse working with blind children knows that they can interpret her moods by the inflection of her voice as other children do by seeing her smile or frown. She should express quiet happiness in her voice. She must let blind children handle all equipment to be used in their examination or treatments, as well as giving verbal explanations.

**Community Action.**   Community action depends upon the attitude of the people in the community toward blindness. Like parents, the community may tend to overprotect the child. Part of the nurse's responsibility for blind children is to channel the community's sympathy for them into helpful activities.

In some communities play groups for children of preschool age have been organized in which blind children can enjoy play with others like themselves. The playground and the equipment are suited to the needs of blind children, and adequate supervision is provided. Such play helps these children to make social adjustments, which serve as a basis for contacts with the sighted and which can be developed into a normal ability to participate in group activities.

**Prognosis.**   The outcome of treatment varies with every case, and no general statements can be made. Great strides are being made in the prevention of blindness from gonorrhea and syphilis, and with improved care of premature infants there are fewer cases of blindness due to retrolental fibroplasia.

The prognosis for mental health is good. The child who is born blind can usually make a happier adjustment to his handicap than a child who becomes blind in the toddler period or later because of an infection or injury to his eyes. Parent-child relations are more important than any measure which the community can take to help the blind child. But it is the community which provides education and gives the blind person a position in industry or uses the services of the blind professional man or woman. Children with impaired vision may become self-supporting adults fulfilling all the roles of a normal adult. The totally blind find it more difficult to function in society. Their success depends to a great extent upon their early training.

### The Chronically Handicapped Child

Parents of chronically physically or mentally handicapped children should be taught that these children need an environment in which they develop their capacities to the limit, and that the most important element in this environment is the sense of security which loving parents give their children.

Parents may need both financial help and the counsel of experts in fulfilling their exacting role. It is not easy to be a "perfect parent" to a crippled child. The children also must be helped to grow up normally. Severe personality handicaps interfere with their social adjustment more than their physical condition limits successful social interaction. A child acquires emotional problems as a result of deprivation of emotional satisfactions and lack of opportunity to use, and so to develop, his capacities.

It takes months or years for parents to recover from the shock and frustration of having a child who is not normal. They also fear the additional responsibilities involved in the care of such a child, and perhaps most of all they fear society's attitude toward them and the child. These feelings of anxiety and hostility conflict with their normal feeling of love for him.

Such a child disturbs not only parent-child relations, but also all other relations between the members of the family. Parents may manage their feelings in various ways with various reactions on the part of the child. They may deny

the existence of his handicap or over protect him to cover up their negative feelings toward him. Since contact with him causes them anxiety, they may openly reject him and thus not give him the love and security he needs, nor the status of a loved child in the home or that part of the community outside his home where he is learning to adjust to strangers.

Parents may ignore his cues for readiness to learn because they cannot regard him as a person or because they overprotect him. The child therefore does not develop to his potential level. He may even regress.

Help to the parents is given by the whole team of specialists in the crippled children's program: physician, social worker, psychologist or psychiatrist, nurse and others, depending on the child's problem. The nurse must understand normal parent-child relations, the normal developmental process and the needs of the child. She must know how to support parents in accepting problems caused by the child's handicaps, and finally she needs to know the parents well enough to give help when they are ready to accept it. To teach a mother techniques of care before she is ready to learn produces frustration and failure.

The nurse can be a great help to parents when they are discouraged. She must believe in their capacity to care for the child and to give him love and a sense of security. She must communicate to them, not necessarily in words, but by her manner, that she understands their feelings and wants to provide support and assistance.

The nurse must help parents see that their responsibility is to help the child to grow up and to develop his capacity, however little it may be, for self-help in the daily activities of living. Other professional workers have the function of educating the child and giving him many of the pleasures which normal children enjoy, e.g. going to camp in the summer. But it is the parents who give the child experience in daily life within a family. In order to help the parents in their task the nurse must know the evaluation which the total team caring for the child makes of his potential ability. Without such knowledge she cannot communicate realistic goals toward which the parents and the child can work.

The child's response to the help given him is the final test of its success. If the handicapped child feels that his parents are anxious and frustrated, he will feel unloved and may withdraw into a world of fantasy, never developing to his potential level. Some of these children feel only pity for themselves, some try to hurt others as they have been hurt, and others seek punishment for their own negative feelings.

Children who feel loved and wanted are motivated to overcome the limitations of their handicaps or to compensate through success in activities within their ability. These children are likely to succeed beyond what could be expected of them. The handicapped child does not need pity or sympathy. He needs understanding and a knowledge that others accept his differences from the normal and accord him status as an equal.

The nurse must be aware of her own feelings. If she feels repugnance or fear, she should not be ashamed, for most people have the same feelings toward these children. The first step in changing these feelings to a more positive attitude is to know that they exist.

## Crippled Children's Services in the United States

There are more than five and a half million crippled children in the United States known to official agencies. Many others are receiving care elsewhere, and still others are receiving no care. Every state and territory has an official program for their help, generally within the health department. Programs are also developing around medical centers, where personnel needed to help the children are being taught by specialists and where research is a principal part of the program. Regional clinics are developed in connection with these centers.

A well run program combines (1) locating crippled children, (2) treatment (correction if possible), (3) management to promote adaptation to their handicaps and to limit the influence of disabilities upon their lives, and (4) prevention of circumstances in which crippling is likely to occur—e.g. safe delivery of the newborn, immunization for poliomyelitis and prevention of accidents. There is also a secondary aim of attempting to prevent the difficulties in physical, mental, social and economic areas of living caused by the condition of the crippled child—difficulties which may involve the entire family and even the community.

The earliest programs for crippled children dealt almost exclusively with orthopedic conditions. These were extended to include plastic surgery. Today these programs are broad, covering almost any condition which is a serious handicap in normal living. Each state decides what types of cases are to be eligible for assistance under the crippled children's program.

Present programs often include the following: hearing defects, rheumatic fever, heart disease (congenital or rheumatic), certain eye defects, and epilepsy. The reasons for the extension of coverage are that there are now fewer orthopedic cases and cases requiring plastic surgery, and new forms of management have been found for children for whom treatment was formerly unknown.

The first phase in these programs is locating crippled children. Necessary treatment follows, either in the agency sponsoring the program or through referral to another agency which can meet the child's needs. Generally the early programs provided a specialist in the treatment of the child's disability, e.g. an orthopedic surgeon for an orthopedic problem. Today the crippled children's team works with the child, and the community is organized to give many forms of assistance. The public not only gives financial aid for crippled children, but also supports, through the vote, the crippled children's program in the state, county and city. The children are provided for in the public school system, and in some localities special teachers may be sent to the home if the child is confined to bed.

The modern type of service may not carry as heavy a total case load as did the older plan, but better total results are achieved. The newer approach brings together all the resources of the community in prevention, treatment and education. Under the newer program the child lives as normal a life as is possible and is helped to form positive attitudes toward himself and his deformity.

### Emotional Disturbances

When a toddler appears anxious, the conflict between his instinctual desires and the demands of his environment is becoming too much for him to endure. Indications of anxiety at his age are refusal to go to bed, "jittery" behavior during the day, restless sleep at night and disturbance of bowel and bladder functioning.

Toilet training problems are an acute source of anxiety to many children. Children who have achieved bowel and bladder control may have accidents or may play with feces after they have discontinued this habit. If a child has been too severely trained, he may become afraid of moving his bowels, with the result that he becomes constipated. Constipation may also develop because he is negativistic toward his mother, who has done something which he dislikes.

Feeding problems may result from a child's anxiety over toilet training. The child may regress to infantile pleasures in feeding, e.g. sucking.

Stuttering may develop as part of this general pattern of regression. The child adopts the infantile way of breathing; his respirations may become irregular, and he catches his breath. This type of respiration produces difficulty in speaking clearly, and stuttering may result. This anxiety reaction has its inception in a sudden fright or shock which produces a startle reflex accompanied by catching of the breath.

Some toddlers, instead of regressing, may appear to grow up suddenly, one evidence of which is masturbation rather than the momentary handling of the genitals seen in infancy. Some toddlers as a result of too severe toilet training become overclean, not wanting to displease mother by soiling themselves in any way.

A toddler who becomes too anxious over the conflicting desires he experiences will not be able to develop satisfying love relations with an adult, nor a sense of autonomy, which is of vital importance. He will, instead, be overcome by shame and by doubt of his own ability. He should be helped to develop a real love relationship with his mother. She should encourage him to take part in activities which he regards as dirty —playing with mud, sand, plasticine and finger paints. She should laughingly praise him for getting dirty when it results from play. If he gets dirty as a means of evincing hostility toward his mother, she should accept this hostility as normal in children of his age, in the same way that she accepts his immature love responses.

Adequate treatment of anxiety should be instituted early in life so that the prevailing mood during childhood may be happy and emotional development may be normal. Untreated, the anxiety of a child is cumulative. It becomes a habitual reaction which may persist into adult life.

### TEACHING AIDS AND OTHER INFORMATION*

*American Public Health Association*
   Services for Children with Cerebral Palsy.
   Services for Children with Cleft Lip and Cleft Palate.
   Services for Children with Hearing Impairment.
   Services for Children with Vision and Eye Problems.

*Children's Medical Center, Boston, Mass.*
   Cerebral Palsy.
   Harelip and Cleft Palate.

*National Paint, Varnish and Lacquer Association, Inc.*
   How to Prevent Lead Poisoning in the Home.
   Painting Toys and Children's Furniture.

* Complete addresses are given in the Appendix.

*National Society for the Prevention of Blindness*
  Kerby, C. E.: Blindness in Preschool Children.
  Young, M. A. C.: The Partially Seeing—Psychological Aspects.

*Public Affairs Pamphlets*
  Abbott, M.: Cerebral Palsy—Its Scope and Management.
  Wishik, S. M.: How to Help Your Handicapped Child.
  Wood, M.: Blindness—Ability, Not Disability.
  Yahraes, H.: Gains for Handicapped Children.

*U.S. Department of Health, Education, and Welfare*
  Emotional Problems Associated with Handicapping Conditions in Children, 1952.
  The Child Who Is Hard of Hearing, 1953.
  The Child with Cerebral Palsy, 1957.
  The Child with a Cleft Palate, 1953.
  The Preschool Child Who Is Blind, 1953.

## CLINICAL SITUATIONS

When Joanne was fifteen months old, Mrs. Wood brought her to the Child Health Conference and complained that her appetite was poor compared with what it had been during infancy. Joanne appeared healthy and was an extremely active child.

1. In discussing Joanne's apparent anorexia with her mother, the nurse would base her comments on the fact that
  a. Since Joanne is not growing as rapidly as she did during infancy, she should not be expected to eat as much.
  b. Probably Joanne's anorexia is due to the fact that Mrs. Wood had stopped giving her vitamins when she was a year old.
  c. Perhaps Joanne should have a complete physical examination by the physician.
  d. Perhaps Mrs. Wood should be more firm in urging her to eat.

2. Joanne must have her basic emotional needs met if she is to develop a healthy personality. During the toddler period she should have
  a. Unlimited opportunity to do whatever she wants and as much independence as she desires.
  b. Recognition as a little child and protection from harm through rigid obedience to parental rules.
  c. Realistic limits set on her behavior by her parents and increasing independence as she is ready for it.
  d. Recognition as a miniature adult who is able to set limits on her own behavior.

3. Joanne's social development is best described by stating that she prefers to play
  a. Alone, but will share her toys and makes friends quickly with strangers.
  b. Alone, but refuses to share her toys and is shy with strangers.
  c. With other children, usually shares her toys and makes friends quickly with strangers.
  d. With other children, refuses to share her toys and is shy with strangers.

4. The accident rate is high during the toddler period because
  a. Parents tend to neglect children at this age.
  b. Their natural curiosity and activity lead them into danger.
  c. They do not comprehend their parents' warnings of danger.
  d. They are negativistic about everything and refuse to listen to their parents.

One day while Joanne was climbing up the cellar steps she fell from the top landing to the cellar floor. On her admission to the hospital the physician made a diagnosis of a fractured right femur and multiple bruises.

5. Joanne was placed in Bryant traction. In order to maintain traction, the nurse's most important responsibility was to make certain that
  a. Joanne's hips were resting on the bed and her legs were suspended at right angles to the bed.
  b. Joanne's hips were slightly elevated from the bed and her legs were suspended at right angles to the bed.
  c. Joanne's hips were elevated above the level of her body on a pillow and that her legs were suspended in a position of comfort almost parallel to the bed.
  d. Joanne's hips and legs were flat on the bed with the pull of traction coming from the foot of the bed.

6. In order to prevent Joanne from turning to watch activity on the unit, the nurse would
  a. Apply an abdominal restraint and have other children come to her bed to play with her.
  b. Apply clove hitch restraints to her arms and move her bed so that she could watch television.
  c. Apply a restraint jacket and move her bed so that she could watch other children.
  d. Apply no restraints, but move her bed near the center of the unit so that she could watch the activities of the unit personnel.

Mrs. McIntyre called her pediatrician and explained that Betty Jane, age 2½ years, had had a slight cold for 2 days, but that within the last few hours she seemed to have increasingly difficult respirations and was extremely restless. After examining the child the physician recommended immediate admission to the hospital. She was admitted with a diagnosis of laryngotracheobronchitis.

7. Betty Jane was placed in a Croupette. Cool moist air is effective treatment of this condition because it
    a. Causes dilatation of blood vessels in the bronchi, thus relieving the congestion.
    b. Increases the cough reflex, thus making it easier to expectorate mucus.
    c. Coagulates the mucus, thus relieving the dyspnea.
    d. Relieves the dryness of secretions, making them easier to cough up.

8. Betty Jane became emotionally disturbed when her mother said she was going home. You as the nurse would suggest that the mother
    a. Omit visiting for a few days until Betty Jane adjusted to the hospital routine.
    b. Visit only when Betty Jane was sleeping so that she would not disturb the child.
    c. Visit as often and as frequently as she could within the hospital visiting policy.
    d. Discipline the child because her crying is harmful to her.

Since Betty Jane's respiratory distress became more severe and she showed signs of increasing prostration, an emergency tracheotomy was performed.

9. Immediately after the operation the nurse aspirated Betty Jane's tracheotomy tube
    a. As often as secretion appeared at the opening of the tube.
    b. Approximately every 15 minutes.
    c. Whenever Betty Jane appeared to have difficulty in breathing.
    d. Whenever Betty Jane requested that it be done.

10. Betty Jane was afraid to try to swallow after the tracheotomy had been done. The nurse
    a. Offered small amounts of her favorite fruit juice or other liquid at frequent intervals and gave approval when she drank it.
    b. Explained to her that she would get a "needle" if she did not take some juice by mouth.
    c. Told her that her father would give her a dime for every cup of fluid she drank.
    d. Told her she would read a long story to her each time she took a cup of juice.

11. When the nurse aspirated Betty Jane's tracheostomy, she cleaned the inner cannula
    a. By running hot tap water through it and aspirating secretions from it with a catheter.
    b. By soaking it in an antibiotic solution and cleaning the outside with a detergent.
    c. By soaking it in hydrogen peroxide and passing tonsil wire and gauze through it.
    d. By running cold tap water through it and wiping it off with petrolatum.

12. The nurse on one occasion found that Betty Jane had torn off the elbow restraints and had succeeded in pulling out the tracheotomy tube. She was cyanotic, and respirations had apparently ceased. The nurse
    a. Went immediately to the telephone to call the physician, held open the incision with a hemostat and gave mouth-to-mouth resuscitation.
    b. Inserted another tracheotomy tube into the trachea, aspirated the trachea, asked another nurse to call a physician, and gave oxygen through a nasal catheter.
    c. Inserted another tracheotomy tube immediately, asked another nurse to call the physician, gave oxygen through a nasal catheter and provided artificial respiration.
    d. Asked another nurse to call the physician, held open the incision with a hemostat, aspirated the trachea, provided oxygen through the incision, and gave artificial respiration.

13. When Betty Jane was well enough to play in bed, the nurse would assume, on the basis of her understanding of growth and development, that Betty Jane would enjoy
    a. Playing with her favorite toy.
    b. Constructing a tower of 20 blocks.
    c. Listening to popular songs on the radio.
    d. Stringing small beads.

Roosevelt Jones, a two-year-old child, was admitted to the pediatric unit with a diagnosis of chronic lead poisoning. His mother stated that he had eaten paint periodically from his crib and from the window sills over a period of several weeks.

14. Roosevelt should be observed carefully by the nurse for
    a. Hemorrhage from the rectum.
    b. Convulsions.
    c. Edema of the extremities.
    d. Respiratory difficulty.

15. Roosevelt responded well to treatment. One day when the nurse was bathing him, he said, "My mommy does it *this* way." His comment indicates that
    a. He does not like the way the nurse gives a sponge bath.
    b. Routines or rituals learned at home are important to him.
    c. His mother gives a bath better than the nurse.
    d. He hates his nurse.

16. The nurse found Roosevelt in the bathroom, splashing in the water in the toilet. The nurse should
    a. Slap his hands and remove him from the room.
    b. Explain that children should not play in such dirty water.

c. Give him a basin of clean water in which to splash.

d. Take him back to his unit and lock the bathroom door.

17. During his nap Roosevelt wet his bed. The nurse would

a. Change his clothes and bedding and make no issue of it.

b. Tell him that he will catch cold if he lies in a wet bed.

c. Promise to give him a piece of candy if he has no further accidents.

d. Explain that only babies wet their beds.

18. Roosevelt had frequent temper tantrums during his hospitalization. The best way to deal with them would be to

a. Punish him by putting him back in his crib for the rest of the day.

b. Reason with him and tell him why he should not become angry.

c. Prevent temper tantrums by pampering him.

d. Protect him during his tantrums and attempt to prevent them by helping him meet necessary frustrations.

19. The care which Roosevelt should have after a temper tantrum is

a. Ignore him for the rest of the day because he has been a "bad boy."

b. Wash his face and hands and provide a toy for him.

c. Make fun of him before other children in his group.

d. Make him apologize for his behavior.

20. After a prolonged period of hospitalization Roosevelt became a quiet, withdrawn child who evidenced little interest in his mother when she visited. The nurse should realize that

a. He has accepted his hospitalization well and has matured because of his experience.

b. He has finally been disciplined, and she would expect gratitude from his parents.

c. He had probably become a very disturbed little boy because of his traumatic experience.

d. He was ready to be toilet trained because he seemed to enjoy playing with his feces.

## GUIDES FOR FURTHER STUDY

1. During your experience in the pediatric unit observe the motor development of as many toddlers as you can. Compare the similarities and differences among the children in each age group: 15 months, 18 months, 2 years and 2½ years.

2. Investigate the resources in your community for the dissemination of information about the treatment of children who have taken poison. If your community has a Poison Control Center, familiarize yourself with its func-tions. If your community does not have such a facility, discuss with your instructor in seminar your role as a citizen and a nurse in meeting this need.

3. Prepare a plan which you could use to teach a mother the home care of a toddler who has had a tracheotomy. In addition to the content and skills she would need to know, investigate the sources and the approximate cost of the equipment she would need to provide this care.

4. Prepare and give a twenty-minute talk on "Accident Prevention" to a small group of mothers of toddlers in your community. Provide pamphlets and a bibliography for them on this subject. Allow time for discussion at the end of your presentation. Make a list of questions which these mothers asked and submit them with your answers to your instructor.

5. What measures are taken to prevent the spread of staphylococcal infections in your hospital?

6. Investigate the programs and services (public and private) offered for crippled children in your state and your community. Discuss in seminar the adequacy of these programs in relation to the need for them.

7. List the functions of the health team members who coordinate their efforts in the care and habilitation of a child with cerebral palsy. If possible, interview the parents of a child having this diagnosis to determine their feelings about this condition and their reaction to the child's treatment. Identify the nurse's specific responsibilities in providing education for the parents and care for this child throughout his growth period. Discuss your findings and conclusions in seminar.

## REFERENCES

Austin, C.: Mass Preschool Vision Screening. Children, 6:58, 1959.

Barckley, V., and Campbell, E. I.: Helping the Handicapped Child Achieve Emotional Maturity. Am. J. Nursing, 59:376, 1959.

Callison, C.: Nephrosis in Children, Nursing Care. Am. J. Nursing, 56:301, 1956.

Cardwell, V. E.: Cerebral Palsy—Advances in Understanding and Care. New York, Association for the Aid of Crippled Children, 1956.

Carr, L. B.: Preschool Blind Children and Their Parents. Children, 2:83, 1955.

Coyle, I.: The Public Health Nurse in the Cerebral Palsy Program. Nursing Outlook, 4:95, 1956.

Cutler, H. M., and Goldstein, R.: Does He Hear You? Nursing Outlook, 3:286, 1955.

Davidson, M.: The Celiac Syndrome. Pediatrics, 21:508, 1958.

Deaver, G. G.: Cerebral Palsy, Methods of Evaluation and Treatment. Rehabilitation Monograph IX. The Institute of Physical Medicine and Rehabilitation, New York University–Bellevue Medical Center, 1955.

Deaver, G. G., and Brittis, A. L.: Braces,

Crutches, Wheelchairs, Mode of Management. Rehabilitation Monograph V. The Institute of Physical Medicine and Rehabilitation, New York University–Bellevue Medical Center, 1953.

DeGutiérrez-Mahoney, C. G., and Carini, E.: Neurological and Neurosurgical Nursing. 3rd ed. St. Louis, C. V. Mosby Company, 1960.

Denhoff, E., and Robinault, I. P.: Cerebral Palsy and Related Disorders: A Developmental Approach to Dysfunction. New York, McGraw Hill Book Company, Inc., 1960.

Gibbons, H., and Cunningham, F.: Finding and Helping the Partially Seeing Child. Nursing Outlook, 7:524, 1959.

Greenberg, M., and others: A Study of Pica in Relation to Lead Poisoning. Pediatrics, 22: 756, 1958.

Gross, R. E.: The Surgery of Infancy and Childhood. Philadelphia, W. B. Saunders Company, 1953.

Harvie, F. H.: Pediatric Methods and Standards. 3rd ed. Philadelphia, Lea & Febiger, 1958.

Hathaway, W.: Education and Health of the Partially Seeing Child. 3rd ed. New York, Columbia University Press, 1954.

Headley, L., and Leler, H.: A Nursery School for Cerebral Palsied Children. Children, 8: 17, 1961.

Heap, B.: Sodium Restricted Diets. Am. J. Nursing, 60:206, 1960.

Hood, O. E.: Your Child or Mine: The Brain-Injured Child and His Hope. New York, Harper and Bros., 1957.

Jackson, C. L.: Blind Children. Am. J. Nursing, 61:52, February, 1961.

Kaplan, S. A.: Nephrosis in Children, Medical Aspects. Am. J. Nursing, 56:300, 1956.

Katz, B. E.: Education of Cerebral Palsied Children. J. Pediat., 53:467, 1958.

Koch, F. P.: A Nursery School for Children with Cerebral Palsy: Five-Year Follow-up Study of Thirteen Children. Pediatrics, 22: 329, 1958.

Kolodny, R. L.: Therapeutic Group Work with Handicapped Children. Children, 4:95, 1957.

Larson, C. B., and Gould, M.: Calderwood's Orthopedic Nursing. 4th ed. St. Louis, C. V. Mosby Company, 1957.

Losty, M. A., and others: A Hospital-to-Home Link for Crippled Children. Nursing Outlook. 5:650, 1957.

Lyons, D. C.: The Dental Problems of Handicapped Children. Children, 8:14, 1961.

MacCollum, D. W., and others: Habilitation of the Cleft-Palate Patient. New England J. Med., 254:299, 1956.

MacCollum, D. W., and Richardson, S. O.: Care of the Child with Cleft Lip and Cleft Palate Am. J. Nursing, 58:211, 1958.

Mackintosh, J. M.: Accidents Are Not Accidental. World Health Organization, World Health, 13:17, May-June, 1960.

McCrory, W. W., Rapoport, M., and Fleisher, D. S.: Estimation of Severity of the Nephrotic Syndrome in Childhood as a Guide to Therapy and Prognosis. Pediatrics, 23: 861, 1959.

Martmer, E. E. (editor): The Child with a Handicap. Springfield, Ill., Charles C Thomas, 1959.

Moor, P. M.: Blind children with Developmental Problems. Children, 8:9, 1961.

Nelson, W. E. (editor): Textbook of Pediatrics. 7th ed. Philadelphia, W. B. Saunders Company, 1959.

Norris, M.: What Affects Blind Children's Development. Children, 3:123, 1956.

Paterson, D., and McCreary, J. F.: Pediatrics. Philadelphia, J. B. Lippincott Company, 1956.

Prinzing, D. M.: Cleft Palate Habilitation. Nursing Outlook, 7:577, 1959.

Randall, P.: The Management of Cleft-Lip and Cleft-Palate Patients. Am. J. M. Sc., 233: 204, 1957.

Robertson, J.: Young Children in Hospitals. New York, Basic Books, Inc., 1958.

Seitock, B. B.: The Deaf Child. Am. J. Nursing, 56:594, 1956.

Sheldon, W.: Celiac Disease. Pediatrics, 23: 132, 1959.

Silver, H. K., Kempe, C. H., and Bruyn, H. B.: Handbook of Pediatrics. 3rd ed. Los Altos, California, Lange Medical Publications, 1959.

Stewart, M.: Role of the Nurse in Pediatric Rehabilitation. Health News, 33:4, 1956.

Terry, F. J., Benz, G. S., Mereness, D., Kleffner, F. R. and Jensen, D. M.: Principles and Technics of Rehabilitation Nursing. St. Louis, C. V. Mosby Company, 1957.

Wallace, H. M.: Coordinating Health Services for Handicapped Children. Children, 5:20, 1958.

Ward, M. M.: Self-help Fashions for the Physically Disabled Child. Am. J. Nursing, 58: 526, 1958.

Idem: Toilet Seats for Disabled Children. Am. J. Nursing, 57:483, 1957.

White, H. H., and Fowler, F. D.: Chronic Lead Encephalopathy: A Diagnostic Consideration in Mental Retardation. Pediatrics, 25: 309, 1960.

Zickefoose, M.: Feeding Problems of Children with Cleft Palate. Children, 4:225, 1957.

# The Preschool Child

# Chapter 18

# The Normal Preschool Child: His Growth, Development and Care

## OVERVIEW OF EMOTIONAL DEVELOPMENT

THE PRESCHOOL child, having learned to trust others and to know that he is a person in his own right, is ready to find out what he can do. He must learn certain things in order to become the kind of person he wants to be. He watches adults and attempts to imitate their behavior. He longs for the time when he can fully share in their activities.

The preschool child is imaginative and creative. Since he cannot really participate in the adult world, he pretends that he can. The simplest equipment may represent articles used in real life. For instance, a series of wooden boxes or blocks can become a train, or a few small cardboard boxes can furnish a doll's house, the boxes becoming a bed, a chest of drawers, a chair and a table.

The child learns quickly that different materials are suited to specific purposes. He understands language well enough to communicate through speech. This increases his ability to learn from the experiences of others and to understand much that he has not personally experienced. He questions others almost constantly, asking about the world, its people and their activities. He may become loud and persistent in his questioning and at times annoying. He is searching for explanations of the phenomena in his environment, which to him are problems of causation and function which must be solved in order to do what he wants and get what he wants without adult help.

**497**

The preschool child is as vigorous in physical activity as in intellectual explorations. He moves freely and violently. He may attack others on purpose or by accident during play. He enjoys gross motor activity, but may also settle down to tasks which develop the finer muscular skills.

The infant and the toddler are guided in their activity largely by the direction of their parents, but the preschool child shows evidence of having a conscience of his own. The "still, small voice" within him guides him or passes judgment on his deeds. Experts state that children may now begin to feel guilty for their errors or wrong doing or even for their thoughts. Their unrestricted thoughts and actions frighten them.

The central problem for the preschool child is to learn about the world and other people. He must also learn to assert his own will in such a way that he will not feel too guilty. If he has the knowledge and the ability to solve this problem, he will develop a *sense of initiative* comfortably controlled by conscience. If he fails to solve this problem, he will emerge from this period feeling overwhelmed and with a *sense of guilt*.

Preschool children may feel guilty because of plans they want to carry out, but may not because of parental disapproval, or because of thoughts or fantasies of which conscience disapproves.

If the child is to develop a sense of initiative and a healthy personality, his parents and other adults in his environment must encourage his plans and the use of his imagination. They must limit punishment to those acts which are dangerous, morally wrong or so socially unacceptable that the result would be unfortunate or harmful to the child or his family.

Preschool children look forward to becoming like their fathers or mothers. They learn adult roles from their parents, who serve as models of behavior. Children enjoy practicing these roles in their play. They begin gradually to learn how to cooperate with their peers

and with adults and gain great pleasure from success in their attempts (see p. 520). Parents should encourage the child's efforts to cooperate and let him share in the decisions and responsibilities of family living. If he is denied this opportunity, if his imagination is curbed and he is frustrated too often in his attempts at growing up, he becomes overanxious and spends too much time and energy in purposeless activity. Such children are apt to develop rigid consciences which exercise strong control over their behavior. At the same time they may feel resentment and bitterness toward the adults who restrict their normal behavior.

The preschool child's sense of initiative must be encouraged throughout childhood and youth. If it is not, the good beginning may end in failure.

### The Preschool Child and His Family

**The Family Romance.** During infancy and the toddler period children of both sexes tend to love, and to be more dependent upon, the mother, who cares for them, than on the father, who is not home during the day and may see little of his children except on weekends. Between the ages of three and six a change occurs. The little girl becomes more interested in her father. The little boy, however, remains in love with his mother. This change in the love-object influences the children's behavior toward their parents and the roles they assume in play. The girl is "Daddy's little girl" and assumes the role of wife and mother in her play. The boy becomes "Mommie's little boy." He gradually becomes more masculine in his play, taking his role from the pattern set by his father.

During this period the little girl may become possessive of her father and may be in competition with her mother for his love. The little boy may likewise become possessive of his mother and may compete with his father for her love. Children feel some aggression toward the parent of the same sex. Usually they keep their feelings hidden, but at times show their attitude in full force, as when they say to the parent of the same sex, "I hate you, go away!" Such feelings make the child feel guilty and anxious, and he may fear retaliation from the parent. The child feels even more conflict within himself, because at the same time that he hates he really loves the parent, though less than the parent of the opposite sex. Children love both parents because of the love and attention which parents normally give their children, irrespective of sex.

The parent of the same sex as the child provides a model for the child to imitate as he develops and matures. This conflict of love and hate is seen in the play of children between three and six years of age.

Parents must give their children much love and understanding during this period of conflict. The child, in order to continue to grow emotionally, must bury his sexual feelings toward the parent of the opposite sex in the unconscious and must identify himself with the parent of the same sex. By the end of this period the boy no longer wants to take his father's place; he simply wants to be like his father. The girl no longer wants to take her mother's place; she wants to grow up to be like mother and to have children of her own one day. The child becomes friends with both parents, not regarding either one as a specific love-object. The *family* then becomes a meaningful love-object. The intensity of response to each member is decreased. The conflict has been resolved.

It is especially important at this stage that the parents be the kind of people that society accepts. If the parents are not acceptable according to society's standards, the child will learn attitudes and feelings which will later be a detriment to his development.

Unfortunately, some children do not make this shift in emotional attachment. The little boy may continue to love only his mother, and the little girl only her father. These children may not then be able to take the next steps in emotional development because of fixation at this preschool level. Such children may in later years need guidance to change this immature relation with their parents.

**The Only Child and the Adopted Child.** The only child is the object of all parental relations in the home; attention is concentrated upon him. The only child of young parents is likely to fare better than one of older parents; he is more likely to have young cousins, and parental attention is less likely to be tinged with anxiety and more likely to be jolly and playful. To put it briefly, he is the object of deep affection, but also a source of fun and amusement.

The first child is an only child until the second comes along. Young parents are more likely to be expecting a second child. Expectation of another child has somewhat the same influence as his actual presence would have, and their first child is not wholly treated as an only child. This is different from the attitude of older parents who over a period of years have longed for a child and cannot expect at their age to have other children.

All that has been said about an only child appears to be reinforced through

**Figure 189.** The preschool child imitates the parent of the same sex. (H. Armstrong Roberts.)

the experience of the death of one or all of the other children.

What has been said of the only child is commonly true of the adopted child. He has in many cases been adopted after the death of a couple's own child or when they find that they are unable to have children. Most child-placing agencies will allow only one child to adoptive parents, since the demand for children to be adopted is greater than the number to be placed. (If twins or siblings are to be placed for adoption, it is customary to give them to parents who desire both children.) The custom of giving adoptive parents only one child works to the detriment of the children, since the life of an only child, lacking contact with brothers and sisters, is not complete.

It is generally considered the best policy to tell the child that he is adopted before this status has any meaning for him. He accepts the parents' attitude that they want him and is satisfied. As he grows older he may feel that he is different from other children and may attribute discipline or punishment to the fact that he is an adopted child whom his parents do not love as they would their own natural child. The increasing number of adoptions during recent years makes the situation more commonplace and less emotionally charged.

**Effect of the Birth of a Sibling.** Any environmental change has a traumatic effect on a child. Even such a change as moving to a new house should be discussed with the child. The birth of a sibling is a change of such magnitude that the child should become accustomed before the baby is born to the idea of no longer being an only child. The birth of another child unavoidably deprives the older child of some parental attention, and a child mistakes this for loss of affection. It is difficult for the toddler or little child of nursery school age to accept the situation, for his love is still centered almost exclusively on his parents.

The child feels rejected and may become jealous. Infantile expression of jealousy is of two types. It may be shown *directly* in open dislike of the baby, or the child may appear to love the baby more than is normal. In so doing he is laying the foundation of a martyr attitude which may persist throughout life. He usually shows his hostility to the new baby openly and directly. He may make derogatory remarks about the baby. If his parents reprove him, he may feel guilty and may rationalize on the childish level. For instance, he may give as an excuse for hitting the baby the fact that the infant has taken his blanket—a blanket which the mother has given to the infant. Later, when the baby is old enough to take his toy, he grabs it back and says, "It's mine." When his mother intervenes, he sulks or hits the baby or her. Such displacement of his anger toward anyone who pets the baby is common.

The child's jealousy may be shown *indirectly* by clumsiness in his contacts with the infant. If his feeling of guilt is great and he is unable to express his jealousy openly, he may drop the baby when given him to hold.

The child handles his hostility toward his mother in different ways. Direct actions against her include physical or verbal attack. On the other hand, he may refuse to have anything to do with her, ignoring her completely because she has brought the new baby home. He may displace his hostility toward her and be hostile to other adults, e.g. his nursery school or Sunday School teacher. He may regress and demand attention similar to that given the baby, refusing to drink from a cup, wanting his milk from a nursing bottle, and soiling himself so that his mother must give him the same toilet care she gives "the baby." The mother should accept such temporary regression. If it is too long continued, however, it may be necessary to obtain professional help for the child. The child may repress any outward reaction, without solving his problem. This reaction may interfere with his successful handling of jealousy in later childhood or even throughout life.

Jealousy may begin when the older

preschool child learns that the mother is pregnant, possibly during the fourth or fifth month of gestation. It is not wise to tell a young preschool child too early of the pregnancy, since he would have too long a wait before the child's birth. Before the birth of the new baby the mother can control the child's jealousy to some extent by giving him as much attention as usual and stressing her pleasure in having him share in loving the coming baby brother or sister. The baby's coming should be discussed with the child even though he is too young to understand the changes which the birth of a new infant will make in the family life. Parents should encourage him to talk about his unborn sibling and either to verbalize or express in play his hostility toward the child.

It is a good plan to send the child to nursery school in order to develop outside contacts. He may be shown a child's picture book about the arrival of a new baby in the family, to help him visualize what his mother means by all the preparations she is making for the coming of the infant.

Jealousy can be handled in a number of ways. A child who shows indications of wanting to hurt the infant

Figure 190. The young child may be given a pet to care for as his mother cares for the new baby. (H. Armstrong Roberts.)

should never be left alone with him. A more positive measure is to give the child a pet so that he has something to care for, just as mother is caring for

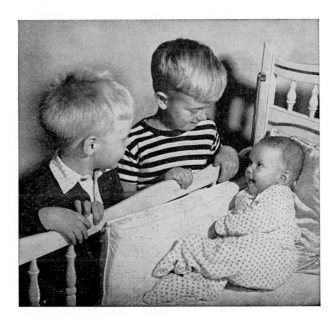

Figure 191. Children are encouraged to identify with the parents and to protect a younger sibling. (H. Armstrong Roberts.)

the baby. He may be encouraged to identify with his parents in lovingly protecting the infant.

All sexual questions should be answered frankly, explanation being adjusted to the child's vocabulary and ability to understand sexual processes. The mother may discuss with him the difference between his needs and those of the infant; this may be done in terms of his being more grown up than the baby. For instance, he can clean his teeth, whereas the baby has no teeth; he can walk, holding mother's hand, or run about and play, but the baby must be carried or go in his carriage; in the car he can be held on the seat between father and mother, while the infant must be in his basket or in mother's arms. The mother should arrange to be alone with the child, or she and his father together with him, while the baby is sleeping in another room. If possible, the child may be with his father when the mother must care for the infant in the evening. Evidences of affection for the infant should be minimized in the presence of the older child.

### Needs of the Preschool Child

The preschool child needs security and independence. He needs the security which comes with the knowledge that he has parents who are daily with him in the home. He needs their love and understanding. Within this circumscribed world of security and love he needs an opportunity to express his hostility and antagonisms. Because of his growing verbal ability he has increasingly less need to use physical expressions of hostility. As he grows he needs opportunities to assume more responsibility and independence. By expressing his hostility and his growing independence he learns what these feelings are like and how he can deal with them.

The child feels love and security when he has two parents with whom he has daily contact. The parents, besides showing love for him, must teach him and guide him toward maturity: (1) From verbal interaction with them

he learns how to express himself so that he can communicate with others on a verbal level. (2) In the home he learns to assume more responsibility and be more independent. (3) He gains from them the knowledge he needs to grow up. Two important aspects of knowledge learned in this age period relate to sex and to religion. More important than the facts he learns are the attitudes he forms toward this knowledge. The preschool child turns his interests to the outside world, to the why's and how's of living.

**Guidance.** There are few, if any, set rules for the guidance of preschool children, but the following suggestions may be helpful. Limits to his behavior must be set and consistently maintained, thereby giving the child a basis for prediction of the reactions of other people to what he does and thus making rational behavior possible.

Limits set by parents give him a feeling of security which he does not have when he is allowed to decide for himself on matters which are beyond his ability to decide wisely. Suggestions— not commands—helpful to the child in achieving what he wants at the time, or in forming good relations with other people, should be made in positive form. Commands are seldom necessary, but when given in positive rather than negative form are more effective. The child should not be spoken to in such a way that he feels guilty or fearful. Rather he should be reassured by the sense that his parents are helping him solve problems as they come up in his activities and social relations. A choice of actions should be given him only when he actually may decide which of two or more lines of behavior he may take. A child does not always understand that redirection of his activities is consistent with his own interests. He learns this gradually by experience with the satisfying results which follow parental redirection.

Adults should not make the mistake of playing *for* the child. Instead, he should be helped to enjoy his own activities. For instance, adults should not make art models for him to copy.

He should be allowed freely to create his own work. He should be encouraged to do as much as possible for himself so that he can grow in independence. Help should be provided whenever necessary, however; this is an important element in his feeling secure in his parents' protecting love. Children live in the present, and suggestion, to be truly helpful, should be provided and reinforced at appropriate times.

**Learning Language.** The preschool child learns to communicate his feelings and ideas through language in a more precise form than he did as a toddler. He constantly asks questions and learns about the outside world by seeking the meaning of what he experiences through sensory stimulation. He asks how, why, what, when and where about everything which interests him.

During the preschool period he uses progressively longer and more complex sentences. This is a period of rapid vocabulary growth. Between the ages of 2 and 6 years the child learns about 600 words a year, chiefly through the answers given by adults to his questions. He also learns by imitating adults and other children with whom he associates. He may acquire words which his parents do not want him to use, such as ungrammatical terms ("ain't"), slang or so-called bad words. Usually if adults in his environment ignore unacceptable words and do not give him attention when he uses them, he will cease to use them in his conversation.

An analysis of a child's questions shows his need for information, for relief from anxiety and for attention. Answers to his questions should give him increased understanding of his environment and of what is going on about him, as well as a secure feeling that adults can and will help him to learn. Through answers to his questions the child gets not only factual knowledge, but also a concept of adult attitudes and feelings about the topics discussed.

The questions of three-year-olds are rather simple when compared with those of four- and five-year-olds, who want to know how things function. These latter questions require more detailed explanations which adults at times may not be prepared to give. All adults should remember the guiding principle about answering questions of children and youths: to tell the truth to the best of one's ability. If a lie is told, the child will lose his sense of trust in the individual, and his trust in all others may be weakened. The answer should be in terms of the child's level of understanding. If an adult does not know the answer, he should tell the child so. Then adult and child are ready to seek the answer together.

**Sex Information.** The child who learns to trust others and to give as well as receive love has already begun his preparation for a satisfactory marriage and rearing children of his own.

Sex education during the preschool years contributes specific knowledge which the child wants to know and also helps him build desirable attitudes toward this aspect of life. This is especially true when parents love and respect each other and so set a good example for the child to follow. In such a family the preschool child will learn that he or she is a boy or a girl and that each sex has its own role to play in life. The attitudes and feelings which children acquire greatly influence their relations to marital partners and to their own children. It is essential that the child understand that sex is important to his own personality as well as to that of others.

Although the extent and method of sex education must be fitted to the individual child's needs, certain general principles are applicable to the sex education of all children. Adults should know the age when a child is likely to ask questions about sex. Children may ask such questions by the time they are three to four years of age, although some may not ask until they are six years old. There are individual differences, of course, depending on factors in the child's environment and his degree of maturation. Information on sex should be given in response to the child's interest in the subject, but never

**Figure 192.** The child who learns early the origins of animals and birds will more easily understand the story of his own creation. (H. Armstrong Roberts.)

as facts which have no connection with the family life. In general the child is old enough for correct answers when he is sufficiently mature to ask questions.

Sex information may be given at home, church or school. The best source of information should be sincere and loving parents. If for some reason this is impossible, the school or church may give the information. Information may also be acquired from acquaintances, but unfortunately is likely not only to be incorrect, but also to give the child a distorted attitude to the whole subject of sexual relations.

Parents should answer the child directly and honestly, basing the amount of information given and the phraseology used on the individual child's physiologic and developmental level. Information should be given promptly when the question is asked. It is not good to tell more about the subject than is involved in the answer to the question. The information should be given

frankly and unemotionally. The child will grasp his parents' attitude toward sex more than their answers, and this will free him from worry and preoccupation with sexual problems.

Some of the questions which preschool children ask concern the birth of a child. They commonly ask, "Where do babies come from?" because curiosity is natural to this age group and because conditions pertaining to sex are obvious in the social life about him. The child sees pregnant women, and mass media treat openly of sex. Household pets deliver their young, and rural children learn early of reproduction in farm animals. When the child asks where babies come from, he should be helped to clarify his fantasies. If his questions are answered frankly and with a positive attitude of acceptance of his interest in the matter, he will receive the information without shame or anxiety. During the preschool period emphasis should be placed on the physical aspects of sex. The preschool child

s too young to understand moral implications, other than the value of doing
what his parents ask of him.

Many of the problems which beset
adolescents arise because they dwell on
sex and have fantasies about many aspects of sexuality. If answers had been
given during the preschool period and
enlarged upon as the child grew older,
there would be less danger of such turmoil during adolescence.

**Religious Education.**   Close parent-child
relations normally extend through the
years during which the child is socialized. The greatest influence in a
child's life is his parents' attitude about
such basic aspects of life as religion,
sex, love of country, economic systems,
and education. In answering questions
parents must be understanding, objective and kind, particularly in regard
to religion, since faith as well as science is involved.

A few general principles pertaining
to religious education may be given. A
child cannot be kept spiritually neutral.
Whatever his parents may desire, he
hears about religion from other children, and he sees churches and pictures
of religious objects.

Whatever the parents tell the child
about religion has the same force as
does information on other subjects. Yet
the child observes what his parents do,
and if their actions are not in accord
with what they teach him, he is quick
to notice it.

A child should be brought up in a
genuinely religious home, for a religious attitude toward life is not just
an afterthought to living. It is the
spiritual atmosphere which pervades
the whole of life.

There are two general methods of
religious education: that of indoctrina-
tion and that of letting the child follow
the religion of his choice. The preschool child does not follow any religion because he understands it.
Rather, he accepts religion because it is

**Figure 193.**  In a genuinely
religious home the spiritual atmosphere pervades all living.
Children learn more by example
than they do from mere verbal
explanations. (H. Armstrong
Roberts.)

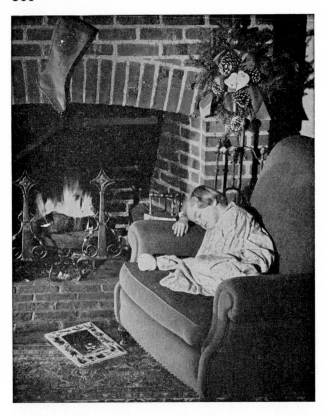

**Figure 194.** A young child truly believes that Santa Claus will come. (H. Armstrong Roberts.)

expected of him, because someone he loves influences him to do so or because it offers some other concomitant pleasures. Both methods have many adherents. Neither, taken alone, meets the real issue.

Suggestions for religious training in the home include early training in the faith held by the parents. The preschool child is old enough to go to Sunday School. Religion should be made attractive to him, but should not be forced upon him. He should be taught that God is within our lives, that God loves him. Parents should not give the child the impression that they are condescending to his level when speaking of religion; the discussion should be a shared experience between parents and child. As the child grows up he will learn about religions other than that held by his parents.

Religious training in the hospital is difficult, since the child's questions must be answered only by persons of the same faith as his parents. This avoids confusion of ideas in the child's mind. Furthermore, what the child is told may be a matter of extreme importance to the parents, since the child is not able to think through conflicting statements about religion. In a nonsectarian hospital there is no organized Sunday School.

Religious holidays raise many questions in a child's mind. The following explanation of the significance of Christmas and Easter may be given unless the policy of the hospital prohibits discussion of the religious concepts involved. The questions most commonly asked are only indirectly of a religious nature.

There is the old question, "Is there really a Santa Claus?" The answer to be given to a very young child is usually, "Yes." He is too young to understand abstract ideas, and Santa stands for the spirit of Christmas. When the child really begins to question this belief, he is already doubting its truth. He should be allowed to discuss his own ideas on the matter. If he actually doubts whether there is a Santa Claus, he is ready for an explanation of what Santa Claus stands for. He may be told that the spirit of Christmas is that of good will. It is a time to make others happy as Santa Claus made him happy on Christmas Day last year and the year before, as far back as he can remember. The origin of Christmas can be told him, and its religious significance, which he probably already knows if his parents are of the Christian faith. Customs which have developed around the celebration of Christmas in different countries will interest him.

The myth of the Easter Bunny can be explained with similar adaptations.

### Anxiety in the Preschool Child

At each age in life certain problems or difficulties may arise which produce anxiety. Problems which may cause anxiety and tension in the preschool child may come from within or may arise from his environment. They may be due to lack of satisfaction of a need or to an increase in the number and intensity of the child's fears. His response to the problem is to mobilize defenses to deal with the dangers.

**Specific Causes.** There are several causes of anxiety which are common during the preschool period. The child may fear being deserted by his parents, that they no longer love him or that he is being punished for misdeeds or thoughts which he should not have held. He has a great fear of physical injury.

These specific causes of anxiety are intensified by the peculiar combination of anxiety-producing circumstances which occur during hospitalization. The main causes of anxiety are separation from his parents and fear of pain.

*Loss of Parental Love.* To a preschool child parental love is manifested in his daily life with his parents. Separation from his parents means loss of their love. Hospitalization is for most children only a temporary separation from their parents. Long-term or permanent separation must now be considered.

The child who has lost his father or mother by death or divorce does not live in a complete home. He may live with the remaining parent or with relatives, or may be placed in an institution. If the parent has died, there is not the sense of shame which is likely to trouble a child of divorced parents. Still, as divorce becomes more common, children may not feel its significance as much as children in past generations did. Divorce is generally preceded by a period of troubled life in which the child may be urged by each parent to love him or her only and to be hostile to the other parent. Generally the court gives the child to the mother, but after the divorce the child may visit his father at times prescribed by the court. The child of divorced parents is confused by the antagonism of each parent toward the other and yet the love of each for him. Of course the child who is loved by only one parent or by neither is deprived of the parental affection which is a child's birthright.

If by death or divorce of his parents a child is without a home, placement in the home of a relative or in a foster home is considered better for the child than life in an institution. An older child who has lost his home and contact with his relatives may find the neutral atmosphere of a well organized institution less of an emotional strain than a foster home where foster parents give him affection and want an affectionate response. Later, however, a foster home may prove successful. The social worker of a child-placing agency may be the only adult with whom the child establishes a satisfying and continuing relation throughout a childhood spent in institutions or foster homes.

An adopted child, particularly if he is a little child, may have the same love relations with adoptive parents which a child under normal circumstances has with his natural parents.

A child may be separated from his parents for business or patriotic reasons. In general this separation is relatively temporary, and he remains with his mother, who speaks to him of his father and builds up in the child a happy expectation of his father's return. If the father is absent for a long time, good parent-child relations may be difficult to establish.

When a boy of preschool age loses his father, he lacks a male in the home with whom he can identify, against whom he can be aggressive and from whom he can learn about the role of a man in the home, community or country. The boy may become a substitute love-object to his mother for her absent husband. He may develop a feminine outlook on life and never learn the typical masculine technique of competition or aggression. The effect upon the boy of absence of his mother is generally less serious than that due to his father's absence because there is usually a mother-substitute in the home, e.g. a grandmother, aunt or housekeeper. The boy of preschool age may regress after his mother has left home until he adjusts to her substitute. He may be deeply hurt by his mother's leaving him when he loves her so dearly and may fear loving a woman who takes her place in the home, lest he be hurt again if she leaves.

The effect upon a girl of absence of the mother is essentially the same as that of absence of the father upon a boy. She will have no one with whom to compete for the father's love, and until a mother-substitute is found she will have no woman with whom she can identify and from whom she can learn the feminine role in life. She may develop a masculine outlook on family and community life.

The effect upon the girl of absence of the father is essentially the same as that of absence of the mother upon the boy. She may become too closely attached to the mother, and also may become afraid of loving a man again and

being hurt by his loss. This feeling, if carried over into adolescence, interferes with normal courtship and marriage.

Separation of a child from both parents has all the effects of the loss of a single parent. The trauma to the child is extreme, and the child goes through a period of mourning for his parents. Since the child is less verbal than the adult, his feelings must be judged from nonverbal behavior. He may show physical symptoms such as vomiting and diarrhea, or a return to more infantile behavior. For instance, although he is toilet-trained, he may soil himself. He may be uncooperative and naughty.

Everyone working with children should know how to help a child who has been separated from one or both parents. No adult should scold or punish a child for his response to parental loss no matter what form it takes. The child should be treated with kindness and helped to express his feelings. He should be encouraged to talk about the parent who has gone away. Preschool children may feel that they have caused the death or departure of the parent of the same sex because they wished him or her to leave and be out of the way. The child must be helped to understand that his wish was not the same thing as a deed of violence against the parent.

Substitute parents should be provided as soon as possible for children who have lost both parents, and should make every effort to win the children's love and confidence. Some children may need psychologic help if the trauma has been too great for them to accept.

**Common General Types.** *Conscience anxiety*, in which the child feels that he has done something wrong and expects punishment, is prevalent among children of overparticular or strict parents. The bogyman of the modern child is the person who will punish him if he is naughty.

A common and almost unavoidable kind of *anxiety* is that *arising out of inconsistency* in the do's and don't's of parents and parental actions. This difficulty is increased when the parents do not lead the kind of life which they teach the child that he must lead. During World War II, for instance, children were taught to sublimate their destructive feelings and direct them to positive ends, and yet they were given toy weapons with which to play soldier and saw adults condoning destructive feelings about war. The children were too immature to understand the difference between personal aggression and that prompted by love of country and group morale. This was a major difficulty in the training of little children during the war.

*Infectious anxiety* is acquired from an adult, generally the mother. If the mother is relatively free from overt anxiety under severe circumstances, the child also is apt to be free. But if the mother is overanxious even in commonly accepted situations, the child is also likely to be anxious. This sort of anxiety is often seen in hospitalized children. If the mother is anxious about the child, he will be anxious about himself. This is one reason why the nurse should make the mother comfortable and secure about the hospitalization of the child.

Real or *objective anxiety* or fear is dependent upon the child's ability to understand the nature of the danger which threatens him. Fear of lightning is a needless fear due to the child's not understanding the cause of the sudden streak of light zigzagging across the sky. In contrast, a child's fear of needles is gained from experience; he knows that they cause him pain.

Objective fears of preschool children must be managed with consideration of

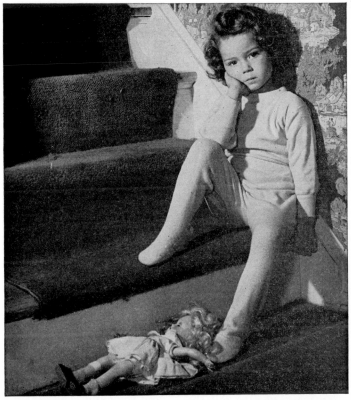

**Figure 195.** A child grieves when her parent has gone away. This overwhelming feeling of loneliness is difficult for her to handle. (H. Armstrong Roberts.)

the child's stage of maturation. Many unreal fears may appear real to little children, and most preschool children have one kind or another of these fears. This is natural, for they have a limited understanding of the world about them. Adults must help a child to handle his fears if they are not to persist, possibly in a compulsive form, in adult life. A real fear of a situation which is dangerous is logical. The remedy is to show the child what may be done in such a situation and how to avoid dangerous situations. Crossing the street is an example. The child should be taught to cross at the corner with, not against, the traffic light.

Ordinary fears include fear of being injured (or seeing people who have been injured or are crippled), being lost or deserted, and being hurt by animals (particularly those which are large or noisy). Some children fear death, but not as adults do. The child may have had a real experience with any one of these fear-producing situations. Children feel most fearful when they are alone or away from their parents among strangers.

Anxiety, in contrast to fear, occurs when a child feels unloved. He may have been punished for masturbation, or deprived of his mother's love because of the arrival of a new sibling. To the child who is anxious many things appear to be dangerous, and vague, unknown dangers appear to be ever present. The adult must understand not only the child's fear of external dangers, but also his inner anxiety, in order to help him.

The frightened child needs, more than anything else, to be reassured and to gain a feeling of safety. His mother should hold him and let him feel her protection and strength. After he has calmed down, his attention may be directed from the source of his fear. When he appears sufficiently secure, he may want to talk about his fear and even to have contact with the feared object or situation. Perhaps, before contact, he may want to play out the fearful situation as a game. The adult's

role in helping a child to overcome fears is to be supportive and understanding, not punishing or threatening.

Common fears can be prevented to a large extent by imagining how new situations seem to a child and talking to him from his point of view. The adult knows that a puppy is only active and playful, not vicious, but to a child the puppy appears to be a monster that cannot be controlled. The adult who protects a child from meeting fearful experiences until he is prepared for them and has sufficient self-confidence will prevent many of the common fears of childhood.

## SPECIAL PROBLEMS OF THE PRESCHOOL CHILD

Although the general causes of anxiety and conflicts in the preschool years have been discussed, the common behavioral manifestations of children's feelings are also so important that they must be given detailed consideration in order that the student may learn to give the child comprehensive nursing care. Children of this age group may have such behavioral problems as continued thumb-sucking, enuresis, selfishness, hurting others, destructiveness and masturbation.

### Thumb-Sucking

The important danger in continued thumb-sucking is not in the habit itself, but in the response of parents and other adults to it. Parents in general tend to feel that if a child sucks his thumb in the preschool period, they themselves have failed in training him. They respond to this feeling of failure by becoming inconsiderate of the child in their handling of the problem. They may alternately punish, love and ridicule him because he does not overcome the objectionable habit.

Mothers need not fear that thumb-sucking will injure the thumb or spoil the shape of the child's jaw unless the habit is continued into older childhood and the child exerts maximum pressure when sucking. In any case the shape of the mouth is likely to return to normal after the thumb-sucking has stopped.

Many of the children who suck their thumbs probably had too little sucking pleasure during infancy. Thumb-sucking may be a sign that the child feels unloved, that he is in danger or is not good enough. It may be an expression of dissatisfaction with life. When parents or other adults exert pressure upon him to give up the activity, his unhappiness is increased.

In order to help the child with this problem, parents and other adults responsible for his care must observe the whole child and try to provide a happier childhood experience for him. Adults should note the occasions when a child sucks his thumb and provide more love and security for him at such times. It is essential to find the basis of the problem. Is the child lonely, too excited or bored? Has he too few toys or does he feel neglected? Although children usually outgrow the habit by the age of five or six years, it is important to find and correct the cause in order to prevent the child from acquiring another habit which serves the same function of giving him pleasure and comfort. The matter may be discussed with a child of five or six years who seems to be trying to overcome the habit. He may be encouraged by assurance that he will probably outgrow the habit.

## Enuresis

Enuresis, or wetting after control should be established (in general about three years of age), is both a source of embarrassment and a nuisance to the mother of an enuretic child. Mothers should remember that a child can be toilet-trained only when he is physiologically and psychologically ready for control of urine and stool.

Some of the causes of enuresis are lack of training, too early training, overtraining or too severe training. If parents would regard toilet training as only a part of the general training of the child—take it in the stride of child training—there would be fewer problems of enuresis. Children who have achieved control of urine and stool may revert to wetting, especially bed wetting, when they meet problems which they cannot solve, such as those connected with the coming of a new baby.

Adults should not make an issue of toilet training. They should not use bribes or punishment or threaten to stop loving a child because he continues this habit. If enuresis is nocturnal only, giving less fluid in the evening may be tried. But the problem is usually more psychologic than physical. Adults should try to be casual and assure the child that he will outgrow this habit. They should help him to achieve a positive attitude toward enuresis—to want to stay dry—and develop confidence in his ability to control elimination. Wetting will not stop at once, but if the child is more relaxed, dryness will be achieved more easily and with less danger to the child's personality development.

A few cases of enuresis may be due to a physical cause. For this reason children who do not respond to parental training should be examined by a physician. A few cases of nocturnal enuresis may be due to environmental factors, such as a dark hall through which the child must walk, or to his reluctance to get out of a warm bed to go to the cold bathroom. Adults should analyze the situation in order to determine his specific problem.

## Selfishness

No child is born with the ability to share with others what is his. He can only slowly learn the joy of giving, or even sharing with others, what he wants to keep for himself. He cannot be forced to share. He must first develop a sense of ownership before he can learn to be generous.

Adults can help him to learn to share with others if they let him have possessions which both they and he recognize as his. He should be allowed to decide whether to give or refuse to give his toy to another child. If a squabble occurs over one child's possession of a toy which another child wants, a substitute toy should be provided so that each has what he wants. Many parents make the mistake of taking a toy from its rightful owner and giving it to a smaller child or to a guest or a girl. In order to learn the difficult and often unpleasant lesson of sharing, a child should be helped to enjoy playing with other children. Group play encourages the habit of sharing. He will learn first that using things together is fun and then to share and take turns with his toys and those of other children.

### Bad Language

Children learn improper words just as they learn all the other words in their vocabularies. Parents are horrified when their children call names such as "stinker," "louse" or "stupid." They may be shocked when their children say unapproved words in connection with toilet training. They may be hurt when their children say, "I hate you!" or "I'll shoot you."

Bad language generally has more meaning for the adult than for the child, who, as a rule, has little understanding of what such words mean or their connotations. He may use these words on purpose to annoy adults and enjoy the sensation he creates.

In such a situation adults should relax and not be worried or shocked. The child should not be punished, for punishment emphasizes the importance of the words. The adult may say the same word back to the child in an unemotional way and thus make the word seem of little importance, or give the child a more difficult word such as "Mississippi" to say. The adult may say to the preschool child, "I'm tired of hearing that," or he may request the child not to use the word again because it may hurt others. Since no one method will work in all situations, more than one method may have to be tried.

In a nursery school the teacher may try the methods of nonparticipation with the group, suggestion of other words, distraction, or playing with other words or sounds. She should not shame or punish the children for using bad language. The less attention is paid to the use of such language, the sooner will it cease.

### Hurting Others

Small children hurt others and are themselves hurt when they play together. Neither outright punishment, shaming nor ignoring the action is a suitable technique to use in such a situation. If the hurting is accidental, the incident should be overlooked. But if a child persistently tries to hurt others, he needs adult help to control his actions or to prevent him from inflicting some serious injury on another child.

The child who repeatedly wants to hurt others by biting, scratching, pulling hair or hitting is a troubled child. He may be jealous or frustrated, and his behavior may result from his mental state. In any case he must not be allowed to hurt other children. He needs to know that someone who loves him deeply will control him and so prevent the unpleasant consequences of his behavior. He needs to feel secure within limits beyond which he is not allowed to go.

The child should not be punished by having the same injury inflicted on him which he inflicted on another child. He should not be told that he is a bad child. He should not be forced to apologize to the child whom he hurt. Under no circumstances should he be made to feel rejected by the adult who is in charge of the children. The adult should take positive action in situations in which the child is likely to hurt others. If it is evident that a child intends to throw a stone or hit or bite one of his playmates, the adult should restrain him, saying, "Sammy does not want to be hurt." If the harm has already been done, the injured child should be soothed and the offender removed to a less emotional environment in which he is helped to control himself. The attention of the other children should be directed to some activity which they all enjoy in order that happy play may be resumed. As soon as practical, the offending child should rejoin the play group.

Toys and other objects with which a child can hurt others should be removed from the environment if a child who is likely to attack others is participating in group play.

In the long run the child who wants to hurt others should be helped to identify with the group, accepting them and being accepted by them. He should be given physical outlets in his play through which to work off some of his excess energy and relieve his feeling of frustration. He should be praised for his achievements in group and solitary play and for kindly acts which he does for others.

## Destructiveness

All children occasionally break things; such is part of the normal life of a child. Parents must learn to differentiate between accidental and intentional destruction of objects which they may value highly. Much of the child's accidental destructiveness is the result of his boundless energy and endless curiosity. In spite of the damage to property, parents should not too severely limit his outlets for energy and curiosity, for these are valuable qualities which must not be destroyed.

To avoid accidental destruction at home, the parents should remove valuable objects that the child might break or damage. They should provide space for him to play in without danger of his breaking or harming the furnishings of the house.

Toys are apt to be given rough use. Parents should realize that material possessions do not mean as much to a child as to adults. In the course of play children give toys a great deal of wear and tear and may break them by using them in ways for which they were not

intended. Adults should set up certain restrictions, however, in the child's use of his toys and of objects belonging to adults. He is then able to learn to value his own possessions and those of others. Progress is slow, however. What he values he will learn to use with care. The child who loves his parents is often intensely sorry if he breaks something which he knows they value, even though he also knows that he will not be punished in any way.

If a child is intentionally destructive, he is usually an unhappy child who is unable to control his feelings of jealousy, helplessness, aggression or anger. He may feel unloved, disliked by his peers, or bored by inadequate playthings. Sometimes such children seem to want to be punished, since it is one way of getting attention. The cause of such destructiveness must be found and appropriate treatment given. The parents should avoid scolding or punishing. They should help him direct his energy into appropriate activities.

## Masturbation

Parents are apt to be confused in their understanding of the practice of masturbation. They find it hard to accept as an almost universal experience in young children. The infant soon discovers that a pleasant sensation accompanies handling of the genitals, which has no other significance to him and of course is not accompanied by fantasies. In the preschool child masturbation may be increased and is commonly accompanied by fantasies. Masturbation is utilized in adolescence to fulfill sexual urges which in our culture do not have socially approved release in heterosexual intercourse outside of marriage. It may have a useful part in the ultimate attainment of heterosexual expression of the sex urge, since it facilitates the fusion of normal psychologic components of sexuality with the normal and socially necessary physical aspects.

The child who masturbates excessively for his stage of maturation should not be punished. Rather, he should be helped to work out the problem which is causing him to masturbate more than is normal. The child who has discovered the pleasure derived from masturbation should be given ample opportunity to find other more socially acceptable pleasures in the environment outside his body.

Sex education does not solve the problem of masturbation. It does help the child, however, to understand his pleasure in the practice and to understand that the true function of the sexual organs is reproduction.

Although we should not scold the child for masturbating, the habit, if excessive, may keep him from other pleasures which are necessary for optimum growth and development in childhood. Like any pleasure which is practiced in solitude, it interferes with social interaction. If masturbation is excessive, it may become so fixed a habit that it interferes with the normal desire for heterosexual intercourse within marriage.

Poor handling of the problem of masturbation in the preschool child is likely to result in fixation at the auto-erotic level, wherein the child seeks pleasure in himself rather than in his relations with others.

Parents should be told that masturbation does not produce nervous diseases or weaken the mind or organs of reproduction, but that parental condemnation of the practice in the child may induce lasting psychologic and emotional harm.

The adolescent who masturbates excessively is failing socially. He is lonely and unhappy. He needs treatment for his social difficulty, not condemnation.

Two important aspects of the problem should be kept in mind. Masturbation focuses feeling in the genital region. This feeling is necessary for the healthy functioning of men and women. Shame and threats related to this activity can force children to repress sexual feelings. This might eventuate in impotence in the male and frigidity in the female. Both conditions tend to unhappiness in marriage and to increased susceptibility to mental illness.

The important fact to remember about preschool children is that masturbation in excess is a symptom of poor mental hygiene and is not a pathologic process in itself.

There is no one way of helping the child to overcome his tendency to excessive masturbation. He should be assured that he is safe in his parents' affection and that he should not be afraid or ashamed. He should not be threatened or punished, because such treatment would increase his fears. He should be given opportunity for happy relations with playmates and sufficient toys to play with. His parents should be particularly careful to answer all his questions about sex, adapting their answers to his level of understanding.

## OVERVIEW OF PHYSICAL, SOCIAL AND MENTAL DEVELOPMENT

### Physical Growth and Development

Children grow relatively slowly in the preschool years, but they change from the chubby toddler to the sturdy child. They gain an average of less than 5 pounds a year. The average child of six years of age has doubled his weight at one year of age. During the preschool period the child gains about 2 to 2.5 inches a year. The average height of the 6-year-old is 40 inches, or double his birth length. Since the child grows proportionately more than he gains in weight during the preschool years, he appears to be tall and thin by the end of his preschool days.

Children in the years from three to six gain muscular coordination which enables them to explore the physical environment, just as they acquire the ability to explore intellectually through constant questioning of adults and older children or even their playmates.

The child of six years has learned to walk more as adults do. The lordosis of the smaller child has disappeared. During the preschool years the constantly overactive child may suffer from persistent fatigue and may therefore develop poor posture unless preventive measures are taken.

In general, after the second year the child's motor development consists essentially in increase in strength and ease of performance. No distinctly new types of muscle activities are seen after early childhood. New kinds of performance are based on the use of skills already learned. By the time a child is five years old his skill in the use of muscles and his accuracy and speed allow him to be increasingly independent of others.

The pulse rate is normally 90 to 110, the respiratory rate about 20 when the child is at rest. The blood pressure is approximately 85 to 90 mm. of mercury systolic, and 60 mm. diastolic.

## Social and Mental Development

The child of this age has developed a conscience and has, more than in the toddler stage, internalized the mores of his group. He has begun to develop for himself such concepts as friendship, acceptance of responsibility, independence (some children of this age show their independence by running away from home), the passage of time, spatial relations, abstract words, and numbers. His attention span has lengthened.

## Specifics of Physical, Social and Mental Development

Chronologic age is misleading as a basis for child care. The development of the whole child must be considered; this requires individual consideration of the child. Yet chronologic age is useful for any discussion of classified group characteristics. By using the average of each of the characteristics as the norm for the child of any given age, it is possible to tell how far any individual child deviates from the norm. No child conforms to the average in all areas of development. He may be far above in one area, behind in another and average in all other areas. For this reason a child's behavior at any time is likely to be that of one age group in certain areas and of another age group in other areas.

*Although development does not proceed at a uniform rate in all areas, it follows a logical, precise sequence.* The rate at which this sequence occurs is an individual matter. This is the most important point to remember in applying the concept of growth and development to the care of any particular child.

**Three Years.**   The three-year-old child is less negativistic and more easily cared for than the toddler. He has fewer temper tantrums, understands words better and can be given simple reasons and explanations of cause and effect in the phenomena occurring in the world about him. He is interested in new activities; hence this is a period when learning from experience is rapid. Mental activity and verbal expression are increasingly substituted for or reinforce physical activity in the expression of emotions. For instance, a three-year-old is likely to say, "I don't like you," rather than hit someone or throw a stone. Or if he does throw the stone, his emotion is verbalized as he throws.

*Motor Control.*   Motor control in the three-year-old is evinced in the following acts:

Rides a tricycle, using the pedals
Walks backward
Walks downstairs alone; walks upstairs, alternating his feet
Can jump from a low step
Can try to dance, but balance may not be adequate
Pours fluid from a pitcher well
Begins to use scissors
Can hit large pegs in a peg board with a hammer
Can string large beads
Builds a tower of 9 or 10 blocks
Tries to draw a picture
Imitates a 3-block bridge
Copies a circle or cross to imitate model
Can undress himself; can unbutton buttons if on front or side of clothing
Helps dress himself
Can go to toilet
Can wash hands
May be able to brush teeth
Can feed himself well
Can help to dry dishes and dust.

*Vocalization, Socialization and Mental Abilities.* The three-year-old child feels safe in his world because his mother gave him security in the toddler period. His accomplishments are as follows:

Has a vocabulary of about 900 words
Uses language fluently and with confidence
Talks in sentences about things. Does not appear to care whether others listen or not
Repeats a sentence of 6 syllables. Uses longer sentence than the 2-year-old
Uses plurals in speech
May attempt to sing simple songs
Knows whether he or she is a boy or a girl
Plays simple games with others. Begins to work through the problem of his family relations with other children in play
Can understand what it means to take turns
Is toilet-trained at night

Can repeat 3 numbers
Begins to be interested in colors
Knows his family name
Has little understanding of past, present or future
Can name figures in a picture.

The three-year-old may continue to be ritualistic in many of his activities, such as arranging toys or going to bed. He is a friendly, laughing child who wants to please others, though he may be jealous of his siblings. He may have some fears, usually visual, of the dark or of animals.

**Four Years.** The four-year-old is not usually as pleasant a member of the group (family, nursery school or play group) as the three-year-old child. He

**Figure 196.** The 3-year-old (*A*) builds a tower of 9 to 10 blocks, (*B*) helps to dress herself, (*C*) can wash her hands, and (*D*) can brush her teeth. (H. Armstrong Roberts.)

**Figure 197.** The 4-year-old (A) can climb well and (B) enjoys cooperative play with other children. (H. Armstrong Roberts.)

is more noisy. It is a stormy age. Parents may expect too much of him and clamp down on his manners and the language he uses. *Do's* and *Don't's* become important. His aggression is turned toward his parents. His emotional tone is likely to change suddenly from gay to unhappy.

*Motor Control.* The four-year-old has the following accomplishments:

Can climb well
Can jump well
Can go up and down stairs without holding the railing, and using his legs alternately like an adult
Throws a ball overhand
Uses scissors successfully to cut out pictures
Copies a square
Can build a 5-block gate when model is given
Can button buttons if on front or side of clothing
Can lace his shoes
Can brush his teeth.

*Vocalization, Socialization and Mental Abilities.* The four-year-old has the following achievements:

Has a vocabulary of 1500 words or more
Exaggerates, boasts, and tattles on others
Tells family tales outside of home with little restraint

Talks with an imaginary companion, usually of the same age and sex. Projects on this imaginary playmate what is bad in himself. The imaginary playmate is usually forgotten by 6 years of age
May be mildly profane if he associates with older children
Is cooperative in playing imaginative games with several children. Group activities are longer in duration
Can go on errands outside of home
Tends to be selfish and impatient
Takes pride in accomplishments
Aggressive physically as well as verbally
May run away from home
Can name 3 objects he knows in succession
Can count to 3
Can repeat 4 numbers. Is learning number concept
Knows how old he is
Knows which is the longer of 2 lines
Can count 4 coins
Can name one or more colors well
Space perception is poor.

**Five Years.** This is usually a comfortable age for the child, and for his parents and kindergarten teacher. He has internalized social norms to the extent that he is likely to want to do what is expected of him. He is less rebellious than at four years. With greater strength, improved muscular coordination and ability to reason, he is less

**Figure 198.** The 5-year-old can roller skate. (H. Armstrong Roberts.)

frustrated by obstacles in the environment.

The five-year-old is beginning to take more responsibility for his actions. He still needs reassurance and guidance from adults in adjusting to the needs of his group. Kindergarten is important to him; the experience in group membership in an environment planned for learning under professional leadership should supplement home training and experience in the play group. The child of this age has developed an individual personality which gives an indication of what he will be like when he is older.

The outstanding physical change is that the child is beginning to lose his temporary teeth.

*Motor Control.* This includes the following abilities:

Can run skillfully and play games at the same time
Can hop well
Can jump rope
Jumps from 3 or 4 steps
Skips on alternating feet
Can roller skate on 4 wheels
Can balance on one foot for about 8 seconds
Puts toys neatly away in a box
Can use a hammer and hit a nail on the head
Can form some letters correctly
Can fold paper diagonally
Prints first name and possibly other words
Draws a fairly recognizable picture of a man
Copies a triangle from model
Can wash himself without wetting his clothes
Dresses himself without assistance
May be able to tie shoelaces.

From this age on the child will learn to be more skillful with his hands if he is given assistance and an opportunity to learn. The five-year-old has good poise and excellent motor control.

*Vocalization, Socialization and Mental Abilities.* These are as follows:

Has a vocabulary of approximately 2100 words
Repeats a sentence of 10 syllables or more
Talks constantly
Can certainly name 4 colors, usually red, green, yellow and blue. Depending upon his intelligence and his environment, he may learn earlier
Is interested in meaning of relatives—e.g. aunts, uncles, cousins
Asks meaning of words
Asks searching questions
Can determine which of 2 weights is heavier
Can identify penny, nickel, dime
Counts 10 coins
Knows names of days of weeks and a week as a unit of time
Can put together a rectangular card which has been cut diagonally into 2 pieces
No longer runs away from home.

The five-year-old is serious about himself and is concerned with his ability. He wants to assume responsibility and glories in his achievements.

### Summary

At the close of the preschool period the child's basic personality is formed. He has internalized ideals and standards taught him by his parents and teachers. For this reason his conscience influences his actions more than in a younger child. He is less dependent upon the emotional support and reassuring physical presence of his parents, and is content away from them for longer periods of time. Since he has internalized their attitudes and normally has a strong desire to please them, he is controlled by their wishes, even in their absence, far more than is the younger child. His socialization, begun in the home, is reinforced by his teachers. He feels guilty if he acts in an asocial way so as to displease the adults whom he loves.

## PLAY

**Importance of Play.** The progress which the preschool child makes in his personality development, ability to deal with reality, and control of his feelings can be seen in his play. Through play the child learns to express his feelings, whether of anger or of love, less by actions and more by words. Children of this age as they play together are less likely to inflict injury on each other than are toddlers. Through play these children develop concern for their playmates; they are sympathetic with a child who is knocked down or falls.

By observing children at play the adult gains a view into the child's world.

**Beginnings of Cooperative Play.** The child gradually shifts from solitary and parallel play to a simple form of cooperative play. He begins to exchange ideas with other children and gradually to interact with them in play activities. Among children between the ages of three and five years a loosely organized play group emerges. The activity of the group may be continuous, but the membership changes as children join or leave the group at will. These children enjoy social play, but still feel the need of solitary play at intervals; in solitary play they can do what they want in their own way. This type of loosely organized play goes on despite the bossiness or aggressiveness of some children in the group.

Toward the latter part of the preschool period a more organized type of play emerges. The membership of the group changes less frequently. It is still, however, neither complex nor stable in

**Figure 199.** The preschool child gradually learns to cooperate with others in varied situations. (H. Armstrong Roberts.)

**Figure 200.** Preschool children enjoy imitating activities which they observe adults doing. (H. Armstrong Roberts.)

its organization. Within such groups the typical child takes temporary roles of leader or follower.

**Characteristics of Play.** Preschool children play actively. They climb, run, hammer, and open doors with a bang and slam them shut. Their developing motor skills require practice so that improvement in skill may be progressive.

These children imitate the social life of adults. They play house, enacting the roles of the different members of the family, or they may imitate firemen, storekeepers, conductors or their teachers. They change from one role to another as their interest shifts with new experiences.

Preschool play is highly imaginative, but the children are always aware of the difference between the real and their imaginary world. When a child pretends that he is an Indian, he knows that he is not. Yet he plays as if there were no distinction between fact and fancy.

The play of preschool children is not only an imitation of the life about them, but also is repetitive. These characteristics are more notable in some groups than in others. Many play themes stem from a confusion in children's minds about experiences they have had in real life, e.g. the death of a grandparent or the birth of a sibling. The theme may arise from a strong feeling the child has about something in his environment, or from the urge to destroy and demonstrate aggression and power.

*The Three-Year-Old.* Three-year-olds enjoy active games, but they also like to listen to nursery rhymes which they may later dramatize. They are increasingly interested in playing with other children in constantly shifting groups of two or three. Activities shift frequently, but not always with the entrance into the group of a new member or the departure of a child who instituted the activity. These children are willing to take turns; this makes co-operative play possible. Such play takes the place of enjoyment in mere physical contact with other children. They enjoy activities with sand and water and playing with toys built for dumping and hauling. Quiet activities which they enjoy are cutting, pasting and building with blocks.

Three-year-olds like to combine playthings to make a more lifelike situation. For instance, playing with dolls brings into use the doll's bed, tea set and baby carriage. Imaginative children make substitutes for bought toys; they will use a box for the doll's bed and bits of paper for dishes.

*The Four-Year-Old.* There is a decided rise in both physical and social activity in the play of four-year-olds. They want to play in groups of two or three and often choose a favorite companion of their own sex. Although they fully accept the practice of taking turns, they are often bossy in directing others.

To be silly in their play, doing things wrongly by intention, is characteristic of this age group.

Four-year-olds have complicated ideas which they are unable to carry out in detail because of lack of skill and also of time. They are not able to carry their plan over from day to day as an older child does. They show an increase in the constructive use and manipulation of materials. They are fond of dramatic play and like to dress up. When playing house, the little girl wears her mother's old clothes. Boys as well as girls play house, and each takes the role played by the parent of the same sex. They like not only to play at household activities, but also to help mother with cleaning, wiping dishes, dusting and even ironing and hanging clothes.

Perception of shape in the four-year-

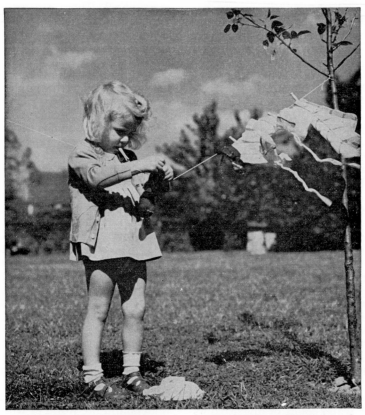

**Figure 201.**    This little girl imitates her mother by washing her doll's clothes, thus preparing for her own adult role in life. (H. Armstrong Roberts.)

old is poor, but he enjoys simple picture puzzles, using the trial and error method of finding the correct place for a piece. He is able to put his toys away, but is not likely to do so unless reminded by his mother or nursery school teacher. (In nursery school or kindergarten where all the children replace their toys on the shelf, they remind each other and do not need the teacher's direction.)

*The Five-Year-Old.*    At this age children enjoy varied activities. They like to run and jump. Such expressions as "I can and you can't" are common. Now the child plays in groups of five or six, and friendship with his playmates is both stronger and continued over a longer time. He is definitely interested in finishing what he starts, even though it takes several days to complete it. He plays house and likes to dress in adult's clothing to make his game more realistic. He is fond of cutting out pictures and of working with colored paper or on a specific project with his large blocks, e.g. making a store or boat.

In this last year of the preschool period he becomes cooperative, sympathetic and usually generous with his toys. He is interested in the world outside his immediate environment, likes to go on excursions and listens to stories of things he has never seen. He maintains interest in stories of greater length than does the three- or four-year-old.

**Selection of Play Materials.**    The choice of play materials for the preschool child should be based on the same general principles of purpose, utility and safety as the selection of toys for earlier age groups. Play materials especially enjoyed during this period are housekeeping toys and playground apparatus such as sandboxes, jungle gyms, slides and swings. Toys for active play, such as balls, wagons, tricycles and other transportation toys, and large blocks for building steps and bridges are valuable in muscle development and for learning some basic facts and principles of physics. Manipulative materials, e.g. plastic for molding, water colors or finger paints and musical toys are needed for quiet

activities. Children need equipment for cutting and pasting, picture books to color and illustrated books, both prose and rhyme, which adults or older siblings will read to them.

**Role of the Adult in Children's Play.** Children need help in learning to find pleasure in being with other children and in learning to share and remember that others have rights which they must recognize. They want to please their mothers or nursery school teachers. If a child fears instead of loving an adult, he may cooperate when the adult is present, but when she is not, he knows no limits to his actions.

# NURSERY SCHOOL

Children from two and a half or three years to five years are accepted in nursery school. There are several reasons why a child is sent to nursery school: when the mother must work outside the home to help support the family; when the child needs the socializing experience of contact with other children and total care under the guidance of well qualified people, and/or educational experience to supplement what he receives at home. Experience is given in nursery school in investigation, experimentation, exercising the imagination, creative activities, problem solving and socializing.

**Values.**    Nursery school experience promotes growth and development and improves the general health of the child. It increases the child's capacity for independent action, his self-confidence, and feeling of security in a variety of situations. Since he is in an environment planned to meet his needs and under the supervision of experts in child care, his understanding of himself and of others develops normally, and he is better able to handle his emotions. Nursery school also broadens his appreciation of the avenues of self-expression through art, music and rhythms. As he learns more about the community in which he lives, he is better able to understand the world of which his daily environment is such a small part.

**Qualifications.** The qualifications for the selection of the individual school include the qualifications of the teacher, the proportion of teachers to the number of children, health policies, physical setup and educational methods.

**Activities.** The activities provided at nursery school are first of all those of

**Figure 202.** Preschool children enjoy active play. *A,* On the sliding board. *B,* On their tricycles. (H. Armstrong Roberts.)

**Figure 203.** Preschool children also enjoy painting with (*A*) finger paints, (*B*) water colors. Note the long smock to protect the child's clothing. Newspapers may also be spread on the floor to protect the floor covering. (H. Armstrong Roberts.)

**Figure 204.** At nursery school and kindergarten young children are given many opportunities to solve new problems and to learn to interact with their peers. (H. Armstrong Roberts.)

daily life—activities which the child would perform at home, e.g. eating, toileting, napping, health practices, and play, both indoor and outdoor. The school has equipment for activities appropriate to the child's size and abilities.

**Preparation for Nursery School.** Even if the child feels secure when separated from his mother for a brief time, she must realize that nursery school, where there are a number of little children, may be a very upsetting experience for her child. Unless he is adequately prepared, the child may defend himself against the experience by uncooperative behavior or by rejecting it entirely. Each child may adjust in a slightly different way to nursery school, because the school does not present the same situation to all children. Each child has his own past experience and interprets nursery school on the basis of this experience.

Gradual preparation for nursery school generally begins with the mother's own confidence in the school she has selected. If she does not have confidence, it will be almost impossible for her to give the child confidence in the school and make it a pleasant experience for him. She should take him to the building when the school is not in session so that he may become familiar with the physical surroundings before he is left with strange adults and with children whom he may not know. He should meet his teacher on these visits and learn to trust her. He may feel more secure if he brings a toy or something else from home to make concrete the continuity of school life with that at home.

After this preparation, decision is made as to whether the child should attend the school. This depends on whether he will be able to profit from the experience, whether he feels at home there, likes his teacher and feels sure that she will take care of him when his mother is not there, enjoys being with other children, knows the routine and is confident that his mother will return and take him back home with her. Children must know these things if they are to feel secure when separated from home and mother for more than a short time. If both the mother and the child feel secure about the nursery school experience, future adjustment will probably be advantageous, and the child will enjoy and profit from the experience.

The mother stays with her child on the first day he enters school and should continue to come until he feels secure without her. The time he is in the school without her may be gradually lengthened. She should always tell him when she is leaving and assure him that she will return for him at the close of the school day. Some children need to have the experience of mother returning after a short period of being without her, to be certain that her return is part of the nursery school routine.

## CARE OF THE PRESCHOOL CHILD

### Physical Care

The preschool child is gaining competency in self-care. A feeling of security in his home environment will help him to become independent in self-care. He learns to feed himself without too much spilling, to dress and undress, to wash his face and hands, to brush his teeth and to toilet himself, but he does not take full responsibility for stopping his play and going to the toilet before urgency makes him unable to control elimination.

Even if it is more convenient for the mother to care for the child than to allow him to be independent, she should encourage him to use his abilities so that he may become steadily more independent and that independence may be the goal he desires. Naturally he is slow and often clumsy in his movements. He needs help in his bath, to tie his shoe-laces and to manipulate buttons or snappers which are almost out of reach. A little child can seldom brush and comb his hair. The straight, short hair of the boy is more easily arranged than the longer and often waved hair of the girl. The mother should plan the child's day to give him plenty of time for self-care before breakfast and before going off to nursery school or kindergarten, and for the general cleaning up before dinner. The daily schedule of activities should include time for active play, quiet play and, for the younger children in this age group, rest periods, if not naps. Time should be set aside for mother's meeting his need for cuddling and reassurance that she likes to have him home with her. She should hold him on her lap while she reads or sings to him, or as they talk together.

Throughout this carefully planned day his mother protects the child from accidents and from frustrating experiences which retard rather than develop independence.

### Sleep

The preschool child is normally so interested in whatever he is doing that he does not know when he needs sleep and rest, and resists going to bed.

The sleep of the three-year-old is frequently disturbed at night. He may have frightening dreams due to his real and imaginary daytime fears. These children may not stay in their beds, but wander around the house or want to sleep with their parents. Sleeping in a room with a brother or sister who is several years older and has outgrown the fears of the preschool period is often reassuring. Children who sleep poorly at night should have naps during the day; otherwise they are restless.

By the time the child is five years old he usually sleeps quietly and peacefully through the night. The child who gets adequate rest at night no longer needs a daytime nap. Most children over four years of age reach a stage at which naptime becomes a battle between mother and child. If the child does not sleep,

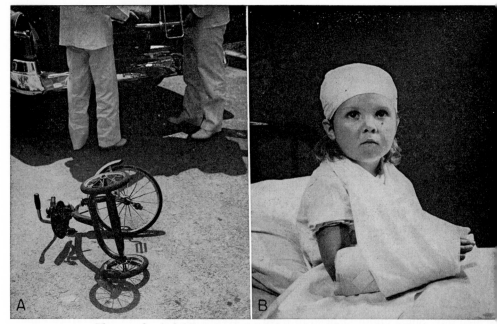

**Figure 205.**   The preschool child's increased freedom of activity coupled with an immature understanding of danger may result in accidents. *A,* The child should not have been riding her tricycle in the street. *B,* Immediate hospitalization may result. (H. Armstrong Roberts.)

he cannot be forced to do so, but his mother should insist on a rest period in a darkened room. A sleepy-time record played on his toy record player may be helpful, and he may have his favorite cuddly toy in bed with him. Before kindergarten age even the rest period may be eliminated for the average child, although overactive, excitable children may require rest in the afternoon. Most nursery schools and kindergartens have brief rest periods when the children lie on mats upon the floor or on small cots which can be folded easily and stored away when activity is resumed.

### Safety Measures

Since preschool children enjoy a wider range of freedom than does the toddler—playing outdoors alone, frequently away from the safe environment of the back yard—more accidents are likely to occur away from home.

Important causes of accidents in this age group are their increased initiative and their desire to imitate the behavior of adults, which leads them into situations hazardous for little children.

Their activities often result in falls, and their interest in new things and investigation of what they can do with them often result in serious accidents. They may play with matches, turn on the hot water faucet or get an electric shock. Their increased freedom, coupled with their immature understanding of danger, results in their playing around motor vehicles, garden pools or swimming pools.

Since preschool children cannot be kept in an accident-free environment, it is important that parents and all adults in charge of children emphasize safety measures to them. They should explain in terms the child can understand the safety measures adults take and why it is not safe for him to attempt all that his parents can do without injury. As he learns what he can do without danger of injury and how to protect himself, the child should be allowed to take greater responsibility for his own safety. Teachers in nursery school and in kindergarten not only provide a safe environment for the children, but also help them to understand the underlying principles of safety measures. The children may play games which teach them the necessary precautions to take in everyday situations such as crossing the street (see Fig. 206).

There are many cases of accidental poisoning in this age group. The children are less rigidly supervised than they were as toddlers and so are able to investigate all kinds of containers in medicine cabinets, in the kitchen, bathroom or basement. Preschool children are apt to take pills, powders or liquids because they have seen their parents take them. They may take a substance which looks like food because they think it will taste good.

The care of the preschool child who has taken poison is similar to that of the toddler (see p. 454). The preschool child, however, is more likely to be able to tell from what container he got the poison and is more cooperative in emergency measures to induce vomiting.

## Health Supervision

Regular visits to a physician are important, at intervals which he recommends, usually every six months or yearly. The physician gives the child a complete examination. He records the growth, gives advice about nutrition and any problems which occur in the management of the child, and instructs the mother on the safety factors which are essential. He may give the child who is between three and four years old a second booster dose of immunizing material against diphtheria, pertussis and tetanus. Revaccination against smallpox is done every five years; hence the child is revaccinated before he enters school.

*Dental care* is important at this age. Caries of the deciduous teeth commonly begins between the ages of three and six years and tends to spread rapidly. Since

**Figure 206.**   Children in kindergarten learn how to differentiate traffic signs and to cross the street at the proper time. (H. Armstrong Roberts.)

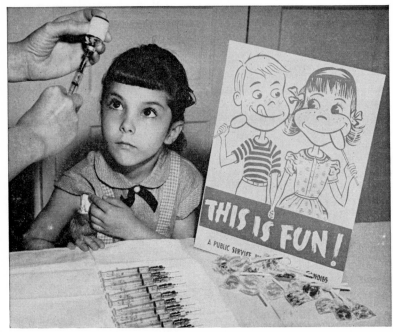

**Figure 207.** Further immunization against childhood diseases is an important part of the health supervision of preschool children. (H. Armstrong Roberts.)

the deciduous teeth act as pathfinders for the growth of permanent teeth, it is essential that the deciduous teeth be kept in good repair until the permanent teeth erupt. If the deciduous teeth are lost, the permanent teeth may drift or be crowded out of position.

Factors in caries formation include a tendency to decay, position of the teeth, the formation of pits or fissures during dental development, the presence of fermentable carbohydrate or acid-producing bacteria which cause decalcification of the teeth, and the fluoride content of the teeth.

Optimal general health reduces the probability of dental caries. Dental supervision should be a part of general health supervision, and daily care of the mouth is necessary. The teeth should be brushed after eating, and the child's intake of refined sugar should be limited.

Much research has been done on the subject of fluorides in relation to dental health. Fluorides are found in foods and in the water supply of some areas in the United States. In localities where the fluoride content is low, fluorine can be added to the drinking water; it can also be applied locally to the teeth to prevent decay. To be effective, fluorine must be available during the period when dental structure is being built up. Fluorine makes the enamel of the teeth more resistant to decay, but does not function in the repair of damage which has already occurred.

### Nutrition

Because of the preschool child's interest in exploring his environment and because of his relatively slow growth, he is less interested in eating than he was during infancy. Attempts to force him to take food that he does not want usually result in failure. Forcing a child to eat usually results in more strenuous refusal and in persistent eating problems in the future. His appetite will increase as he nears school age. Measures which have proved helpful in increasing his food intake include serving the meal in a quiet environment where there are few distractions, providing a rest period before meals, using pretty dishes, providing a comfortable chair and table, and giving small servings.

These children like plain food served attractively in separate dishes. Each child has his definite likes and dislikes. New foods should be added gradually so as to increase the variety of his intake. A small amount, e.g. a teaspoonful, should be served and a second helping given if he likes the food. If he refuses the new food, it should be offered again after he has forgotten its taste.

Children of three and a half years use a spoon, and those of four or five years use a fork. They often prefer to eat with their fingers, however. Foods which can be picked up in the fingers should be served at every meal.

By the time the child is five or six years old he can eat a simple adult diet. Even at this age, however, most children dislike creamed or highly flavored food.

Preschool children are influenced by the example and expectations of their parents in eating as in other activities. In an atmosphere in which everyone is enjoying the meal children are likely to eat more than when the father appears critical of the food and the mother is eating sparingly for fear of gaining weight. Children should not be coaxed, bribed or forced to eat. Distractions should be avoided, and the child should be allowed sufficient time to eat without having attention paid to what he has and has not eaten. He should not be permitted to nibble between meals, although midmorning and afternoon snacks of wholesome food may be given. Children are good imitators and will

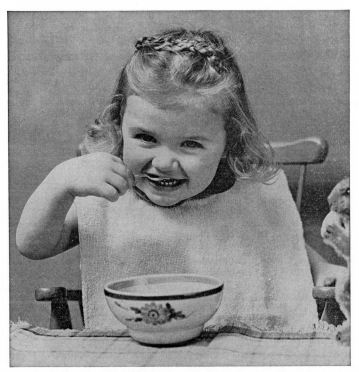

**Figure 208.** Children between 3 and 4 years still prefer to eat with a spoon, although some may show interest in using a fork. (H. Armstrong Roberts.)

copy bad eating habits from their parents or siblings just as readily as they follow good habits.

The child identifies with his family. He enjoys eating with them and joining in the conversation. Talk should include the child and not be focused on adult interests alone. It is a good time for parents to answer children's questions, provided this does not distract the child from eating.

Children of four or five years generally have acceptable manners, but too much emphasis should not be placed on details, and accidents should be accepted without causing the child embarrassment. It is more important that he eat his meal than that he have perfect table manners. The older preschool child wants to help with setting the table and washing the dishes, and should be encouraged to do so. Often helping mother at mealtimes results in the child's taking more interest in food and eating more wholesome food, rather than asking for packaged cookies, cakes, potato chips or pretzels.

Table 7 lists the food requirements of the preschool child.

*Table 7. Recommended Daily Dietary Allowances for the Preschool Child*

| | |
|---|---|
| Calories | 1700 |
| Protein | 50 gm. |
| Calcium | 1.0 gm. |
| Iron | 8 mg. |
| Vitamin A | 2500 I.U. |
| Thiamine | 0.9 mg. |
| Riboflavin | 1.3 mg. |
| Niacin equivalents | 11 mg. |
| Ascorbic acid | 50 mg. |
| Vitamin D | 400 I.U. |

From the Food and Nutrition Board, National Research Council: Recommended Daily Dietary Allowances (1958).

If the child actually refuses to eat sufficient food at mealtimes to keep him healthy, the following factors should be considered: eating too much between meals, an emotional disturbance, overfatigue or imitation of adults who have poor appetites. If the child is ill or has dental caries, he may refuse food because it nauseates him or gives him a toothache. Some children use poor eating habits as a means of getting attention or to express sibling rivalry. These causes are likely to be manifested in other behavior than simply refusal to eat. The cause must be removed to prevent trauma to the child's physical and mental health. He needs reassurance that he is loved.

## EFFECTS OF SEPARATION

The four- or five-year-old child still shows distress when his mother leaves him with strangers, but he has sufficient intellectual maturity to understand her explanation of the separation. He knows enough about the passage of time—the meaning of "soon," "this afternoon" and "tomorrow," or even "the day after tomorrow"—to realize that if he waits, his mother will come back at some fairly definite time.

A child of this age after being separated from his mother may cry when he sees her again. This is because seeing her causes his suppressed emotions to be released in tears now that she is there to comfort him. His distress is decreased by crying even if he cries again when she leaves. The child left by his mother in a child care center, nursery school or hospital is reassured by her visit because it shows that she loves him and will come back to take him home.

## TEACHING AIDS AND OTHER INFORMATION*

*American Dental Association*

Tommy's First Visit to the Dentist, 1954.
Your Child's Teeth, 1952.

*Bureau of Publications, Teachers College, Columbia University*

Baruch, D. W.: Understanding Young Children.
Hymes, J. L.: Being a Good Parent.
Hymes, J. L.: Discipline.
Neisser, E. G.: Children in the Family.
* Complete addresses are given in the Appendix.

*Child Study Association of America*

Atkin, E. L.: Aggressiveness in Children.
Wolf, A. W. M.: Helping Your Child to Understand Death, 1958.

*Hart Publishing Company, Inc.*

Blaine, A.: Play Ideas for Tots, 1957.
Lane, C. M.: Three-Minute Bedtime Stories, 1957.

*John Hancock Mutual Life Insurance Company*

Between One and Five, 1958.

*National Association for Mental Health, Inc.*

Ridenour, N., and Johnson, I.: Some Special Problems of Children: Aged 2–5 Years.

*National Dairy Council*

McEnery, E. T., and Suydam, M. J.: Feeding Little Folks.

*Public Affairs Pamphlets*

Baruch, D. W.: How to Discipline Your Children.
Dietrich, H. F., and Gruenberg, S. M.: Your Child's Safety.
Dublin, L. I.: Water Fluoridation: Facts, Not Myths.
Hymes, J. L.: How to Tell Your Child about Sex.
Hymes, J. L.: Three to Six: Your Child Starts to School.
LeShan, E. J.: The Only Child.
LeShan, E. J.: You and Your Adopted Child.
Wolf, A. W. M., and Stein, L.: The One-Parent Family.
Wolf, A. W. M.: Your Child's Emotional Health.
Yahraes, H.: Your Teen—How to Save Them.

*Ross Laboratories*

Your Children and Discipline.
Your Children's Quarrels, 1957.
Your Child's Fears, 1960.

*Science Research Associates*

Escalona, S.: Understanding Hostility in Children.
Kirkendall, L. A.: Helping Children Understand Sex.
Leonard, C. W.: Why Children Misbehave.
Mohr, G. J.: When Children Face Crises.
Montagu, A.: Helping Children Develop Moral Values.
Neisser, E. G., and others: How to Live with Children.
Puner, H. W., and others: Helping Brothers and Sisters Get Along.
Ross, H.: Fears of Children.

*U.S. Department of Health, Education, and Welfare*

Accidents and Children, 1959.
A Healthy Personality for Your Child, 1952.
Day Care Services, 1960.
Food for Family with Young Children, 1955.
Food for Groups of Young Children Cared for during the Day, 1960.

Foods Your Children Need, 1958.
Home Play and Play Equipment for Young Children, 1961.
Protecting Children in Adoption, 1955.
When You Adopt a Child, 1958.
Your Child from One to Six, 1956.
Your Children's Feet and Footwear, 1957.

# REFERENCES

American Public Health Association: Health Supervision of Young Children. New York, American Public Health Association, 1955.
Ast, D. B., and Schlesinger, E. R.: The Conclusion of a Ten-Year Study of Water Fluoridation. Am. J. Pub. Health, 46:265, 1956.
Austin, C.: Mass Preschool Vision Screening. Children, 6:58, 1959.
Badgeley, E. W.: Making Friends with Children. Am. J. Nursing, 57:1558, 1957.
Bain, K.: What Makes a Good Adoption? Am. J. Nursing, 57:306, 1957.
Bakwin, H., and Bakwin, R. M.: Clinical Management of Behavior Disorders in Children. 2nd ed. Philadelphia, W. B. Saunders Company, 1960.
Baruch, D. W.: New Ways in Sex Education. New York, McGraw-Hill Book Company, Inc., 1959.
Brauer, J. C., and others: Dentistry for Children. 4th ed. New York, McGraw-Hill Book Company, Inc., 1958.
Breckenridge, M. E., and Murphy, M. N.: Rand, Sweeney and Vincent's Growth and Development of the Young Child. 6th ed. Philadelphia, W. B. Saunders Company, 1958.
Cooper, L. F., Barber, E. M., Mitchell, H. S., and Rynbergen, H. J.: Nutrition in Health and Disease. 13th ed. Philadelphia, J. B. Lippincott Company, 1958.
DeSchweinitz, K.: Growing Up. 3rd ed. New York, Macmillan Company, 1953.
Douglas, T. S.: Religion Begins at Home. Parents' Magazine, 31:34, July, 1956.
Downing, B.: A Preschool Vision Screening Program. Nursing Outlook, 4:351, 1956.
Erikson, E. H.: Childhood and Society. New York, W. W. Norton and Co., 1950.
Fink, R. M.: How Children Tell Us They Are Afraid. Childhood Education, 32:264, Feb., 1956.
Fraiberg, S. H.: The Magic Years. New York, Charles Scribner's Sons, 1959.
Gans, R.: Eight Important Things Children Learn from Play. Parents' Magazine, 30:46, Nov., 1955.
Gesell, A., and others: The First Five Years of Life. New York, Harper and Brothers, 1940.
Harlan, H. R.: Nursing in Dental Health Programs. Nursing Outlook, 5:80, 1957.
Hudziak, B.: The Nurse's Role in Preventive Dentistry. Nursing Outlook, 9:80, 1961.
Hurlock, E. B.: Child Development. 3rd ed. New York, McGraw-Hill Book Company, Inc., 1956.
Josselyn, I. M.: The Happy Child. New York, Random House, 1955.

Kesel, R. G., and Sreebny, L. M.: Toothbrushing. Am. J. Nursing, 57:186, 1957.

Knutson, J. W.: Fluoridation: Where Are We Today? Am. J. Nursing, 60:196, 1960.

Krause, M. V.: Food, Nutrition and Diet Therapy. 2nd ed. Philadelphia, W. B. Saunders Company, 1957.

Lerrigo, M. O., and Southard, H.: Parents' Privilege. New York, E. P. Dutton and Co., Inc., 1956.

Moore, B. M.: Adults Look at Children's Values. Childhood Education, 32:257, Feb., 1956.

Moore, B. R.: When Johnny Must Go to the Hospital. Am. Nursing, 57:178, 1957.

Murphy, L. B.: Learning How Children Cope with Problems. Children, 4:132, 1957.

Nelson, W. E. (editor): Textbook of Pediatrics. 7th ed. Philadelphia, W. B. Saunders Company, 1959.

Read, K. H.: Discipline in the Nursery School. Childhood Education, 32:322, March, 1956.

Idem: The Nursery School: A Human Relationships Laboratory. 3rd ed. Philadelphia, W. B. Saunders Company, 1960.

Recommended Dietary Allowances. Revised 1958. Washington, D.C., National Academy of Sciences, National Research Council.

Schwarz, B. E., and Ruggieri, B. A.: Parent-Child Tensions. Philadelphia, J. B. Lippincott Company, 1958.

Settlage, C. F.: The Values of Limits in Child Rearing. Children, 5:175, 1958.

Spock, B.: Baby and Child Care. 3rd ed. New York, Duell, Sloan and Pearce, Inc., 1957.

Watson, E. H., and Lowrey, G. H.: Growth and Development of Children. 3rd ed. Chicago, Year Book Publishers, Inc., 1958.

Witmer, H. L., and Kotinsky, R.: Personality in the Making: The Fact-Finding Report of the Midcentury White House Conference on Children and Youth. New York, Harper and Brothers, 1952.

Woods, R. L. (editor): The Catholic Concept of Love and Marriage. Philadelphia, J. B. Lippincott Company, 1958.

# Chapter 19

# Conditions of the Preschool Child

# Requiring Immediate or Short-Term Care

## HOSPITALIZATION OF THE PRESCHOOL CHILD

THE SEPARATION anxiety brought about by hospitalization of the preschool child is likely to be less severe than that in the toddler. Children who have made a satisfactory adjustment to nursery school and have become accustomed to their mothers' being away from home for a time generally make a better adjustment to hospitalization than those who have never left their mothers' side for any length of time. Nevertheless preschool children who are ill need the security of mother's presence. The more the mother can be with the child during unrestricted visiting hours or stay night and day with him in his room, the less emotional disturbance will he suffer during and after hospitalization. If she cannot be present, the child may show an excessive desire for affection and even revengeful behavior after hospitalization.

**Preparation for Hospitalization.** The preschool child, because of his increased understanding of language, can be prepared for hospitalization in a much better way than can the toddler.

Preparation is most likely to be successful when given by the parents. They should assure the child that they will see him as often as they can and will take him home again as soon as he is well enough to leave the hospital.

The child should be told why he must go to the hospital. A detailed explanation may be beyond his understanding; what he is told should be the truth expressed as simply as possible. Young children may feel that they are ill because they have done something their parents had asked them not to do. This may be literally true as when a child is burned while playing with matches, when he knew that his parents would not permit it. He needs to be reassured that his pain is not a punishment, but the result of dangerous play. Some par-

**533**

ents appear to use this childish concept to threaten the child with illness or injury if he is disobedient. For example, a mother may say, "If you do not drink your milk, you will not grow big and strong. You will be sick." When such a child is sick, he may believe that he is to blame and that he is being sent to the hospital in punishment, possibly forever. A child should never be threatened in this way, and when hospitalization is necessary, the true reason for it should be given him.

The child pictures the hospital as very different from any previous experience he has had. He has heard adults speak of hospitalization, and always with sympathy for the sick. What he sees on entering the hospital may not be alarming in itself, but it stands for a life so different from what he knows at home that he is frightened by ideas of what may happen there.

A few days or even a week before hospitalization the mother should tell her child about the pediatric unit and stress the similarity with his daily life rather than the points of difference. Then he will ask questions as they occur to him; e.g. when he is going to bed, he can be led to ask about nighttime in the hospital and be reassured by his mother's explanation. It is not well to talk too much about the hospital far in advance of his admission, since his attention should not be centered on the experience to the point that anxiety is built up rather than relieved by what he is told.

The mother can tell the child that he will have a bed in the pediatric unit like his crib at home, but of a different color; that meals will be served him, but that he may eat his meals in bed or perhaps at a table with other children. The use of bedpans and urinals often troubles the child just admitted to the unit. This source of anxiety would be relieved if the mother had explained that they are used when children must stay in bed rather than go to the toilet.

The uniforms of nurses and physicians often frighten children because uniforms make the people about him look different from the adults he knows

at home or sees elsewhere. Much of the anxiety over these details of hospital life can be eliminated if a picture book showing the physical and social environment is given the child. Such books can be obtained from a children's library and are often routinely shown to well children by librarians or by nursery school teachers.

If older siblings have been hospitalized, they often reassure a child because he sees that they really did come back home. They may tell him that he will have ice cream there or that a child care worker or Play Lady will bring toys to him, or that a nurse made a paper cap like the one she wears for a little girl in the bed next to his. Siblings know the details of hospital life which really interest a child.

The parents should prepare the child for unpleasant experiences. If he is going to have an operation, the parents may play through the experience with him, or a sibling who has undergone surgery may enter into the game. A child should be told about going to the operating room and be reassured that his parents will be in his room when he is brought back to it. The parents should know something about the type of anesthesia to be used. If the anesthetic is to be given through a mask, this may be enacted. A towel may be used for the mask, and the child should be told to take deep breaths and then pretend to go to sleep. Depending on his age, the concept of deep breathing may be explained by telling him to pant like a dog running, to breathe as though he were blowing up a balloon or as he does when he runs rapidly. The parents may breathe with him to demonstrate how it is done. He should understand that some discomfort will be involved.

It is not advisable to explain all the procedures that might be done. The important thing is that he feels that his parents know what will happen to him. After his admission such procedures as injections should be explained to him by his mother or, if she is not present, the nurse immediately before they occur.

Visiting the children's unit before admission has few advantages for the child of four or five years. The child may enjoy packing his own toothbrush and other articles he will take to the hospital and selecting clean clothes to wear on his return from the hospital. This provides additional assurance that he will be returning home.

If the child has a toy or a blanket which he prizes and which provides a feeling of security when he is afraid or tired, it should be taken with him to his bed in the pediatric area. It will be a link with home and will give him comfort in the strange situation. Nursing personnel on the unit should recognize the importance of such a possession and protect it from being lost or damaged by other children.

All too often parents are unable to carry out such preparation because of their own anxiety over the hospitalization of the child. They may not prepare him at all, or perhaps through their ignorance they may give him a misleading impression of what he may expect. These parents might be helped if some member of the health team—the pediatrician, head nurse, supervisor, social worker or psychologist—were to explain both the life of the children in the particular area where he would be placed and the treatment necessitated by the child's condition. A little time spent in this way might save much anxiety on the part of the parents and the child, and also time of the nursing personnel.

**Response of the Child to Hospitalization.** The degree to which a preschool child responds to acute illness with anxiety and fear depends on the extent of parental anxiety and on how well he has been prepared by previous experiences for separation. Parents react differently when a child is ill than they do when he is well, because of their anxiety. They are not able to hide this feeling completely, and a complete denial of it confuses the child. The parents should master their own anxiety by a full understanding and a full acceptance of the situation. Only then can they build up confidence and courage in the child himself.

Children also feel differently toward their parents because, as the child sees it, the protecting role of the parents has weakened. Parents cannot shield the child from the discomfort or pain caused by his sickness, and he does not understand the reason for this. In the hospital he cannot understand fully why they let physicians and nurses hurt him. He becomes frightened at his parents' impotence and often angry with them for their failure. The parents must understand his feelings and provide support and comfort through meeting his total needs, even if they cannot relieve his pain. The sick child needs to feel the warmth of parental empathy, not only to hear it expressed in words.

The child's level of understanding has an important bearing on his response to illness. Because of his lack of knowledge of time sequence, he may believe that he will be ill forever. Furthermore, he cannot understand the pain or his feeling of being lost. Because of both his physical and emotional state he may have nightmares and lose the ability to evaluate reality as he could when he was well. The very unfamiliarity of his environment arouses fear that new dangers are imminent. These unaccustomed feelings and fears may cause him to become increasingly dependent. He may lose his interest in former activities and center his attention on the part of his body which is most involved in the pathologic process.

It is important first of all to help the parents handle their own anxiety and then with their aid to assist the child to face reality, understand and accept his illness, and maintain his normal interests in spite of the distraction caused by his condition. The nurse must understand her responsibility in providing emotional support to both the parents and the child. She must realize that the recovery of an unhappy, anxious child is retarded by his emotional state, that his progress is not the same as that of a happy child who is neither severely frustrated nor depressed.

**Parental Role during Hospitalization.** If the mother is not permitted to participate in giving care to the child, she may feel guilty and think that she has somehow failed as a mother. She may long to have her child back home with her, thinking of all his lovable traits and forgetting a few which are undesirable. When he is discharged from the hospital, he may be anything but lovable at home with her. His behavior is likely to make her feel even less adequate, especially when she remembers how cooperative he was with the nurses. (If he was not cooperative, she may be subconsciously glad.) She should understand that he is not reacting to her, but to the separation experience as a whole. She must not become irritable and too demanding. Rather, she should give him the love and reassurance he needs, and wait until he has recovered from his hospital experience before expecting the pleasing mother-child relations which existed before his hospitalization.

If the mother is permitted to help with the child's care, little of the reaction just described is likely to occur. If maximum contact is kept between mother and child, she will remain realistic about his illness and the kind of child he is. On discharge from the hospital the child will not find it necessary to unload his feelings of anger on his mother, for these will have been kept to a minimum during hospitalization. Children whose mothers have stayed with them during hospitalization have a low incidence of disturbances afterwards.

### Physical Care of the Child

**Bathing and Dressing.** The basic physical care of each child, with the exception of therapeutic procedures, should be similar to what he was accustomed to in his home. It should be based on the information obtained from the answers in the questionnaire which was completed at the time of the child's admission (see Fig. 9).

On the basis of the questionnaire the nurse can learn to what extent the child can bathe himself and brush his own teeth. If he is physically able, she should let him care for himself as he did at home. If he expresses his dependency needs by wanting the nurse to carry out these procedures, she should do so until he wants to do them himself. The nurse has an excellent opportunity to help the child improve his health habits on the basis of what he has already learned about such procedures.

If the child is old enough to make choices, he should be allowed to choose what daytime clothes he would like to wear. Bright-colored clothing which resembles the kind he wears at home is preferable to the hospital gown that opens down the back. It is disturbing to a preschool child to be dressed inappropriately. The nurse should make certain that such clothing fits so that the little boy does not trip over pant legs that are too long or the little girl be made uncomfortable by a dress or panties that are too tight.

**Nutrition.** Nutrition of the child who is ill may present a challenge to the nurse. While he is confined to bed it is particularly important that food be made easily available to him and that he be positioned comfortably while eating. If he is permitted to sit up, his back should be supported by a backrest or by a pillow placed against the head of the crib. His tray should be placed before him on a bed table. (These tables are attractively colored and made with collapsible legs.) The nurse should help him if he finds it difficult to feed himself. Any problems about eating which the nurse cannot solve should be referred to the head nurse or to the nutritionist.

The serving of meals for the child who is able to be out of bed should follow the pattern used in child care centers and those nursery schools which provide meals for children. Regularity is important. A bell may be rung some time before the meal is served. At this warning bell the children stop playing, and preparations for the meal are made. Following the same routine each day makes it habitual, and mealtime is orderly. The meals should be preceded by a quiet period of perhaps fifteen

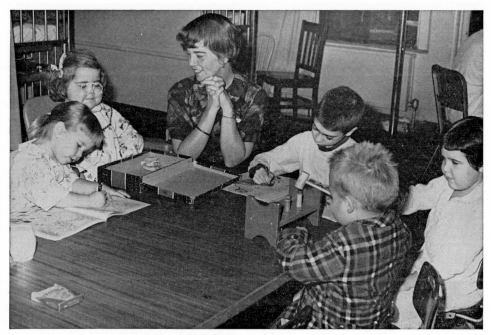

**Figure 209.**   Children enjoy playing together under the guidance of the Play Lady. As soon as the child is able to be out of bed, he should be encouraged to play with other children in a group just as if he were at home.

minutes, during which the children relax, stories are told, and they sing or listen to a record player. A positive attitude toward meals stimulates good eating habits. The children in bed should be given bedpans and urinals, and their hands should be washed. Children who are up and about the unit should go to the toilet and then wash their hands with soap under running water. Paper towels are used for drying.

Children whose condition permits should have their meals served at a table. Usually several can be seated at one table. Those with special diets or whose activities are limited may need individual service.

The chairs should be of suitable height for the table and also suited to the individual child so that his feet touch the floor. Dishes should be attractive and forks and spoons of a size appropriate for the child. All equipment which is not disposable should be sterilized. Brightly colored straws encourage a child to take fluids.

Meals should be well prepared, and a wide variety of wholesome food should be served. Small servings are preferable, and the nurse should prepare the food so that the child can eat it. Bread and butter may be served in sandwich form so that the child can handle it more easily. His meat and vegetables should be cut up so that he can take a suitable mouthful on his fork or spoon. If the food is served from a cart set up in cafeteria style which can be brought to the child's table or bed, he may have a choice of foods and, if able, help himself to what he wants. A meal served in this way is likely to be a happier experience than if a tray is set before him and he has no active participation in deciding upon the foods which will give him a balanced meal. For instance, he may choose between string beans and carrots, ice cream and custard, cookies with pink and those with white icing.

The atmosphere of the dinner table should be happy, the children talking pleasantly with one another. It is a good plan to have an adult eat with the chil-

**Figure 210.** Angry feelings which may result from hospitalization can be worked off through the use of (*A*) a bang board, (*B*) equipment peculiar to the hospital such as a "play" hypodermic injection for his nurse.

dren, to give help to those who need it and to provide a more homelike atmosphere.

### Rest

Nap time and bedtime may present problems in the hospital. The individual child's needs for sleep and his routine at home must be considered in planning his schedule in the hospital. The room should be darkened and each child prepared for either sleeping or playing quietly in his crib. A child may like to hold one of his toys. If the nurse demands that all children sleep at nap time, one or two may keep all the others awake by their rebellion against such an unreasonable order.

### Activity

Children need play activity in the hospital just as they do at home. They need it for entertainment to fill lonely hours and, by expressing their feelings through it, to reduce the trauma caused by hospitalization. While the child is confined to bed it is important for the nurse or child care worker (Play Lady) to provide toys selected on the basis of his interests and his physical state. As

soon as he is able to be out of bed he should be permitted to play with other children in a group.

Some hospitals have a special nursery school room where the children can play together under the guidance of a nursery school teacher. If no other provision has been made, the children should have a place in the unit such as a sun porch away from the acutely ill children and out of the way of the physicians making rounds. One of the unit personnel should be designated to provide the guidance which such a group needs. In the play area children should be free to develop mental, motor and social skills and to express themselves in a variety of art media, such as finger painting or molding with clay. Even in the hospital children enjoy playing with household equipment. They also like equipment peculiar to the hospital which will allow them to work out their feelings about hospitalization.

Children frequently select toys such as doctor or nurse dolls, play syringes and stethoscopes with which they can imitate the activities they see around them. Old cloth can be used in such play to restrain a doll, to make a doll's sheet, to make bandages or to improvise a sling for a supposedly broken arm.

Much of the equipment which is of value in the play of normal children is also necessary in the hospital play area, particularly simple craft materials, blocks, puzzles, story books and phonograph records. Play telephones are enjoyed because children can pretend that they are calling home.

Children's play areas cannot be kept clean and orderly when judged by adult standards. If the nurses are too concerned about the physical appearance of play areas during playtime, the children feel that the unit personnel do not approve of their play and are likely to enter only half-heartedly into their make-believe, creative work or games.

The children should be taught to take care of their personal toys which they brought from home or had given them by their parents. They may and indeed should let other children play with them if their social growth is to go forward in the hospital as it normally would in their homes, but a place must be provided where their toys can be safely stored. As a child learns to take care of his own toys he also learns to respect those of other children.

Nurses should have an opportunity to participate in the play programs for hospitalized children. In this way they not only learn about children and their play, but also have an opportunity to appreciate the contribution of the play supervisor, child care worker (Play Lady) or occupational therapist to the comprehensive care of their patients.

## Communicable Diseases

Because of the preschool child's expanding world, his participation in activities with other children in nursery school and play groups, and his exposure to environmental conditions unlike those of his home, he comes in contact with organisms which cause communicable disease more frequently than do younger children. Some of these diseases are preventable, and primary immunizations and booster doses have been given him in infancy (see p. 291), during the toddler period (see p. 425) and during his preschool years (see p.

527). Other communicable diseases are not preventable and occur more frequently in this age group than in any other. The serious complications common in past years are less frequent today, however, because of early recognition of the disease and prompt treatment.

The morbidity and mortality rates of communicable diseases have declined dramatically during recent decades, but in order to maintain this record, continued research and its application in preventive and curative medicine are necessary.

The diseases discussed in this chapter are those common in young children or against which immunizations are commonly given. The student is referred to medical textbooks for data on other communicable diseases.

**Definitions.** In order for the student to understand any discussion of communicable diseases, she must comprehend the meaning of certain terms.

A *communicable disease* is an illness caused by an infectious agent or its toxic products which can be transmitted from one person to another by

**Figure 211.** Immunization helps to check the spread of communicable diseases. All states include in their maternal and child health programs immunization against diphtheria, whooping cough, tetanus, smallpox and poliomyelitis. The incidence of pertussis, diphtheria and poliomyelitis has decreased as a result of these immunization measures. (Interdepartmental Committee on Children and Youth, Golden Anniversary White House Conference on Children and Youth: Children in a Changing World, 1960, p. 61.)

direct contact with an infected person, by indirect contact with material containing the causative agent or by contact with an intermediate host, vector or inanimate object in the environment. *Sources of infection* may be man, insects, animals or environmental factors such as dust and contaminated water or food. *Causative agents* include bacteria, yeasts, molds, protozoa, viruses and rickettsiae.

Communicable diseases may be endemic, epidemic or pandemic. An *endemic* disease is that in which the disease occurs in a proportionately limited number of people in a given area and at a relatively constant rate. *Epidemic* disease is that in which a sharp and sudden rise occurs in its incidence in a given area. A disease is *pandemic* when many cases occur over a large geographic area.

*Virulence* indicates the ability of the infecting organism to overcome the defenses of the *host*, the body which is involved. The recent habitat of an organism to a large extent influences its virulence. The *incubation period* of a contagious disease is the period between exposure to the disease and the appearance of initial symptoms. The *period of communicability* (communicability period) is the time during which the infected person can transmit the disease directly or indirectly to another person.

A *carrier* is a person or animal harboring an infectious agent without manifesting symptoms, although he or it may infect others. A *contact* is a person or animal exposed to an infection by being in contact with an infected person or animal.

*Immunity* is the ability of the body to resist the infecting agent. Such protection against specific diseases is due to the presence of antibodies which can weaken or destroy the disease-producing agent or neutralize its toxins. *Natural immunity* is present when immunity exists, although the person has not had the disease or been given any form of immunization against it. *Acquired immunity* may be either active or passive. *Active immunity* may be acquired by having had the disease or by inoculation with antigens such as dead organisms, weakened organisms or toxins of organisms. The antigens produce active immunity by stimulating the production of antibodies which protect the body against the infecting agent. Active immunization against common communicable disease has been discussed in relation to health supervision in the various age groups (see pp. 291, 425, 527). *Passive immunity* is relatively short-lived and is acquired by transference of antibodies from mother to child or by inoculation with serum which contains antibodies from immune persons or animals. Passive immunization is used to modify the disease if a person has been exposed or is already infected. Although various types of serums may be used to produce passive immunization, gamma globulin is the most frequently used source of human antibodies.

*Skin tests* may be done to determine a person's immunity against certain diseases. The most reliable and commonly used skin tests are the *Dick test*, which determines a person's susceptibility to scarlet fever, and the *Schick test*, which determines susceptibility to diphtheria.

The *treatment* of communicable disease involves helping the body to resist the invading organisms. *Prevention* is dependent on the establishment of immunity and the prevention of contacts with the causative organism. *Quarantine* means the limitation of freedom of movement of those persons or animals that have been exposed to a communicable disease for a period of time equal to the longest usual incubation period of the disease.

Children having a communicable disease are hospitalized only if they require the kind of care which necessitates hospitalization. They may be admitted to a *general hospital* if proper facilities for *isolation* are available (see p. 53). All personnel caring for such children must be instructed in isolation technique and conscientiously carry it out as a part of medical or nursing care.

**Classification.** Communicable disease entities may be classified into one of

**Figure 212.** Purpuric rash of measles. (Joseph Stokes, Jr., in Nelson: Textbook of Pediatrics. 7th ed.)

**Figure 214.** Tripod sign: characteristic position associated with stiffness of the spine in poliomyelitis. (Alex J. Steigman, in Pediat. Clin. North America, Vol. 1A.)

four groups: *upper respiratory* such as pneumonia (see pp. 302, 446), measles and diphtheria; *gastrointestinal* such as dysentery and typhoid fever; *dermal* and *membranous* such as impetigo (see pp. 190, 626) and venereal diseases (see pp. 554, 709); and *parenteral* such as serum hepatitis and malaria. If these diseases are to be controlled, the combined efforts of all personnel in medicine, nursing, dietary department, laundry, housekeeping and other departments must be available. Cleanliness is essential in preventing the spread of infection.

Table 8 presents in brief form the common communicable diseases found in the pediatric age group and those against which immunization is given.

### Acute Tonsillitis

**Incidence and Etiology.** Acute tonsillitis is common after the first year or two of life. Tonsillitis may occur with any upper respiratory tract infection or with some of the acute contagious diseases listed above. It is caused by either viruses or bacteria. Group A hemolytic streptococcus, the pneumococcus or type b *Hemophilus influenzae* may be responsible.

(*Text continued on page 550.*)

**Figure 213.** Purpuric eruption in meningococcal meningitis. (William L. Bradford, in Nelson: Textbook of Pediatrics. 7th ed.)

*Table 8.   Communicable Diseases*

| Disease | Incubation Period | Communicability Period | Causative Agent | Method of Spread | Clinical Manifestations |
|---|---|---|---|---|---|
| Chickenpox (varicella) | 10–20 days | One day before onset to 6 days after first vesicles appear | Virus | Airborne–droplet infection Direct or indirect contact | General malaise, slight fever, anorexia, headache. Successive crops of macules, papules, vesicles, crusts. These may all be present at the same time. Itching of skin. Generalized lymphadenopathy |
| Diphtheria | 2–5 days or longer | Several hours before onset of disease, until organism disappears from respiratory tract | *Corynebacterium diphtheriae* (bacillus) | Droplets from respiratory tract of infected person or carrier | Local and systemic manifestations. Membrane over tissue in nose or throat at site of bacterial invasion. Hoarse brassy cough with stridor. Toxin from organisms produces malaise and fever. Toxin has affinity for renal, nervous and cardiac tissue |
| Encephalitis | Dependent on type | Dependent on type. Types: 1. Virus encephalitis 2. Postinfectious a. Encephalitis occurs with infectious diseases; measles, German measles, mumps, smallpox and following vaccination; pertussis and following immunization 3. Toxic encephalitis Occurs with acute infections or with lead poisoning | | Transmitted by insects and mites from horses to man. Occurs with infectious disease. Cannot be transmitted to others | Encephalitis is an inflammation of the brain. Several types of virus encephalitides, depending on location in which they were found: (St. Louis, Western [U.S.], Eastern [U.S.] and others). Onset is abrupt with vomiting, fever, stiff neck, convulsions, coma. Symptoms may appear early or late. Mild symptoms include headache, stiff neck, fever, delirium. More severe manifestations include convulsions, coma, paralysis. Clinical manifestations may be produced by toxin during the course of illness. Child may be very irritable, have muscle twitching or convulsions and abnormal ocular movements |

**Table 8.    Communicable Diseases (continued)**

| Treatment and Nursing Care | Complications | Immunity |
|---|---|---|
| Symptomatic. Prevent child from scratching. Keep fingernails clean. Use soothing lotions to allay itching. If secondary infections occur, antibiotics or chemotherapy may be given | Secondary invasion of pathogenic organisms. Erysipelas, abscesses may occur | *Active immunization:* none<br>*Passive immunization:* none<br>*Tests:* none |
| Aims of treatment are to inactivate toxins, to kill the organism and to prevent respiratory obstruction. Antitoxin is given against toxin. Toxoid is given to immunized contacts. Prevent exertion. Observe for respiratory obstruction. Liquid or soft diet. Oxygen and emergency tracheotomy may be necessary | Vary with severity of disease—bronchopneumonia, circulatory or cardiac failure. Degenerative changes may occur in kidneys | *Active immunization:* one of suitable antigens may be given as part of diphtheria, pertussis, tetanus immunization.<br>*Passive immunization:* (1) newborn obtains it transplacentally from immune mother. (2) Subcutaneous injection of 1500 units of antitoxin. Immunity lasts about 3 weeks.<br>*Test:* Schick test—intracutaneous injection of diphtheria toxin. In susceptible persons, discoloration does and vesiculation may occur at site. If immune, no reaction occurs |
| No specific treatment can be given. Symptomatic care, adequate nutrition and control of convulsions are essential. Nursing care includes providing a quiet environment, aspiration of nasopharyngeal secretions, gavage or intravenous feedings, oxygen, oral hygiene, good skin care, catheterization and enemas. Sedation and broad-spectrum antibiotics to prevent secondary infection are used. Parents must be helped to understand the prolonged convalescence needed for these children | Incidence of behavioral and neurologic disturbances is higher in young children than in adults. Mental deficiency may occur | Immunization is dependent on type of organism involved. Vaccines have not proved effective against anthropod-borne types of encephalitis. Insects such as mosquitoes and mites should be destroyed by insecticides |

*Table 8.   Communicable Diseases (continued)*

| Disease | Incubation Period | Communicability Period | Causative Agent | Method of Spread | Clinical Manifestations |
|---|---|---|---|---|---|
| Epidemic influenza | 24–72 hours | Not known— possibly during early and febrile stages | Virus types A and B and sub-types | Airborne, droplet infection, direct contact | Manifestations are seen in respiratory tract. Sudden onset with chills, fever, muscle pains, cough. If infection is severe and spreads to lower respiratory tract, air hunger may develop |
| Measles (rubeola) | 7–18 days | Onset of coryza to 5 days after appearance of rash | Virus | Direct contact and airborne by droplets and contaminated dust | Fetus may contract measles in utero if mother has the disease. Coryza, conjunctivitis, photophobia are present before rash. Koplik spots in mouth, hacking cough, high fever, rash and enlarged lymph nodes are present. Rash consists of small reddish-brown or pink macules changing to papules; fades on pressure. Rash begins behind ears, on forehead or cheeks, progresses to extremities and lasts about 5 days. |
| Measles— German (rubella) | 12–22 days | Not known. Perhaps 1 or 2 days before and after appearance of rash | Virus | Direct contact or by contaminated dust particles in air | Slight fever, mild coryza. Rash consists of small pink or pale red macules closely grouped to appear as scarlet blush which fades on pressure. Rash fades in 3 days. Swelling of posterior cervical and occipital lymph nodes. No Koplik spots or photophobia as in measles |
| Meningococcal meningitis (cerebrospinal fever) | 2–10 days | Until meningococci are no longer present in mouth and nasal discharges | Meningococcus or *Neisseria intracellularis* | Direct contact | Sudden onset. Fever, headache, chills, convulsions, irritability, stiff neck and vomiting. Petechial and purpuric areas are seen in skin and mucous membranes in meningococcal septicemia. General muscular rigidity and opisthotonos are seen. Delirium, stupor or coma may occur |

Table 8. Communicable Diseases (continued)

| Treatment and Nursing Care | Complications | Immunity |
|---|---|---|
| Symptomatic. Provide bed rest and increased fluid intake. Antibiotics and sulfonamides may prevent secondary infection. Antipyretics, drugs to control cough, and analgesics for pain may be given | In severe cases pulmonary edema and cardiac failure. Secondary invaders may produce bacterial infections of respiratory tract | *Active immunization:* vaccines *Passive immunization:* none *Test:* none |
| Symptomatic. Light in room should be dimmed. Keep hands from eyes. Irrigate eyes with physiologic saline solution to relieve itching. Increase humidity in room to relieve cough. Tepid baths and soothing lotion relieve itching of skin. Encourage fluids during fever. Immune serum or gamma globulin may be given to modify illness and reduce complications. Antibacterial therapy given for complications. | Vary with severity of disease: otitis media, pneumonia, tracheobronchitis, nephritis. Encephalitis may occur | *Active immunization:* none, although research on a vaccine is in progress. *Passive immunization:* pooled adult serum, pooled convalescent serum, placental globulin, and gamma globulin of pooled plasma. Newborn obtains immunity transplacentally from mother *Test:* none |
| Symptomatic. Bed rest until fever subsides | Chief danger of disease is damaging effect on fetus if mother contracts infection during first trimester of pregnancy. Severe complications are rare. Encephalitis may occur | *Active immunization:* none *Passive immunization:* gamma globulin, pooled adult serum or plasma *Test:* none |
| Sulfadiazine and penicillin may be used. Intravenous therapy is usually necessary. Symptomatic care includes adequate nutrition (gavage if necessary), prevention of decubiti, stomatitis, and drying of conjunctivae. Sedatives may be needed for restlessness | Otitis media, ophthalmia or pneumonia may occur. Infection may extend to ventricles and cause obstructive hydrocephalus. Subdural collections of fluid may occur. Headache may persist. Intellectual faculties may be impaired. Child may have paralysis, spasticity, contractures | *Active immunization:* none *Passive immunization:* infant may have protection from placentally transferred humoral antibodies *Test:* none |

*Table 8. Communicable Diseases (continued)*

| Disease | Incubation Period | Communicability Period | Causative Agent | Method of Spread | Clinical Manifestations |
|---|---|---|---|---|---|
| Mumps (infectious parotitis) | 17–21 days | Two days before first symptoms appear until swelling disappears | Virus | Contact with salivary secretions | Salivary glands are chiefly affected. Parotid glands, sublingual and submaxillary glands may be involved. Swelling and pain occur in these glands either unilaterally or bilaterally. Child may have difficulty in swallowing, headache, fever and malaise |
| Pertussis (whooping cough) | 5–14 days | Four to 6 weeks from onset | *Hemophilus pertussis* | Airborne | Coryza, dry cough which is worse at night. Cough occurs in paroxysms of several sharp coughs in one expiration, then a rapid deep inspiration followed by a whoop. Dyspnea and fever may be present. Vomiting may occur after coughing. Lymphocytosis occurs |
| Poliomyelitis (infantile paralysis) | 5–35 days | During period of infection, latter part of incubation period and the first week of acute illness. | Virus types 1 (Brunhilde), 2 (Lansing) and (3) (Leon) | Oral contamination by pharyngeal and intestinal excretions | Acute illness. Initial symptoms of upper respiratory tract infection, headache, fever, vomiting. Types of poliomyelitis include abortive, nonparalytic, spinal paralytic and bulbar paralytic forms. Clinical manifestations may vary from mild to very severe after symptomless period following initial symptoms. Later symptoms may include intense headache, nausea, vomiting, muscular soreness, nuchal and spinal rigidity, changes in reflexes, paralysis. Tripod sign is indicative of spinal rigidity (See Fig. 214) |

**Table 8. Communicable Diseases (continued)**

| Treatment and Nursing Care | Complications | Immunity |
|---|---|---|
| Local application of heat or cold to salivary glands to reduce discomfort. Liquids or soft foods are given. Bed rest until swelling subsides | Complications are less frequent in children than in adults. Meningoencephalitis, inflammation of ovaries or testes, or deafness may occur | *Active immunization:* parenteral injection of formalized virus is being studied. Placentally transferred immunity is possible for newborns. *Passive immunization:* Gamma globulin from convalescents or unfractionated convalescent plasma or serum is of doubtful value. *Test:* complement fixation test |
| Symptomatic. Gamma globulin or hyperimmune serum may be given. Protect child from secondary infection. Provide mental and physical rest to prevent paroxysms of coughing. Provide warm humid air. Oxygen may be necessary. Avoid chilling. Offer small frequent feedings to maintain nutritional status. Refeed if child vomits. Sulfonamides and antibiotics may be given to prevent secondary infection. Small amounts of sedation may be given to quiet the child | Very serious disease during infancy because of complication of bronchopneumonia. Otitis media, marasmus, bronchiectasis and atelectasis may occur. Hemorrhage may occur during paroxysms of coughing. Encephalitis | *Active immunization:* vaccine. May be given as part of diphtheria, pertussis, tetanus immunization. *Passive immunization:* gamma globulin prepared from hyperimmune human serums. *Test:* Agglutinin titer and by complement fixation and mouse protective tests. |
| Avoid overfatigue. Both parents and child need support and reassurance. Place child on firm mattress with support for feet. Maintain good body alignment. Change position frequently. Physiotherapy may be necessary. Encourage oral intake of food and fluids. Applications of moist heat to alleviate muscular pain. Respirator, tracheotomy and oxygen therapy may be necessary in severe cases. Rehabilitation may be required. Antibacterial prophylaxis may be ordered | Emotional disturbances may occur. Gastric dilatation, melena, hypertension or transitory paralysis of bladder may occur as complications. Tonsillectomy should not be done during epidemic because of possibility of bulbar poliomyelitis. Immunizations should not be done during epidemic because of possibility of paralysis in the injected extremity | *Active immunization* may be acquired from apparent or nonapparent infection. 3 approaches are being studied: (1) killed virus vaccine, (2) living nonvirulent mutant strain of virus, (3) live virus under protective cover of antibody. *Passive:* newborn obtains it transplacentally from mother if immune. Pooled adult gamma globulin. *Test:* none |

*Relief - pain but no barbiturate*

*Isolation*

*Bland Hi Protein Diet*

*Bulbar - higher spinal; respirator*

*1952    57 thousand cases of polio    20 thou paralyzed*

*Table 8. Communicable Diseases (continued)*

| Disease | Incubation Period | Communicability Period | Causative Agent | Method of Spread | Clinical Manifestations |
|---|---|---|---|---|---|
| Rocky Mountain spotted fever | 1–10 days | Not communicable from man to man | *Rickettsia rickettsii* | Spread by wood ticks or dog ticks from animals to man. (If tick is found, it should be removed without crushing it) | Sudden onset of nonspecific symptoms—headache, fever, restlessness, anorexia. One to 5 days after onset, pale, discrete rose-red macules or maculopapules appear |
| Scarlet fever (scarlatina) | 2–3 days; rarely 1–7 days | Onset to recovery | Beta hemolytic streptococcus, group A strains | Droplet infection or direct and indirect transmission may occur | Initial symptoms are seen in pharynx. Toxin from site of infection is absorbed into blood stream. The typical symptoms of scarlet fever which result are headache, fever, rapid pulse, rash, vomiting, lymphadenitis and delirium. Throat is injected and cellulitis of throat occurs. White tongue coating desquamates and red-strawberry tongue results. Other manifestations may include otitis media, mastoiditis and meningitis |
| Smallpox (variola) | 8–18 days | One to 2 days before symptoms until crusts all drop off; usually 3 to 4 weeks | Two types of virus: variola major and variola minor | Direct or indirect contact; possibly airborne. Crusts are infectious | Abrupt onset with vomiting, headache, high fever and generalized aching. Skin eruption occurs a few days after onset, changing from macules to papules, vesicles, then pustules. Umbilication is characteristic of vesicles. Prostration or convulsions may occur. Individual lesions appear in single crop and progress at same rate. Mucous membranes of mouth and eyes become involved. Degree of scarring depends on severity and extent of eruption |

Table 8. Communicable Diseases (continued)

| Treatment and Nursing Care | Complications | Immunity |
|---|---|---|
| Early diagnosis and prompt use of broad-spectrum antibiotics. Supportive therapy, parenteral fluids, oxygen and sedatives may be necessary for seriously ill patients | Central nervous system symptoms, electrolyte disturbances, peripheral circulatory collapse, and pneumonia may occur as complications | *Active immunization:* vaccine<br>*Passive immunization:* none<br>*Test:* none |
| Penicillin, tetracyclines, sulfonamides, immune serum and antitoxin, may be given. Adequate fluid intake, bed rest, drugs to relieve pain, and mouth care are important. Diet should be given as the child wishes; liquid, soft or regular. Increased humidity for severe infection of upper respiratory tract. Cold or hot applications to painful cervical lymph nodes | Complications are caused by toxins, the streptococcus, or secondary infection. Complications of glomerulonephritis or rheumatic fever may occur | *Active immunization:* conferred by series of injections of toxin<br>*Passive immunization:* convalescent serum, whole blood from an immune donor, or antistreptococcal serum<br>*Test:* Dick test—intradermal injection of streptococcal toxin. In susceptible persons erythema occurs at site of injection. In immune persons, no reaction occurs |
| No treatment except antibiotics and sulfonamides for secondary infections. Eye care, oral hygiene, local applications to control itching, and diet as tolerated are given. Severe cases may require sedation and parenteral fluid therapy | Laryngitis, bronchopneumonia and encephalitis. Infants having eczema may develop generalized vaccinia, if vaccinated | *Active immunization:* vaccination, using either multiple pressure method or scratch method<br>*Passive immunization:* vaccinia hyperimmune gamma globulin may modify disease<br>*Test:* none |

*Table 8. Communicable Diseases (continued)*

| Disease | Incubation Period | Communicability Period | Causative Agent | Method of Spread | Clinical Manifestations |
|---------|-------------------|------------------------|-----------------|------------------|-------------------------|
| Tetanus | 4–21 days | Not comminicable from man to man | *Clostridium tetani* bacillus | Organisms are found in soil and enter body through a wound. Deep puncture wounds are ideal for growth of this anaerobic organism. Burns are ideal because of presence of necrotic tissue | Acute or gradual onset. Bacillus produces a powerful toxin having an affinity for nervous system. Clinical manifestations include muscle rigidity and spasm, hyperirritability, headache, fever. *Trismus* or inability to open the mouth is present. Spasm of facial muscles results in *risus sardonicus*, or the sardonic grin. Urine may be retained due to spasm of urethral muscles. Cyanosis and asphyxia may occur due to muscle spasms of larynx and chest |

**Clinical Manifestations.** *Nonbacterial* tonsillitis is a mild disease of gradual onset and short duration. The temperature is not usually above 102° F. There is headache, anorexia, sore throat and cough. There may be vascular injection of the throat and an exudate. Cervical lymphadenopathy is present. There are no complications.

In *bacterial* tonsillitis the onset is rapid, the temperature rising to 102 to 105° F., causing in the younger child convulsions, in the older child chills. There is headache, vomiting and pharyngeal pain. The throat may be mildly injected or may become very red and swollen, with patches of exudate. Cervical lymphadenopathy is present.

Serious conditions may follow or be precipitated by bacterial tonsillitis due to the streptococcus, e.g. scarlet fever, acute glomerulonephritis and rheumatic fever. Urinalysis should be made weekly for about a month, and the child should be observed for a rash and for manifestations of rheumatic fever.

**Diagnosis and Complications of Bacterial Tonsillitis.** The *diagnosis* is made by bacterial cultures, and treatment is based on the results of this laboratory study.

*Complications* which may occur include abscess formation in the cervical lymph nodes, and ulcerative throat lesions which may be found in debilitated children. Pneumonia, otitis media and meningitis are possible complications. An acute mesenteric adenitis, which may simulate appendicitis, may also follow the acute attack of tonsillitis.

**Treatment and Nursing Care.** The *treatment* of nonbacterial tonsillitis is symptomatic. Penicillin is given in bacterial tonsillitis if the infection is caused by group A beta hemolytic streptococcus. Other antibacterial drugs given depend on the type of organism involved. Isolation is necessary, and bed rest essential. Aspirin may be given to relieve pain, and cold or hot compresses and/or an ice collar or hot-water bottle may be placed around the neck. An adequate fluid intake is essential. Cold or hot fluids are preferable to those at room temperature. When the throat is extremely painful, the child should not be encouraged to eat, but if he desires food, a soft diet may be given.

| Treatment and Nursing Care | Complications | Immunity |
| --- | --- | --- |
| After injury and during illness toxins should be neutralized with antitoxins. Wound should be cleaned thoroughly. Antibiotics should be given to prevent infection of wound. Place child in darkened, quiet room. Avoid any stimulation which may cause spasms. Sedation may be used to control spasms. Tracheotomy may be necessary if laryngospasm occurs. Parenteral fluids, oxygen, respirator, gavage feedings and indwelling catheter may be necessary | Obstruction of larynx, anoxia, atelectasis, and pneumonia | *Active immunization:* toxoid is a potent antigen. May be given as part of diphtheria, pertussis, tetanus immunization. *Passive immunization:* newborn has placentally transmitted antitoxin, but it is inadequate for protection. Passive immunization results from injection of antitoxin within a few hours after wound occurs *Test:* none |

Warm saline throat irrigations may be ordered for the older child. He should sit up and hold his head forward over a basin. If the child is prepared for the procedure and instructed how to cooperate, he is not likely to choke or gag.

If the child has had rheumatic fever at some time, penicillin should be given prophylactically to prevent recurrence, and the child should be kept from contact with children who have throat infections.

## Acute Glomerulonephritis

**Incidence, Etiology and Pathology.** Acute glomerulonephritis is the most common form of nephritis in children, but the least common among adults. Approximately 66 per cent of the cases of this disease occur in children under the age of 7 years. It is seldom seen under three years of age and is more common in boys than in girls. The condition does not appear to run in families.

Acute glomerulonephritis is an antigen-antibody reaction following an infection in some part of the body—usually due to a group A beta hemolytic streptococcal infection of the upper respiratory tract. Nephritis may follow scarlet fever or a streptococcal infection of the skin such as impetigo or infected eczema. Nephritis may occur from one to three weeks after the onset of the infection.

The kidneys become enlarged and pale. On the cortical and cut surfaces there are small punctate hemorrhages. The glomeruli appear large and relatively avascular. The glomerular capillaries permit blood protein and cells to pass into the glomerular filtrate. The cells of the tubules appear granular and swollen. Capillary damage occurs. (Kidney tissue can be obtained by needle biopsy during life and can provide some information about the pathologic process occurring.) There may be generalized edema of the body with cerebral edema. Cardiac involvement may occur.

**Clinical Manifestations and Diagnosis.** Attacks of glomerulonephritis may vary from a mild illness which may go unnoticed to a severe illness having a sudden onset. *Clinical manifestations* in severe cases may include headache, malaise, high fever, hypertension, oliguria or anuria, and possibly cardiac decompensation leading to death.

In the usual case the child is not

critically ill, but has hematuria. The urine may appear grossly bloody or may have a smoky color. There may be mild edema around the eyes; only rarely is there generalized edema unless the child has cardiac decompensation. The temperature at first may be elevated to 104° F., but within a week falls to 100° and continues at this level until the kidneys heal. The child may have a headache, anorexia, vomiting, constipation or diarrhea. Hypertension may occur. The systolic blood pressure may be elevated to 200 mm. of mercury; the diastolic pressure may be 120 mm.

Cerebral symptoms may occur when the blood pressure rises, owing to cerebral ischemia as a result of vasospasm. The child complains of headache, may be drowsy, may have diplopia and convulsions and may vomit. The pulse is slow. The cerebral symptoms disappear when the blood pressure is reduced.

The urinary output is usually less than normal. The urine contains albumin, red blood cells, some white blood cells and casts, and has a high specific gravity. The blood urea nitrogen value is elevated. Anemia may be present. The corrected erythrocyte sedimentation rate is rapid.

Clinical improvement can be noted between one and two weeks after the onset. The urine becomes normal in approximately six weeks to four months.

Approximately three quarters of all children having glomerulonephritis have cardiac involvement. Cardiac failure may cause death, but if the child recovers, there is complete restoration of cardiac function.

Renal function is seldom normal early in the disease. With clinical recovery renal function may return to normal immediately or gradually over a period of several months.

The *diagnosis* is based on the history of previous infection, the presence of hematuria, slight edema and albuminuria. If cardiac failure occurs early in the disease, nephritis may not be the initial diagnosis.

Other diagnoses which must be considered are acute pyelonephritis (see p. 338), scurvy (see p. 349) and blood dyscrasias.

**Treatment.** The treatment is symptomatic. Bed rest is ordered during the acute stage of the disease and until urinary findings are nearly normal. After that, activity does not affect the course of the disease. The urine should be examined at frequent intervals. The child must be protected from chilling, fatigue and contact with other children and adults having respiratory infections. The diet during the first few days should consist of milk and sweetened fruit juices. After the acute phase the child may have a soft and then a regular diet. If edema is severe, the salt in the diet may be limited. During the acute phase protein may be restricted to some extent.

Penicillin should be given during the acute phase because of streptococci found on pharyngeal cultures.

If the blood pressure is elevated, indicative of vasospasm, cardiac failure or hypertensive encephalopathy may develop. If the systolic blood pressure is above 140 mm. and the diastolic above 95 mm., magnesium sulfate may be ordered for intravenous or intramuscular administration as a hypotensive agent. This drug, given to relax the vasospasm, may sometimes produce toxic manifestations of severe respiratory depression and affect the heart muscle. These manifestations may be counteracted by giving calcium gluconate or calcium chloride intravenously. Fluids should be restricted if the child has severe hypertension, unless the urinary output is large. Recently it has been found that a combination of reserpine and hydralazine hydrochloride (Apresoline) given intramuscularly reduces the blood pressure. Reserpine and hydralazine hydrochloride may be given orally in divided doses after the initial dose.

If the child has hypertensive encephalopathy with convulsions, he may need sedation. A lumbar puncture and oxygen therapy may also be ordered. If the child has cardiac failure, sedation with opiates, digitalis and oxygen may be indicated. It is necessary to follow the cardiac status after the symptoms have disappeared.

If the urinary output is decreased, acidosis, edema and uremia may develop. The need in therapy is to increase the urinary output and the excretion of waste products of metabolism, but there are no known therapeutic measures by which this can be done. Enough water should be taken so that the kidneys can excrete at their maximum capacity. If the child is vomiting, fluids can be given intravenously or subcutaneously to prevent dehydration and acidosis. Solutions containing potassium should not be given when oliguria or anuria is present. Sodium lactate and 10 per cent glucose solution may be given. When nitrogen retention is severe, it may be necessary to eliminate protein from the diet.

If anuria persists for five to seven days, the artificial kidney or exchange transfusions may be used.

Tonsillectomy and adenoidectomy should not be done for several months after the acute phase, and administration of penicillin should precede and follow the operation to prevent bacterial spread.

**Nursing Care.** The nurse should prevent chilling of the child by dressing him warmly and, when he is in bed, covering him with light but warm blankets. He should be kept in a well ventilated, warm room away from children with infections. During the acute phase of the illness he should be in bed, and when he is allowed up, he should avoid fatigue. He should have sufficient play activities to keep him quiet and contented.

Vital signs should be noted as ordered; the blood pressure should be taken frequently because of sudden changes which may occur. Any rise should be reported at once. The nurse should observe indications of cerebral manifestations due to hypertension. When these occur, the child should be placed in his crib with the gates raised. If he is in a bed, side bars should be applied to prevent him from falling. When the blood pressure is elevated, the nurse should have equipment on hand to give magnesium sulfate or other medications which the physician may order.

Good skin care is necessary. The skin should be kept clean and dry. The diet and fluid intake should be as ordered by the physician, and any limitation of salt, fluids or protein followed exactly. If the fluid intake is restricted, the amount allowed in twenty-four hours should be divided throughout the day. The fluid intake and output should be measured. The child should be weighed daily to determine progress.

To prevent these children from becoming disciplinary problems when they feel better, all the nurses caring for them should establish limits to behavior and be consistent in their care. They should allow the child as much independence within limits as he is able to assume. If he is sent home for convalescence, the nurse should help the mother plan ways to keep him happy while on prolonged bed rest.

**Prognosis.** The prognosis is guarded. Glomerulonephritis is usually benign in childhood, and the prognosis is good, but it is unpredictable for the individual child. Second attacks are uncommon, but if healing is not complete, the child may again have symptoms if he has another upper respiratory tract infection or a tonsillectomy. The course of glomerulonephritis may last from ten days to a year. Chronic nephritis may develop in a small number of children, or they may die as a result of their illness.

### Vulvovaginitis

Vulvovaginitis occurs with some frequency in childhood, especially after the toddler period. There are two types: nongonorrheal vaginitis and gonorrheal vaginitis. Nongonorrheal vaginitis is common, whereas gonorrheal vaginitis is decreasing in frequency.

Prepubescent girls tend to acquire vaginal infections more readily than do adolescents or adult females because the mucosa of the immature vagina is covered with a very thin epithelium in comparison with that of the adult, and the vaginal secretions are neutral instead of acid as in the adult. Since a thick vaginal epithelium and an acid medium are protective devices against infections, the child is relatively open to infection in this area.

### Nongonorrheal Vulvovaginitis

**Etiology, Clinical Manifestations, Treatment and Prognosis.**   Practically any pathogenic organism can cause nongonorrheal vaginitis. It may be caused by organisms producing thrush, varicella, measles or diphtheria at the same time that the systemic disease occurs. It may occur when the child has an upper respiratory tract infection or may be caused by organisms commonly found in the colon.

If the child is not kept clean, if she masturbates, inserts a foreign object into the vagina or has pinworms, vulvovaginitis may result. If the vaginitis does not respond to therapy, the physician should look for a foreign object causing irritation with subsequent infection.

The *clinical manifestations* are red and swollen genitals and a vaginal discharge of varying amount and consistency. In some cases a foul odor is present.

The *treatment* is both systemic and local. The child's general health should be improved and the underlying cause of the infection found. The genitals must be kept clean. If the causative agent is that which produces thrush, Mycostatin or 1 per cent aqueous solution of gentian violet may be applied locally. Mycostatin may also be given systemically. Antibiotic therapy should be given as needed for specific infections. Douches may be ordered, but usually are unnecessary. Removal of the cause and appropriate treatment assure recovery in most cases.

### Gonorrheal Vaginitis

**Etiology, Clinical Manifestations and Diagnosis.**   Bacteria causing gonorrhea may gain entrance into the child's vagina during the birth process, from the contaminated hands of the attendants

or, later, the hands of the mother. Infection may be transmitted by a rectal thermometer or by contact with contaminated articles such as bathtubs or, with older children, the toilet seat.

The discharge may vary from a thin watery type to a thick, yellow, purulent discharge, depending on the severity of the infection. There is redness of the vulva and vagina. Although in some cases there is little or no discomfort, there may be dysuria, fever, and excoriation of the skin of the thighs.

The *diagnosis* is made by laboratory analysis of a sample of the discharge obtained from the vagina or the cervix of the uterus. Bacterial studies, including a culture and a direct smear, should be made.

**Complications and Treatment.**   *Complications* are much less frequent in children than in adults and usually consist of inguinal adenitis, proctitis or urethritis.

The *treatment* generally consists in extreme cleanliness. Penicillin is the drug most frequently used. The child should be examined bacteriologically two weeks after therapy has been completed.

**Nursing Care.**   The nurse should examine the genitals when bathing all children for evidence of a discharge of any kind. If a discharge is present, she should report this to the physician. Individual bedpans and thermometers should be provided for all children. U-shaped toilet seats with paper protectors should be used for each child. Showers or spray baths are preferable to tub baths.

The child should be isolated until cured, and the nurse should be careful in carrying out isolation technique that she does not transmit infection to other children or herself become infected. The child should not return to kindergarten or nursery school until the infection is completely cured, because of the danger of spreading gonorrhea among the other children.

**Prognosis.**   The prognosis is good with adequate treatment; without treatment, infection continues for a long time, possibly until puberty.

## Strabismus (Squint, Cross-Eye)

**Significance and Etiology.** Strabismus is a condition in which the extraocular muscles do not balance; therefore the eyes cannot function in unison. The child seems to be looking in two directions at once. The normal newborn many times appears to have a squint at birth, and this may continue until approximately the age of six months, when his eyes become normal. Other young infants appear to have strabismus when they have epicanthal folds and a broad nose. This latter condition is termed *spurious squint*, and no treatment is necessary.

The importance of strabismus in the pediatric age group is that (1) one eye is generally not used as much as the other, and therefore poor vision in that eye results from disuse; (2) there is absence of fusion of vision; and (3) emotional problems occur when the child is taunted by other children about his deformity. Since in strabismus the eyes do not maintain parallelism, the image seen by the deviating eye is suppressed. As a result there is progressive diminution of vision on the affected side leading to loss of vision (amblyopia).

There are several causes for strabismus, and one or more may be found in any case. In some cases it is difficult to ascertain the cause. Strabismus may be congenital or familial, or it may be caused by an acute illness such as encephalitis or diphtheria. It may be due to paralysis of certain muscles or may occur because, although they are not paralyzed, the muscles do not function together.

**Clinical Manifestations and Treatment.** The child with strabismus may be able to fuse when he looks in certain directions, but not in others. He may not be able to describe to his mother what he sees, but he may tilt his head to bring the images together or close one eye to block out an undesired image. He may appear clumsy and may stumble, or be unable to pick up objects with accuracy. There are various types of strabismus, each producing slightly different effects on the eyes.

The first step in *correction* of strabismus is to prevent double vision and to hide the defect by placing a patch over the good or fixating eye. The patch should be kept on all day and cover the eye completely. The patch may be necessary for weeks or months while the child is forced to develop the deviating eye. Small children, even as young as fourteen months, may wear corrective glasses. Orthoptic treatment or muscle exercises may also be effective in developing fusion.

Surgical treatment is carried out on children who do not benefit from exercises or glasses. Operation must be

| A | B |

**Figure 215.** Strabismus. *A*, Demonstrating the squint of congenital nonaccommodative esotropia of the left eye. There is also a hemangioma of the left upper eyelid. *B*, The internal strabismus is bilateral and symmetrical. At operation both internal rectus muscles were found to be short, fibrous and ropelike in consistency. (From the collection of Dr. Arnall Patz of Baltimore.) (Schaffer: Diseases of the Newborn.)

done by the age of three or four years if parallelism of the eyes and binocular vision are to be achieved. Surgery consists in lengthening or shortening extraocular structures.

Strabismus should be corrected before the child goes to school, because other children will laugh at his defect, and he will in consequence suffer emotional trauma.

**Nursing Care.** The nurse should help both the mother and the child to understand the importance of eye exercises and of wearing glasses prescribed by the ophthalmologist. The child who wears glasses must be taught how to protect them when he plays and how to keep them clean. A broken lens should be replaced immediately. The child's glasses should be brought with him when he is hospitalized and kept in their case, in the bedside table, when he is not wearing them.

The child who is scheduled for operation for strabismus should be hospitalized a few days before the day of operation. He should be prepared by his mother not only for hospitalization, but also for the postoperative period when his eyes will be covered and his arms restrained. The reasons for this type of treatment should be explained to the child before he goes to surgery. He should also experience having his eyes covered and his arms restrained by his mother or nurse so that he will not be frightened when this is done after his return from the operating room. The child should know that as soon as possible the eye dressings and restraints will be removed. The child's mother should be encouraged to remain with him postoperatively to provide the sense of security he needs when he cannot move or see. His mother or nurse should read stories to him, play phonograph records or turn on the radio, and play simple games with him so that the hours of blindness pass more quickly. The mother or nurse should speak before touching him so that he is not startled.

A regular diet may be given postoperatively as soon as the child is no longer nauseated. These children enjoy being told about their food while the mother or nurse feeds them. Postoperatively the nurse can help the mother understand the exercises recommended by the ophthalmologist. She can also notify the nursery school or school nurse so that the same exercises may be continued regularly.

**Prognosis.** Usually, the earlier treatment is given, the better are the results to be expected. Early surgical correction usually cures the deviation and prevents personality disorders from occurring. If visual acuity has been affected, permanent reduction of sight may be expected.

### Tonsillectomy and Adenoidectomy

Not all children need to have their tonsils and adenoids removed. These tissues act as a definite defense against occurrence and spread of respiratory infections. The physician considers the necessity for removal in the individual case. Operation was done in the past for many reasons in no way connected with these lymphoid tissues. Today the conservative approach to this problem is becoming widespread. Antibiotic treatment for respiratory infections has obviated the need for tonsillectomy and adenoidectomy in many cases.

**Indications.** Indication for removal of tonsils and adenoids is based on clinical manifestations related to pathology in these tissues. The usual indication is recurrent or persistent sore throat. The child may have chronic infection with hypertrophy of the tonsils and adenoids. In considering hypertrophy, it must be remembered that tonsils are normally relatively larger during early childhood than in later years. Hypertrophy may be due to chronic infection, and the cervical glands may also be enlarged. In some children, however, the tonsils may be small and embedded behind the faucial pillars.

Obstruction to breathing or swallowing is more often due to enlarged adenoids than to tonsils. The adenoid structure which is normally present, especially on the posterior wall or roof of the nasopharynx, may become hypertrophied and interfere with the passage of air through the nose and also obstruct the eustachian tube.

The clinical manifestations of the condition include mouth-breathing, rhinitis and sometimes a dull facial expression. The voice may be muffled and nasal in quality. A persistent cough may be present. Chronic otitis media may occur, and the child may become permanently deaf unless the obstruction to the eustachian tube is removed.

Infection of structures near the tonsils may be an indication for tonsillectomy. Such infections include retro-tonsillar and peritonsillar abscesses and suppurative cervical adenitis.

The decision for performing tonsillectomy and adenoidectomy must be based on problems connected with these tissues. Usually the tonsils and adenoids are removed at the same time; the child's condition may indicate that separate removal is advisable, however. Operation in the past was sometimes done in a blind search for the source of an infection. It is warranted only if the physician attributes clinical manifestations directly to a pathologic condition of the tonsils and adenoids. Other symptoms, such as fever or anorexia, it must be remembered, may be due to many other causes.

If removal of the tonsils and adenoidal tissue is indicated, but operation is contraindicated, as when a child has hemophilia, the physician may recommend radiologic treatment which results in shrinkage of the tissue.

**Age for Operation.** The tonsils and adenoids seldom need to be removed in infancy or the toddler period, but during the preschool period tonsillectomy and adenoidectomy may be necessary. The operation should be postponed as long as possible for two reasons: (1) the condition may correct itself in a year or more as the tissues normally become smaller, and (2) the operation is psychologically more traumatic to a younger child because of fears prevalent in this age group.

**Time for Operation.** Tonsillectomy and adenoidectomy should not be done during the summer or early fall because of the increased danger, created by the raw surface, of the child's contracting poliomyelitis should he be exposed to the disease. This precaution is advisable even if the child has been immunized against poliomyelitis. He is more likely to suffer the dangerous bulbar type after operation than at any other time. Colds and sore throats are more prevalent in the winter and spring than at any other time of the year, but antibacterial agents are given to reduce the danger of such a secondary bacterial infection.

Tonsillectomy and adenoidectomy should not be done until about fourteen to twenty-one days after an acute infection has subsided. If the child has a chronic infection and surgical removal of the tonsils and adenoids is necessary, an antibiotic should be given for a few days before and after operation. When a child has a history of rheumatic fever, penicillin or sulfonamides, or both, should certainly be given.

**Preparation for Operation and Preoperative Care.** The child's parents should be told of the nature of the operation. The child should be prepared for admission to the hospital as are all children brought in for treatment. He should also be told something about the operation he is to have. He should know that it will be in his throat. The nurse in the clinic or physician's office may help the mother if she does not know how to prepare the child in terms he will understand. If the mother has not prepared the child before he comes to the hospital, she is probably incapable of doing so. The nurse must then explain to the child in a general way what will be done in the operating room, particularly with reference to how he will feel when he comes out of anesthesia.

Since these children are of an age when the first teeth are loosened and fall out, the nurse should observe for loose teeth and report them to the physician so that they may be removed before the child is given the anesthetic.

One of the barbiturates, together with atropine, is used for preoperative sedation. Food and fluids are withheld for several hours before operation.

**Postoperative Care.** Immediately on his return from the operating room the child is placed in a prone position with a pillow under his abdomen and chest to facilitate drainage of secretions and to prevent aspiration of vomitus. He should be observed constantly until he is awake and frequently thereafter for several hours. His pulse—rate and quality—degree of restlessness, frequency of swallowing and vomiting should be noted, since these are symptoms indicative of hemorrhage.

Bed rest is indicated for the remainder of the day, and rest periods are necessary for several days after.

Chipped ice may be given when the child wakens. Soft foods and fluids may be started as soon as the nausea following anesthesia is over. Milk and synthetic fruit juices are given at first, and later the natural fruit juices. The synthetic juices are less irritating to the throat than are most natural juices. All contact with infection should be avoided. Aspirin may be ordered for discomfort and ice bags applied to the throat to relieve pain.

**Complications.** Possible complications are postoperative hemorrhage, lung abscess, septicemia and pneumonia. The most common complication is hemorrhage. This may be controlled by packing or ligation. If the hemorrhage is severe, anemia, fever and possibly cardiac dilatation may develop. A transfusion may be indicated.

**Reaction of Child to Operation.** Children who are able to integrate this experience into their personality structure and who have few, if any, emotional ill effects later are those who have been able to transfer positive feelings from the mother to the nurse, to direct their interest away from themselves to other children and to toys and games, and to express themselves freely, either verbally or by crying.

The children who are the most likely to have emotional problems are those who fail to establish positive relations with the nurse, possibly because the mother-child relations are inadequate, who withdraw from the situation or react with panic to it, who are concerned only with their own discomfort and who cannot express their feelings about surgery or hospitalization. Parents and nurses may consider these children good during hospitalization, but they are likely to show trauma on their return home.

**Discharge of the Child from the Hospital.** Written instructions should be given parents about the care of the child after discharge and about symptoms which would indicate that he should be seen at once by a physician. Such symptoms are transient earache, frequent swallowing or the vomiting of blood. The instructions should include (1) suggestions for his care, such as keeping him quiet for a few days, fluids and foods to be given, and the necessity of protecting him from infection; (2) information about the giving of medications ordered by the physician; and (3) if the child is not under the care of a private physician, the name and telephone number of the physician to be called in case the mother needs his advice or emergency care for the child, and the location of the place where the child should be taken for the follow-up examination.

## TEACHING AIDS AND OTHER INFORMATION*

*Children's Medical Center, Boston, Mass.*
> Sever, J. A.: Johnny Goes to the Hospital, 1953.
> Sever, J. A.: Johnny's First Visit to His Dentist, 1957.
> Sever, J. A.: Johnny Visits His Doctor.

*Equitable Life Assurance Society of the United States*
> Larimore, G. W.: Home Health Emergencies, 1956.

*F. A. Davis Company*
> Shane, S. M.: Anesthesia for Frankie, 1955.

*John Hancock Mutual Life Insurance Company*
> Home Care of Communicable Diseases, 1957.
> Diversions for the Sick, 1954.

*Mental Health Division, Department of National Health and Welfare, Ottawa, Canada*
> Preparing Your Child for Hospital.

* Complete addresses are given in the Appendix.

*Science Research Associates*
Josselyn, I. M.: Emotional Problems of Illness.

*State of Illinois, Department of Public Welfare*
Going to the Hospital.
You and Your Child—Getting Sick.

*U. S. Department of Health, Education, and Welfare*
Meningococcal Meningitis, 1960.

*Wonder Books*
Berger, K., Tidwell, R. A., and Haseltine, M.: A Visit to the Doctor, 1960.
Chase, F.: A Visit to the Hospital, 1958.

## REFERENCES

American Academy of Pediatrics: Care of Children in Hospitals. Evanston, Illinois, American Academy of Pediatrics, Inc., 1960.
Idem: Report of the Committee on the Control of Infectious Diseases. Evanston, Illinois, American Academy of Pediatrics, Inc., 1957.
Barker, S. M.: Pediatrics, Family Style. Am. J. Nursing, 58:1123, 1958.
Blom, G. E.: The Reactions of Hospitalized Children to Illness. Pediatrics, 22:590, 1958.
Bower, A. G., Pilant, E. B., and Craft, N. B.: Communicable Diseases. 8th ed. Philadelphia, W. B. Saunders Company, 1958.
Boyd, T. E.: How the Present Poliomyelitis Vaccine Was Discovered. Am. J. Nursing, 57:722, 1957.
Brooks, M.: Constructive Play Experience for the Hospitalized Child. Journal of Nursery Education, 12:7, Winter, 1957.
Burian, H. M.: Strabismus. Am. J. Nursing, 60:653, 1960.
Carter, F. H., and others: Hemodialysis in Children. J. Pediat., 51:125, 1957.
Coleman, L. L.: Children Need Preparation for Tonsillectomy. Nursing World, 130:8, May, 1956.
Dimock, H. G.: The Child in Hospital. Philadelphia, F. A. Davis Company, 1960.
Doran, S. L.: About Polio. Children, 6:194, 1959.
Dull, H. B., and Rakich, J. H.: Tetanus Today. Nursing Outlook, 7:464, 1959.
Erickson, F. H.: Play Interviews for Four-Year-Old Hospitalized Children. (Monographs of the Society for Research in Child Development, Inc.) Lafayette, Indiana, Child Development Publications, Purdue University, 1958.
Erickson, F.: Reactions of Children to Hospital Experience. Nursing Outlook, 6:501, 1958.
Flugge, M., and others: A Good Time for All. Am. J. Nursing, 56:1540, 1956.
Gross, R. E.: The Surgery of Infancy and Childhood. Philadelphia, W. B. Saunders Company, 1953.
Harvie, F. H.: Pediatric Methods and Standards. 3rd ed. Philadelphia, Lea & Febiger, 1958.
Krugman, S., and Ward, R.: Infectious Diseases of Children. St. Louis, C. V. Mosby Company, 1958.
Maclean, M. M., Creighton, H., and Berman, L. B.: Hemodialysis and the Artificial Kidney. Am. J. Nursing, 58:1672, 1958.
Mauksch, I. G.: Larry Has His Tonsils Out. Am. J. Nursing, 57:903, 1957.
Moore, B. R.: When Johnny Must Go to the Hospital. Am. J. Nursing, 57:178, 1957.
Moos, M. S.: More than Child's Play. Am. J. Nursing, 58:1679, 1958.
Nelson, W. E. (editor): Textbook of Pediatrics. 7th ed. Philadelphia, W. B. Saunders Company, 1959.
Paterson, D., and McCreary, J. F.: Pediatrics. Philadelphia, J. B. Lippincott Company, 1956.
Paul, J. R.: Poliovirus Vaccines: Killed and Alive. Am. J. Nursing, 60:60, 1960.
Reed, H.: Squint or Strabismus. The Canadian Nurse, 55:16, 1959.
Riley, R. L.: Air-Borne Infections. Am. J. Nursing, 60:1246, 1960.
Robertson, J.: Young Children in Hospitals. New York, Basic Books, Inc., 1958.
Ross Pediatric Research Conference. Report of the Twenty-seventh, Nov. 14, 15, 16, 1957. The Nonoperative Aspects of Pediatric Surgery. Columbus, Ohio, Ross Laboratories, 1958.
Silver, H. K., Kempe, C. H., and Bruyn, H. B.: Handbook of Pediatrics. 3rd ed. Los Altos, California, Lange Medical Publications, 1959.
Smendik, P., and Kurtagh, C. H.: Isolation in the Home. Am. J. Nursing, 56:575, 1956.
Steigman, A. J., and Epting, M. H.: Diphtheria in Children. Am. J. Nursing, 57:467, 1957.
Thompson, LaVerne: Viruses—Old and New. Am. J. Nursing, 59:349, 1959.
Top, F. H.: Communicable and Infectious Diseases. 4th ed. St. Louis, C. V. Mosby Company, 1960.

# Chapter 20

# Conditions of the Preschool

# Child Requiring Long-Term Care

## MEANING OF LONG-TERM ILLNESS TO THE PRESCHOOL CHILD AND HIS FAMILY

THE ACUTELY ill child usually requires a brief period of bed rest, but the chronically ill child requires either a prolonged period in bed or frequently recurring, briefer periods of complete rest. This need for rest is trying to the preschool child, for his need for physical activity and interaction with other children is curtailed. The care of the chronically ill child in the hospital is difficult enough, but in the home it poses a problem which often seems to be too great for the mother to handle.

It is the mother who is hardest hit when a sick child is cared for at home. She must nurse him, carry on with her usual household tasks and also manage the needs of her husband and the other children. Eventually she becomes overtired and irritable; she is no longer able

to provide the love and support her family needs.

The nurse can often offer suggestions to ease her burden. The mother must accept the fact that she needs rest and that it is useless for her to attempt the impossible. Perhaps she can rearrange the household duties so that the father has a greater share of the responsibilities and the other children give more help about the house. Neighbors may come in at mealtimes or on wash days and take over the care of the child, so that she can serve the meals and eat undisturbed at the family table or finish the washing and ironing without interruption.

If the child can spend the day on the living room couch instead of in his room on the second floor, the mother does not constantly have to go up and down stairs.

The mother cannot be with the child at all times, and it is good for him to amuse himself. If he is able to sit up, a bed table placed over his bed makes a play area on which he can draw, color in his picture book or play with small toys.

It is difficult for the mother, in the midst of housework, to remember when medicine is due. An alarm clock set for the time of the next dose may help. One-dish dinners that are easily prepared are just as nourishing as more complicated meals, and there are thus fewer dishes and cooking utensils to wash and dry. A medicine table near the child's bed with plenty of clean spoons and a pitcher of water saves needless errands to the kitchen or bathroom.

Chronic illness also creates difficulties for the child and for his siblings. The sick child often seems to the others to be favored and to get more attention than they do. This heightens the normal sibling rivalry. The children should be helped to understand that the sick child needs extra attention, but is not loved more than they are. Outings with a neighbor, small gifts or special treats may help to relieve their feeling of neglect.

Siblings as well as the sick child may have fears which parents find it difficult to understand. Illness frightens children and makes them fear pain. If they are old enough to associate sickness with death, they may develop a real fear of death, not only for the sick child, but also for themselves. Parents should be truthful with the children about the condition of the sick child, within the limits of what children can understand. If restrictions must be placed upon the sick child's activities, the siblings should be told why this is necessary.

Sibling jealousy may sometimes be so strong that the well children may have passing or relatively fixed wishes that something "bad" would happen to the sick child. Such thoughts make children feel guilty. If the sick child's condition becomes worse, it seems to them as if their wish were responsible for his plight. Then their feeling of guilt may reach disturbing proportions. They need the help of an understanding mother who accepts such feelings as a natural result of the disturbed emotional relations in a household where the sick child's needs often take precedence over those of his siblings.

As the sick child improves, he may have to make a difficult adjustment. He may look back longingly to the time when his condition secured for him constant attention. He may be demanding and easily upset if he does not get what he wants. His readjustment to healthful living may take weeks. Parents must be patient and understanding and give adequate love, although less attention, while he adjusts to the real tasks of living.

If disability follows a child's illness or if his activity must be curtailed in any way, the family members should understand the reason for this, and teachers and other adults with whom he comes in contact should be told. Then all persons in his environment can exert a consistent influence on the child. He should be encouraged firmly but kindly to derive pleasure from things he can do for himself and for others. Overconcern about the disability must be reduced; the child must be helped to live with his problem. Emphasis should be put on the assets he still has rather than on his liabilities, even though these are recognized.

## CHRONIC OR LONG-TERM CONDITIONS

### Leukemia

**Incidence and Etiology.** Cancer is outranked only by accidents as a cause of death in childhood, and leukemia is the principal type of cancer in children. More than 50 per cent of cases of childhood leukemia occur in children below 5 years of age.

Leukemia is a malignant neoplasm involving all blood-forming organs and causing an overproduction of any one of the types of white blood cells. The normal white blood cell count is 5000 to 10,000 per cubic millimeter. In leukemia the cell count may be more than 50,000 per cubic millimeter.

Leukemia may occur at any age; in children it is most common between the ages of three and eight years. Acute leukemia is the more common form, but chronic leukemia may occur. The disease has no relation to racial, geographic or regional factors or to socioeconomic status. The *etiology* is unknown.

**Types, Pathogenesis and Clinical Manifestations.** The type of white blood cell involved offers a basis of classification, but it is sometimes difficult to distinguish which type of leukemia is present in children. The acute undifferentiated or stem-cell type is common, as is acute myeloblastic leukemia. Subacute or chronic forms are rare in childhood.

The number of leukemic cells circulating in the blood is not always high, even though there is overproduction of a single cell type. When a high percentage of blast cells is present and the white blood cell count is high, the blood picture is termed "leukemic." When a low percentage of blast cells is present and the white cell count is low, the blood picture is termed "aleukemic." For a diagnosis of aleukemic leukemia a sample of bone marrow, obtained by aspirating marrow fluid, must be examined.

Pathologic changes are related to the increased number of white blood cells and to secondary changes due to disturbed function of the involved organs. Immature white blood cells multiply rapidly, but do not develop into or function as mature cells. The production of normal blood cells is rapidly reduced. The low platelet count is largely responsible for hemorrhagic manifestations of the disease. The liver, spleen and all lymph nodes are enlarged. Renal and osseous changes are seen. Areas of ulceration and secondary infection may be found anywhere in the body.

There are certain common *clinical manifestations* regardless of the type of leukemia. The onset may be rapid or gradual. Widespread petechiae appear. The child is pale and has anorexia, vomiting, weight loss, weakness and fatigue. The temperature is elevated.

Palpitation of the heart and dyspnea are distressing symptoms. Episodic abdominal pain may occur, owing to the enlarged lymph nodes. Anemia becomes severe as the condition progresses. When the platelet count drops, the child bleeds easily, and a slight bruise results in large ecchymotic areas; necrotic lesions develop which are apt to become secondarily infected. There are also hemorrhagic areas of the mucous membranes and vital organs.

Clinical manifestations depend on which organ or tissue of the body is invaded by leukemic cells. If the kidney is affected, hematuria results. Necrotic ulcerative lesions may occur around the rectal and perirectal areas, and there is ulceration of the gums. The liver and spleen become enlarged, and lymphadenopathy, especially of deep lymph nodes, develops. The child suffers from leg or joint pain caused by the extensive osseous involvement.

Other clinical manifestations vary, owing to the fact that the disease primarily affects the blood-forming organs; it affects body tissues by infiltration or by blood changes within them.

**Diagnosis and Treatment.** The *diagnosis* is made on the basis of the clinical manifestations. A differential blood smear is done if immature cells are present in the peripheral blood. Anemia is present. Examination of aspirated or surgically removed bone marrow is necessary for a diagnosis of leukemia. The bone marrow of the leukemic child shows abnormal leukopoietic tissues and few normal hematopoietic elements. Roentgenograms of the long bones show osseous changes.

*Treatment* begins as soon as the diagnosis is made. The characteristics of the disease and its treatment should be discussed with the parents. The child with leukemia is happiest at home, and periods of hospitalization should be minimal. Parents should help the child to live as normal a life as he can, doing the things he enjoys. As his condition retrogresses, parents are no longer able to give him the care he needs, and hospitalization becomes necessary.

At present no cure is known, and treatment is palliative. With adequate treatment the child may live one or two years after the onset of leukemia.

Folic acid antagonists, adrenal cortical hormones and 6-mercaptopurine are used in treatment. The folic acid antagonists given are Aminopterin, Amethopterin and Methotrexate. These drugs interfere with folic acid metabolism (folic acid is essential to the synthesis of nucleoproteins required by rapidly multiplying white cells). These drugs are toxic and may cause depression of bone marrow and gastrointestinal bleeding. Adrenal cortical hormones used include ACTH, cortisone and hydrocortisone. All produce a remission of symptoms for a few weeks or months, but side effects develop when heavy doses or prolonged therapy is given. Nevertheless when symptoms recur after a remission, further therapy can be given. 6-Mercaptopurine (Purinethol) acts differently from the folic acid antagonists; it is a purine analogue. Toxic symptoms include anorexia, nausea, vomiting, and thrombocytopenia with possible hemorrhage.

Antibiotics are given to prevent or control intercurrent infection. Blood and blood derivatives are used for transfusions, whether given during a brief or long-term hospital admission, to correct severe anemia and to stop bleeding. Sedatives are given whenever needed to make the child comfortable.

Bone marrow aspiration is necessary in the diagnosis and treatment of leukemia. Marrow is obtained from the sternum or iliac crest. The child should be told the purpose and something of the details of the procedure. He will feel the restraint necessary to hold him in position, the cleaning of the area, the injection of procaine and the pressure of the needle as it enters the tissue.

In *chronic leukemia* urethane, roentgen therapy or a type of nitrogen mustard therapy may be used.

**Nursing Care.** The nursing care of the leukemic child is difficult in many ways. The child and his parents should be helped to make a positive adjustment to the frequent periods of hospitalization.

The nursing care is similar to that for anemia (see p. 362). The nurse should handle the child's body gently, since the extremities are painful when touched. Oral hygiene is needed and must be done with the utmost care to prevent trauma to the sore and bleeding gums. An adequate fluid intake is important. To prevent nausea, small amount of fluids which he likes should be offered frequently. The intake and output are routinely charted.

Well balanced meals can be planned from foods which he likes, and should be served when he is awake. He should not be wakened at mealtimes, since he needs his rest.

Accurate charting is important. The nurse should watch for bleeding and report both the site and the amount. It is difficult to get these children to say how they feel, but any complaints should be charted, together with the circumstances bearing upon the complaint.

The child is irritable because he is extremely uncomfortable. All who care for him should be patient and try to provide a quiet but happy atmosphere in which there are as few frustrations as possible. The mother should be with him as much as possible, both to give him the constant loving care he needs and to learn how to nurse him during his periods at home. Parents have a natural and positive outlet for their affection when they are allowed to help in the nursing care of their child while he is in the hospital.

During his illness the child may be nauseated, lonely and easily tired. The company of parents who have accepted his fatal illness and adjusted to it helps him also to accept and adjust to his condition. The child may at times appear to be anxious. This may be partly the result of anxiety which his parents were unable to conceal from him. Since the child may be ill for months, with remissions and exacerbations, the parents will need emotional support from physicians and nurses who they know have cared for such cases before. Parents may know intellectually that the child will die, but emotionally they continue to hope for a cure.

Terminal nursing care is difficult. The child must be given physical and emotional support, for he is most uncomfortable as long as he is sufficiently conscious to be aware of his sensations. His nose and throat should be kept clean, and his lips and mouth moist. Frequent bathing is necessary to keep the skin clean, and his position should be changed as often as is possible without disturbing him, in order to prevent bedsores. Sedatives may be given when necessary.

To minister successfully to the dying child and his parents, the nurse must be able to accept the way in which they express their fear and grief. To do this she must face her own feelings about death. The children in the unit sense her tension and that of the other personnel. They need her emotional support. When the child lapses into unconsciousness, the nurse must remain with the parents at his bedside so that they know that everything possible is being done for his comfort. Parents need emotional support, and if the nurse leaves them alone with the dying child, she may thereby indicate to them rejection of their grief. If parents cannot be present, the nurse must remain constantly with the dying child to prevent loneliness and the feeling that there is no one to help him when he is suffering and afraid of the change that is coming over him.

**Complications and Prognosis.** *Complications* arise as a result of lack of normal white blood cells. Intracranial and visceral hemorrhages may occur. Intracranial hemorrhage is the most common immediate cause of death. The mouth and pharynx may become infected and ulcerated and may hemorrhage. The anemia present throughout the course of the disease becomes relentlessly worse. Death results from the disease itself or from intercurrent infections, or both.

Without treatment the course of acute leukemia is usually that of constant deterioration. No cure is known,

and the disease is eventually fatal. Acute leukemia may, however, be changed into a chronic form with treatment, and the survival time lengthened.

## Tetralogy of Fallot

**Preoperative Care and Treatment.** Tetralogy of Fallot was described in connection with congenital defects in the newborn infant (see p. 210). Since operation is usually postponed until the child is between three and five years of age, preoperative and postoperative nursing care and a description of the types of operation are included in this chapter.

If the mother has followed the suggestions previously outlined for admission of a child to a hospital (see p. 533), the child admitted for heart surgery will probably be able to adjust to the new situation without great difficulty. If she has not prepared him, he will be irritable, emotionally unstable and overdependent on adult care.

The child should be admitted a few days before operation for diagnostic procedures such as the exercise tolerance test, roentgen examination and fluoroscopic examination. Oxygen saturation tests, electrocardiography, cardiac catheterization and angiocardiography may be done. Parents must understand the seriousness of cardiac surgery, especially open-heart surgery.

Since many children are in poor condition preoperatively, adequate diet and fluid intake, rest and controlled exercise are needed to bring them to optimum condition for operation. If cardiac failure is present, absolute rest, digitalis, diuretics and oxygen therapy may be needed. Antibiotics are given prophylactically before operation. The child must be protected from patients and personnel having infections.

Fluids may be given parenterally before and during operation to prevent dehydration. During operation transfusions of plasma, rather than whole blood, are usually given because, if the surgical result is good, the child will have sufficient red blood cells, owing to his polycythemia.

The nurse who cares for the child preoperatively should care for him postoperatively so that changes in his condition can be easily noted and the child may feel secure in her presence.

Before and during operation the nurse must give the parents support by answering their questions and preparing them for the child's appearance after operation so that their anxiety may be reduced.

**Surgical Correction.** One of several types of surgical correction may be done. In closed-heart surgery (palliative surgery) there are the Blalock-Taussig operation, the Potts operation and the Brock procedure.

*Closed-Heart (Palliative) Surgery.* In the *Blalock-Taussig operation* a branch of the aorta is anastomosed to the pulmonary artery. In children under two years the innominate artery is used; in children over two years the subclavian artery is preferred. The result of this operation is that a connection is made between a systemic artery and the pulmonary artery, thus increasing the blood flow to the lungs, improving exercise tolerance and reducing cyanosis.

In the *Potts operation* a direct connection is made between the aorta and the pulmonary artery. The same results are achieved as with the Blalock-Taussig operation. None of these operations is corrective. The operative risk with anastomotic procedures is low. Although the immediate clinical improvement is good, some incapacity may remain.

The *Brock procedure* is a direct operation for the pulmonary stenosis and is done through a right ventricular approach. This operation increases the flow of blood to the lungs, but does not correct the ventricular septal defect.

*Open-Heart (Corrective) Surgery.* This method of surgical therapy would seem to be best for the child, since it affords relief of the pulmonary stenosis and closure of the ventricular septal defect. It can be done with the aid of a pump oxygenator. During operation the circulation of the blood is maintained temporarily by an artificial heart-lung machine. Under direct vision the ventricular septal defect is closed and the pulmonary stenosis resected. The operative risk is higher at present than that of the anastomotic procedures. The results are spectacular, however, in successful cases.

During these operations a thoracotomy tube is usually inserted into the pleural space and attached to a gravity suction bottle placed lower than the chest. The pleural space is thus kept free from drainage. The fluid in the tube oscillates with respiration, indicating that there is an airtight seal at the site where the thoracotomy tube is inserted.

**Postoperative Treatment and Care.** The child requires extremely close observation by experienced nurses. They must note the degree of cyanosis and exercise intolerance and watch for signs of tracheal irritation if intratracheal anesthesia was used—namely, restlessness, dyspnea and increased pulse rate. Treatment of tracheal irritation is by steam inhalations, use of the Croupette and possibly a tracheotomy.

The postoperative treatment ordered by the physician must be carried out with skill and exactness. Oxygen is given to prevent dyspnea. Intrapleural drainage tubes are used. The thoracotomy tube may be removed the day after operation if the lung is expanded normally. For a child with a thoracotomy tube in place the nurse must observe the amount and kind of drainage, proper functioning of the tube and also the child's condition. If fluid accumulates in the chest, the child will appear listless and have diminished breath sounds and increased pulse rate. His hands should be restrained if he attempts to pull out the thoracotomy tube. He should be turned frequently.

Parenteral fluids are given slowly as ordered. Too rapid injection adds to the strain on the heart. Oral fluids are started when the child regains consciousness. Soon a soft, and then a regular, diet is given.

Antibiotics are given to prevent infection, analgesics to control pain and sedatives to promote rest. The intake

Figure 216. Cardiopulmonary bypass. Cannulation of venae cavae for withdrawal of venous blood and of aorta for perfusion with oxygenated blood from apparatus. The sucker for collecting blood from the open chamber of the heart is placed beneath the tricuspid valve, returning this blood to the apparatus. (Courtesy of American Heart Association. Adapted from Ventricular Septal Defects with Pulmonary Hypertension, by James W. DuShane and others: J.A.M.A., Vol. 160.)

and output are measured to detect anuria.

The vital signs should be recorded every fifteen minutes to one hour as ordered by the physician, including the rhythm, rate and volume of the pulse beat, depth and rate of respiration and the blood pressure. There will be no pulse on the side of the heart on which closed-heart surgery was performed until the collateral circulation compensates for the changed route of blood flow. If the Blalock-Taussig operation was done, blood pressure readings must be taken on the arm opposite the side on which operation was performed. The child should be encouraged to cough and breathe deeply to clear the airway. Gentle suction may be necessary to prevent atelectasis.

The child must be observed closely for postoperative hemiplegia which can occur because of spontaneous clotting of the blood as a result of dehydration. If a thoracentesis is done, the kind and amount of fluid withdrawn and the color and appearance of the child after the treatment must be recorded in detail.

The child recuperates rapidly, but requires rest. Return to activity must be gradual in order to prevent strain upon the heart. Before he is discharged the physician, parents, social worker, school teacher, visiting nurse and hospital nurse must work out together a plan of care for the child. His personality may change completely after operation. He is usually more active, aggressive and independent. These changes may frighten the parents because they fear that he will overexert himself. The nurse can help them by pointing out his obvious enjoyment of new activities and his new freedom from dyspnea and fatigue.

**Complications and Prognosis.** Because circulation is sluggish and the viscosity of the blood increased, cerebrovascular thrombi form easily and can cause death. The *prognosis* is good after operation; that with closed-heart surgery is better than that with open-heart surgery at present, but with research the prognosis in all types of cardiac surgery will be improved.

### Hemophilia

**Incidence.** Hemophilia is not a single disease entity, but a syndrome which represents distinct inborn errors of meabolism. There are defects in any one of several substances needed for thromboplastic activity.

*Hemophilia A* is due to deficiency of antihemophilic globulin; *Hemophilia B,* of plasma thromboplastin component; and *Hemophilia C,* of plasma thromboplastin antecedent.

Hemophilia A is the true or classic form of the disease. Since the nursing care is approximately the same in all types, the others will not be considered in this text.

Hemophilia A is inherited as a sex-linked recessive trait. Though it appears only in males, it is transmitted by symptom-free females. Male hemophiliacs can transmit a latent form of the disease to female children, however. It is a congenital defect in the blood-coagulating mechanism leading to severe bleeding.

The disease is seldom diagnosed in early infancy unless the newborn bleeds from the umbilical cord or after circumcision. As children grow older and become more active the condition is apparent, for even a slight injury produces continued bleeding.

**Pathogenesis, Clinical Manifestations and Treatment.** The disease is characterized by a tendency to prolonged bleeding caused by an extremely delayed clotting time. Normal blood clots in three to six minutes; hemophiliac blood may require an hour or more for clotting.

The prothrombin time and the bleeding time are normal when a test cut is made because the cut is smooth and small; the incised surfaces are approximated, with the result that adequate thromboplastin becomes available from damaged cells. But hemorrhage may be spontaneous or result from a slight injury. In children hemorrhage frequently occurs from the nose or into the knee, where repeated hemorrhage may result in permanent crippling. Hemorrhage into the joints is known as *hemarthrosis.* Anemia, moderate elevation in platelets and leukocytosis may occur if hemorrhages have been extensive.

Immediate *treatment* of an open wound consists in cleansing it thoroughly and placing in the laceration fibrin foam or absorbable gelatin foam with thrombin. Bleeding may also be stopped by pressure on the area, cold applications, blood transfusions and administration of plasma. Antihemophilic globulin in stored blood loses its activity rapidly; therefore transfusion of fresh whole blood or plasma is essential for treatment of hemorrhage. Anticoagulant substance may form in the blood of the hemophiliac, and subsequent administration of fresh blood or plasma may be less effective in controlling hemorrhage. Therefore local measures for control should be tried before blood or plasma is used. Sedatives may be required if the child must be kept extremely quiet during treatment. If repeated hemorrhages cause the joints to become involved, orthopedic treatment may be necessary.

**Nursing Care.** Because of repeated hospitalization for transfusions and treatment, it is necessary for the nurse to understand the attitude of the child and of his family toward the disease and his hospitalization. Careful handling of the child is necessary, and the nurse must be alert to symptoms of pain or pressure, since bleeding may occur anywhere in the body.

If the condition is diagnosed in infancy, the child's toys must be soft and the sides of his crib and play pen padded to protect him from injury. When learning to stand and walk, the child must be protected from falling. He may wear sponge rubber pads on his knees and buttocks and a football helmet on his head. As he grows older, both he and his parents must understand the danger of trauma in his more active life. His teachers and the school nurse should be informed of his condition and the problems it creates. While they supervise his activities they must guard against assuming an overprotective attitude and allow the growing child some activity within the limits of safety.

The nurse must provide continued emotional support. During periods of freedom from bleeding his parents may become less conscious of the necessity for medical follow-up. The nurse should emphasize the necessity of medical supervision.

Parents, especially the mother, may feel guilt at having given birth to the child and resentment at having to care for him. Their problem is increased by the necessity of providing experiences for him which will promote his emotional growth. If they are too anxious, the child will become self-centered and fearful. As a result he may withdraw from other children and become overdependent on adults. He may use his disease to control his parents and purposely do things that are dangerous for him. The parents must undertake the difficult task of preparing him for a satisfying role in adult life, both for himself and for his community.

**Prognosis.** The prognosis is uncertain. A cyclic pattern may be noted in which periods of little bleeding and of severe bleeding occur. Death may follow intracranial hemorrhage or exsanguination from a serious hemorrhage elsewhere in the body.

### Purpura

Spontaneous hemorrhages are characteristic of the condition known as purpura. These hemorrhages may occur in the skin, mucous membranes or internal organs. Such hemorrhages may develop in any condition in which there is a decreased number of platelets in the blood, defective capillary walls or in which damage is done to normal capillary walls beyond the point at which platelets can stop the bleeding. Petechiae, or minute hemorrhages into the skin, may also occur as an allergic manifestation when a local specific tissue reaction results in capillary stress.

Two specific types of purpura are discussed in this text: idiopathic thrombocytopenic purpura and anaphylactoid purpura.

### Idiopathic Thrombocytopenic Purpura

**Etiology, Incidence, Clinical Manifestations and Laboratory Findings.** Purpura is associated with a deficit in the number of circulating blood platelets. This deficiency is caused by factors outside the platelets themselves.

The disease has its greatest *incidence* in the age group between three and seven years. It is uncommon in Negro children. The most frequent form of the disease during childhood is the acute self-limited type.

The onset of the acute type is sudden. It may follow a mild respiratory infection or measles. There is fever and prostration. Characteristic, spontaneous small hemorrhages into the skin, mucous membranes or other tissue occur. Large ecchymoses may result from trauma. In the severe form of the disease there may be hemorrhages from the vaginal and nasal mucous membranes and from the urinary and gastrointestinal tracts. Cerebral hemorrhages are to be feared.

In the chronic form, infrequently seen in children, the onset is gradual. The child may have a history of prolonged bleeding following injury and of ready bruising. Periods of good health alternate with periods of excessive bleeding.

The *laboratory findings* confirm the diagnosis made upon the clinical manifestations. The platelet count is always below 100,000 per cubic millimeter of blood (normal is between 200,000 and 500,000). In the chronic form of the disease iron deficiency may occur from loss of blood. The bleeding time is usually prolonged. The clotting time is normal, but the clot fails to retract in the usual manner. The bone marrow is studied in order to rule out leukemia.

**Treatment, Course and Prognosis.** Supportive *therapy* includes transfusions of whole blood to replace blood loss, antibiotic therapy to treat infections, bed rest for moderate or severe bleeding, a well balanced diet and vitamin therapy. If severe bleeding occurs, an infusion of platelet-rich plasma or whole blood is necessary. ACTH or cortisone can control severe bleeding, but the effect upon the platelet count cannot be predicted. Splenectomy may be performed if the disease continues for six to twelve months or if hemorrhaging is severe. Splenectomy may induce lasting missions in children with the chronic form of the disease. The operation modifies symptoms in children who are not cured.

The majority of children who have the acute form of purpura recover in about two months under supportive therapy. Intracranial hemorrhage is uncommon, but it is responsible for most deaths from purpura. About 10 per cent of the children with purpura have the chronic form with remissions and exacerbations.

## Anaphylactoid Purpura (Schoenlein-Henoch Syndrome)

Schoenlein-Henoch syndrome is the term used for anaphylactoid purpura because the illness is a polymorphic systemic disease. Skin and visceral lesions are manifestations of the condition.

**Incidence and Etiology.** The disease is not uncommon; it affects all races. It has its highest *incidence* between the ages of three and seven years, the average being about five years.

The *etiology* is unknown. The onset may occur after contact with a specific substance. In such cases allergy seems to be important. It is possible that this is one type of hypersensitivity response to a variety of antigenic stimuli. The onset may follow an upper respiratory tract infection with beta hemolytic streptococci.

**Clinical Manifestations and Laboratory Findings.** A series of *clinical manifestations* take place, possibly following an infection. Abdominal pain or arthralgia, or both, may occur. After the initial symptom a skin rash appears on the lower extremities and the buttocks, and spreads to the face, arms and trunk. There is usually malaise and a low-grade fever. The skin rash consists at first of urticarial wheals; then a variety of maculopapular erythematous lesions appear. The lesions may finally become petechial or purpuric, changing from red to purple, to rust, and then fading. Several types of lesions may be present at the same time. Hemorrhage

and edema may occur in the gastrointestinal and urinary tracts.

Other manifestations are acute, colicky abdominal pain, vomiting and melena. In cases with renal involvement there may be albuminuria and hematuria. About half of the children with kidney involvement also have hypertension or azotemia. The joints, usually of the knees or ankles, may be involved. If so, they are painful and swollen, and motion is limited. These symptoms may be confused with symptoms of rheumatic fever. Cerebral edema and hemorrhage may cause convulsions and coma.

*Laboratory findings* show no change from the normal in clotting time, platelet count, bleeding time, clot retraction or in the blood and blood-forming organs. Anemia results if the blood loss is great. The erythrocyte sedimentation rate is elevated.

**Treatment, Complications, Course and Prognosis.** There is no specific *treatment*. If a specific allergen (food substance, bacteria, drug or pollen) is involved, the child should be kept from contact with it. If purpura follows a bacterial infection, antibacterial treatment should be given to eliminate pathogens. During the acute phase bed rest is necessary, and the child should be observed closely for signs of involvement of the kidneys or brain. Corticosteroids may give relief from symptoms and reduce hemorrhage, but they do not shorten the course of the illness. They are usually given on an experimental basis only, since adverse effects may occur. Blood transfusions are given as needed.

Renal *complications* may occur, and renal insufficiency may manifest itself several years after the acute phase of the illness.

The *course* and *prognosis* are extremely variable. The condition may last from about six weeks to one or two years. Usually it is mild and lasts for only a few days. Death, however, may occur from gastrointestinal and kidney changes, from hypertension or intracranial bleeding.

## Allergy

**Etiology and Predisposing Factors.** The term "allergy" means that the individual has an altered tissue reactivity to one or more substances. When an antigen or a foreign substance enters the body, the individual defends himself by creating an antibody to destroy the foreign material or change it into a harmless substance. Histamine is produced in large amounts by these reactions in allergic persons and is responsible for causing unfavorable allergic effects on body tissues. In nearly all cases the antibody is already present because of the body's responses to previous doses of antigen. Such sensitization may result from inhalation, absorption through the skin, ingestion or parenteral injection.

The antigen most frequently responsible for the allergic state is a foreign protein, a protein from a different animal species than man. Carbohydrates, lipids or chemicals may be protein-linked and may act as antigens in the production of antibodies.

The development of allergic manifestations depends partly on inheritance, in which case the term to be used is *atopy*, partly on the nature of the allergen and partly on the degree and duration of exposure. Although all persons are potentially allergic, susceptibility to allergy varies in degree. Approximately 75 per cent of allergic children have a positive family history of allergy. The child's allergens and his allergic manifestations need not, however, be exactly the same as those of his parents.

The fetus may be passively sensitized in utero, but does not develop manifestations of the sensitivity until his first exposure to the allergen. Infants and children who have had severe gastrointestinal disturbances may develop sensitivities due to unchanged protein which enters the blood stream because of increased permeability of the intestinal wall. Psychologic factors involved in stress are important in the development of allergy.

**Clinical Manifestations, Diagnosis and**

**Laboratory Findings.** *Clinical manifestations* may differ, depending on the age of the child. An infant who has eczema (see p. 373) may suffer allergic rhinitis or asthma as a child. New sensitivities may appear in children, while old ones may continue or be lost.

Infants and children having allergic manifestations should be skin-tested in order to determine the offending substance. Although they react to test allergens as do adults, reactions must be interpreted in the light of clinical findings. The intensity of the reaction does not necessarily indicate the importance of the particular test substance in the etiology.

The *diagnosis* of an offending allergen may also be made by giving the child an elimination diet. This is effective in determining the etiologic agent in an infant whose diet includes only a few foods. The mother should understand that certain foods must be eliminated completely from the diet and that the child's reactions to other foods must be accurately observed.

Except in acute asthma, in which it may be absent, eosinophilia of the peripheral blood is usually present in allergic persons. Eosinophilia of the mucous membranes of the nose may be present in any kind of allergic manifestation.

**Treatment, Prognosis and Prophylaxis.** To treat an allergic child satisfactorily the physician must obtain a detailed history of the child and his family, and the parents must be willing to cooperate in a long-term program of treatment. Three methods of treatment may be attempted: the offending allergen may be removed; sensitization to specific known allergens may be decreased or the individual response toward the offending allergens may be altered.

Probably the most effective way to manage food allergies is to eliminate the particular food from the diet. In the growing child care must be taken that the subsequent diet is adequate for a child of his age.

There is no exact method of determining the dosage necessary for desensitization to a known allergen. Densitization to inhalants is usually one by injection of extracts of the material in gradually increasing doses. he initial dose is usually the smallest mount which, given subcutaneously, ill produce a positive intradermal test. ubsequent doses are given at three- to ve-day intervals, and each is larger an the preceding dose. At no time is n amount given which will produce ymptoms. Desensitization to foods is ccomplished by giving a gradually increasing amount of the substance hich causes symptoms.

The third method of treatment for llergic conditions is altering the reponse of the body to the offending llergen. Disturbing emotional factors ould be corrected, since the emotional ate influences the response of the ody. Any endocrine imbalance should e treated. Certain drugs may be beneicial in treatment, including antihisimines, epinephrine and ephedrine. orticotropin (ACTH) and the cortiones may also be used. Any respiratory fection should be treated, since it may redispose to an allergic state. Dehyration depresses the allergic response. llergic manifestations may be reuced by provision for adequate rest nd improvement in the general health f the child.

An allergy to a substance cannot be ured, but it may be kept sufficiently nder control so that no symptoms are roduced. Partial or complete removal f the allergen from the environment of ensitive persons should be attempted. is important that infants and children hose parents are known to have alrgies avoid contact with substances hich may produce allergy. If one or oth parents are allergic, the newborn hould not be given cow's milk before e begins breast feeding, since sensitiation to cow's milk may occur. Furiermore, during infancy and childhood dditions to the diet should be in the orm of single, simple foods. If a comination of new foods were given at the ame time, and an allergic manifestaon developed, it would be difficult to now which food was the cause. Chilren of allergic parents should not be

given foods which commonly cause an allergic response. Among such foods are cow's milk, eggs, chocolate, wheat and oranges.

**Types of Allergy in Children.** The most important clinical manifestations of allergy in children include eczema (see p. 373), asthma, allergic rhinitis (hay fever) and serum sickness. Chronic conditions of the nose, throat and gastrointestinal tract may also be caused by allergy.

## Asthma

**Incidence, Etiology and Pathology.** Asthma is a pulmonary disorder caused by an allergy. Infantile eczema is a common forerunner of asthma. The disease is uncommon in infancy; its *incidence* increases in children three years of age and older.

Asthma may be evoked by particular foods, inhalants or infections, particularly those of the respiratory tract. It may also follow vigorous activity, exposure to cold or an emotional upheaval. Asthmatic attacks often occur at night after the child has been put to bed, because of his contact with a feather pillow, a wool blanket, a fuzzy, stuffed toy or even dust in the area.

The smallest bronchioles undergo the greatest change. Initially the bronchiolar musculature goes into spasm, and the mucous membrane becomes pale and edematous. Then thick, tenacious mucus collects, and there is further obstruction of the air passages. During the attack not all the inspired air can be expired, and some collects in the alveoli, thereby causing obstructive emphysema. Wheezing and rales, due to the presence of bronchial secretions, are heard. Atelectasis may develop, caused by obstruction of a bronchus.

The attack may last for a few hours or continue for a few days. The child eventually coughs up the mucus, and the spasm relaxes. If infection is present, further respiratory embarrassment is observed.

**Clinical Manifestations and Treatment.** Asthma is characterized by paroxysms of an expiratory type of dyspnea with wheezing and generalized obstructive emphysema. The onset may be gradual with sneezing, nasal congestion, a watery discharge, and a slight cough before the attack. In other cases the onset may be sudden, and often at night. The child may sit up in bed to breathe more easily. He perspires profusely and appears anxious. The wheezing occurs largely on expiration. He may cough almost continually. If a bronchus becomes plugged with mucus, atelectasis occurs in that lobe, and the mediastinum then shifts toward the involved area. The neck veins become distended, and cyanosis is common. During the asthmatic attack the child often prefers to be left alone and to struggle by himself with the problem of breathing. The parents become extremely anxious, and their anxiety may further alarm the child, who then becomes increasingly emotionally disturbed.

With treatment such an attack may be over quickly. Untreated, it may last several days. If the child has *status asthmaticus* (refractory asthma), the attack may continue for several days, both day and night. Death may occur during status asthmaticus.

The most effective way to treat asthma is to eliminate the offending allergen, whether it be food or an environmental allergen. If this cannot be done, hyposensitization to the allergens involved may be carried out. The child should avoid fatigue and chilling and should be kept calm and emotionally at ease.

The most effective drug used in the *treatment* of asthma is epinephrine. Long-acting preparations of epinephrine in oil may be used. Epinephrine may also be administered by a pharyngeal spray; it should be sprayed deeply into the pharynx as the child inhales.

Other drugs frequently used are ephedrine sulfate or hydrochloride, aminophylline (ethylenediamine), which is a bronchodilator and may be used when epinephrine has lost its effectiveness, and antihistamines. For status asthmaticus a corticosteroid may

provide relief quickly. Potassium iodide is of some value because it liquefie bronchial secretions and enables th child to cough them up. Although atro pine would decrease bronchial spasm it is not used because it tends to dr up secretions.

The asthmatic child should have generous fluid intake in order to liquef secretions in the bronchi. Sedation ma be needed if the child shows indica tions of becoming exhausted. Sedative which may be given include phenoba bital, chloral hydrate and paraldehyde Morphine is not used because it de creases the cough reflex and makes difficult for the child to get rid of se cretions.

Oxygen may be given to reduc anoxia and cyanosis. Increased humid ity in either an oxygen tent or in th air of the room tends to liquefy secre tions and enables the child to expec torate. If a bronchus becomes plugge and atelectasis results, bronchoscopi aspiration may be necessary to open th airway.

Antibacterial therapy should be give when the child has an infection alon with an asthmatic attack. To prevent respiratory infections he may be move to a warm, dry climate during the win ter months. Some physicians have rec ommended giving the child small dose of an antibiotic as prophylaxis agains infection during the winter months Other physicians have recommende the use of bacterial vaccines to reduc the incidence of respiratory infections

In the treatment of an asthmati child the services of an allergist and child psychologist or psychiatrist ma be necessary.

**Nursing Care.** The nurse, besides co operating in the therapy, should als make accurate observations of th child's behavior when he is with othe children or hospital personnel, as wel as the interaction between the child an his mother during her visits. A con tinuous record of observations is o great importance to the physician o psychiatrist in determining the emo tional factors involved.

It is important that the asthmati

hild be kept in good health. He should
eceive a balanced diet with vitamins.
ince he may eat slowly because of his
espiratory difficulty, sufficient time
hould be permitted for meals. Smaller
neals at frequent intervals may be less
ring than large meals at longer in-
ervals. The child should have adequate
est. He will probably be more comfort-
ble sitting up than reclining. He should
e kept as emotionally calm as possible.
imple amusements and quiet play are
ecessary to keep him happy.

Although the nurse should be patient
vith the child, she must set limits for
is behavior. Inconsistency tends to
reate emotional conflicts which in-
rease the respiratory difficulty. These
hildren should be permitted to attend
ursery school and, later, school, pro-
ided the teachers and school nurses
nderstand their problem, so that they
an live as normal a life as possible.

**Prognosis.** The prognosis is most
avorable if treatment is begun early.
Many children will cease to have asth-
natic attacks at puberty, though others
vill continue having them into adult
fe. If the asthmatic attacks cease, the
hild may exhibit some other allergic
nanifestation.

## llergic Rhinitis (Hay Fever)

**Etiology and Incidence.** Hay fever is
n allergic manifestation involving the
pper respiratory tract. Attacks may be
erennial. Allergic rhinitis may be
aused by pollen or by exposure to
ther inhalants. Ragweed and roses
ause allergic rhinitis in susceptible
ersons. The condition is seldom seen
n children under three or four years
f age.

**Clinical Manifestations and Treatment.**
linical manifestations include sneez-
ng, which may be paroxysmal, rubbing
he nose to relieve itching, and nasal
tuffiness. Itching and erythema of the
onjunctivae may also occur. The mu-
ous membrane of the nose is pale and
wollen. The nasal discharge may at
rst be clear and profuse, but as sec-
ndary infection occurs, it becomes
urulent.

Allergic rhinitis is milder than other
allergic diseases and requires less
dramatic *treatment*. The most effective
method of treatment is elimination of
the allergen from the environment if
that is at all possible. Air-conditioning
and filtering devices may be used. Desensitization may be attempted if the
allergen cannot be eliminated.

Antihistamines such as Benadryl or
Pyribenzamine are frequently used for
seasonal hay fever. Agents to constrict
the nasal mucous membranes, such as
ephedrine, are helpful. Epinephrine is
seldom used unless asthma is also a
problem.

## Serum Sickness

**Incidence and Etiology.** All persons
may potentially get serum sickness if
the amount of injected foreign serum
is sufficient. It may occur at any age in
both sexes.

The most common cause of serum
sickness is the prophylactic injection of
horse serum, although other serums
may also produce clinical manifestations. Injection of the serum incites the
production of antibodies, which unite
with the rest of the serum to produce
the allergic reaction.

The first injection of minute amounts
of serum may sensitize a person for
years. Total reactions may resemble
anaphylactic shock and may occur in
persons sensitized to horse serum.

**Clinical Manifestations, Prognosis and
Prevention.** The *clinical manifestations*
vary from mild to severe. The onset is
usually about two days after the injection of serum, although it may vary
from a few hours to a month. The skin
eruption, an urticarial wheal, occurs
first at the site of the injection, but
spreads over the entire body. In more
severe cases purpura and exudative
eruptions may occur. Angioneurotic
edema involving the eyelids, lips,
tongue, hands or feet may occur, and
generalized edema may be present.
Itching is intense. Generalized lymphadenopathy and enlargement of the
spleen may be present. The joints may
be swollen and red. Muscular pain,

headache, fever and malaise are frequent. In severe cases neurologic and cerebral complications may be seen. If the person has been sensitized previously, clinical manifestations appear early after serum injection.

When the skin test is done for serum sensitivity or when serum is given, epinephrine should be available to control anaphylactic symptoms and urticarial eruption. Ephedrine may also be used, as may antihistaminic drugs and corticosteroids. Cold compresses, starch baths and antipruritic lotions may be used to relieve itching. Sedatives and salicylates may be ordered to make the child more comfortable.

The reaction to serum is a self-limited condition. It usually lasts from one to three days, but may last a week or longer.

*Prevention* of serum sickness requires sensitivity tests. It is important that the nurse understand the purpose of this procedure, because serum is frequently used in the prevention of disease.

Before any foreign serum is injected the child should be tested for sensitivity. An intradermal injection of horse serum, for instance, is made, especially if the child has a history of allergic eczema, asthma or hay fever. If the child is known to be sensitive, a very weak testing solution should be used at first. If the area becomes red after twenty minutes, the reaction is considered positive. The ophthalmic test may also be used as a guide in determining sensitivity to serum. If the eye becomes red in a few minutes, the test is considered positive. An antihistaminic drug may be given prophylactically to prevent serum sickness.

### Epilepsy (Chronic or Recurrent Convulsions)

Convulsions in infancy have already been discussed (see p. 379). Convulsions during the preschool period may indicate that the child has epilepsy.

Epilepsy is characterized by paroxysmal, recurrent attacks of impaired consciousness or of unconsciousness. Tonic or clonic muscular spasms or another type of abnormal behavior occurs. Epilepsy is not a specific disease entity in itself, but rather a general term which includes a variety of recurrent seizure patterns.

People in the community as well as family members sometimes fear children and adults who have epilepsy, or they consider the disease socially disgraceful. Physicians, nurses, social workers and other team members must educate the public to the real meaning of the disease as a chronic illness. A large amount of information should not be given at once, but slowly so that it does not pose too great a threat.

There are two types of epilepsy—idiopathic and organic.

**Idiopathic Epilepsy.** The cause of the seizures in idiopathic epilepsy cannot be found. More than half of the children who have recurrent seizures before puberty have idiopathic epilepsy. The onset is commonly between four and eight years of age. Treatment to control the seizures is possible in about 85 per cent of the cases. Heredity may be a factor in the disease, but this can seldom be clinically demonstrated.

**Organic Epilepsy.** Organic epilepsy may result from a number of focal or diffuse injuries to the brain which have left residual damage. Such injuries may be caused by direct laceration of brain tissue due to trauma, hemorrhage due to trauma or the hemorrhagic diseases, anoxia (asphyxia neonatorum), infections (e.g. meningitis, encephalitis) or toxic manifestations due to kernicterus or lead poisoning. Degenerative changes may take place in the brain. Congenital problems such as hydrocephalus or diseases such as syphilis or toxoplasmosis may result in organic abnormalities in the brain. Children with organic epilepsy usually have abnormalities shown on electroencephalograms.

**Clinical Manifestations and Diagnosis.** The *clinical manifestations* are used as the basis for the classification of seizures; grand mal, petit mal, psychomotor, focal and infantile myoclonic seizures.

*Grand mal* seizures in little children

are not likely to be preceded by a period of aura such as is common in adults. Older children may have a headache, may be irritable and lethargic or may have digestive upsets before seizures. The seizure is a generalized convulsion; a tonic and a clonic phase are usually seen.

A *tonic* spasm is an involuntary, violent, persistent contraction. In the tonic phase the child falls to the ground, the pupils dilate, and the face is distorted. The neck, abdominal and chest muscles are held rigidly. The limbs stiffen. As the air is forced out of the lungs, a brief cry may be heard. The child may bite his tongue and may void or defecate as the result of contracture of the abdominal muscles. Since respiratory movements are arrested, cyanosis occurs. This phase usually lasts up to forty seconds.

The *clonic* phase, which consists of alternate contraction and relaxation of muscles, lasts for an indefinite time. After this the child goes into a deep sleep. When he wakens, he may complain of headache and may appear confused or stuporous. A child may have seizures at night (*nocturnal epilepsy*) and in the morning find his bed wet or discover that he has bitten his tongue.

A child who has grand mal seizures may become egocentric and negativistic, owing to the attitudes of others toward him and his illness.

*Petit mal* seizures consist of transient loss of consciousness with possibly rolling of the eyes, lip movements or slight movements of the head, limbs or trunk. The child does not fall. He usually stares into space. After the age of three years petit mal occurs more frequently in girls than in boys. These attacks last up to thirty seconds. The child may not realize that he had a seizure. He may have as many as a hundred or more in a day or as few as one a month. He is usually confused after an attack.

There is a third type of seizure— *psychomotor seizures*—which cannot be recognized easily because there seem to be purposeful but repetitive inappropriate muscular acts. Usually no tonic or clonic movements are noted. The child may have a slight aura and may sleep after an attack. He is usually not confused.

*Focal seizures (jacksonian epilepsy)* may be either motor or sensory. The kind of manifestation depends on the location of the focal area in the brain which has the abnormal neuronal discharge. Unilateral jacksonian attacks are usually clonic, indicating that their origin is in the motor cortex. The muscles involved are usually those of the hand, tongue, face and foot. A focal seizure beginning in one area such as the hand spreads to areas of the body on the same side in a fixed pattern. Consciousness may or may not be disturbed.

*Infantile myoclonic seizures* are seen before the age of two years and involve one group of muscles. The child may lower his head and flex his arms innumerable times a day. He may also flex his legs on his abdomen. This type of convulsion usually disappears by the third year, and grand mal seizures appear. The condition is usually accompanied by mental retardation.

*Diagnosis* of epilepsy is made on the family history and the child's record of convulsive seizures. Different types of epilepsy show a variety of electroencephalographic abnormalities. For diagnostic purposes, therefore, whenever a convulsive disorder is present, an electroencephalogram is made. Roentgen studies of the skull are also necessary in some cases. Other tests such as pneumoencephalography and examination of the cerebrospinal fluid may be done if indicated.

**Treatment.** During an attack the child should be protected from injury. His clothing should be loosened around the neck, and he should be turned to one side so that he does not aspirate secretions. Oxygen should be given if cyanosis occurs and if the convulsion is prolonged.

A prolonged series of grand mal seizures is termed *status epilepticus*. Oxygen is given and phenobarbital sodium is administered intramuscularly. The environment should be quiet while the child is recovering from a prolonged convulsion. He and his parents need reassurance.

Prolonged therapy has three purposes: control of the convulsions, education of the child's family and others in his environment to accept him, and help so that he may function to full capacity. The treatment consists of anticonvulsant drugs, good care of the whole child, diet therapy and psychotherapy if necessary. The family and the child should have a positive attitude toward his illness. He should lead as normal a life as possible. Anxiety tends to increase the occurrence of seizures. If the child appears anxious, the social worker or child psychiatrist may help the family find the sources of his anxiety. The child should be kept at home rather than institutionalized if his capacities permit home care.

The choice of drugs and the dosage needed to control convulsions depend upon the individual case and the type of seizure. Phenobarbital is often used over a long period for grand mal seizures. If the child has an idiosyncracy to phenobarbital, a maculopapular skin eruption, drowsiness and fever may be noted. Mebaral (mephobarbital) is also used in some cases of grand mal seizures. Dilantin (diphenylhydantoin sodium) is also used. This drug is an effective anticonvulsant, but does not produce excessive drowsiness as barbiturates may. Nonhemorrhagic, painless hypertrophy of the gums may follow administration of Dilantin. No special treatment is required. Drowsiness and ataxia may occur if the child receives too large a dose.

Tridione (trimethadione) is effective in the treatment of petit mal seizures. This drug may increase the occurrence of grand mal attacks if the child also suffers from such seizures. Phenobarbital or Dilantin may also be ordered. Prolonged or excessive use of Tridione may produce drowsiness, nausea, photophobia or skin eruptions. Aplastic anemia may also occur. Mysoline (primidone) is given for grand mal and psychomotor seizures. Side effects include drowsiness and ataxia.

Diet therapy is important. A fasting diet, ketogenic diet and a reduction of fluid intake tend to prevent seizures. Diet therapy may be used with the older child who cooperates with treatment, but is usually more difficult than with the little child. The diet should be varied so that it is palatable, since a ketogenic diet containing large amounts of fat is not appetizing when taken over a long period.

**Nursing Care.** The nurse must record and report her observations of a convulsion. This is important because the physician is seldom present when the child has a seizure. Although the child must be closely watched, he should not be made to feel that he can never be left alone. The physical aspects of the nursing care of the child are similar to those of the infant during a convulsion (see p. 379). Prevention of injury to the child is a principal concern.

The nurse should keep the child in the hospital as free from anxiety as possible. Unnecessary stimulation should be avoided. Diversion appropriate to his age and ability should be provided. His play equipment should be such that it will not cause injury during a seizure.

The nurse assists with the diagnostic tests. All procedures should be explained to the child in a way that he will understand. The nurse must see that he swallows his anticonvulsant medications and must observe for side effects of the drugs.

Parent-child relations should be observed for indications of rejection or overprotection of the child. He should be watched for traits of egocentricity, emotional instability and selfishness and what is noted should be reported to the physician. These traits develop as a reaction to adult attitudes toward the child and his illness. The parents and the child must understand the need for continued medical care and supervision to control convulsions.

**Course and Prognosis.** Since the child is better off at home than in the hospital if the mother can give him the care he needs, it is important that she learn how to care for him. The child should have as normal a life as pos

ble. Outdoor activity should be pro-
ided. If the convulsions are not too
evere and the child is mentally able
o profit from the experience, he should
o to nursery school and later to school.
he attitude of adults and their treat-
ient of him when he has a seizure in-
uence the attitude of other children
ward him

The role of parents of an epileptic
hild is difficult; the child's role is even
ore difficult. Parents and child need
motional support, reassurance and
raise for their achievements. The sei-
res can be reduced in frequency so as
ot to interfere too much with the
hild's activity. Personality changes
an be minimized if parents treat the
hild as though he were essentially
ormal. They must prevent him from
ecoming overdependent on them.

The *prognosis* depends on the degree
f mental and physical handicaps the
hild has and on the adequacy of medi-
al and environmental management. If
he child has adequate treatment and
vas mentally normal at the beginning
f his illness, he can be expected to
emain essentially normal throughout
is life.

## Mental Deficiency

**Incidence and Etiology.** Mental de-
ciency is any interference with intelli-
ence that causes a limitation in the
ay the child is able to adapt to his
nvironment. It is not a disease entity
self, but is a complex of symptoms
ue to a variety of causes. Between 3
nd 4 per cent of all children born in
he United States will at some time in
heir lives be classified as mentally
etarded.

Heredity may be the cause; in some
ases mental deficiency can be traced
hrough generations and an incidence
bove average among relatives proved.
here are so many other factors, how-
ver, that it is difficult to single out
eredity. Some of these factors may
e classified as follows: (1) *prenatal*
auses, including metabolic disorders
uch as phenylketonuria (see p. 371)
r hypothyroidism (cretinism) (see p.

369), mongolism (see p. 227), cranial
malformation (see p. 383), maternal
infections such as German measles or
syphilis, maternal irradiation, anoxia
and iso-immunization (kernicterus)
(see p. 160); (2) *neonatal* causes, including intracranial hemorrhage (see
p. 166), anoxia (see p. 184) or birth
trauma; (3) *postnatal* causes, including intracranial injury or hemorrhage
(see p. 381), infections such as meningitis (see p. 544) or encephalitis (see
p. 542), poisoning such as with lead
(see p. 473), cerebrovascular thrombosis, anoxia, neoplasms (see p. 654)
or recurrent convulsions.

**Diagnosis.** Such factors as epilepsy
(see p. 574), cerebral palsy (see p.
476), severe malnutrition (see p. 342),
emotional disturbances (see p. 581),
blindness (see p. 485), deafness (see
p. 483) and speech disorders (see p.
403) may lead to an incorrect diagnosis
of mental deficiency which may result
in the child's being treated as a mental
defective and deprived of the opportunity to attain his potential mental development.

A definite diagnosis of mental deficiency should be made only after a
thorough study of the family and the
child has been done. Such a study
should be done by a team composed of
a pediatrician, a psychologist, a psychiatrist, a social worker and public
health and hospital nurses. In recent
years centers have been established,
usually in connection with medical
schools of large universities, for research and diagnosis and for the development of plans of care for individual
retarded children.

Mental deficiency of a severe degree
may be recognized as early as birth. It
is indicated by failure of the infant to
learn to suck at the breast or from a
bottle. If a three-month-old infant who
has lived in an adequate environment
fails to develop normally, mental deficiency must be considered. Throughout
infancy, before the child learns to talk,
rough estimates of his mental ability
may be made by testing his motor abilities. Does he sit, stand and walk
within the usual age limits for a physi-

cally and mentally normal child? Mentally defective toddlers may be slow in trying to help themselves, in speaking, in feeding themselves or in toilet training. Until the child is of preschool age, slowness of development may not be recognized. It becomes a very disturbing problem, however, as soon as the child is with normal preschool children living in the same environment as he. A child who is only mildly mentally retarded may pass through infancy and even the preschool years with no indication of his retardation. When he enters school, however, and is expected to understand abstract concepts, his handicap may become apparent.

Causes of delayed development should be sought whenever a child has retarded physical and motor development. The infant or child should have a thorough examination to determine whether there is a physical cause for which therapy can be given. The child may be malnourished, have a chronic illness, be blind or deaf or be emotionally disturbed and thus appear retarded.

Intelligence tests and other evaluation devices should be given to provide an estimation of mental capacity. A study of emotional reactions and social adjustment should be made. Personality characteristics of mentally deficient children vary; some children are pleasant and get along well with other children and with adults, but others are restless, irritable and disobedient. These traits interact with mental capacity in social adjustment. Children of low intelligence are usually clumsy in their movements and slow to respond to stimuli.

**Classification and Clinical Manifestations.** Mentally retarded children may be classified in three groups. (1) Those children who are *mildly retarded but educable*, who have an intelligence quotient between 51 and 75 can reach a mental age of 8 to 12 years (usually known as *morons*). (2) Those children who are *moderately retarded but trainable*, who have an intelligence quotient between 21 and 50 can reach a mental age of 3 to 7 years (usually known as *imbe-

*ciles*). (3) Those children who are *severely retarded and are completely dependent on others for their care*, who have an intelligence quotient between 0 and 20 can reach a mental age of 0 to 2 years (usually known as *idiots*).

Morons may learn to function fairly well in the home if they are able to care for themselves, and in the community by learning to perform simple manual services or trades. Imbeciles may learn to talk fairly well and understand what is said to them. Their ability to concentrate varies, but is not long upon any one task. They may be able to dress themselves, to acquire socially acceptable toilet training and to feed themselves without assistance. Some idiots may not be able to speak or walk until five years of age, and others may never learn. They require constant care and supervision. Although they may make some progress slowly, they are usually institutionalized.

**Management.** Management of the mentally deficient child is the responsibility of the home, school, community and state. The initial step is for the physician to inform the parents of the problem. They should not be told, however, until the diagnosis is definitely established. Although parents may have suspected the diagnosis, they face it with great anxiety and, when it is confirmed, may have a feeling of guilt. Parents need sympathetic understanding of their problems and acceptance of their attitudes in order to free themselves from their feeling of guilt, or at least responsibility for the child's condition, for lack of normal parental love and the feeling that he is a burden. As soon as possible they should be included with other health team members in making realistic plans for the child's care based on the parents' reaction to the handicap, the degree of the child's retardation and the community facilities in the area in which they live.

If the cause of the deficiency can be found and is amenable to treatment, every effort should be made to help the child. Thyroid extract is given for cretinism, operation is performed for subdural hematoma, hydrocephalus or

:aniosynostosis, and dietary management is provided for phenylketonuria.

Parents should be educated as to a child's potential and should have a realistic concept of his ability. They should offer affection, approval and acceptance. This is particularly necessary, though difficult, when there are other children in the family. Parents and teachers should not use pressure in an attempt to force a retarded child to learn. Such pressure leads only to frustration, which causes further emotional problems. The retarded child needs from parents and teachers the same kind of love, security and help that a normal child needs, but he needs them over a longer period because his dependence extends beyond the usual age.

The plan of management should include environmental arrangements in which the child can utilize his capacities to the best advantage. For some children institutional care is best. For other children special training can be given at home. Some children may profit from attendance at special nursery schools and grade schools. They should be taught to care for themselves and should learn a vocation if possible.

Before realistic plans can be made the parents of retarded children must accept the diagnosis. If they do not, they may continue to search for a medical reason for the problem and cure of the condition. Once they have accepted the diagnosis and plan for the child's care, they may gain confidence and emotional support by joining a group of parents whose children have the same problem as theirs.

**Nursing Care.** The nurse may be the first to detect early signs of mental deficiency in young patients. She may see the child in the outpatient department,

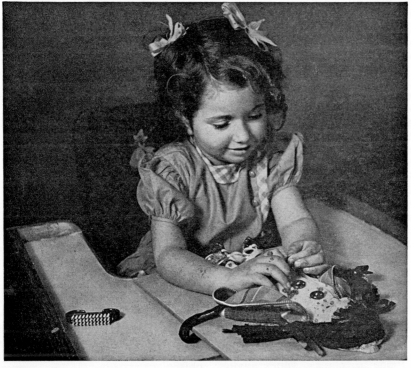

**Figure 217.** One aim of the occupational therapist is to estimate the child's ability to use the hands in daily activities such as buttoning, zippering and other dressing skills. (From Mary Stewart: Role of the Nurse in Pediatric Rehabilitation. Health News, Volume 33.)

hospital or his home. Often, because of her understanding of normal growth and development, she can observe lack of development which the parents are unaware of. She should report her observations to the physician, who, with the other team members, can determine the degree of retardation and its possible cause.

The nurse should be a member of the team which plans and carries out recommendations for the care of the child at home and for his education and training. To do this the nurse should have a good knowledge of community and state resources for such children. She may also help interpret the advice of the team to the parents and may be a sounding board for their problems.

When such a child is hospitalized, the nurse's specific functions are provision of physical care as for a normal child and supervision of the child to prevent self-injury. Close restraint is not good for such children. They should be given constructive play activity so that their attention is focused on acceptable behavior.

The nurse may help the parents select toys on the basis of the child's mental, not chronologic, age. She should help them to understand that his attention span is short, and that they should give approval for his successes and provide for him simple responsibilities at home.

**Prognosis, Prevention and Planning for the Future.** Unless the child is severely retarded, the outlook for length of life is about that of normal children. His adjustment to society will depend on the extent of his retardation and on the extent to which he has learned to use his mental resources.

Great strides are being made in the *prevention* of the causes of and the problems due to mental deficiency. Research is being done to find means to reduce the incidence of mental retardation. Many communities are making strides in providing special services for retarded children. Even greater efforts must be made to increase funds available for research, for the preparation of personnel to care for retarded children, for the organization of more parent groups and for comprehensive programs to help these children.

## EMOTIONAL PROBLEMS

Two emotional disorders that occur most frequently during the preschool period are phobias, or irrational fears, and temper tantrums.

### Phobias

Children usually have many fears of dangers in the real world. They learn fear of such things as fire, sharp knives, or a busy street from their parents, who wish to protect them from accidents or harm. But children also fear things which could not possibly cause them harm. They may be afraid of the dark, of the dead, of noises or of ghosts. Boys are more commonly afraid of injury to their bodies, and girls of the dark and of strange noises. The incidence of these fears is greatest during the preschool period.

When an unreasonable fear produces panic in a child, he is said to have a phobia. Not even the reassurance of a loving adult can reduce the emotional feeling toward the dreaded object. If the cause of the phobia is close to reality—e.g. fear of a dog which actually is capable of harming a child—the phobia is not too serious. If the cause is not close to reality, the child is emotionally ill. The real problem is not the phobic object, but an insoluble emotional conflict. Most children recover from their phobias, but they may need help to do so.

The most effective way to help a child rid himself of a phobia is to help him slowly cope with the situation or object. The adult should gradually give him an opportunity to be near the feared object and have a chance to inspect or ignore it. The adult should also help him actively to participate in the dreaded situation or with the feared object.

Sometimes reassurance and demonstrations that the object is really harmss or that other children do not fear will help the child to master his own ear. Under no circumstances should is fear be ignored, nor should he be orced to contact the object.

The child should be encouraged to be nore self-helpful and to spend more me with other children instead of with is parents. He should be permitted to xpress his hostility verbally or to en-age in active games in order to work ut his feelings.

Children whose activity is seriously mited because of a phobia or whose hobic object is not close to reality hould have psychiatric treatment.

### emper Tantrums

Temper tantrums are normal during he toddler period, but if they continue nto the preschool period and become nore severe, the child has not learned ow to handle the normal frustrations f growing up.

During a severe temper tantrum the hild is unconscious of his surround-ngs and of reality. He uses a great leal of muscular energy, striking out gainst his surroundings or himself, arely against the adult who was re-ponsible for his frustration. The child's eaction is usually out of all propor-ion to the apparent cause.

In taking his frustration out on him-elf the child is, in effect, angry with imself. When he becomes exhausted s a result of so much physical activity, e is remorseful because he allowed imself to act like a baby or toddler.

Temper tantrums occur in every hild's life. If they are serious or pro-onged or recur too frequently, the hild's development is probably not proceeding as it should do. Possibly a hild having pathologic temper tan-rums has been overindulged and has not learned to control his impulses or to eact within normal limits to frustra-ions. Treatment consists in helping uch children to gain more control of heir infantile desires and to get pleas-re from more mature forms of satis-action. A nurse can help by causing a child to feel more pleasure in pleasing her than in giving way to every im-pulse.

*Pathologic temper tantrums* may also occur if the child has been forced too early to be independent and to exert too rigid controls on his behavior. Such a child tries hard to behave in a way that will make his parents approve of him. Treatment consists in helping such a child to lower his own stand-ards of behavior so that he can act in accordance with his age. Under psy-chiatric care such children learn to control themselves and to function at their age level.

## EMOTIONAL ILLNESS

### Autism (Childhood Schizophrenia)

**Incidence.** The incidence of autism appears to be increasing. More child care units for these patients are being opened in both general and psychiatric hospitals. With better diagnosis, chil-dren with mental retardation and those with a schizophrenic illness are being separated and treated in more appro-priate ways. The need for nursing per-sonnel in children's psychiatric units is desperate.

**Clinical Manifestations.** These children have an arrest of personality develop-ment, usually accompanied by a return to earlier, more primitive thinking, be-havior and ways of communicating with others. They usually appear to develop normally until the deviant symptoms appear.

Generally these children begin to withdraw from contact with people in their environment between their second and fifth years of life. Even though they may have learned to talk, they refuse to do so.

These children cannot distinguish what is real from what is unreal, nor differentiate themselves from objects or other persons in the environment. The ability to test what is real develops in the first year of life in a child who receives mature, loving maternal care. In childhood schizophrenics this ability either has not fully developed or has been lost.

Autistic children wander about, hiding in places such as closets where they have little human contact. They enjoy oral activity, mouthing various objects, and must be protected against swallowing harmful substances.

Attempts to fit such children into organized routines result in increased temper tantrums, masturbation, preoccupation and anxiety. When they are permitted to remain by themselves, they enjoy solitary play or bodily preoccupations such as sucking or headbanging.

**Management.** The autistic child should in most cases be removed from the inadequate mother who could not provide mature maternal love during her child's infancy. If such a child is hospitalized, it is the function of his nurse to provide the love, security and permissive acceptance that he desperately needs. Nurses thus become therapeutic agents who act in close cooperation with the child psychiatrist.

Further treatment includes helping the children to identify their own bodies as separate from those of other people, helping them to integrate their concept of self, and protecting them from their own destructive impulses. The nurse must try to see the world as the autistic child sees it, thereby increasing her ability to understand the child and his behavior. As the autistic child improves, routines can be gradually introduced. The aim of routines is to provide a cycle of rest and activity and to help the child learn to help himself with such functions as bathing, dressing and eating.

**Prognosis.** The earlier a schizophrenic illness begins, the more guarded is the prognosis. Young children who do not develop strength of personality before the psychotic symptoms occur have nothing to return to after their symptoms have abated. The psychiatrist must then help them to develop their personalities from the earliest foundation. The older the child when his withdrawal occurs, the better is the prognosis.

Most younger autistic children are considered extremely mentally ill, and only concentrated therapy and care can provide hope for their recovery.

## CLINICAL SITUATIONS

Mrs. Rashofer brought her three-year-old son Barry, to the pediatric clinic. Although her other four children were well, Barry had recently become pale, had been losing weight and seemed to be tired constantly. On physical examination the physician found that the child had widespread petechiae of his skin and ulcerations of his gums. The tentative diagnosis of acute leukemia was made and was later confirmed when a sample of bone marrow was examined.

1. Methotrexate was ordered for Barry. The nurse should know that this drug is
   a. A folic acid antagonist.
   b. An adrenal cortical hormone.
   c. A salicylate.
   d. A purine analogue.

2. When the nurse cares for Barry, she should observe him especially for
   a. Vomiting and diarrhea.
   b. Tinnitus.
   c. Cyanosis.
   d. Hemorrhage.

3. The physician has told Barry's parents that although he may have periods of remissions, the eventual prognosis of a child having leukemia is extremely poor. During Barry's illness the nurse would encourage Mrs. Rashofer to assist her in giving him care because
   a. No nurse has time on a busy pediatric unit to provide all the detailed care a child having leukemia requires.
   b. Barry cries whenever his nurse cares for him. He would probably be happier if his mother gave him care.
   c. His mother apparently is not satisfied with the care the child is receiving since she has several times discussed the possibility of employing private duty nurses for him.
   d. His mother needs help in expressing her affection for him and also in learning how to care for him when he is discharged from the hospital.

4. Barry has had a remission of his illness and the physician has decided to send him home. Just before Barry's discharge from the hospital he and Dickie (three years old also) were playing with blocks in the hospital play area. Barry took one of Dickie's blocks, and Dickie began to cry. The nurse would
   a. Encourage Barry to return the block to Dickie.
   b. Tell Dickie that he cannot play with the blocks unless he can share them.
   c. Take the blocks away from both children.
   d. Give Dickie another block similar to the one Barry took.

5. In a few weeks Barry was readmitted with his initial symptoms. Mrs. Rashofer assisted the nurse in giving him care as she had on his previous admission. One afternoon the nurse found her crying in the hall outside the pediatric unit. Mrs. Rashofer explained, "I just cannot satisfy Barry any more. Every time I touch him he cries." The nurse would show her understanding in this situation by saying,
   a. "I think Barry probably would stop crying if you bought him a new toy. What do you think he would like?"
   b. "Perhaps he misses his father. Could he come to care for him awhile this evening?"
   c. "Barry is very uncomfortable now. Perhaps you could help him most by just holding his hand and reading his favorite story to him."
   d. "Children sometimes cry when they are feeling better. Why don't you get a cup of coffee? He will be happy to see you later."

6. Barry had lapsed into unconsciousness, and the physician had told the parents the gravity of his condition. Mr. and Mrs. Rashofer sat quietly sobbing beside his crib. To comfort these parents the nurse said,
   a. "After Barry dies you'll have to forget him and devote your lives to your other children. They have probably missed you since you have been spending so much time in the hospital."
   b. "All of us have done everything possible for Barry. In helping to care for him I have learned to love him too. I believe I can understand to some degree your feelings about your son."
   c. "I know you would prefer that I leave you alone with Barry. Please call me if you need me."
   d. "I just cannot understand why little children have to suffer. What sin did Barry commit to deserve punishment such as this?"

Martin Schleer, a four-year-old boy, has been admitted to the pediatric unit with a diagnosis of acute glomerulonephritis. Mrs. Schleer said that all three of her children had recently been ill with scarlet fever. Martin's clinical manifestations on admission included slight edema of the face, hematuria and hypertension.

7. When Martin was admitted to the hospital, the head nurse purposely did *not* put him to bed near
   a. Barry, who has leukemia.
   b. Susan, who is mentally retarded.
   c. Wanda, who has a streptococcal tonsillitis.
   d. Marsha, who has rheumatic fever.

8. After the nurse had given Martin an intramuscular injection he said, "I hate you. Go away." The nurse should answer
   a. "I hate you, too."
   b. "You should not say that. You are a naughty boy."
   c. "I am sorry you hate me. I like you."
   d. "I won't let your mother come to see you if you say that again."

9. When the nurse took Martin's blood pressure, she found it to be 150 mm. systolic over 110 mm. diastolic. She reported this finding to the head nurse, who said that the physician would probably want to give the child
   a. Ammonium chloride.
   b. Magnesium sulfate.
   c. Aminophylline.
   d. Diamox.

10. One day during visiting hours Martin's mother told him that he had a new baby cousin, Doris. Martin asked his mother where his baby cousin "came from." His mother should
   a. Give him a complete description of the normal birth of a baby.
   b. Tell him that he must not ask questions like that.
   c. Tell him her mother bought Doris at the hospital.
   d. Tell him the baby came from inside her mother's body.

11. Martin was in the hospital during the Christmas season. His mother had told him about Santa Claus. Some time during the next few years Martin will question the truth of this myth because Santa could not possibly fit through their chimney. At that time his mother should
   a. Insist that there is a person named Santa Claus.
   b. Tell him truthfully about the spirit of Christmas.
   c. Tell him that Santa will forget him if he persists in asking questions.
   d. Feel ashamed that she had told the child a falsehood.

12. Martin was discharged from the hospital. On his first return visit to the outpatient department his mother told the nurse that he had recently become fearful of dogs. In this situation Mrs. Schleer should
   a. Force him to touch a dog so that he would get over his fear.
   b. Tell him that dogs will not hurt him, that it is a very unusual dog that will bite children.
   c. Encourage him to talk about his fear and to play with a small dog in his mother's presence.
   d. Ignore the fear because he will outgrow it in a few years anyway.

Mrs. Rinell thought that Susan was slow in developing motor skills in comparison with her other two older children, but she did not become too concerned about her until she observed her behavior with other five-year-old children in kindergarten. Although her family doctor had said that Susan was a healthy child, she consulted a pediatrician who admitted her to the hospital for diagnosis.

13. After a thorough study of the family and the child by the health team members

Susan was found to have an intelligence quotient of 65. The nurse should know that she is
  a. Within the lower limits of the range of normal intelligence.
  b. Mildly retarded, but educable.
  c. Moderately retarded, but trainable.
  d. Severely retarded and will be completely dependent on others for her care.

14. The nurse should realize that one of her major objectives in the care of this child is to
  a. Help the parents gain a realistic concept of Susan's ability.
  b. Encourage her parents in their persistent efforts to have Susan learn something new each day.
  c. Help her parents to develop a *laissez-faire* attitude toward Susan's training.
  d. Encourage her parents to be lenient in their setting of limits on Susan's behavior.

15. Mrs. Rinell, who lives in a community where there is a poliomyelitis epidemic, called the public health nurse and told her Susan was not feeling well. The nurse's advice to her was to
  a. Take Susan and her siblings to her grandmother's home in another town so that she would not be exposed to poliomyelitis in her weakened condition.
  b. Take Susan to the isolation unit of the local hospital for treatment.
  c. Ignore her symptoms since her complaint seemed indicative of an upper respiratory tract infection.
  d. Put Susan to bed and call her pediatrician.

## GUIDES TO FURTHER STUDY

1. Compare the development of three children during your observation in nursery school according to the following: their motor ability, independence in dressing, toileting and eating, selection of playthings, sociability with adults and children, and ability to rest. Discuss in seminar the similarities and differences in behavior and abilities of these children.

2. During your observation in nursery school observe the behavior of the same three children as in Question #1 as they part from their parents. Note the age of each child and the length of time they had been attending nursery school. Answer the following questions for each child. Did the child hang his outer garments in the coatroom in the parent's presence? Did the parent wait until the child was inspected? Where did the parent actually leave the child? What words did the parent use when parting? Did the child appear unhappy when the parent left the school? What could have been done to make the parting more happy if it was unhappy?

3. Observe the health inspection in nursery school and plan to discuss the following in seminar: the purpose of the daily health inspection, the time it occurred, the procedure of examination, and the way the nurse gained the children's cooperation. Did the children learn anything from this routine? If the nurse encountered any difficulties in gaining the children's cooperation, discuss each situation as it occurred and make suggestions as to how the problem(s) could have been resolved.

4. As the nurse in The Little Friend's Nursery School it is your responsibility to inform both teachers and children about Rhonda Evans's illness. She has recently been hospitalized with a diagnosis of epilepsy. Discuss what you believe both groups should know about this illness so that positive attitudes can be formed toward this child.

5. Billy Jeffries, three years of age, has been admitted to the hospital for treatment of hemophilia. Describe the role and responsibility of the nurse in relation to both parents and child from the time he is brought to the hospital to the time of his discharge. What guidance should the parents have had by the time of discharge?

6. Preschool children fear bodily injury. During your experience in caring for children collect incidences in which children have shown such fear, expressing it either verbally or nonverbally. How could these manifestations of fear have been prevented? What was your role in reducing these fears?

## TEACHING AIDS AND OTHER INFORMATION*

*American Cancer Society*
  A Cancer Source Book for Nurses—Reprinted 1959.
  Cancer in Children, 1957.

*Children's Medical Center, Boston, Mass.*
  Asthma.
  Hay Fever.
  Seizures and Epilepsy.
  The Mentally Retarded Child.

*Federal Association for Epilepsy, Inc.*
  Duggins, V. A.: Epilepsy, Its Causes, Effects and Treatment, 1959.

*Mental Health Division, Department of National Health and Welfare, Ottawa, Canada*
  The Backward Child, 1955.

*National Association for Retarded Children, Inc.*
  Now There Is Hope.
  The 3 R's for the Retarded.
  Zwerling, I.: Initial Counselling of Parent with Mentally Retarded Children.

*Public Affairs Pamphlets*
  Hart, E.: How Retarded Children Can be Helped.
  Jacob, W.: New Hope for the Retarded Child.

  * Complete addresses are given in the Appendix.

Jacob, W.: The Retarded Child.

Osborne, E.: When You Lose a Loved One.

Yahraes, H.: Epilepsy—The Ghost Is Out of the Closet.

*U.S. Department of Health, Education, and Welfare*

Child with Epilepsy, 1952.

Dittman, L.: The Mentally Retarded Child at Home, A Manual for Parents, 1959.

Hormuth, R. P.: The Public Health Nurse in Community Planning for the Mentally Retarded, 1957.

Motor Characteristics of the Mentally Retarded, 1960.

The Child Who Is Mentally Retarded, 1956.

# REFERENCES

Auvil, D. L.: Danny: A Nursing Care Study. Am. J. Nursing, 60:241, 1960.

Bakwin, H., and Bakwin, R. M.: Clinical Management of Behavior Disorders in Children. 2nd ed. Philadelphia, W. B. Saunders Company, 1960.

Beck, H. L.: Counseling Parents of Retarded Children. Children, 6:225, 1959.

Begab, M. J.: Child-Welfare Service for the Mentally Retarded. Children, 5:105, 1958.

Bieck, C.: Tetralogy of Fallot. Am. J. Nursing, 59:384, 1959.

Brodish, M. S.: The Nurse's Role in the Care of Children with Acute Leukemia. Am. J. Nursing, 58:1572, 1958.

Burr, A. M.: Learning to Care for Mentally Retarded Children. Am. J. Nursing, 60:1000, 1960.

Caplan, G. (editor): Emotional Problems of Early Childhood. New York, Basic Books, Inc., 1955.

Clark, H. V.: Music, Mobiles, and Cardiac Catheterization. Am. J. Nursing, 57:1026, 1957.

Clark, M. W.: Accepting a Child—for a Lifetime. Nursing Outlook, 5:279, 1957.

Clarke, A. M., and Clarke, A. D. B. (editors): Mental Deficiency. Glencoe, Illinois, The Free Press, 1959.

Clise, M. H.: Disturbed Children Are Disturbing Children. Nursing Outlook, 5:638, 1957.

Cobb, B.: Psychological Impact of Long Illness and Death of a Child on the Family Circle. J. Pediat., 49:746, 1956.

Cooley, D. A.: Open Heart Surgery in Children. Am. J. Nursing, 58:200, 1958.

Craig, E. S., and Pack, S.: Nursing Care of the Child after Open Heart Surgery. Am. J. Nursing, 61:78, Feb. 1961.

Dimock, H. G.: The Child in Hospital. Philadelphia, F. A. Davis Company, 1960.

Erickson, F. H.: Play Interviews for Four-Year-Old Hospitalized Children. (Monographs of the Society for Research in Child Development, Inc.) Lafayette, Indiana, Child Development Publications, Purdue University, 1958.

Feifel, H.: The Meaning of Death. New York, McGraw-Hill Book Company, Inc., 1959.

Finch, S. M.: Fundamentals of Child Psychiatry. New York, W. W. Norton Co., 1960.

Flory, M. C.: Helping Parents Train a Retarded Child. Nursing Outlook, 5:426, 1957.

Idem: Training the Mentally Retarded Child. Nursing Outlook, 5:344, 1957.

Folck, M. M., and Nie, P. J.: Nursing Students Learn to Face Death. Nursing Outlook, 7:510, 1959.

French, E. L., and Scott, J. C.: The Child in the Shadows: A Manual for Parents of Retarded Children. Philadelphia, J. B. Lippincott Company, 1960.

Garrison, M. J.: Research Trends in Mental Deficiency. Children, 6:10, 1959.

Golbey, R. B.: Chemotherapy of Cancer. Am. J. Nursing, 60:521, 1960.

Hallas, C. H.: The Nursing of Mental Defectives. Baltimore, Williams & Wilkins Company, 1958.

Hardy, W. G., and Pauls, M. D.: Atypical Children with Communicative Disorders. Children, 6:13, 1959.

Harris, C. E.: A Decade of Research Concerning Children. Children, 6:145, 1959.

Hartmann, J. R., and Bolduc, R. A.: Hemophilia. Am. J. Nursing, 56:169, 1956.

Harvie, F. H.: Pediatric Methods and Standards. 3rd ed. Philadelphia, Lea & Febiger, 1958.

Holt, K. S.: The Home Care of Severely Retarded Children. Pediatrics, 22:744, 1958.

Hormuth, R. P.: Community Clinics for the Mentally Retarded. Children, 4:181, 1957.

Jubenville, C. P.: Day Care Centers for Severely Retarded Children. Nursing Outlook, 8:371, 1960.

Kirk, S. A., Karnes, M. B., and Kirk, W. D.: You and Your Retarded Child. New York, Macmillan Company, 1955.

Koch, R., and others: Attitude Study of Parents with Mentally Retarded Children. Pediatrics, 23:582, 1959.

Lesser, A. J.: New Program for Mentally Retarded Children. Am. J. Pub. Health, 48:9, 1958.

Michal-Smith, H.: The Mentally Retarded Patient. Philadelphia, J. B. Lippincott Company, 1956.

Mulder, D. W., and others: Treatment of Epilepsy. Postgrad. Med., 25:404, 1959.

Nelson, W. E. (editor): Textbook of Pediatrics. 7th ed. Philadelphia, W. B. Saunders Company, 1959.

Nixon, N.: A Child Guidance Clinic Explores Ways to Prevent Mental Illness. Children, 4:9, 1957.

Parsons, M. H.: A Home Economist in Service to Families with Mental Retardation. Children, 7:184, 1960.

Paterson, D., and McCreary, J. F.: Pediatrics. Philadelphia, J. B. Lippincott Company, 1956.

Peay, R.: The Emotional Problems of Children Facing Heart Surgery. Children, 7:223, 1960.

Richmond, J. B., and Waisman, H. A.: Psychologic Aspects of Management of Children with Malignant Diseases. A.M.A. J. Dis. Child., *89:*42, 1955.

Rosen, H. G.: Camping for the Emotionally Disturbed. Children, 6:86, 1959.

Schwarz, B. E., and Ruggieri, B. A.: Parent-Child Tensions. Philadelphia, J. B. Lippincott Company, 1958.

Silver, H. K., Kempe, C. H., and Bruyn, H. B.: Handbook of Pediatrics. 3rd ed. Los Altos, California, Lange Medical Publications, 1959.

Stanley-Brown, E. G.: Pediatric Surgery for Nurses. Philadelphia, W. B. Saunders Company, 1961.

The Woods Schools—Proceedings of the 33rd Spring Conference. Counseling Parents of Children with Mental Handicaps. Langhorne, Penna., The Woods Schools for Exceptional Children, May 2–3, 1958.

Watson, E. H.: Counseling Parents of Mentally Deficient Children. Pediatrics, 22:401, 1958.

Weiss, R. C.: A Creative Workshop for Retarded and Emotionally Disturbed Children. Nursing Outlook, 7:716, 1959.

Wellin, E., and others: Community Aspects of Mental Subnormality—A Local Health Department Program for Retarded Children. Am. J. Pub. Health, 50:36, 1960.

Wilson, H. E., and Price, G.: Leukemia. Am. J. Nursing, 56:601, 1956.

Wortham, E. D., and Ritchie, G.: Nursing Care of Children after Open Heart Surgery. Am. J. Nursing, 58:203, 1958.

Wortis, J.: Mental Retardation in the Soviet Union. Children, 7:219, 1960.

Wright, S. W., and others: Etiologic Factors in Mental Deficiency. A.M.A. J. Dis. Child., 95:541, 1958.

# The School Child

# Chapter 21

# The School Child:

# His Growth, Development and Care

## OVERVIEW OF EMOTIONAL DEVELOPMENT

BY THE TIME a child reaches his sixth birthday he should have learned to trust others and should have developed a sense of autonomy. He should also have learned the fundamentals of getting along in his particular environment, through experience in living and through questioning his parents and other adults. He should have developed a sense of initiative, but his activities should be controlled to some degree by his conscience.

These stages which the child passes through before he is six years old are probably the most important for his healthy personality development. They are the foundation for further development. Children whose personality growth has been warped are likely to remain handicapped unless help is given them. There are exceptions to this, of course, for experiences in later childhood and in adolescence influence the trend in emotional development.

**Sense of Industry.** Between the ages of six and twelve years the child develops a *sense of industry* and a desire to engage in tasks in the real world. He should no longer be involved in the imaginative fantasy life of the pre-school years. Even before he is six years old a child may show evidence that he enjoys doing socially useful tasks for others, that he wants to do things and to learn to do them well.

These years are usually a calm period, and few overwhelming upheavals in the child's life are apt to occur. The child continues in a steady growth toward learning how to attain the goal of becoming a responsible citizen. He acquires knowledge and skills which will help him to make a worth-while contribution to society. He learns how to cooperate with others, to play fairly and follow the rules of the game, and to conform to social norms so that his life

**589**

Figure 218. The school child wants to learn to do things and to do them well. (H. Armstrong Roberts.)

with others will be a positive experience for him and for those with whom he interacts.

Instead of developing a sense of industry, the child may acquire, or intensify earlier, *feelings of inferiority* and inadequacy. This is more likely to happen if he has not successfully passed through the previous stages of personality development.

**The Child and School.** At school the child has a task, one that will continue throughout childhood. If he is not adequately prepared, if his needs as a growing individual are disregarded or if for any other reason he is not successful at school, the experience may have a negative rather than a positive influence on personality development. If he is not successful in school because he is dull, his self-image is that he is stupid. If he is too maladjusted to make friends among his peer group, he feels that nobody likes him. He may stay in school, passively accepting his inferiority, or leave school as soon as the law permits.

Out of school he may find a job and attempt to secure a sense of accomplishment through this activity. To succeed, he needs the sense of industry which he failed to develop during his school years when it was a major developmental task. If he fails in the job, he may turn to delinquency to gain the status and recognition among his peers which he failed to gain in school and at work. If his delinquency is extreme, he also gains attention from adults which he could not secure by legitimate means.

The importance of adapting the school experience to the needs of the growing child is evident.

School is not the only place where a child may gain a feeling of mastery and acquire a sense of industry. The child who is unable to master his studies may be given useful tasks at home. Parents may delegate to him responsibilities which contribute to the happiness and well-being of all the family. Such tasks and responsibilities should not be those which adults do not want to do themselves, but rather should be based on a division of labor in which the child's tasks are suited to his abilities. The child's work should not be so time-consuming that he has no opportunity to study, to take on status-giving tasks outside the home and to play with his siblings and friends.

Community organizations for children stress both recreation and work— e.g. the 4-H Clubs and the Girl Scouts and Boy Scouts of America.

The school child must grow out of the dependence upon his family which was natural for the younger child, and must find satisfaction in the company of his peer group and adults outside the home. He must develop neuromuscular skills so that he can participate in work and games with others. He must acquire sufficient knowledge to interact with adults outside of school and thereby learn from them about the social life of his society. He must gain some understanding of adult concepts, logic and ways of communicating.

More specifically, during the school years the child should develop wholesome attitudes toward himself as a person and should learn his or her appropriate masculine or feminine social role. He should learn how to get along with his age mates, yet should be able to act according to his conscience and his scale of values. The child should achieve independence in caring for himself. He should learn the fundamental skills of reading, writing and calculating, and the physical skills necessary for ordinary games. By the time he is twelve years old he should have developed positive attitudes toward his own and other social, racial, economic and religious groups, and have learned the concepts necessary for participation in daily living with adults in his environment.

## The School Child and His Family

**Relations with Parents.** The child between six and twelve years should have widened his social horizons beyond the confines of his own home. Although he is still dependent upon his parents' love, companionship with his peers and adults outside the home has become of increasing importance.

The child's relation with the parent of the opposite sex which existed during his preschool years has been resolved. He has come to respect and love that parent, but now identifies with or tries to be like the parent of the same sex. By imitating that parent's role he learns his own social role.

Children gain increasing ideological as well as physical and emotional independence from their parents. They gain new ideas from adults outside the family: school teachers, Sunday School teachers, parents of their friends, policemen, television performers, newspaper writers and authors of textbooks and of fiction. Often these ideas and attitudes conflict with those of their parents. This is likely to be so if the parents are immigrants or of a low socio-economic status. The adults who teach these children must help them to understand this conflict so that they do not become impatient with their parents and lose respect for them.

Health education is a part of modern general education in the public schools. Health measures such as taking a bath every day, accepted by the children, may seem foolish to their parents, who went to school twenty to thirty years ago. Daily baths may be almost impossible in a crowded tenement flat. There is then a conflict between what the child is taught at school and at home, a conflict which places a serious strain on parent-child relations.

The school child learns to think of himself as a person in his own right and may resent rigid limits which parents continue to impose on his behavior. Furthermore, he dislikes a show of affection. He often pulls away from the adult's embrace and turns his face from kisses. The parents may be confused and thrown into emotional conflict by the new concepts which children bring home, by their efforts at independence and by the apparent disinterest in a physical show of parental affection.

Parents need help in understanding the normal growth and development of their children when such conflicts arise. They may discuss these matters with the child's teacher, alone or during parent-teacher conferences, with their physician, religious advisor or a nurse who visits in the home or cares for the child in the hospital.

**Relations with Siblings.** Whether the school child is an only child or one of a group of siblings has more and more effect upon his personality. If he is an only child, he tends to cling longer to his concept of being the center of the family. When he goes outside the family to make friends in his peer group, he still expects to be the center of the group and becomes frightened when he finds that he is not. He finds it difficult to learn the give and take of social living with other children. An only child who does not succeed in establishing himself as a group member may find that being home in the evening with his parents, or playing by himself on rainy days, is a lonely kind of existence. He may come to resent being an only child and long desperately for siblings such as his friends have. In addition, since he is the recipient of the undiluted force of his parents' attitudes and feelings, he is likely to be limited in his freedom.

Children in a large family are of different ages. They find adjusting to children outside the family and sharing with the group easier than does the only child. They learn early that some are given opportunities and restrictions, while others are not. They learn that no one of them, unless it is the youngest child, is singled out as being the center of interest, although each in his own way is loved by his parents. Although they may disagree among themselves, each sibling has a deep affection for the other children in his family.

Children in large families have problems, however, which the only child does not have to face. Sibling jealousy is a problem even in families in which all the members love one another. Although it is more acute in preschool children than among children over six years of age, it still exists. An older child may envy the attention which the younger siblings receive; he may resent the fact that his discarded toys are being broken by a younger child. He may resent the fact that, despite his feelings, he is expected to love and often to take care of his siblings.

If the school child is a younger sibling, he may envy the older child his freedom and his skills. He may strive to be like the older child and be defeated in his attempts. The school child's jealousy of his siblings, younger and older, may actually increase as he strives to keep ahead of the younger child or to catch up with an elder brother or sister. Scholastic ability is a principal cause of sibling jealousy among school children, particularly in a child who is mentally inferior to his siblings.

School children often prefer to be with their friends rather than with their siblings. Relations with a friend are less emotional and freer from parental interference. A child chooses his friends; the sibling relationship is one he is born into and cannot be discontinued when he wishes to be free of it. Ideally, experience with siblings should facilitate a child's social adjustment outside the family, but it does not take the place of friendships of his own choice.

## The School Child and His Friends

**Relations with Friends.** As the child psychologically moves slowly away from home, his friends become increasingly important to him. He learns to take his place as a member of a group, and his social life begins. In making this adjustment children tend to avoid the company of the opposite sex. During this period boys consider girls sissies, and the girls think boys too rough. Each sex tends to develop its own language and its own activities and behavior.

Children of school age can be exceedingly cruel to each other. They want to control or feel that they are able to control another person. The state of being "picked on" is common during the school period. Some children are excluded from friendship groups and verbally are made to feel uncomfortable. School children can also be cruel to adults whom they dislike. This may be because the parent-child relations in their home are poor. They may attempt to hurt those in authority because they do not wish to remain submissive as they were when younger, or because their parents have not shown them the proper pattern of behavior to follow in relation to adults who have temporary control over them.

**Gangs or Groups.**   Since school children have learned that their parents are not omnipotent, that they make mistakes and are sometimes afraid, they tend to confide not in them, but in their friends. They form close friendships and ultimately join a group of other children of their own sex. Such a group may be merely a friendship group or it may be a secret society or an antisocial gang, depending upon the needs of the children who form it. Among themselves the children discuss the problems they face. They discuss their own theories about life, death and sexual matters; they share attitudes, values and beliefs with the peer group.

Much of a boy's hostility and aggression is worked off in his peer group through fighting, either in a supervised, organized game such as baseball or football or while playing "cops" and robbers or cowboys and Indians. Unfortunately some of these juvenile gangs turn their hostility not against their own age group in play, but against other youths or adults in deadly earnest. When this occurs, the pattern is laid for delinquent behavior against society.

Girls also form their own groups and discuss their own problems. They do not, however, as a rule engage in the

**Figure 219.**   During school years friends become increasingly important. Each sex enjoys its own language and its own kinds of activity. (H. Armstrong Roberts.)

aggressive and hostile activities common in the boys' gang.

Toward the end of the school period children have learned to compete with others, to compromise with others and to cooperate so that they can accomplish something in their group which no one child could do without adult help. They have learned how to get along with their own and other groups and to follow the rules of the larger society. They have developed a sense of responsibility about matters which they know are important.

Parents should be understanding and accepting of the activities of their school children and willing to give independence when it is needed. All too often only the mother is interested, and she seldom understands the boy's interests. The father often appears disinterested in his children's individual or group activities. This is unfortunate because the boy especially needs his father's loving interest at this time.

## OVERVIEW OF PHYSICAL, SOCIAL AND MENTAL DEVELOPMENT

**Physical Development.** During the school years the child shows a progressively slower growth in height, but a rapid gain in weight. As a result he tends to lose the thin, wiry appearance of the earlier years. General growth is slow until the spurt just before puberty. Muscular coordination improves steadily; the child's posture should be good (the earlier lordosis has disappeared). The lymphatic tissue reaches its height of development in the early school period. The frontal sinuses are fairly well developed by six years of age. From this time on all the sinuses are potential foci of infection.

This is the period of eruption and growth of the permanent teeth. The six-year molars are the first to erupt and are the keystone for the permanent dental arch. The receding mandible, characteristic of the younger child, has extended forward to allow room for the permanent teeth.

The temperature, pulse and respiration approach the adult type. The normal temperature is 98.6° F. The average pulse rate is from 85 to 100 per minute; the blood pressure is 90 to 108 systolic and 60 to 67 diastolic. The rate of respiration is 18 to 20 per minute.

The physical changes which indicate pubescence may begin to appear toward the end of the school age. Normal children may show the first evidence of change two years before or after the average date of expectancy. The average age of onset of puberty in girls is thirteen years, in boys fourteen or fifteen years.

**Social and Mental Development.** In attending school the child has an opportunity to widen his social contacts while he develops his mental abilities. The school hours of the six-year-old in many places are shorter than those of older grade school children. This makes the transition from home to school life and the adjustment to new experiences easier for the child.

## SPECIFICS OF PHYSICAL, SOCIAL AND MENTAL DEVELOPMENT

The older a child becomes, the less is it possible to set norms as standards for his behavior or abilities. Such norms illustrate merely the kinds of behavior that often occur at a certain age. Individual differences and the effects of home, school and community environment become more and more pronounced as the child grows older.

### Six Years

The sixth year is a year of transition, a year of physical and psychologic changes which society has taken as the criterion for readiness to enter school. It is a difficult period for parents, and also for the child because he wants to assume increased responsibility and self-direction and yet lacks the basis for making wise decisions. Typically, he is upset and tense, self-centered and a show-off. He enjoys bossing others, but is easily hurt by the criticism he evokes. He is ready to start anything, but not anxious to finish the task. He may be defiant and rude with adults as a result of his unstable emotional reactions.

Six-year-olds feel tension because they are growing up and because they are leaving the security of home to go to school. They want the role of the little child again. Parental love and praise are important to them.

Boys and girls play together. Their play is apt to end in chaos. There are disputes and physical battles in which boys and girls take equal parts. The individual child is still more important than the play group as a whole.

The six-year-old may still be troubled by some of the sex questions he asked in the preschool period. He may indulge in sex play. Although he looks forward to marriage, he pays little attention to the sexual aspect and may invite one of his relatives to be his marital partner. He is likely to want his mother to have a baby even if there is already one in the family.

**Physical Development and Motor Control.**
Physical development and motor control are seen in the changing characteristics and abilities of the six-year-old. The loss of the temporary teeth continues, and the first permanent teeth, the six-year molars, erupt. In school, if he did not go to nursery school or kindergarten, he is exposed to infection more frequently than he was at home, and ear, nose and throat problems are common. He appears to be in constant motion. He enjoys physical activity, but his movements may be clumsy because of his fatigue from overactivity—wrestling, playing tag, tumbling, and jumping with other children. His balance is improving; he climbs, skips, hops and gallops well. Girls jump rope, a single rope, but not double. Both sexes can walk steadily on a chalk mark and learn to skate. Some children can ride a bicycle.

These children can throw and catch a ball. They are aware of their hands as tools, cutting and pasting well. They can hammer, build simple struc-

**Figure 220.**    Six-year-olds enjoy physical activity, but their movements are not as coordinated as those of older school children. (H. Armstrong Roberts.)

tures, manipulate fasteners on clothing with the aid of sight to guide their hands, and tie shoelaces.

**Vocalization, Socialization and Mental Abilities.** The six-year-old has command of practically every form of sentence structure. Speech is fixed, and he is no longer experimenting with its use. He asks questions which show thought and uses language as a tool and less for the pleasure of talking as he did during the preschool age. He may use language aggressively, expressing himself in slang and even swearing. He uses language to share in the experience of others and is interested in learning more about his relatives and his own and their place in the family tree. He still defines objects in terms of their use: a chair is something to sit on, and a spoon is what he eats with. But he has some concept of abstract words; he knows whether it is morning or afternoon. He knows his right hand from his left, can count to twenty or more, but when printing, he may reverse one or two of the digits. His printing is limited to capital letters. There are some which he cannot produce, and he may print others in reverse. Since he can now recognize shapes, he can read, and describe objects seen in pictures. He can draw a man with hitherto absent features such as hands, neck and clothing, and he can distinguish between what he has been taught is attractive and what is ugly when shown a series of faces. He is able to obey three commands given in succession, e.g. "Wipe your hands, put the dishes on the table, and close the door."

Probably his greatest achievement in abstract thought is his beginning interest in the concept of a power greater than himself or his parents, God.

### Seven Years

Seven is an assimilative age, a quieting-down period. The child is less of a problem than he was at six years, more often quiet than boisterous. Many teachers find the second-grade group the easiest to teach in elementary school. He has less intense relations with others; he does not ask for trouble. But he enjoys teasing, and this often gets him into difficulty with children younger than himself and with adults who take their part. He likes to play alone, although he prefers group play. When playing, he is more passive than the six-year-old.

The seven-year-old sets high standards for his family and feels both a personal inferiority and anger over even their minor failures, as he sees them, in living up to their respective roles. His ethical sense is developing; he is conscious of right and wrong in the conduct of others and in what he himself does. He may tattle on other children from a sense of justice. On the whole he is now a cooperative member of the family and wants the approval of his parents. Parents must respect his inner life, his strains of sadness and his uncalled-for periods of shyness. It is during these periods that he is becoming aware of himself and thus of others.

The seven-year-old is more modest about sexual matters and indulges in less sex play. Many seven-year-olds would like to have a baby brother or sister. The seven-year-old may become involved in an elementary love affair with someone of the opposite sex.

**Physical Development and Motor Control.** The general level of activity is lower at seven years than at six, but varies widely in individual children. The child has a trait which annoys his elders, but fascinates him and other children— wiggling a loose tooth.

The books he reads need no longer be printed with type larger than average, for his eyes become fully developed between seven and eight years of age. His posture is now more tense and ready for motion than that of the younger child.

Boys and girls enjoy skating and other active sports. There begins to be a division, however, between boy and girl sports. Girls jump rope and play hopscotch, games which boys are likely to participate in only in a teasing way. Although seven-year-olds are active, they enjoy games in which they can sit down and rest.

**Vocalization, Socialization and Mental Abilities.** The child is becoming oriented in time as well as space. He knows which month it is and the season of the year, particularly months in which some event in which he is intensely interested takes place—Christmas or his birthday. He begins to read the clock, both the hours and the minutes.

His hands are becoming more steady, and he often prefers a pencil with an eraser to a crayon. He can print several sentences, though the letters become smaller toward the end of the line. Reversal of letters is less common, and he is likely to correct such errors. He can repeat five numbers in succession and three numbers backward, count by two's and five's, grasp the basic idea of addition and subtraction, copy a diamond without confusing it with a square, and tell what parts are missing from an incomplete picture of a man. His attention span is lengthening, and he enjoys repeating activities that afford him satisfaction. He is more self-helpful, needing little assistance in dressing, undressing and going to bed. He is increasingly interested in God's place in the world and wants to know where heaven is and what it is like.

## Eight Years

The eight-year-old is at an expansive age and wants to do everything. This is an age of broadening experiences and intellectual exploration. He is more creative and active in his solitary play and work, but he needs other children and their approval, and he actively seeks their company. He is full of enthusiastic energy and wants to be considered important by adults. He wants to assume responsibility and to spread his influence in the culture of his group by putting on dramatic shows and inventing new ways of doing tasks.

He tries to understand adult ideas and standards by listening to what is told him. He learns by experience and from others what is necessary for group living. If his mental ability is average or above average, he becomes very much interested in reading, group activities and school, especially in science as he sees it pictured in space ships and machinery. He likes science fiction. Hero worship begins at this age.

He likes to join clubs if they are not too rigidly organized and takes group fads seriously. Eight-year-olds appear to be sex-conscious, choosing playmates of their own sex. Boys are usually secretive about girl friends, especially if *she* is a new girl in the neighborhood. They show less active interest in sex questions which are beyond their comprehension than does the younger child, but they may ask questions at appropriate times. Mothers should suggest to their children that it is better not to discuss the answers to sex questions with siblings or friends.

The eight-year-old has company manners and behaves best when strangers are present or when he is away from home.

**Physical Development and Motor Control.** There are subtle changes in the body of an eight-year-old; the arms are growing longer in proportion to the body, and the hands are also proportionately larger. His movements are becoming smoother, more graceful and perfected. His amusements change as he matures. He now likes hiking, playing ball and such games as follow-the-leader. The boy wants to improve his skill in boxing and wrestling, and the girl in jumping rope, hopscotch and roller skating. Both boys and girls are dramatic in their activities and accompany speech with descriptive gestures.

**Vocalization, Socialization and Mental Abilities.** In school the child of eight is writing rather than printing, and enjoys his new skill. In mental tests for his age group are found questions such as naming from memory similarities and differences between two objects— e.g. ball and block—and counting backwards from twenty. In school and daily life he has new abilities. He is beginning to understand perspective in drawing. He can repeat the days of the week and has some concept of the number of days which must pass before some pleasant event will take place—a holiday, his birthday or, in the hospital, visiting day and that eventful day when he goes home.

Some children enjoy going to Sunday School and are interested in hearing about heaven as "the place you go to when you die."

### Nine Years

The nine-year-old is no longer a child, nor is he a youth. He is only beginning to take part in family group discussions. He is not as restless as the eight-year-old and is more interested in family activities. He is impelled to show others that he is an individual and resists or ignores adult authority when it conflicts with ideas or values of his peer group. Teachers find the children in fourth grade difficult to teach. In broadening his experiences outside the home he grows toward independence. He is better able to accept blame for his acts and assumes responsibility for care of younger siblings and for keeping his room in some sort of order. He is motivated, as well as more likely, to complete the tasks he begins.

He fluctuates between childhood and youth in his actions and thoughts. Hero worship is becoming pronounced. Girls still prefer to play with girls, and boys with boys. They are usually less concerned with the reproductive aspect of sex than when they were eight. This depends, however, on whether their desire for information about the conception and bearing of children was satisfied when they first asked for it. The nine-year-old is in a state of constant urgency, as though he were in a contest with time.

**Physical Development and Motor Control.** These children have more individual variation in skills than they had during their first three years of school. Normally, hand-eye coordination is devel-

oped, and the child becomes skillful in manual activities. In general, children of this age can use both hands independently.

The child works and plays hard and enjoys displaying his motor skill and strength; he shows great interest in competitive sports such as baseball.

**Vocalization, Socialization and Mental Abilities.** New abilities, which show his mental development, include describing common objects in detail not in terms of use as he did when he was six years old, repeating the months of the year in order, knowing the date, telling time correctly, writing (usually with small, even letters), matching the material which he reads with reality, making correct change from a quarter, arranging five weights according to their heaviness, multiplying and dividing (simple division) and repeating four numbers backward (this is one item in a commonly given mental test).

The child can take care of his bodily needs completely; this is a great step away from early childhood and toward adult self-reliance. He has developed acceptable table manners and shows them without coaching from his parents. Although he has fewer fears than when he was younger, he has become a worrier. His advance toward adult attitudes is shown in his rejection of the Santa Claus myth, and yet he does not intentionally destroy it for a younger sibling. In contrast to the two preceding years, he may show a lack of interest in God and in religion.

### Ten Years

The average child of ten years is at the beginning of the preadolescent period. The girl is further advanced than the boy toward puberty. The ten-year-old is even more reasonable than the nine-year-old, for he has acquired greater mastery of himself and his environment. He is courteous and well mannered with adults, and shows more self-direction in his actions. He wants to measure up to a challenge, defined in the social norms of the group. He has broad interests and is beginning to think clearly about social problems and social prejudices. Special talents appear in this age group.

The child adjusts better than before to home routines; he can live by rules and tolerates frustrations. He is entering the age when the need for group activities is at its highest point. To him, attaining a goal for the group is more important than his own ideas or desires. He is capable of great loyalties and intense hero worship; both are qualities making for successful group membership.

The ten-year-old is interested in matters of sex, but is more likely to discuss the subject with his peer group than with his parents. Children of both sexes investigate their sexual organs. Some children are modest, but others present problems of sex play.

Outside the classroom the two sexes rarely mix. Although kissing games may be played in children's entertainments arranged by adults, they are seldom played spontaneously. Children tease each other about friends of the opposite sex.

The ten-year-old wants to be independent. For this reason requests should be made positively and with tact. Negative requests affront his sense of personal worth. The power of suggestion is important at this age and can be used to help the child develop a good character.

**Physical Development and Motor Control.** As the child's body matures sex differences are more pronounced. Both boys and girls have perfected most of the basic small motor movements. They desire perfection in their complex abilities. Girls have more poise than boys, partly because of their earlier maturation.

**Vocalization, Socialization and Mental Abilities.** The child now thinks of situations in terms of cause and effect. He has some insight into the fundamentals of human relations and wants to accomplish great things in life.

His education is more advanced, and he uses what he knows and the skills he has acquired in his daily life. He can write for a relatively long time and maintains good speed. He likes mystery stories, science fiction and practical magic. He can use numbers beyond 100 with understanding and can do simple fractions.

### Ten to Twelve Years (Preadolescence)

The years between ten and twelve are known as the preadolescent period. It is a time of rapid growth and development, a period when many problems occur. As he approaches adulthood the child may become overcritical of adults, comparing them with the self-image of the man or woman he or she intends to be. The child wavers between dependence and independence and is likely to withdraw when he is frustrated instead of voicing his anger. He may rebel against parental standards of bathing and dressing.

Friends in his peer group are extremely important to him; he shares their attitudes and tells them his thoughts rather than confiding in his parents. He enters with enthusiasm into group community projects such as collecting worn clothing for charity or old newspapers for the Boy Scouts.

He is critical of what he does. He wants to become somewhat financially independent of his parents; he is happy to do small jobs after school or during vacations. He seeks an adult friend of the same sex with whom to identify and interchange criticism of his parents. The composure and control of the ten-year-old gradually vanish at eleven to twelve years. He becomes annoying, sloppy, exhibitionistic and negativistic. He tries hard to master reality in preparation for adolescence. He is interested in how things work and curious about the world in general, but his interest in acquiring academic knowledge may lag.

As an individual he needs to gain strength of personality so as to be able to make healthy solutions to the conflicts of adolescence. The adult who is responsible for the preadolescent at home, in the community or at school must accept the fact that the child needs to rebel and depreciate others

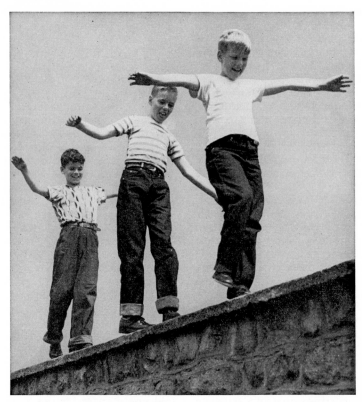

**Figure 221.** Preadolescents have good muscular control and balance. (H. Armstrong Roberts.)

in order to work through his conflict between dependence and independence. He is still dependent, but he does not wish to be made to feel infantile. He rejects his parents because he does not want to feel dependent on them; he meets his dependency needs by relations with other adults. The adult whom the preadolescent selects to fill this role must handle the child through democratic guidance. He must accept the child, yet provide limits to his behavior as the parents did when the child was younger. The preadolescent needs help to channel his feelings and energy in the proper directions—sports and work suitable to his stage of growth and development. The child needs help in accepting himself in his new role of preadolescent. Adults in his environment should help him to build up his self-esteem and strengthen his personality in order to prepare him adequately to meet the problems of adolescence.

**Motor Control and Physical Development.** Children in this age group are filled with energy and are constantly active. They need to assert themselves and impress others with their independence. Their muscular control is good, and manipulative skill almost equals that of the adult. They appear to be under tension, which is relieved by foot-tapping on the floor or finger-drumming on table tops.

The twelve-year molars erupt; they are the last teeth to erupt during childhood. The preadolescent spurt in growth comes earlier in girls than in boys, but girls lag behind boys in endurance and physical strength.

**Vocalization, Socialization and Mental Abilities.** Before he is twelve years old the average child is able to define some basic abstract terms such as honesty and justice. His development of vocabulary and diction depend upon his intelligence, experience and environmental opportunities. Children in this age group can see the moral of stories. Their individual interests and intellectual pursuits vary. Intellectual growth is seen in their interest in world affairs, both past and present, and their attitude toward social problems, especially those which touch their daily lives.

They are eager to learn about health. They want to know why the mouth should be covered when coughing. They are capable of self-care in ordinary life situations, but should still be under some supervision of sympathetic adults. They can assume some responsibility for the care of younger children. Their contact with children and adults goes well beyond the limits of home.

The peer group is very close to the eleven-year-old. This is a period for sharing secrets. Even a secret language may be devised and used strictly with the close peer group. These children still prefer to play with their own sex

group, but accept the opposite sex in their activities.

## SCHOOL

Attendance at school is an important part of the growing child's life. It is especially important that school contribute to his developing sense of industry. For this reason schools for all children, irrespective of their socioeconomic group and intelligence level, should be planned to meet the children's needs. The course of instruction should be such that every child will be able to get a feeling of successful accomplishment in some area.

All children should feel that they can accomplish something both in school and, later, in community life. This does not mean that all children should be passed along with their group in school whether they do well or not. They do not want to be rewarded when

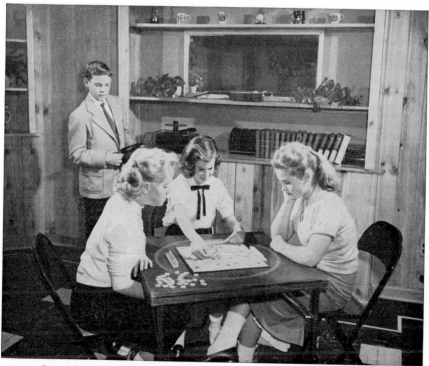

**Figure 222.** Preadolescents still prefer to play with others of their own sex, but accept the opposite sex in their activities. (H. Armstrong Roberts.)

**Figure 223.** Attendance at school is an important part of the child's life. In school children should be helped to develop their sense of industry. (H. Armstrong Roberts.)

they know that they have failed. They do not desire praise which they know they do not deserve. They need opportunities for success on their individual level of achievement.

Not every child is capable of excelling intellectually in academic courses, but the school should help each child to realize his potential ability and find real satisfaction in his achievement in other areas of living—areas in which the child who does not do well at school may be more successful than those who excel in class work.

**Preparation for School.** Just as not all children are ready for nursery school or kindergarten at the same age, so not all children are emotionally ready for school at the same chronologic age. If the preschool child has attended and adjusted well to nursery school, he probably will have little difficulty with adjustment to school. If he has not attended nursery school, he will need special preparation for school experience, an experience which is one of the highest hurdles a child has to conquer.

As soon as school starts there is an enforced separation of the child from his home. The unprepared child, more than those who are prepared, may be uncertain of the expectations of the teacher, a new adult in charge of part of his life. He may be frightened by leaving his parents and by the demands of a group of children different from those he has known before. In general, however, if he has attended kindergarten in the public school of his neighborhood, he will have friends in the first grade and will be accustomed to the school building. If a younger sibling is entering kindergarten, he is protective and tells him all about it. He will go to and from school with siblings or neighborhood friends.

Preparation for school experience is much like preparation for attendance at nursery school. The child will, of course, know his full name and address before entering school. He should have a physical examination and must meet school requirements for immunization. The mother should take the child o school the spring or summer before school starts in order to orient him to the physical environment and to meet his teacher. If he has gone to kindergarten in the same school, he is already familiar with the environment and many features of school life. Parents should talk positively about school experience at all times, but particularly to the child entering school. Older siblings will present school as a matter-of-fact experience for all six-year-olds and as something to brag about to younger children. After school has started if the child appears afraid of the school experience, the mother may stay with him in the classroom for a while until the teacher has established a positive relation with him. Before parents allow a child to go to school alone they must be certain that he knows the way or, if he must take a bus, which bus to ride. Generally the school is either in easy walking distance or sends a school bus to collect the children who live too far away for them to walk to school.

A problem may arise after the child has become familiar with school life in that he pays more attention to the job of gaining friends than to gaining knowledge. This is to be expected, especially if none of his old friends from home, kindergarten or nursery school are in his class at school.

Parents should not expect too much from children upon their return from school. Children have put in a day of school work and recreation under supervision, both of which are planned to promote growth and development. Nevertheless the child should gradually assume some home responsibilities, planned so that he has time for play with his siblings and friends and also to be by himself. This last is a need often overlooked even by thoughtful parents.

During the orientation period as well as during all his school life the child's parents should be willing to listen to his tales about his school experiences. This strengthens his ability to use language and also helps him to become more of a person in his own right.

Parents' unflagging interest in school and the child's activities does more than anything else to invest education with its real importance.

If the child refuses to attend school, is chronically unhappy there or is not learning at the rate he should, his parents should investigate the situation in conjunction with his teacher or other school personnel.

**Role of the Teacher.** Teachers play a definite role in helping children develop a sense of industry through their assignments, stimulation of group activities and their suggestion that children accept responsibilities for nonacademic duties in the classroom. In addition, teachers can also deepen their students' sense of trust, autonomy and initiative, or encourage the growth of these personality traits in children whose emotional growth has been stunted.

The teacher also has the responsibility of helping her pupils achieve certain developmental tasks such as learning mental skills, and the masculine or feminine role and getting along with age mates. Teachers can also do much to foster creative ability and help the child develop as an individual.

A teacher has a profound influence because, next to the parents, she is the most important person in a child's life. This is especially true during the grade school period when the child needs an older person of his own sex to "worship." This is one reason why it would be beneficial to have more male teachers; the grade school boy is apt to lack this model. The teacher should be the kind of person whom the child can profitably imitate. Unfortunately some parents want the teacher to take too much responsibility for their children; they want relief from their own duty of rearing their children. They want the teacher to solve all the child's problems while he is in school. These parents should be helped to understand the proper function of the school and to recognize their own responsibilities as parents.

Parents may seek guidance from teachers or school counselors as individuals or collectively. Parent-teacher groups are especially valuable for interpreting the function of the school in the child's life, growth and development at various age levels, and problems such as discipline, sibling rivalry, sex education and special health problems of children. The leader of such a group may not always give advice; she should let the group solve the mutual problems facing its members.

## PLAY AND WORK

Play is a child's tool for learning, and his play changes with his developmental needs. Adequate play materials should be provided.

In general, time spent in play and the number of play activities decrease as the child matures. Nevertheless the time spent upon different specific activities increases because the attention span becomes longer and the child has a deeper interest in what he is doing. Play during the school years becomes more formal than it was during early childhood, more organized, more competitive and to some degree less physically active. The child begins to have an interest in hobbies or collections of various kinds.

As the child participates in more organized, competitive sports such as football, baseball or running matches he needs the help of adults in learning the rules. Parents should spend more time with their children. The adult should not be the leader, however. Children tend to respond best when they plan their own play experiences. In this way they learn self-government and self-direction of activities.

Another responsibility of the parents during the school years is helping the child learn to work. He should be permitted and encouraged to assist with duties in or around the house. Allowing him to help may take more time than doing the work without him, but ultimately the adult's time is saved and the child has developed his sense of industry. If he is not allowed to help when he is young, he may not be interested in helping later in life. The work he is asked to do should definitely contribute to the welfare of the group and should not be a task given him merely to keep him occupied.

As soon as the child shows interest in earning his spending money—this will be during his later school years—he should be helped to decide the kind of work he would like to do, whether it is delivering papers, mowing lawns or baby sitting. The attitudes toward work which he develops in these early years will be important in shaping the kind of workman he is during adult life.

### Six to Eight Years

From six to eight years of age the child is interested chiefly in the immediate environment and the immediate present. He needs, in play, an opportunity to express his feelings and find acceptance. Play must be suited to his interests and concentration span. Since he knows more about family life than any other kind of living, he enjoys playing house. A child also takes the role of a member of various occupational groups which he comes in contact with: storekeeper, milkman or trainman. What a child pretends to be gives the adult insight into his personality.

**Six Years.**   The child six years of age plays with spreading scope and movement. Sex differences in play are defining themselves more clearly. Both sexes, however, enjoy many activities in common. For instance, both girls and boys like to paint and color and to cut out and paste. Boys enjoy drawing airplanes, trains and boats; girls are more likely to draw people and houses. Boys enjoy digging more than girls do, though it is a favorite activity of both sexes. Boys are more likely to have bicycles than girls are, but all children of this age want to learn to ride. If they have none of their own, they borrow the bicycles of their older siblings and friends. Both sexes enjoy running games, tag, hide-and-seek, roller skating and swimming. Girls enjoy jumping rope.

Both boys and girls like to pretend,

out there is a sex difference. Boys pretend that they are conductors, motormen or soldiers or imitate some other masculine role in which there is plenty of activity. Girls dress up in costumes and play at being mothers or teachers, with younger children or dolls as their children. Irrespective of sex, these children start collections of miscellaneous items such as bits of fancy paper, pictures or anything that takes their fancy.

Children six to eight years old like to "read stories from memory," look at comic books, play simple table games and listen to radio and television programs. This is the age when doll play is at its height, and every toy pertaining to the mother role adds to the child's pleasure.

Boys and girls may play school and house together, but boys do not do so when playing only with boys. Boys particularly enjoy games characterized by getting under cover and shooting the enemy. They are interested in construction and transportation games.

Suitable toys for girls include dolls, doll clothes, wash baskets, doll strollers or baby carriages, swings, stoves, suit cases and make-up equipment. Boys like electric trains, airplanes, boats, trucks and automobiles.

**Seven Years.** Play at seven is approached more cautiously than at six years, and there are fewer new ventures. The child is more obsessive in his play interests. He enjoys funny books and coloring in books with pictures suited to his age. He likes table games, jigsaw puzzles, magic and tricks. He reads simple books fairly well, and enjoys reading. He is content to play by himself when no companions are about and is better able than the six-year-old to plan what he wants to do next. He listens to the radio and watches television programs of adventure in which there is plenty of shooting and wild horseback riding. Boys like to invent and then construct playthings and gifts for mother, using cereal boxes, fruit crates and even packing boxes. Girls enjoy designing dresses for paper dolls.

These children enjoy collecting in quantity, not for quality; they collect stones, bottle caps and almost anything they find which is out of the ordinary.

They demand more realism in their play. They need guns and caps to play cowboys and Indians or "cops" and robbers. All seven-year-old "mothers" want dolls the size of a real baby, which can "suck" from a bottle and wet the diaper. These "mothers," who want a realistic family of "children" whose ages range from newborn to four, also love "older" dolls with hair which can be brushed and combed. They like large "sister" dolls, but find them too big for mothering.

Both sexes enjoy active games. Girls like hopscotch, jumping rope and the quiet game of jackstones. Boys play ball, climb trees, race and play marbles. Both sexes ride bicycles well, and learn to swim under supervision. If they have the opportunity, many learn to ski. Girls enjoy almost all forms of play which boys engage in, but are not likely to be as proficient as the boys in active sports.

**Eight Years.** Eight years is an active age, one in which there is a wide variety of interests. Unsupervised play among eight-year-olds becomes noisy and may end in a quarrel. They do not enjoy playing alone. If they are with an adult, they demand his complete attention; if they are with other children, they demand full participation. Their drawings are full of action.

Girls like to mix dough for cookies, make Jell-o in fancy molds, frost cakes and experiment with simple cooking. Boys enjoy simple chemistry sets and equipment for making telegraph sets and performing magic tricks. They are fond of dramatics, staging air raids, fighting and rushing to fires. Girls also enjoy dramatics, though of a less masculine type, and always want an audience.

Boys and girls of this age make collections, but are now conscious of quality, and they classify and organize the items. Boys collect stones and rocks, marbles, cards of baseball stars or cars. Girls collect paper dolls, valentines and Christmas cards or similar items.

**Figure 224.** Dramatic play is important in the life of the 8-year-old. *A,* Girls enjoy dressing up in their mother's old clothing. *B,* Boys enjoy putting on a "show." (H. Armstrong Roberts.)

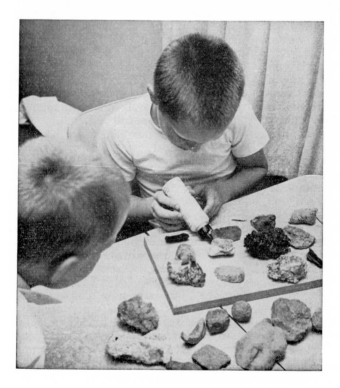

**Figure 225.** School age children enjoy making collections. This 8-year-old has classified and organized his collection of rocks. (H. Armstrong Roberts.)

These children enjoy active games. In spite of their fondness for exuberant activity, they respond well to supervision.

Eight-year-olds begin to form loosely organized, short-lived clubs. They have secret passwords which must be given before permission is granted to enter the club house, hut or hang-out.

They enjoy various sports in season. They are interested in table games such as checkers and dominoes. They may invent their own rules for an old game, often to such an extent that it is virtually a new game. Rules may be short-lived, but must be adhered to by all participants while they are in effect. Children of this age do not accept losing a game easily, they argue about decisions, and they often walk out of the group if they are beaten.

Most eight-year-olds can read well enough to enjoy childhood classics such as books on travel and geography. Comic books are still prime favorites. These children are at the peak of want-ing prizes and objects given with coupons from breakfast cereals plus a small sum of money. They are thrilled to receive mail as adults do. Radio and television are extremely important in their lives. They like stories of adventure and mystery. Science fiction is becoming a prime favorite.

### Nine to Twelve Years

The interest of children in this age group expands to distant places, backward into history and forward into the jet age. They like tales of King Arthur and of Robin Hood—tales which do not point a moral, but give examples of courage, kindness, endurance and adventure. They feel responsible for performing some service as part of their day's activities. They are developing a sense of satisfaction from contributing to group activity, and the beginning of group loyalty which characterizes the gang age of older siblings. They are now able to receive help in understand-

**Figure 226.** Young school-age children enjoy sports in season. Boys enter enthusiastically into sand-lot games of baseball. The youngest boy in this group has been assigned the job of holding the bats. (H. Armstrong Roberts.)

**Figure 227.**   Members of this 10- to 11-year-old "gang" have built their own tree house. (H. Armstrong Roberts.)

ing the advantage of mature behavior, although they can seldom live up to their ideal of a self-image. They are interested in their future as they say, "What I'm going to be . . ." Parents should be observant of the natural inclinations of the child, although vocational decisions should not be made until he reaches adolescence.

**Nine Years.** The nine-year-old plays and works hard, often to the point of fatigue. He is busy with his chosen activities; he enjoys reading, listening to the radio and viewing television for prolonged periods. Boys play football or baseball, and girls play with dolls for hours on end.

Both boys and girls enjoy active sports. They are old enough to want to improve their skills, and there is a purpose in their play which they seldom had when younger. Boys often disturb the peace of the home by rough-housing.

Nine-year-old girls and boys are great readers, reading their favorite books over and over again. They often read the junior classics, but comic books and books on adventure, war and slapstick domestic humor still fascinate them.

Many children are interested in music and take music lessons in school or from a private teacher. They often apply themselves well to music study and acquire skill through hours of practice. Talents appear at this age, especially in the creative arts. Children have an opportunity to hear good music on the radio, television and record players at home or at school. They still have favorite programs on the television, but are not as rigid about viewing only these as when they were younger. They all want to go to the motion pictures.

**Ten Years.** Sex differences in play are pronounced among ten-year-olds. Boys and girls are developing the skills which each sex needs in our society. At school the boy works with speed and likes the challenge of mental arithmetic.

The ten-year-old is so conscious of

...eeding the support of his peers that ...e often esteems the opinions and attitudes of his gang or club more than those of his family. He is interested in ideas of social welfare and social justice. He is loyal to his group and does not divulge group secrets. He may indulge in hero worship.

On the radio and television the likes of the ten-year-old are much the same as those of the nine-year-old. Boys spurn romance and love stories. The two sexes are well separated.

Girls enjoy dramatizing life situations, and the subjects they choose are likely to deal with engagements and weddings. They still play with dolls, however, taking the role of mother and "bringing up their children." They are becoming much more interested in their appearance.

**Eleven Years.** The eleven-year-old is filled with energy and activity. He ex-

periments with various projects and is intensely interested in the activities of his group. His interest in school may diminish, particularly if he is not a good student. Play is no longer paramount in his life; companionship has become more important than play.

Although these children may seem bungling in motor skill at home, they have acquired new types of agility in play. Everything interests them. This is the gang age, and the gang enjoys meeting in its own hut or tree house. The child's interest in reading and motion pictures has increased; the characters he learns about appear to be alive, people he would like to know or perhaps punish in some way.

**Twelve Years.** The twelve-year-old is enthusiastic, so much so that he acts without consideration of consequences. Although he is very much a part of his group, he also likes to be alone. He

**Figure 228.** Twelve-year-olds enjoy earning their own money. This youth has assumed the complete responsibility for his paper route. (H. Armstrong Roberts.)

engages in sports with more team spirit and less wandering of attention to some other factor in the environment which is of personal interest to him. He has not the same need for individual praise that he had a year before. His broader interests are seen in his wanting a pen-pal from a foreign land.

Twelve-year-olds are becoming interested in earning money not for running errands or little jobs for their parents, but in some form of organized project, especially a twosome project, in which they are heavily motivated to succeed. They may be interested in publishing a news bulletin, and many boys have paper routes. Boys and girls still tend to stay apart.

## CARE

### Physical Care

**Bathing, Dressing and Toileting.** Children between six and twelve years of age are fairly self-sufficient in bathing, dressing and toileting, but they need some help with the niceties of manicuring, neatness and even cleanliness. There are, of course, individual differences. Some children resent having their ears kept clean, and others do not like to have their hair combed and brushed. Sex differences are apparent. Girls are generally more careful of their appearance than boys are.

The six-year-old needs help, though he does not readily accept it. He dawdles and needs management. In undressing he drops his clothes on the floor or flings them aside. The seven-year-old still dawdles, but tends to complete his tasks. The eight-year-old is more efficient in caring for himself. From nine years to the end of the school age children show increased responsibility in selection of clothes, adapted to the occasion and the weather, hanging them up and disposing of soiled garments. They can take care of toileting and bathing, but may still need reminders to brush their teeth or wash their hands thoroughly, and girls need help with long hair.

### Sleep

The sleep of the school child is rarely quiescent. Fears in the form of night terrors or nightmares prevent his sleeping peacefully. The bedtime hour should be a quiet time when the parent and the child feel greater interdependency. It is a good time for confidences, questions and answers, and discussions. Routine prayers may be said.

The older child may become self assertive about the time when he wishes to go to bed. Parents must judge the amount of sleep the child needs and see that he is in bed in time for sufficient sleep. The amount needed decreases with age. The six-year-old may need eleven to twelve hours of sleep, while the twelve-year-old generally needs only ten hours.

### Safety Measures

With the broadening scope of activity among children during the elementary school years, parents cannot hope to be with them constantly in order to prevent accidents. If parents and nursery school and kindergarten teachers have emphasized safety measures, a child should be ready to build on the foundation of past experience and develop further his ability to meet the accident hazards common to school children.

Between the ages of six and twelve years the most common cause of accidental injury and death is *motor accidents*. Children may cross a street against the light or from between parked cars, or be injured while riding bicycles in traffic. Little children sit in the mother's lap or in their special chair while she drives, toddlers stand beside her on the seat, and school children like the rear section of an automobile or a station wagon and sit facing the back window. If the car is hit children are in greater danger than adults. Children resent the use of the safety belt which some manufacturers of cars introduced as a safety measure.

The second most frequent cause of accidental death is *drowning*. Children should be taught to swim as early as possible.

Figure 229.  Motor accidents cause the death of many children each year. This 11-year-old boy is a member of the Safety Patrol in his school. He takes his responsibility of protecting other children very seriously. (H. Armstrong Roberts.)

Accidents also occur when children are skating, riding the school bus, or playing with other children or with animals.

## HEALTH OF THE SCHOOL CHILD

Responsibility for the child's health rests with the parents. The health of the school child is influenced by the health supervision the child receives from the family physician and the dentist, by the health instruction given by his parents and teachers, by the environment of his home and school, by the community public health program and by the direct services he receives in school.

### Preschool Health Examination

Every child should have a preschool health examination. His height, weight, posture, hearing and vision should be checked carefully in this examination. Beginning problems of school children may be due to faulty hearing and vision. A dental examination and correction of defects are essential. If the child is to gain the optimum benefit from school, he needs to be physically well.

Immunization and booster doses should be given as necessary against diphtheria, pertussis, tetanus, poliomyelitis and smallpox. Such immunization is essential just before school if the child was not immunized when an infant and did not receive booster doses against diphtheria, pertussis and tetanus when he was four years old and revaccination against smallpox when he was five. Immunization against pertussis is not given after the latter part of the preschool period because the danger of the disease is greatly reduced as the child grows older.

**A**

AMERICAN ACADEMY OF PEDIATRICS, INC.
©1959

STANDARD HEALTH EXAMINATION RECORD
THIS PART TO BE FILLED IN BY PARENT BEFORE PRESENTATION TO PHYSICIAN.

ORGANIZATION OR SCHOOL

NAME _____ PARENT OR GUARDIAN _____ PHONE _____
LAST      FIRST

ADDRESS _____ BIRTH DATE _____ AGE _____ SEX _____

RELIGION

| PAST ILLNESSES. (CHECK – GIVING APPROX DATES | | DISEASES DATE | SUGGESTIONS FROM PARENTS. |
|---|---|---|---|
| FREQUENT COLDS | STOMACH UPSETS | CHICKEN POX | |
| FREQUENT SORE THROATS. | KIDNEY TROUBLE | MEASLES | |
| SINUSITIS | HEART TROUBLE | MUMPS | |
| ABSCESSED EARS | RHEUM FEVER | SCARLET FEVER | |
| BRONCHITIS | CONVULSIONS | POLIOMYELITIS | |
| ASTHMA | TUBERCULOSIS | WHOOPING COUGH | |
| ALLERGIES | DIABETES | | |
| OPERATIONS OR SERIOUS INJURIES | | | |
| SERIOUS IVY POISONING | | | |

OTHER DISEASES OR DETAILS OF ABOVE

COMMENTS FOR CAMP

BEHAVIOR _____ SLEEP WALKING _____ BED WETTING _____ NIGHT TERRORS _____
FAINTING _____ MENSTRUATION _____ CONSTIPATION _____ OTHER _____
ANY CONTRA-INDICATION TO SWIMMING? _____ TO DIVING? _____
ANY SPECIFIC ACTIVITIES TO BE ENCOURAGED? _____ ANY RESTRICTED? _____
IS STUDENT UNDER ANY SPECIAL MEDICAL OR DIETARY REGIMEN TO BE CONTINUED? _____

**B**

| IMMUNIZATIONS | | | PHYSICAL EXAMINATION (BY LICENSED M D) |
|---|---|---|---|
| IMMUNIZATIONS | DATE PRIMARY SERIES COMPLETED | DATE OF LAST BOOSTER | DATE OF EXAMINATION |
| WHOOPING COUGH | | | HEIGHT _____ WEIGHT _____ |
| DIPHTHERIA | | | MUSCULOSKELETAL |
| TETANUS | | | |
| POLIOMYELITIS | | | SKIN |
| SMALLPOX | | | SCABIES |
| OTHER | | | ATHLETES FOOT |
| | | | IMPETIGO |
| | | | OTHER |
| TUBERCULIN TEST _____ DATE _____ RESULT | | | |

EYES _____ VISION: R 20/ _____ 20/ _____
EARS _____ HEARING _____

PHYSICIANS COMMENTS AND RECOMMENDATIONS

THIS PERSON IS IN SATISFACTORY CONDITION AND MAY ENGAGE IN ALL USUAL ACTIVITIES EXCEPT AS NOTED

NOSE
THROAT
TEETH
HEART
LUNGS
ABDOMEN
  GENITALIA
  HERNIA

_____ M.D

ADDRESS _____

URINALYSIS _____

Figure 230. This Standard Health Examination Record has been approved by the American Academy of Pediatrics for use with children of school age. (Courtesy of American Academy of Pediatrics.)

The preschool examination should be done in the spring before the child enters school in the fall, so that treatment for any defects or problems can be given before school opens.

Parents should see that the child receives a thorough physical examination every year. If he is not well, he should be taken to a physician. Dental examinations should be made twice a year or as often as the dentist recommends.

### School Health Program

The school health program is an important part of the national health program. The main purpose of the school health program is to maintain, improve and promote the health of every school child. Adequate supervision of the physical, mental, emotional and social aspects of school life should be included in the program. The program also includes planning the course content in health education and nutrition, and putting it into effect through instruction and the routine life of the children during school hours. Accident prevention, recreation and physical education should be included.

The school nurse and other personnel in the program should see to it that routine health appraisals are done on all children, with follow-up on children who need care to see that they receive it. Parent education and parent counseling are also necessary. Teamwork by parents, teachers, nurses, and private and school physicians is essential. Local physicians should understand the school health program and wherein it supplements their service to children. Other personnel who may cooperate include the child's personal dentist and school dentist, the principal of the school, the school counselor, the school custodian and engineer, school psychologist, social worker, physical education teacher and special education staff. Preventive services should be used to control tooth decay, accidents, emotional disorders, poor nutrition, infectious diseases, unhygienic environment and insufficient care after an illness.

### Health Problems during School Age

Among the most important health problems of the school child is greater exposure to communicable diseases. Diseases against which he is immunized or which he had in the preschool period present no problem. The mother should be informed of the school regulations about keeping the child home from school when he has a fever, cold, rash or other symptoms of communicable disease, to prevent exposing other children.

Another function of the school is to meet the needs of the handicapped child on entrance to school. His condition poses a special problem for the school personnel. They should be kept informed of the total rehabilitation program being carried out and their specific part in it.

A third problem is presented by the older children, who should be told something about the physical changes they will experience at puberty. Both sexes should be informed of this. Although parents should talk over these matters with their children in order to maintain good parent-child relations, the school nurse or a teacher may also discuss them individually or in class. Stressing the universality of the experience gives it a less personal and a more objective nature. Parents should know what the children are taught in school. Pictorial presentation should be supplemented with discussion. The material should be selected according to the interests, chronologic age and level of understanding of the children. It should be factual and presented unemotionally. The child who is unprepared for the physical changes which accompany puberty may be terrified when they occur.

### NUTRITION

During the school age caloric requirements per unit of body weight continue to decrease, but the nutritional requirements remain relatively greater than in a mature person. A good basic diet is important.

Table 9 gives the nutritional requirements for children of school age.

School children usually eat well and have fewer food fads than preschool children. Eating problems relate more to the time of eating—e.g. whether it interferes with television programs or group activities—and the manner of eating than to the content and amount of food consumed. Since a school child

Figure 231. The sense of industry is further developed as the child learns to assume responsibilities at home. (H. Armstrong Roberts.)

Table 9. Recommended Daily Dietary Allowances for Children of School Age

|  | 7-9 Years | 10-12 Years |
|---|---|---|
| Calories | 2100 | 2500 |
| Protein | 60 gm. | 70 gm. |
| Calcium | 1.0 gm. | 1.2 gm. |
| Iron | 10 mg. | 12 mg. |
| Vitamin A | 3500 I.U. | 4500 I.U. |
| Thiamine | 1.1 mg. | 1.3 mg. |
| Riboflavin | 1.5 mg. | 1.8 mg. |
| Niacin equivalents | 14 mg. | 17 mg. |
| Ascorbic acid | 60 mg. | 75 mg. |
| Vitamin D | 400 I.U. | 400 I.U. |

From the Food and Nutrition Board, National Research Council: Recommended Daily Dietary Allowances (1958).

may be hungry after school, nourishment is necessary. Milk and fruit should be given in preference to candy and cookies.

Because the child wants to be like his peers, the kind of lunch he wants will depend on whether his friends take a lunch box to school or eat in the cafeteria. If the noon meal is not adequate, the breakfast and dinner should make up for the deficiency.

School children can be helpful to their mothers at mealtime. They can help plan menus, set the table, shop for food and wash dishes. Although these activities develop a sense of industry and responsibility, parents should not ask too much of young children, who spend many hours in school and require outdoor play to keep them well.

**Eating Habits.** Mealtime should be a pleasant, restful period in the day, but many parents do not keep it so because of overemphasis on manners. The child's eating habits will gradually improve as he grows older.

The six-year-old stuffs his mouth, spills food and grabs for it and may be very talkative while eating. He is more interested in eating at the beginning than at the end of the meal. His appetite is good. He may refuse to use a napkin.

The seven-year-old talks less during

the meal. He may bolt his food, but he is quieting down. His napkin may not remain in place.

Eight- and nine-year-olds eat more neatly, using napkins as their elders do. They are apt to have better table manners in public than at home.

The ten- to twelve-year-olds eat an adult meal and have table manners similar to those of their parents, whether at home, in the school cafeteria or elsewhere.

Children's eating habits would improve more rapidly if less stress were laid on table manners. A friendly atmosphere and enjoyment of the meal are the best aids to appetite.

## EFFECTS OF SEPARATION

If the child has experienced good parent-child relations, he will probably suffer little trauma due to separation from his parents for short periods. The school child has learned to relate to adults and children outside his family and so is not emotionally disturbed when he is left with strange people. He knows the meaning of time gradations and is better able to tolerate separation from his parents. He knows when they will return. Prolonged separation, however, for weeks or months, as during hospitalization, is likely to produce emotional trauma. If his parents do not visit him frequently, particularly if he knows that they are able to come, he feels a sense of rejection which interacts with the physical strain of his illness or injury. The reasons for prolonged separation should be explained to the child in a factual, realistic way by a sympathetic adult, preferably one of his parents. Other evidences of parental love besides visiting should be shown the child.

**Figure 232.** The older school age child can eat an adult meal and has table manners similar to those of his parents. (H. Armstrong Roberts.)

## TEACHING AIDS AND
## OTHER INFORMATION*

*Bureau of Publications, Teachers College, Columbia University*

Gans, R.: Reading Is Fun.
Hymes, J. L.: Discipline.
Theman, V.: A Good School Day.

*Child Study Association of America*

Redl, F.: Pre-adolescents—What Makes Them Tick?

*Equitable Life Assurance Society*

Looking Forward to School, 1956.

*Hart Publishing Company, Inc.*

Jollison, M.: Play Ideas for Girls, 1957.
Lewis, R.: Play Ideas for Boys, 1957.
Thompson, J. E.: Best Riddles, 1957.

*John Hancock Mutual Life Insurance Company*

From Six to Twelve, 1957.

*National Education Association*

Gudridge, B. M.: Happy Journey, Preparing Your Child for School, 1953.

*Personal Products Corporation*

Educational materials on menstrual hygiene.

*Public Affairs Pamphlets*

Baruch, D. W.: How to Discipline Your Children.
Dietrich, H. F., and Gruenberg, S. M.: Your Child's Safety.
Frank, J.: Comics, Television, Radio, Movies—What Do They Offer Children?
Lambert, C.: Understand Your Child—From 6 to 12.
Larrick, N.: Your Child and His Reading.
Neisser, E. G.: Your Child's Sense of Responsibility.
Osborne, E.: How To Teach Your Child about Work.
Ross, H.: The Shy Child.
Yahraes, H.: Your Teeth—How to Save Them.

*Science Research Associates*

Goodykoontz, B.: Helping Children Get Along in School.
Grant, E. H.: Parents and Teachers as Partners.
Landis, P. H.: Helping Children Adjust Socially.
Strang, R.: Helping Children Solve Problems.
Thurstone, T. G., and Bryne, K. M.: Mental Abilities of Children.
Witty, P.: Helping the Gifted Child.
Witty, P., and Bricker, H.: Your Child and Radio, TV, Comics and Movies.

*U.S. Department of Health, Education, and Welfare*

Accidents and Children, 1959.
A Healthy Personality for Your Child, 1952.

*Complete addresses are given in the Appendix.

Day Care Services, 1960.
Food for Families with School Children, 1954.
Foods Your Children Need, 1958.
Screening School Children for Visual Defects, 1954.
Your Child from Six to Twelve, 1949.
Your Gifted Child, 1958.

## REFERENCES

American Academy of Pediatrics, Committee on School Health: School Health Policies. Pediatrics, 24:672, 1959.
Bossard, J. H. S., and Boll, E. S.: The Sociology of Child Development. 3rd ed. New York, Harper and Brothers, 1960.
Brauer, J. C. and others: Dentistry for Children. 4th ed. New York, McGraw-Hill Book Company, Inc., 1958.
Breckenridge, M. E., and Vincent, E. L.: Child Development. 4th ed. Philadelphia, W. B. Saunders Company, 1960.
Cooper, L. F., Barber, E. M., Mitchell, H. S., and Rynbergen, H. J.: Nutrition in Health and Disease. 13th ed. Philadelphia, J. B. Lippincott Company, 1958.
Cromwell, G. E.: School Nursing Is Pediatric Nursing. Nursing Outlook, 5:73, 1957.
Cunningham, F., and O'Neil, J. E.: Eye Safety in Schools. Nursing Outlook, 5:522, 1957.
Etienne, B.: Health Education in the School. Am. J. Pub. Health, 50:64, 1960.
Erikson, E. H.: Childhood and Society. New York, W. W. Norton and Co., 1950.
Gesell, A., and Ilg, F. L.: The Child from Five to Ten. New York, Harper and Brothers, 1946.
Grout, R. E.: Health Teaching in Schools. 3rd ed. Philadelphia, W. B. Saunders Company, 1958.
Harlan, H. R.: Nursing in Dental Health Programs. Nursing Outlook, 5:80, 1957.
Hurlock, E. B.: Child Development. 3rd ed. New York, McGraw-Hill Book Company, Inc., 1956.
Josselyn, I. M.: The Happy Child. New York, Random House, 1955.
Kangery, R. H.: Children's Answers. Am. J. Nursing, 60:1748, 1960.
Krause, M. V.: Food, Nutrition and Diet Therapy. 2nd ed. Philadelphia, W. B. Saunders Company, 1957.
Larrick, N.: A Parent's Guide to Children's Reading. Garden City, New York, Doubleday and Company, Inc., 1958.
Lerrigo, M. O., and Southard, H.: A Story About You. New York, E. P. Dutton and Co., Inc. 1956.
McAleer, H.: Promoting the School Health Program. Am. J. Nursing, 59:370, 1959.
Nelson, W. E. (editor): Textbook of Pediatrics. 7th ed. Philadelphia, W. B. Saunders Company, 1959.
Obert, J. C.: When The Bell Rings at Noon. Am. J. Nursing, 61:89, Feb., 1961.

# Chapter 22

# Conditions of the School Child

# Requiring Immediate or Short-Term Care

## HOSPITALIZATION OF THE SCHOOL CHILD

CHILDREN of school age should have much the same kind of preparation for hospitalization as that given the preschool child (see p. 533). Because of his greater verbal ability the school child usually understands more readily the explanation given him. School children can read booklets prepared by the hospital personnel for children who are to enter the hospital. The parents will adapt this material to the needs of the individual child. He should be told the truth about the experience which is before him. Careful preparation should especially be given if a friend of the child has recently died at the hospital as a result of illness or an accident.

The school child is usually able to accept his illness and separation from his parents better than does the preschool child. The parents should visit him as often as possible, send cards

and telephone him so that he knows that they are thinking of him. He also needs nurses who understand his level of growth and development, his needs and the experiences he should have for continued personality growth while in the hospital. The nurse, like his teacher, should be warm, friendly and fair, yet able to set reasonable limits to his behavior. She should try to understand each child as an individual. He is having many unavoidable frustrations due to his sickness or injury, and the entire health team should try to provide satisfactions which make his situation more endurable.

The convalescent child in many hospitals is taught by a visiting teacher, either at his bedside or in a group of children in a classroom made to accommodate wheelchairs and even beds on rollers. The classroom should have the usual equipment, including blackboard and movable tables and chairs. The child feels that he is still part of his group in the school which he attended and will be able to continue with them when he is discharged from the hospital. The hours spent in study are short, and no child is under pressure to learn. His program is suited to his condition. Attendance at the hospital school helps him to relax and thus promotes his recovery. The school teacher will provide lessons related to activities outside the hospital, since she gives him the textbooks used in his grade at school. This keeps him in touch with his friends and gives him a sense of living a normal life with them even while hospitalized. The nurse may also help the child acquire or improve such skills as reading by encouraging him in his efforts.

A few children may resist going to school in the hospital, and no child is compelled to study. The nurse should try to discover why a child who resists has no interest in school. She and his teacher should try to help him understand the interrelation of academic learning with the activities he enjoys. The nurse and the school teacher should keep each other informed of the progress each child is making.

Children have preconceived notions of what the school teacher or the nurse will be like. If the child perceives qualities of his parents in his nurse, he may react to her as he does to them. For this reason a child may not react to his nurse in terms of how she reacts to him, but rather as he is accustomed to react to his mother. Such behavior on his part gives a clue to his past experience and to his needs for guidance. When the nurse understands the child's background, she is able to accept his behavior and show her approval of improvement even if he has much to learn.

A child's self-image is influenced by

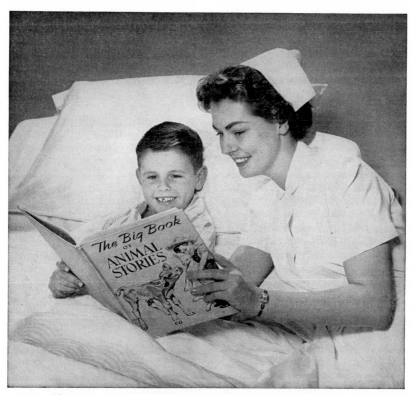

**Figure 233.** The nurse encourages this early school-age child to improve his reading skill while he is hospitalized. Her enthusiasm about his reading encourages him to take increased interest in his school work. (H. Armstrong Roberts.)

the evaluation of his behavior by significant persons in his environment. Hence it is important that evaluation of his behavior be based on his advance toward normal behavior for a child of his age. The nurse's evaluation of his behavior must be relative to what can reasonably be expected of the individual sick child. She recognizes his abilities in self-direction such as caring for himself and doing his school work. She should provide him with opportunities to use initiative and his intellectual capacities—creative ability and judgment—in the hospital situation. This is necessary in addition to the stimulus given by his teacher in the hospital school.

Hospitalized school children miss not only school, but also many opportunities for learning which other children have. They should be given what opportunities are available in the hospital setting. They may be shown the kitchen, porches and laboratories. They can also learn facts about their own bodies and something about preventing disease. Convalescent children may be taken on picnics and sightseeing trips. Those who cannot leave the hospital may have motion pictures and exhibitions brought to them. School children become bored and withdrawn if they are not given an opportunity to learn.

Hospitalized children become anxious about their condition and the experiences they have had, as well as those they expect to undergo. Since they have sufficient verbal ability to master their anxiety by talking with some understanding adult, they should have an opportunity to talk out their problems. The nurse can then help the child to understand what really happened after he has told her what he thinks happened. She can thus prevent him from repressing or suppressing the events and feelings that went with them.

School children have learned the terminology of their group, especially in connection with urination, defecation and the organs of reproduction— terms which may be repulsive to the nurse. She should understand that the child learned his attitudes and ex-

pressions in his home and from his friends. To make him feel ashamed of the only terms which sound familiar and natural to him would cause a younger child to feel that he was among strangers who did not love him. He might be afraid to tell the nurse when he again needed to relieve himself. In school he asks to be excused, but that request does not fit the hospital situation. The older child feels that the nurse rejects him because he comes from a low socio-economic class. His sense of worth, his self-image, is hurt, and he is likely to become withdrawn and earnestly want to be among people like his family and the neighbors.

If the nurse shows no repugnance and quietly says the terms which the child should use when referring to elimination or his genitals, he is likely to accept her terminology as part of hospital life. The nurse may add, "We want to understand you so that we can help you. You can remember, can't you?" When he uses the correct terms, she can show her approval by smiling.

School children who have become fairly independent in caring for themselves become embarrassed when they are ill because they are physically cared for by the nurse. This is especially true of boys ten years old or older. The nurse should help the child to accept the situation and cooperate rather than feel that he is forced to submit because it is the custom in the hospital. The child associates such care with being a baby and feels threatened by his loss of power. It is a good plan to speak casually of the care adult patients receive, asking a little girl whether she would like to be a nurse when she grows up or telling a boy of nursing in the service. The child should be encouraged to regain his independence as soon as he is physically able to do so. Normally he is anxious to do all that he can for himself.

If the child feels too threatened by his illness, he may manifest his anxiety by being aggressive, demanding and uncooperative about following the physician's orders for inactivity and rest. The nurse should listen to the child and find out the basis of his fear. She should help him to understand his illness and why he must stay quiet. She can permit him to help plan his daily schedule, thereby building up his self-confidence. The nurse should visit him frequently. If the physician permits, another child's bed can be brought close enough to his for them to play together. The child may also enjoy making his own rules for keeping himself quiet. If he continues to be aggressive, his behavior should be brought to the attention of the physician, who may recommend further psychologic help or treatment.

When school children have many frustrations during the day and are forced to keep strict self-control, they often release their aggression and tension during the evening hours. If rigid control has been placed on their activities during the day, either because their condition requires that they be kept very quiet or because the nurse in charge has too strict a concept of hospital order and discipline, their need to release their feelings finds vent when they see the evening nurse alone in the unit. She may be faced with pillow fights, arguments, toys thrown on the floor or paper wads hurled from bed to bed.

The best way to handle this situation is by prevention. The children should have opportunity during the day to use their aggression in constructive activities. They can have self-directive physical activity under supervision in the playroom or on the sunporch. This may be free play or recreational therapy under trained leadership. Bed patients also must be helped in the same way. Volunteer Play Ladies are valuable in working with these children.

Nurses in the hospital and in the community should learn ways to help convalescent children to be constructively happy. Nurses are too apt to create some toy for the child, rather than letting him create his own toy or a gift for mother. They are also apt to show a child how to use a toy, put together a puzzle or manipulate a mechanical outfit, rather than letting him

have the pleasure of exploring by himself the possibilities of these interesting objects.

Hospitalized children enjoy continuing the collections they started at home (see p. 605), and starting new collections better adapted to items found in the hospital. They may collect empty antibiotic bottles, paper cups or greeting cards. They may enjoy reading, playing table games, listening to the radio and watching television. The nurse must supervise these activities so that they will not be too exciting for the children.

Some children in the hospital are unusually aggressive. They may attack others, and be cruel, domineering and unable to make friends with other children or with adults. Such children are extremely unhappy. They have not achieved the emotional maturity or received the guidance they needed to help them become more sociable. They need individual psychotherapy given by a physician, psychologist or psychiatrist.

Other children may be too quiet, shy and withdrawn. They are emotionally lonely, afraid, preoccupied and repressed. They also need professional help if they are to develop normally.

School children who enjoy assuming responsibility and caring for younger children may help in the hospital unit during convalescence. This will help them gain confidence and recognition and acquire skills. They may cooperate in cleaning up the playroom and the schoolroom in the afternoon. They may help to put away supplies, pass nourishment and stamp stationery. Often they can help feed younger children, read to them or play with them. This enables the older children to identify with adults in the unit and gives them a feeling of self-confidence.

## ACUTE CONDITIONS

### Epistaxis (Nasal Hemorrhage, Nosebleed)

**Incidence, Etiology, Clinical Manifestations, Treatment and Nursing Care.** Epistaxis is common throughout childhood, especially during the school age, but the incidence decreases after puberty. It is caused by external trauma, foreign bodies, forcible blowing of the nose or picking the nose. Rhinitis may also lead to nosebleed. The strain of physical exercise or emotional excitement may be enough to start nasal bleeding if the child has a local lesion. If there is a circulatory, renal or emotional condition which produces an elevation of blood pressure, nasal hemorrhage may result. It may also occur when a blood dyscrasia or an infection is present. As girls reach puberty, epistaxis may occur as vicarious menstruation.

The onset is sudden. Blood may flow from both nostrils. Bleeding is usually minimal and stops spontaneously, but it may be fatal if the child has a hemorrhagic disease.

The child should be kept in a semierect position. His clothing should be loosened around the neck. He should not blow his nose. An ice bag over the bridge of the nose is helpful, and pressure may be made on the bleeding point if it is just inside the nasal vestibule, by pinching the nose. A solution of epinephrine may be applied to the nasal mucous membrane with a cotton applicator (epinephrine is a vasoconstrictor). The physician may cauterize the point of bleeding with silver nitrate. In more severe cases packing the nares with thromboplastin or Gelfoam may be necessary. In hemorrhagic disease blood transfusion may be required if much blood is lost.

### Respiratory Infections and Communicable Diseases

**Incidence and Care.** If the child has not had the common communicable diseases in the preschool period, he is likely to get them when he goes to school because of close contact with many children. For the same reason the child is prone to respiratory infections. This is especially true if he comes from a small family in which he is overprotected or has been brought up in a rural area where infections are less common. The greatest *incidence* of infections is in the first grade.

Health teaching should begin in the early grades. The child should be taught to cover his mouth with his handkerchief when coughing and to turn his face toward the floor. This is particularly necessary at the table, where coughing would spread droplets on food. He should not contaminate his hands and then contaminate toys, books, door knobs and other objects which others touch.

Children should be dressed according to the temperature and protected from rain and snow with slickers, hoods and boots. They should be taught to come home to change their clothing if they get wet. (If the mother scolds them for getting wet, they will not come home at once, but will wait, hoping to dry off before she sees them.) Teachers should make provision for children caught in the rain on the way to school.

Every teacher should tell her class to report symptoms of a cold, sore throat or other illness. The children should be taught by precept and by practice to wash their hands when contaminated and always before eating. It is essential, but difficult, to teach them not to offer each other bits of candy, apples, laps of ice cream cones and sucks of pop from the bottle or common straw, because they think it friendly and generous to share what they have with another child.

Children should be kept away from others who have respiratory infections. The child with an infection should not be sent to school. If he comes and the teacher finds that he is sick, she or the school nurse may send him home, provided there is someone there to care for him, or should telephone for his mother to come for him. If there is no adult at home to receive him, the child may be kept in the infirmary. If the school has no infirmary, and his condition permits, he should be placed in the rear of the classroom away from other children. If someone comes for the child, she should be told how to care for him. Such instruction includes home isolation technique and how to make paper bags to receive the child's paper handkerchiefs. Immunization techniques should be recommended if necessary. If the child is so sick that he will need considerable nursing care, the mother should be helped to schedule her time so that she gets enough rest.

## Ringworm (Tinea)

Ringworm or tinea is a superficial fungus infection of the skin. Ringworm is classified according to the area of the body affected or the shape of the lesion produced. Since several fungi may cause ringworm, laboratory examination is often necessary before adequate treatment can be carried out. All types of ringworm are contagious.

## Ringworm of the Scalp (Tinea Capitis)

**Incidence and Etiology.** This condition is practically limited to children and is common among neglected children. It is a serious problem in schools of disorganized, low-income urban areas.

The most common etiologic agent is *Microsporum lanosum*. It is transmitted to the child from cats and dogs and is not infectious through contact of an infected child with other children. *Microsporum audouini* infections are transmitted by human beings and are highly infectious. These conditions tend to disappear spontaneously at puberty.

Infection may begin at the base of a single hair, but it spreads in a circular fashion, forming lesions up to 2 inches in diameter. The spores of the fungus invading the hair at the base cause the hair to break off close to the skin, leaving a bald area. The scalp of this area becomes red, and grayish scales appear. A secondary infection may occur. The child may complain of mild itching.

**Diagnosis, Treatment and Prognosis.** The *diagnosis* of fungus infection is proved by examination of the scalp under a beam of ultraviolet light passed through a Wood's filter. Microscopic examination of extracted hairs may also be made.

The response to *treatment* is slow. The hair should be shaved from the infected areas and the lesions washed thoroughly each day with soap and water. Local applications such as tincture of iodine, sulfur ointment, 10 per cent ammoniated mercury or other fungicide should be made to the areas. Recovery is hastened if the hair of the area is not shaved, but completely removed by forceps or x-ray irradiation. (Permanent baldness may result if irradiation is not used with caution.) The head should be covered with cloth or a stockinet skull cap. This is washed and boiled each day to prevent spread of the infection.

The *prognosis* is good, but even with treatment the condition may exceed three months in duration.

## Ringworm of the Skin (Tinea Circinata or Tinea Cruris)

There are two types of ringworm of the skin—tinea circinata and tinea cruris.

The lesions of *tinea circinata* are on the neck, face, forearms and hands. The lesions begin as rounded or slightly irregular, reddish-pink, pea-sized, slightly raised scaly patches. The centers of the patches clear, and the periphery spreads. The outline takes on the form of a ring. Mild itching is present.

The lesions of *tinea cruris* occur on the inner and upper surface of the thighs, the scrotum and the buttocks. Lesions appear as in tinea circinata, but local warmth in the affected area causes inflammation, itching and infection, with small pustule formation.

**Treatment and Prognosis.** *Treatment* depends upon the degree of inflammation. For edematous, exudative lesions wet dressings of Burow's solution or potassium permanganate are used. For dry lesions antifungal agents such as Whitfield's ointment or sulfur ointment are used.

With treatment the *prognosis* is excellent.

**Figure 234.** Pediculosis capitis. *A,* Numerous nits are visible. *B,* Impetiginous lesions frequently develop secondary to scratching, especially in children. (Lewis: Practical Dermatology. 2nd ed.)

### Ringworm of the Feet (Tinea Pedis)

**Incidence.** This condition is common among school children during the summer months. The infection comes from other children and adults. It is acquired at swimming pools and other places where people go barefoot. The infection usually appears between the toes. There is no scale formation, but the superficial epithelium is macerated and desquamates. The raw surface is often covered with fissures. Itching is intense, and pain may follow if the child rubs or scratches the area.

**Treatment and Prevention.** Ointment such as Desenex or half-strength Whitfield's ointment should be applied. The feet may also be soaked in 1:4000 hot solution of potassium permanganate. Stockings and other foot coverings contaminated by the fungus should be sterilized or discarded. Light shoes which reduce sweating are less aggravating to the condition than are heavy footwear.

As a preventive measure children should wear shoes when walking where others are going barefoot and, if infected, are contaminating the area. In-fected persons should stay away from swimming pools and gymnasium dressing rooms and all such places where they may spread infection.

### Pediculosis

**Types, Etiology and Incidence.** There are three types of pediculosis in children: (1) pediculosis capitis, or infestation with the head louse, which is exceedingly common among neglected children; (2) pediculosis corporis, or infestation with the body louse; and (3) pediculosis pubis, or infestation with the crab louse. The second and third types of lice are uncommon. Since pediculosis capitis is the most common type in children, only this will be discussed here.

*Pediculus capitis,* or head louse, is present on the scalp, and the ova (eggs) or nits are attached to the hair. The ova are grayish, translucent, oval bodies which adhere to the shaft of a hair. They hatch in three or four days. The lice are usually seen on the heads of neglected, unclean children. They are easily transferred from child to child in schoolrooms and in homes of

Figure 235.    Scabies. *A*, Interdigital burrows and excoriations, with some secondary pyoderma. *B*, Excoriations over abdomen and lesions in the umbilicus. (Lewis: Practical Dermatology. 2nd ed.)

**Figure 236.** Neglected diffuse impetigo in the older child. (Pillsbury, Shelley and Kligman: Dermatology.)

tenement areas. They are more common among girls than among boys because of the girls' long hair.

**Clinical Manifestations, Treatment and Nursing Care.** There is severe itching of the scalp. Scratching leads to excoriation with serous, purulent or sanguineous exudation. Crusts form, and the hair is matted together.

The posterior cervical lymph nodes become infected from the scalp lesions. Excoriations may also be present on the face and neck.

*Treatment* and *nursing care* are effective. The aims of therapy are to kill the pediculi, devitalize nits and bring relief to the child. All inflamed areas must be healed. Clothing should be dry cleaned or laundered and ironed, and hats should be dusted with 5 per cent DDT in talcum powder. Various preparations containing DDT (chlorophenothane) powder, Kwell (benzene hexachloride) or other types of synthetic pesticides are used on the child's head. Treatment may be repeated as often as necessary on the physician's order. Nits may be removed by combing the hair with a fine tooth comb dipped in hot vinegar. If the hair is heavily infested, it may be advisable to cut it close to the scalp. If pustules are pres-

ent on the neck and face, bacitracin ointment may be used. Children should be cautioned not to exchange hats with other children.

### Scabies

**Etiology and Clinical Manifestations.** Scabies is caused by *Acarus scabiei,* or itch mite. The female acarus burrows under the skin to deposit her eggs. The itch mite is easily transmissible from person to person. The body is involved where the skin is moist and thin, between the fingers or toes, on the wrists, in the axillae and around the abdomen and genitals. The path where the mite burrows under the skin, about ½ inch in length, but superficial, may be seen easily. Secondary infections with papules, vesicles or pustules may occur. Itching is intense.

**Treatment and Nursing Care.** The objectives of care are to kill the parasite and to relieve the itching. Five per cent sulfur ointment may be used. Benzyl benzoate emulsion, 10 to 30 per cent, is effective. Treatment should include all infected persons in the household so that all mites are killed simultaneously. All contaminated clothing and bed linen must be dry cleaned or boiled.

For *impetigo contagiosa* and *furunculosis* see pages 190 and 191.

### Burns

**Incidence and Classification.** A burn is any destruction of tissue caused by heat, chemical agents, electricity, overexposure to ultraviolet or roentgen rays and radioactive substances. Burns are one of the most frequent accidental injuries of infants and children. Younger children are apt to be burned at home, while older children may be burned at home or school or during play away from home.

Classification of burns is made according to the degree (depth of tissue destroyed) and percentage of body surface involved. A *first-degree* burn, involving only the epidermis, is superficial. There is redness of the skin, without blistering, but with pain and swelling. A *second-degree* burn destroys superficial skin layers and damages deep tissues. The area is red and blistered and extremely painful. Some scarring may result. A *third-degree* burn produces destruction of the epidermis and some of the dermis. The burned area may appear charred. Sweat glands and hair follicles are destroyed.

Any child having a burn of 5 to 12 per cent or more of his body surface should be admitted to the hospital for treatment. Figure 237 shows the Rule of Nines. This is approximately correct for the older child or the adult, but body proportions in the infant or younger child are different. In infants and young children the head and neck should usually be counted as 18 per cent and each leg 14 per cent of total skin surface.

**Figure 237.** "Rule of Nines." Simplified chart of percentage of body surface according to Wallace. (From B. W. Haynes, Jr., in Ochsner and DeBakey: Christopher's Minor Surgery. 8th ed.)

**Problems Associated with Burns, Immediate Treatment and Later Treatment.** Fluid and electrolyte imbalance presents a serious problem. Shortly after a burn has occurred there is a decrease in the circulatory plasma volume. Electrolytes, water and protein leave vessels and go to the interstitial space around the burned area. The rest of the body is dehydrated. There is increased concentration of the red blood cells. Erythrocytes are destroyed by hemolysis and bleeding into the burned area. Large amounts of sodium enter the edema fluid of the burned area, where there is consequent replacement of intracellular potassium with sodium. The patient may be in negative sodium balance. Acidosis often develops. Infection is a problem and may delay reabsorption of edema fluid in the burned area.

*Immediate treatment* of a small, superficial area of burned skin consists in cleaning the area and applying sterile ointment such as white petrolatum (U.S.P.) or an ointment containing a local anesthetic. In second- and third-degree burns the first problem is to combat shock. The child should be placed on a sterile sheet and the burned area covered with sterile towels. Morphine, codeine or another pain-relieving drug is given. Plasma and other fluids are administered intravenously as needed to replace electrolytes. The child should be kept warm. Excessive heat, however, may cause dilatation of peripheral blood vessels and aggravate the circulatory disturbance. The hematocrit and hemoglobin levels should be determined as a guide to fluid therapy.

Typing and crossmatching of blood should be done to prepare for transfusion therapy. A urinalysis is also done. If there is to be débridement, adequate anesthesia is essential. Oxygen should be given to combat anoxia. A tracheotomy may be done as an emergency procedure if respiratory difficulty occurs. The foot of the bed is elevated in case of shock. Tetanus antitoxin is given if the patient has not had tetanus toxoid. A booster dose of tetanus toxoid may be given if the child had previous immunization. Gas gangrene antitoxin

**Figure 238.** Anesthesia for changing of dressings of a severely burned child. With removal of the bandages, the subject is placed on a sterile sheet. Afterwards cleansing or skin grafting and application of fresh dressings are done. (From Gross: The Surgery of Infancy and Childhood.)

may also be given. Antibiotics should be given to control infection. A retention catheter is inserted into the bladder so that an accurate output record is possible.

A high protein diet with vitamins, especially vitamin C, and iron for tissue repair is necessary. If the child has a poor appetite, gavage feeding may be necessary. An increased fluid intake aids in elimination of toxins and maintains the body fluid requirements.

There is a difference of opinion among physicians about local treatment, and the nurse naturally follows the orders of the individual physician. In the *open technique* of treatment there is no dressing. The burned area is open to the air, so that an eschar forms. The advantages of open treatment are that the child has less fever, there is less odor, and the patient may be ambulatory if the burned area is not extensive.

The *closed* or *pressure bandage method* is the second commonly used method of treatment. In this method the burned area is débrided and gross contamination is removed. Fine mesh

gauze is used to cover the entire area, which is then covered with several layers of coarse, dry mesh gauze. Absorbent cotton or mechanic's waste covers this. Pressure is then produced by tightly bandaging the entire dressing. This helps to control plasma loss into the tissues. These bandages should be removed in two or three weeks for grafting, or earlier if the temperature is elevated or there is a foul odor from the dressings indicating infection. Some surgeons apply a light plaster of paris cast instead of the pressure dressing.

If a civilian disaster occurred, the best method of treating burns would be to expose the area to the air, elevate and immobilize a burned limb, and give the patient prophylactic antibacterial drugs.

With severe burns, anemia may appear by the fifth day or earlier. Transfusions and iron therapy may be given.

The *later treatment* of a burned child includes skin grafting and other types of plastic surgery. Skin grafting is successful only if a clean, uninfected granulating base can be obtained. Skin is removed from another portion of the body or from a donor and placed on the burned area. Skin from a donor is used only to cover extensive burns until the patient is in sufficiently good physical condition to have a graft of his own skin. Eschar formed from open treatment must be softened with sterile wet saline dressings to prepare the wound for a skin graft. All infection must be cleared before grafting. Necrotic tissue can be soaked off in a tub or by applying wet dressings.

There are three types of skin grafts. To make a *pedicle graft,* a piece of skin is freed from its attachment on three sides, but left in position on one side. The free end is sutured over the burned area. Later, when the sutured portion is attached, the pedicle is freed at its base. *Patch grafts* are small skin grafts. *Split skin grafts* may also be used. Other types of reconstructive plastic surgery may be done after the area has healed and the child's condition has improved.

**Nursing Care.** The plan of nursing care depends on the location and extent of the burned area, on the needs of the child and on the kind of treatment ordered. The nurse should observe, report and record indications of shock (subnormal temperature, low blood pressure, rapid pulse rate, rapid, shallow respirations and extreme pallor) and evidence of toxicity. Toxicity commonly appears in one or two days and is accompanied by high fever, prostration, vomiting, cyanosis, rapid pulse rate and decreased urine output. Unless toxicity is combated, coma and death may result.

The child should be protected from infection and injury to delicate epithelium which grows to replace dead tissue. Sterile gown and mask technique should be used. Thorough hand washing is essential. All linen used for the child should be sterilized. Pain is relieved by medication ordered by the physician. A Stryker or Bradford frame may be used for a child with extensive burns.

An accurate intake and output record is essential. The urinary output should be 25 to 50 ml. per hour. The nurse should report to the physician if it falls below this minimum, since urinary output is a valuable guide to the regulation of parenteral fluid therapy.

Body alignment is important to prevent deformity through contractures. If the anterior surface of the neck is burned, a roll placed under the shoulders will prevent contracture. A footboard may be used to prevent foot drop. The child should be turned every two to four hours, and skin care should be given to prevent pressure areas. The child should be kept dry to prevent discomfort and contamination of the burned areas. Contracting scars and keloids must not be allowed to form during the healing stage.

Ingestion of fluids and nourishment may be a problem; the child should be encouraged to take sufficient food and fluids. Unless his arms and hands are burned, the child should be given toys and equipment for independent play. The nurse should make a sling out of a sheet under the Bradford frame and pin it to the crib sides to support the child's arms and toys. He should be read to, and the pictures in the book shown him. His bed should be placed so that he can see the other children playing. A record player, radio or television is enjoyed.

**Rehabilitation, Response of Parent and Child, Prognosis and Prevention.** The goal of *rehabilitation* in the treatment of a burned child is to help him develop and live to his maximum capacity within the limits of his disabilities.

The *response of the parent and the child* to his trauma varies in every case. The child may be fearful and anxious because of the fright caused by the accident, his extreme pain and his separation from his parents for a prolonged time. The child may also feel guilty if he was hurt while engaged in some activity which was forbidden by his parents or against which they had warned him. Parents may feel guilty because of lack of supervision of the child—supervision which would have prevented his injury. They may show excessive sympathy for or overprotection of the child.

Both the child and his parents need reassurance and understanding. The nurse should discover their fears and give them comfort. She should help them to accept the possibility of residual handicaps. If the child must return to the hospital for plastic surgery, he should have encouragement to face another painful period of hospitalization.

In general, the *prognosis* depends on the extent and depth of the burn. Death during the acute phase of the burn results from shock, alterations of blood volume and also from changes in the electrolyte composition of the blood. Death after the acute phase is the result of toxemia, local or intercurrent infection or debilitation.

The *prevention* of such painful, often fatal, accidents to children is a broad program of education of adults and children in prevention of fire hazards. Kitchens where young children are likely to be hurt should be made safe. Preschool and school children should be taught not to use matches, or to use them with safety, and to stay away from the stove or any open fire until they are sufficiently mature to take reasonable precautions. Adults should keep inflammable materials away from children and teach them how to put out their burning clothing should they become ignited.

### Osteomyelitis

**Incidence, Etiology and Pathogenesis.** The *incidence* of osteomyelitis is highest among children five to fourteen years of age and twice as frequent among boys as among girls. Acute osteomyelitis is due to deposition in the bone of bacteria from some primary source, usually on the skin, as furunculosis, impetigo or infected burns.

The causative organism commonly is hemolytic *Staphylococcus aureus*. Bacteria enter the blood stream and are carried to the metaphysis of a bone. Infection spreads laterally along the epiphysial plate, penetrates the cortex and locates under the periosteum, causing an abscess. The medulla of the bone may become infected. Dead bone forms a sequestrum which may be extruded or absorbed. The periosteum forms new bone and may completely cover the dead shaft with an involucrum.

**Clinical Manifestations and Diagnosis.** The first *clinical manifestation* is a furuncle or other infection of the skin. One or two weeks later malaise, septicemia, fever, chills and vomiting develop abruptly. The child suffers from a sharp localized pain in the affected bone. Signs of inflammation—swelling and redness—are present over the affected bone. The child may become very ill with fever and toxic symptoms.

The *diagnosis* is made on a leukocyte count of 15,000 to 25,000 or more cells. A blood culture is usually positive. If so, the causative organism is located. Roentgenograms may be made after changes in the bone have occurred, i.e. in eight to ten days after the onset of the symptoms.

**Treatment and Prognosis.** *Treatment* consists in giving antibiotics according to the organism found. Usually antibiotics effective against several strains of *Staphylococcus aureus* are used until the specific organism is proved. A splint is applied to the affected extremity to immobilize the limb and lessen the pain. Analgesics are given for pain. If an abscess forms, it is drained immediately.

The course and *prognosis* of osteomyelitis depend on early therapy and its continuance over an adequate time. If the condition is treated early and adequately with antibiotics, the prognosis is excellent. The mortality rate has decreased greatly since specific antibacterial agents have become available.

### Supracondylar Fracture of the Humerus

**Incidence, Etiology, Pathology and Clinical Manifestations.** Supracondylar fractures are common injuries of childhood and are most likely to occur when the school child is climbing or engaged in a competitive sport that requires physical skill. Supracondylar fracture of the humerus occurs just above the elbow and is due to direct trauma to the arm.

There is enormous swelling of the elbow which interferes with the circulation. The distal fragment is displaced posteriorly and presses on the brachial artery, thus interfering with the circulation to the forearm. The swelling and bleeding in the area also hamper the return of venous blood from the forearm. The combination of these two factors can produce serious ischemic paralysis.

**Diagnosis, Treatment and Nursing Care.** The *diagnosis* is made by roentgenogram. It is essential to reduce the fracture promptly and adequately and re-establish the circulation and drainage to and from the forearm. The surgeon may manipulate into place bones with only slight displacement. A splint is applied to hold the elbow in flexed position. The arm is placed in an overhead suspension apparatus to reduce edema. X-ray films should be taken to check the position of the fragments. The arm should be immobilized for three weeks, after which the child may wear a sling. Exercises are done at regular intervals.

If swelling was great at the time of injury, traction and suspension are used to reduce the fracture. The color of the skin and the quality of the radial pulse must be checked with both kinds of treatment.

Upon admission to the hospital the child is usually apprehensive, unhappy, and perhaps feeling guilty because the injury occurred while he was doing something he should not have done. Since there was no time for preparation for hospitalization, he needs a nurse who is a friend.

The nurse should check the radial pulse and the color of the skin of the injured arm frequently—usually every thirty minutes. The nurse should continue her observations for the first twenty-four to forty-eight hours after the injury. If the child complains of numbness or if the fingers are discolored or cold or if the radial pulse is weak, the physician should be notified immediately.

Upon admission the child should be placed on a firm mattress. Proper positioning is important and depends on the kind of treatment to be given. Ice bags may be ordered to aid in the control of swelling and to relieve pain. The bags should be well covered and only partially filled with small pieces of ice. They should be placed under, not over, the arm, since their weight should not rest on the injured area.

To prevent a feeling of dependency, the child should be encouraged to do as much as possible for himself. Various kinds of activity appropriate to his physical limitations should be provided.

## Appendicitis

**Incidence, Etiology, Pathology and Clinical Manifestations.** Appendicitis is rare during the first two years of life, but the *incidence* increases throughout the school years and adolescence.

Obstruction, especially with fecal concretions, is the principal factor in the majority of cases. Obstruction may also be caused by infection or allergy. Organisms found in the appendix include streptococci, *Staphylococcus aureus* and coliform bacilli. Pinworms may be an initial cause of inflammation.

The mucosa is inflamed and ulcerated. The lumen becomes distended, thereby impairing the blood supply. Bacteria may escape through the wall and cause diffuse peritonitis or an abscess confined by adjacent intestine and omentum.

The *clinical manifestations* may be variable. The onset may be abrupt or may follow gastroenteritis. The manifestations may include nausea, vomiting, abdominal pain, constipation or diarrhea, localized tenderness, and absence of peristalsis unless diarrhea is present. Abdominal pain in children may not be localized in the lower right quadrant. The child may not be able to report accurately the site of the pain.

Other manifestations are anorexia, mild leukocytosis (12,000 to 15,000 cells), fever of 99 to 102° F., flushed face, increased pulse and respiratory rates, restlessness, irritability and sleeplessness.

*A*             *B*             *C*

**Figure 239.** Meckel's diverticulum of the ileum. *A*, Ordinary blind sac. *B*, Diverticulum continued to umbilicus as a cord. *C*, Diverticulum with fistulous opening at umbilicus. (Arey: Developmental Anatomy. 6th **ed.**)

**Diagnosis, Treatment, Nursing Care, Complications and Prognosis.** The *diagnosis* of appendicitis in childhood is difficult, since a number of other conditions produce somewhat similar symptoms. If the child has a respiratory infection, abdominal pain may be due to incipient pneumonia or mesenteric adenitis. Inflammation of a Meckel's diverticulum or gastroenteritis may also cause symptoms suggestive of appendicitis. Irritation of the peritoneum may occur in rheumatic fever and resemble appendicitis. Repeated examinations may be necessary before a definite diagnosis is made.

Appendectomy—surgical removal of the appendix—should be done as soon as possible after the diagnosis has been made and the child is in condition for operation. Preoperative preparation is routine and consists in withholding of food, establishment of hydration, reduction of temperature below 102° F. (rectally) and administration of antibiotics to prevent or minimize the danger of peritonitis. Enemas may be ordered, but cathartics are not given.

Recovery after appendectomy is rapid, and the child usually returns to school in two weeks. If he had peritonitis or a peritoneal or appendiceal abscess, continuous gastric suction, chemotherapy and parenteral fluids may be ordered. Recovery, naturally, will be slower than in the uncomplicated case.

The *nursing care* of a child undergoing an appendectomy is usually simple and similar to that of adults.

*Complications* include a localized abscess and diffuse secondary peritonitis. The appendix may perforate, thereby causing complications, because the parents gave the child a cathartic (lay treatment for any abdominal pain in childhood) or because the child, interested in his play and not wanting a cathartic, did not tell his mother of his discomfort.

The operation is practically without risk if it is performed before perforation occurs. Even after perforation has occurred the risk is relatively slight.

### Meckel's Diverticulum

**Etiology, Pathology and Clinical Manifestations.** When the intestinal remnant of the omphalomesenteric duct from the terminal ileum to the umbilical cord persists and does not close, a Meckel's diverticulum is formed. It arises from the ileum, but usually does not have a connection with the umbilicus. A Meckel's diverticulum may be ½ to 3 inches in length and may be lined with intestinal mucous membrane. In some cases it may also contain gastric mucosa.

The diverticulum usually is not responsible for symptoms. When its gastric mucosa secretes gastric ferments, complications do arise. It may produce ulceration in the ileum or in the diverticulum which may lead to massive hemorrhage, to perforation and to peritonitis. The diverticulum may cause intestinal adhesions, strangulation or intussusception, and this may result in intestinal obstruction.

When hemorrhage occurs, the stools may be black at first, and then bright ed. With hemorrhage there will be pallor and an increased pulse rate. If transfusions are not given immediately, collapse and death may occur.

**Treatment and Nursing Care.** Transfusions are given for hemorrhage, and surgical excision of the diverticulum is necessary. Finding the diverticulum is the only way of confirming the diagnosis.

*Nursing care* after removal of a diverticulum is similar to that given after other abdominal surgery.

## Cryptorchidism (Undescended Testicle)

**Pathogenesis, Treatment and Prognosis.** Cryptorchidism is absence of one or both testicles from the scrotum. Early in fetal life the testicles develop in the abdomen below the kidneys. During the last two months of intrauterine life they descend into the scrotum. If they have not descended by birth, they may descend at any time until puberty. The missing testicle or testicles may be in the abdominal cavity or inguinal canal.

At puberty testes normally increase in size and develop increased androgenic and spermatogenic activity. Since an undescended testicle is kept at a higher degree of temperature within the abdomen than in the normal location—the scrotum—the sperm-forming cells degenerate. If both testicles are undescended, sterility results.

Normal secondary sex characteristics develop even though both testes are undescended. If the testicle is in the inguinal canal, it may be injured more easily that if it were in the scrotum. Emotional disturbances may occur, especially during the school age, when the testicles are not descended and the young boy finds that he is different from his peers.

Preservation of fertility is the most important factor to be considered in the *treatment.* There is lack of unanimity about the plan of treatment. Either medical or surgical treatment may be used. Some physicians believe that endocrine therapy should be tried during the preschool period. Such therapy is thought to be successful when no hernia is present (hernias are found in more than half of the cases). Gonadotropic hormone is used. If excessive amounts of this hormone are given, precocious puberty may result.

Surgical treatment is essential if medical treatment is not warranted or is unsuccessful. Many physicians believe that *orchidopexy* should be done in all cases of mechanical interference and prefer to operate on children below three years of age, because of the problem of preservation of fertility and also because of increased fears during the preschool period. Other surgeons prefer to delay operation until the school age.

When the child returns from the operating room, there will be a suture in the lower portion of the scrotum fastened to a rubber band which is

| A | B |

**Figure 240.** Cryptorchidism. *A,* Bilateral undescended testes in a 10-year-old boy. The scrotum is underdeveloped. *B,* Postoperative picture. The testes lie within the scrotum. (Gross: *The Surgery of Infancy and Childhood.*)

attached to the upper inside aspect of the thigh by a piece of adhesive. After about a week this attachment is removed. The nurse should not disturb this tension mechanism in caring for the child and must prevent contamination of the suture line. Antibiotics are given to prevent infection. An indwelling catheter may be left in place after operation to prevent soiling the suture line.

If one testicle is absent or if a testicle must be removed, plastic surgery can be carried out so that the boy will resemble normal boys; thereby no psychologic problem will be induced.

The *prognosis* is good if the testicle is successfully placed in the scrotum and if no changes have occurred in the testicle before treatment.

## REFERENCES

Baker, T. J.: Open Technique in the Management of Burns. Am. J. Nursing, *59*:1262, 1959.

Barnett, C.: This, to ME, Is Nursing. Nursing Outlook, *8*:72, 1960.

Blocker, T. G. and others: The Care of Patients with Burns. Nursing Outlook, 6:382, 1958.

Caldwell, J. A., and Seymour, P.: Supracondylar Fracture of the Humerus in Children. Am. J. Nursing, 57:1177, 1957.

Clatworthy, H. W., and Stewart, M. M.: Intravenous Therapy for Infants and Children. Am. J. Nursing, 57:630, 1957.

Dimock, H. G.: The Child in Hospital. Philadelphia, F. A. Davis Company, 1960.

Ferguson, L. K., and Sholtis, L. A.: Eliason's Surgical Nursing. 11th ed. Philadelphia, J. B. Lippincott Company, 1959.

Foley, A. J.: More than Skin Deep. Am. J. Nursing, *60*:1266, 1960.

Gross, R. E.: The Surgery of Infancy and Childhood. Philadelphia, W. B. Saunders Company, 1953.

Harvie, F. H.: Pediatric Methods and Standards. 3rd ed. Philadelphia, Lea & Febiger, 1958.

Kangery, R. H.: Children's Answers. Am. J. Nursing, *60*:1748, 1960.

Koop, C. E.: Undescended Testicle. M. Clin. North America, *36*:1779, 1952.

Lewis, G. M.: Practical Dermatology. 2nd ed. Philadelphia, W. B. Saunders Company, 1959.

Longino, L. A., Holder, T. M., and Gross, R. E.: Appendicitis in Childhood. Pediatrics, *22*: 238, 1958.

Markley, K., and others: Clinical Evaluation of Saline Solution Therapy in Burn Shock. J.A.M.A., *161*:1465, 1956.

Minor, C. L.: The Empty Scrotum. Pediat. Clin. North America, *6*:1137, 1959.

Nelson, W. E. (editor): Textbook of Pediatrics. 7th ed. Philadelphia, W. B. Saunders Company, 1959.

Ochsner, A., and DeBakey, M. E. (editors): Christopher's Minor Surgery. 8th ed. Philadelphia, W. B. Saunders Company, 1959.

Osment, L. S.: Tinea Capitis. Am. J. Nursing, *60*:1264, 1960.

Paterson, D., and McCreary, J. F.: Pediatrics. Philadelphia, J. B. Lippincott Company, 1956.

Pillsbury, D. M., Shelley, W. B., and Kligman, A. M.: Dermatology. Philadelphia, W. B. Saunders Company, 1956.

Rhodes, V. A., and Shannon, A. M.: Nursing Care of the Burn Patient. Am. J. Nursing, *59*:1265, 1959.

Sarvajic, J.: Principles in the Treatment of Burns. Nursing World, *131*:19, June, 1957.

Silver, H. K., Kempe, C. H., and Bruyn, H. B.: Handbook of Pediatrics. 3rd ed. Los Altos, California, Lange Medical Publications, 1959.

Swenson, O.: Pediatric Surgery. New York, Appleton-Century-Crofts, Inc., 1958.

Terry, F. J., and others: Principles and Technics of Rehabilitation Nursing. St. Louis, C. V. Mosby Company, 1957.

# Chapter 23

# Conditions of the School

# Child Requiring Long-Term Care

## REHABILITATION OF THE SCHOOL CHILD

FREQUENTLY in this text mention has been made of habilation or rehabilitation of children. Rehabilitation in our culture is based on the belief that all persons should be helped to maintain or regain their best possible physical or mental health. Thus rehabilitation becomes one goal in the comprehensive care of patients. The nurse must work closely with other members of the health team to achieve this end. The process of rehabilitation begins as soon after recognition of the illness as possible and continues throughout the child's illness until he is rehabilitated to the total extent possible for him.

As the child grows—certainly by school age and adolescence—he must assume increasing responsibility for his rehabilitation after illness. His cooperation must be gained through understanding the necessity for this. The nurse has an important role in interpreting this need to him and in helping him to assume this responsibility.

In order to help the child achieve the goal of rehabilitation, his own goals must be considered. Thus the nurse has the responsibility to investigate the nature of these goals through discussions with him. She must relay pertinent information to other members of the health team.

Besides working closely with members of the health team, the professional nurse must also guide other members of the nursing team by instruction, supervision and correlation of the efforts of the health team to meet the needs of the child and his family. The nursing team also can contribute to rehabilitation of the child by helping him obtain adequate rest, diet, comfort and recreation and by providing emotional support, health teaching and instruction as necessary throughout his illness.

**635**

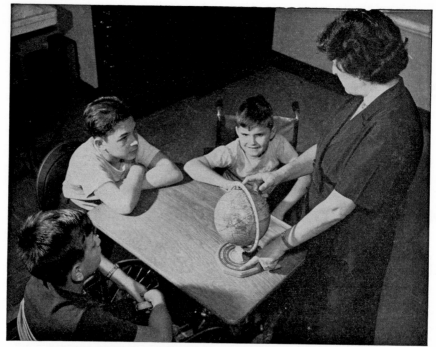

**Figure 241.**  Schooling is an essential part of the rehabilitation program. (From Mary Stewart: Role of the Nurse in Pediatric Rehabilitation. Health News, Vol. 33.)

Only through the combined efforts of the members of the health team and nursing personnel can the individual child be habilitated or rehabilitated to the greatest extent possible for him. In our society it is our privilege and responsibility to help prepare each child, whether normal or handicapped, to take his rightful place in the world of tomorrow.

## LONG-TERM CONDITIONS

### Rheumatic Fever

**Collagen Diseases.** Collagen diseases are a group of diseases characterized by damage to the ground substance of connective tissue, followed by changes in collagen fibrils. The connective tissue of all organ systems is usually affected, and the small blood vessels also are frequently involved. The following are collagen diseases (they are heterogeneous from the clinical point of view, but have certain symptoms in common): rheumatic fever, rheumatic arthritis, periarteritis nodosa, disseminated lupus erythematosus, scleroderma and dermatomyositis. All these diseases respond symptomatically to corticotropin (ACTH) or cortisone during some stage. The basic problem in these conditions is the deposition of fibrinoid material in the tissues. Histopathologically, fibrinoid is extensively deposited in the lumen and walls of blood vessels and in the surrounding connective tissues.

**Etiology, Incidence and Pathology.** Rheumatic fever is a general systemic disease characterized by frequent recurrences following infection with group A beta hemolytic streptococcus. The common origin of infection is in the throat (possibly followed by scarlet fever) or skin owing to group A beta hemolytic streptococcus. The disease may be a hypersensitivity reaction to one or more antigenic components or metabolic products of this organism.

The pathologic sequence in rheumatic fever is (1) the initial infection with group A beta hemolytic streptococcus, (2) usually a latent or non-symptomatic period lasting one to three weeks, and (3) the onset of rheumatic fever.

Rheumatic fever is one of the leading causes of chronic illness and death in children. It has its highest *incidence* between the ages of five and fifteen years; the majority of first attacks occur between six and eight years. It is most prevalent in the temperate zones. Climate is a more important factor than racial susceptibility. The incidence varies with the season and geographic location, but it always follows the curve of incidence of streptococcal infections. It is most common in the spring months. Overcrowded living conditions and general lack of hygiene among the lower socio-economic groups in large cities are predisposing factors. The disease has a high family incidence; hereditary predisposition is possible.

The characteristic lesions of rheumatic fever are found in the connective tissue of the heart, subcutaneous tissue and in the arteries. Collagenous structures become edematous and may form granulomas or Aschoff bodies. These bodies are usually found in the wall of the left ventricle and interventricular septum. Structures resembling Aschoff bodies may also be found as subcutaneous nodules under the skin. These lesions may develop exudative manifestations. Such rheumatic effusions are usually absorbed, but adhesions may be found, especially in the pericardium. They are found in the hearts of the majority of children who succumb to acute carditis. Valvular lesions which form scars as they heal may result in thickening of the leaflet and shortening of the chordea tendineae. Such deformities of the valves result from repeated attacks of infection.

The heart is impaired after rheumatic fever, owing to damage to the myocardium, the endocardium (including the valves), or the pericardium. The effects of the contracting scar tissue may not be evident for several years after the initial attack of rheumatic fever. Chronic valvular heart disease results.

**Clinical Manifestations.** The symptoms

and course of the disease are variable. The three principal clinical manifestations, however, are carditis, migratory polyarthritis and Sydenham's chorea. The typical attack may present any one of the clinical manifestations, which tend to recur at varying intervals. The onset may be acute or insidious with symptoms of "growing pains," pallor, nosebleed, malaise, and attacks of abdominal pain. Attacks last from one to three months, and recurrence may follow if the child acquires a streptococcal infection.

*Carditis* tends to occur in younger children. It is a more serious manifestation than arthritis or chorea, since it may lead to permanent disability or death. The pathologic changes include exudation and proliferation. The pericardium, myocardium and endocardium may be affected with subsequent scarring (see Fig. 242). The temperature may rise to 104° F. Leukocytosis, ane-

**Figure 242.** Acute fibrinous pericarditis. (From Disease Panorama on Rheumatic Fever. Courtesy of the Schering Corporation.)

mia and severe pallor may occur. The respirations are rapid, and the cardiac lesion results in tachycardia, especially during sleep, and a pulse of poor quality. In severe cases the following manifestations may be seen: prostration, weakness, orthopnea, cyanosis, precordial pain and cardiac decompensation and dilatation. Cardiac murmurs are present and may change in quality.

_Arthritis_ of a migratory polyarthritic type is usually seen in older children. The larger joints—hips, knees, ankles, shoulders, wrists and elbows—may be involved. The duration of involvement of any one joint varies, and the pain moves from one joint to another. In older children the affected joint is hot, tender, red and swollen. Permanent deformities do not follow this type of arthritis.

There is moderate leukocytosis, and the erythrocyte sedimentation rate is increased. The child's temperature usually runs from 101 to 102° F. Cardiac involvement may follow polyarthritis. So-called "growing pains" may be distinguished from migratory polyarthritis because they tend to occur only at night and are not associated with other manifestations of rheumatic fever.

_Sydenham's chorea_ (St. Vitus's dance) is a disorder of the central nervous system. It usually occurs in older children. See page 645 for a discussion of this condition.

There are other clinical manifestations of rheumatic fever (see Fig. 243): (1) subcutaneous nodules of varying size which may be found on the extensor tendons of the hands and feet, on elbows, scapulae, scalp, patella and vertebrae. The skin moves freely over these nodules; they are not painful, and they disappear gradually. (2) Pericarditis, in which there is pain in the precordial area and a friction rub heard over the precordium. (3) Muscle and joint pains (the so-called growing pains) may indicate rheumatic fever, and the child should be examined to rule out this disease and also orthopedic problems. (4) Epistaxis is a common manifestation of the onset of rheu-

**Figure 243.** Sites of involvement in acute rheumatic fever. (From Disease Panorama on Rheumatic Fever. Courtesy of the Schering Corporation.)

matic fever. (5) Abdominal pain may be severe and may be mistaken for appendicitis. It is usually located in the epigastrium and may be due to enlargement of the mesenteric lymph nodes or to inflammation of the peritoneum. (6) There may be low-grade fever in the afternoon. If the diagnosis is uncertain, the erythrocyte sedimentation rate should be determined. (7) There may be skin manifestations. Various types of erythema may appear, e.g. erythema marginatum (see Fig. 244) or erythema multiforme. Erythema marginatum is a pink eruption with serpiginous outline, occurring mainly on the trunk. These lesions may appear and disappear for years. (8)

Pleurisy and rheumatic pneumonia may be complications. (9) The child tires easily, loses weight, and is pale and anorexic.

**Diagnosis.** The diagnosis may be difficult because many other conditions show clinical manifestations similar to those of rheumatic fever. Each laboratory test must be interpreted in the light of other test results and of the child's total clinical picture.

Two laboratory tests are of value in diagnosing rheumatic fever and in evaluation of the disease. (1) C-reactive protein is never present in normal blood. It appears in the serum of patients ill with various inflammatory diseases, including rheumatic fever. This protein disappears as the child's condition improves. (2) The erythrocyte sedimentation rate is almost always elevated in children who have rheumatic carditis and polyarthritis, thereby indicating the presence of an inflammatory reaction. The sedimentation rate may remain elevated after clinical manifestations have subsided, showing that the rheumatic process is still active.

The rheumatic process should not be considered over until the white blood cell count is below 10,000 per cubic millimeter. Leukocytosis indicates inflammation. As long as anemia persists, the infection is probably still active.

Streptococci may be present in the upper respiratory tract of the child, a member of his family, or others whom he contacts. The organism may not be present if treatment has been given, but certain antibodies formed against streptococcal products may be present. Laboratory examinations may detect antifibrinolysin, antistreptolysin or antihyaluronidase.

Electrocardiograms may provide evidence of carditis. The P-R interval is often prolonged in the presence of carditis.

**Treatment.** No specific treatment will stop the rheumatic process. Bed rest is essential until the C-reactive protein is negative, the pulse rate normal and the erythrocyte sedimentation rate normal. Bed rest is necessary until the pain is gone and the hemoglobin is normal. The child should have begun to gain in weight before activity is permitted. If the work of the heart is reduced until the healing process occurs, a minimum of scar tissue in the heart will result.

Penicillin is given only to eradicate group A streptococci from the body. It does not alleviate symptoms. Salicylates quickly relieve fever, joint pains and swelling. Symptoms of toxicity such as tinnitus, hyperpnea, purpuric manifestations, nausea and vomiting should be reported and recorded. Salicylates are usually given orally. Aspirin (acetylsalicylic acid) or sodium salicylate is given. This therapy should be continued until C-reactive protein is negative and the erythrocyte sedimentation rate is decreasing. If the child cannot tolerate salicylates, aminopyrine or phenylbutazone (Butazolidin) may be used.

Therapy with corticoids produces the same effects as salicylates. ACTH, prednisone or cortisone may be used. Prednisone is preferred because it may be given orally and causes less sodium retention than cortisone. Laboratory findings tend to return to normal more quickly than with salicylates. Corticoids are especially beneficial in treating rheumatic carditis. These drugs do not terminate the rheumatic process, but suppress it. Congestive heart failure

**Figure 244.** Erythema marginatum rheumaticum. (From Disease Panorama on Rheumatic Fever. Courtesy of the Schering Corporation.)

**Figure 245.** Method of holding a child up in Fowler's position with a knee roll. (From Gross: The Surgery of Infancy and Childhood.)

may be controlled by these drugs. Patients may have a mild recurrence of symptoms when the drug is discontinued.

Steroid therapy masks symptoms; thus it is necessary to watch the child closely for symptoms of infection or complications. These children do not have a fever when they have infections. The blood pressure should be taken daily and the drug discontinued if the diastolic pressure rises to 100 mm. or above. The salt intake should be moderately restricted. Potassium may be added to the diet.

*Cushing's syndrome* is a side effect of steroid therapy and disappears when the therapy is discontinued. It is characterized by acne, moon face, increased pigmentation, hirsutism and abnormal fat distribution.

Morphine is given to control precordial pain, and sedatives such as phenobarbital to allay apprehension. Oxygen may be necessary. Digitalis may be indicated if cardiac failure is present.

**Nursing Care.** *Acute Phase.* In the acute phase of rheumatic fever rest is

all-important in order to reduce the work of the heart. His need for absolute bed rest should be explained to the child, and he should be reassured that it is only a temporary restriction. The bed must have a firm mattress, since this promotes good posture and is less painful for the child than a mattress which sags. During the period of complete bed rest the child's arms should be supported at his sides with pillows to reduce their weight from the shoulders. If the child is dyspneic, the head of the bed may be elevated.

Nursing care should be given at appropriate times so that the child can have long periods of complete rest without being disturbed. Since bodily movement causes pain, he should be moved as little as possible. The nurse's movements must be smooth, sure and unhurried; this helps to inspire confidence of the child in his nurse. If he is hurt by his nurse, he becomes anxious and does not want to be touched. The nurse should explain what she is going to do, e.g. insert the thermometer or lift him. What the child may be permitted to do for himself depends upon the physician's orders. If the child becomes irritable and more restless in bed than he would be out of it, the physician may permit a limited amount of activity in spite of the fact that laboratory findings are not normal.

The child with rheumatic fever who is on bed rest should have frequent skin care, especially of the back and buttocks. If he breathes through his mouth, good mouth care is essential. His position should be changed frequently and his body kept in good alignment. If his joints are sore, they should be handled carefully when he is moved. The child should be helped to use the bedpan as necesary.

Small frequent feedings of light, nourishing food are better than meals served at the usual intervals. It may be necessary to cater to the child's appe-

tite; he should not be forced to eat, nor allowed to overeat, since without exercise he might become obese. When food is brought him, he should be placed in a comfortable position for eating and, if he is unable to help himself, should be assisted by the nurse.

If oxygen is ordered, it is usually given in a tent (see Fig. 247). The procedure should be explained to the child. The school child is not likely to be frightened as is the younger child.

Nursing records must be full and specific. The rate and nature of the pulse are indicative of the child's progress. If the physician so orders, the pulse should be taken when the child is sleeping as well as when he is awake. The pulse rate should be counted for a full minute, before the thermometer is inserted. The temperature and respira-

SUPPORT FOR FEET     SMALL PILLOW     SMALL PILLOW     LARGE PILLOW TO SUPPORT ARM

SMALL PILLOW     SUPPORT FOR FEET

**Figure 246.**   Methods of positioning a child for good body alignment. *A*, Flat in bed. *B*, in a sitting position.

**Figure 247.** A satisfactory type of oxygen tent for administration of a high concentration (90 per cent) of oxygen. (Gross: The Surgery of Infancy and Childhood.)

tion rate should also be taken as ordered and accurately recorded. In general, an intake and output record is required. If possible, the child should be allowed to keep his own record. If fluids are limited, he should have a schedule which he may follow. The reason for limiting fluid intake and for keeping the intake and output chart should be explained to the child. The amount and kind of food taken should also be charted.

Other symptoms to note and record are the degree of fatigue, orthopnea, dyspnea, cough, skin lesions and edema.

The personnel caring for the child should understand the parents' attitude toward the child and his illness. The nurse and the physician should begin early in the child's illness to evaluate the family's attitude toward the child. These attitudes may vary from apparent unconcern to extreme anxiety. Parents must be helped to a more positive approach to the illness if the child is to be successfully rehabilitated.

*Convalescent Care.* Probably the first requisite in successful nursing of the convalescing child is to keep him happy and contented. These children become depressed because they see other acutely ill children admitted, recover and be discharged, while they themselves remain in the hospital. The child's activities must be confined to the limits permitted by the physician. There is a gradual increase in the child's ability to care for himself (bathing, feeding, and so on) as he improves.

If schoolwork is permitted, the child has this interest and the satisfaction of feeling that he is keeping up with his class. This helps him to look forward to the time of his discharge from the hospital. Recreational and occupational therapy helps him by teaching him new skills which he is interested in learning and which are related to the physician's plan for his care while in the hospital. Activities suitable for these children include finger painting, making beads from macaroni and stringing them, or making other types

f jewelry, making puppets or cuddly
oys, soap carving, spatter prints, spool
mitting, making model airplanes and
boats, leather construction, clay model-
ng, knitting, and so on. Making col-
ections of items which interest children of his age is also appropriate.
These children enjoy guessing games,
many of which have educational value.
This acceptance of activities within the
limits set by the physician helps the
child to understand and accept quiet
games or a physically inactive role in
an active game when he plays with his
friends after his discharge.

The play period in the hospital
should be short and should be followed
by periods of music, story telling or
reading, during which the child relaxes.

The time out of bed is gradually increased. A comfortable chair (not a
wheelchair) may be placed by the window, and the child may be given playthings which interest him and ensure
quiet activity. A wheelchair is used
when the nurse pushes him about to
explore his environment. After several
weeks or months he is allowed to walk,
but must be closely supervised so that
he does not overdo it.

Home is the best place for the convalescent child, but if this is not possi-

ble because of overcrowding and general lack of facilities, he may be sent
to a convalescent hospital where the
environment is planned to give him the
emotional security he needs, opportunities for play, education, work and
group life, as well as continued supervision of his physical health. In some
cases the child may be sent to a foster
home, but it is extremely difficult to
find such a home.

Resumption of normal activities is
gradual over a period of several weeks
to months.

If the child is sent to a convalescent
hospital or a foster home, he should
help to make plans, know about total
plans and meet his foster parents before
he leaves the hospital. His parents
should remain in contact with him,
since such arrangements are only temporary.

It is necessary to work out a plan
with the parents or foster parents for
the child's care when he leaves the
hospital. Not only his physical but also
his psychologic needs must be met.
Gradual independence must be given
and behavior disorders prevented. All
aspects of his care should be discussed
with his parents. If any item of equipment is needed, e.g. overbed table,

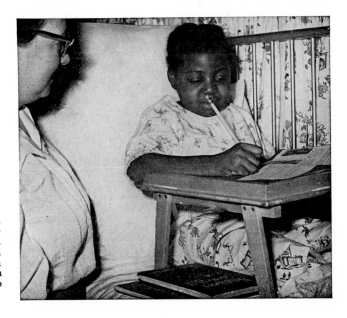

**Figure 248.** This child is on
bed rest and cannot be taken to
the classroom in the hospital
with other children. The school
teacher therefore visits her in
her room and helps her to gain
the satisfaction of keeping up
with her class.

back rest or footboard, the parents may be shown how to make these from orange crates and suitcases, or, if they cannot be made at home and the parents cannot afford to buy them, they may be provided through some agencies.

The home atmosphere should be cheerful. The child should have the same kind of quiet recreation which was provided in the hospital. In some cities a visiting school teacher will be sent by the school board, or a telephone connection may be made between his room and the classroom of the school he has attended. This enables him to hear the instruction given his class and their responses.

Not too much attention should be directed toward the child's heart condition. The whole child should be helped to develop confidence. He should learn how to set his own standards for activity. The ultimate aim should be kept in mind: to restore the child to his place in society with the least possible emotional trauma. When he returns to school, the health team, including teacher and school nurse, must know the health plan to be carried out in the school situation. They should understand his illness and thus help other children to understand and accept the difference in his routine; e.g. he will use the elevator, but they will not; his hours in school may not be as long as theirs.

The parents and the child should be helped to understand the need for visits to the clinic or his private physician for prophylactic medications and dental care. They should understand and accept his daily routine and also be able to recognize respiratory infections and skin infections, possibly caused by streptococci, and to get adequate medical care when these occur.

**Prognosis and Prevention.** The mortality rate seems to be declining from both initial attacks and recurrences of rheumatic fever. Recurrences are most common during childhood and decline after puberty.

Serious cardiac damage results from repeated, severe rheumatic atacks (see

**Figure 249.** The single site of chronic involvement—the heart. (From Disease Panorama on Rheumatic Fever. Courtesy of the Schering Corporation.)

Fig. 249). The *prognosis* for children who have their first attack before six years of age is graver than for those who have it at a later age, because they usually have carditis with residual cardiac damage. Often the residual heart condition may be so severe that it handicaps the adolescent or adult in his home and community life. (The child, of course, may not live to puberty.) (See Figure 250.)

The prognosis is good for children who have no evidence of cardiac involvement. Death in childhood is apt to be due to further rheumatic infection rather than to mechanical failure of the heart.

Rheumatic polyarthritis results in no permanent joint changes, and chorea results in no changes in the central nervous system.

The *prevention* of rheumatic fever lies in the prevention of infection with group A beta hemolytic streptococci. Prevention of the first attack is through elimination of streptococci from the upper respiratory tract when the child has pharyngitis or scarlet fever. Penicillin is given for ten to fourteen days. Intramuscular injection is probably better than oral medication because the patient may discontinue taking his medication as soon as he feels better and therefore may not get an adequate dose.

Recurrent attacks must be prevented, since each attack increases the threat of additional cardiac damage. The child should be kept from persons with upper respiratory tract infections. Ideally, he should live in a warm climate and an uncrowded environment. As a prophylactic measure, benzathine penicillin is given monthly by intramuscular injection, or penicillin or sulfadiazine is given by mouth daily indefinitely after the initial attack.

If it is necessary for the child to have a tonsillectomy and adenoidectomy or undergo dental work, an increased dose of penicillin should be given to prevent bacterial endocarditis.

**Public Health Aspects.** There is need for a community program of control, case finding and preventive work. There should be long-range programs for the care of these children. Improved living conditions of the lower-income group and better health programs in the schools would do much to prevent this serious disease of childhood. In some cities the coordination of team efforts for the benefit of these patients needs to be improved.

### Sydenham's Chorea (St. Vitus's Dance)

**Incidence, Clinical Manifestations and Diagnosis.** Sydenham's chorea is one of the clinical manifestations of the rheumatic process. It is primarily a disorder of the central nervous system. It is most common in girls during later childhood and early adolescence—from seven to fourteen years of age. The highest *incidence* is at eight years. Some authorities believe that the disease occurs in

**Figure 250.** Chronic rheumatic heart. *A,* Superior view of chronic rheumatic heart showing aortic insufficiency and mitral stenosis. *B,* Dissection of chronic rheumatic heart showing fibrosis of mitral valve and thickened chordae tendineae. (From Disease Panorama on Rheumatic Fever. Courtesy of the Schering Corporation.)

certain families more than in the general population (thus heredity would appear to be important) and that nervous persons are most apt to have the disease. It is seldom seen after puberty.

Sydenham's chorea is characterized by involuntary, purposeless, irregular movements involving any part or all of the voluntary musculature.

The *clinical manifestations* may vary from mild to severe. The onset is gradual. The child becomes increasingly nervous, and his jerking, spasmodic, purposeless, incoordinated, irregular movements cause him great discomfort. These movements are different from, and more severe than, those of tic. The first symptom of the condition may be clumsiness, and the child may be reprimanded for dropping something or spilling food at the dinner table. The movements of the facial muscles produce grimaces which often may appear to the adult as rude and to other children as silly. The child's handwriting shows lack of muscular control and may become almost illegible. The child cannot suppress his spasmodic movements, which become worse with excitement and embarrassment, but cease when he is asleep. Muscular weakness may become so great that he is unable to walk or even sit up. He talks with difficulty, and it is often impossible to understand his speech. He is "jittery," and slovenly in his personal habits, and may be unable to dress himself, having greatest difficulty in buttoning his clothes and tying his shoelaces. He may be unable to feed himself and may have difficulty in swallowing. Some children become incontinent. The child's emotional instability is shown in giggling, crying, fretfulness and rapid shifting from depression to elation. Usually the child does not have fever.

The *diagnosis* is based on the clinical manifestations, the most important of which are increase of choreiform movements when tense, increased dysfunction of speech and rapid changes of facial expression from a grin to tears.

**Treatment, Nursing Care and Prognosis.** Both *treatment* and *nursing care* are based on the relief of symptoms. Since there is no really effective treatment, nursing care is of central importance.

Drugs are given as ordered. Neither salicylates nor hormones have a therapeutic effect. The child should have absolute mental and physical rest. He should have a private room or be with a few carefully chosen children who meet his need for companionship. Prolonged, warm baths may have a sedative effect, and sedatives such as tranquilizers and phenobarbital may be given. He cannot feed himself and must be fed by his nurse. He should be protected from injury by padded sideboards for his bed. Blankets, sheets or pillows may be used for this purpose. His toys should be those with which he will not hurt himself. The nurse must anticipate the child's needs. Waiting for a bedpan or urinal increases his nervousness.

Gradual exercise, both physical and mental, is given in accordance with the physician's orders as the child's condition improves.

Since these children move constantly, they need adequate nourishment. They should be fed frequently with a light, nourishing diet, high in protein and iron. Vitamin supplements should be provided. The child should be fed with a spoon rather than a fork, because he might injure himself upon the prongs of the fork.

Skin care is important. Soothing baths given to relieve his nervousness are also part of good skin care. Constant motion is likely to produce abraded skin surfaces on his elbows and knees which will require special care. If he is incontinent, the bed should be changed as soon as it is soiled or wet, and the skin of the buttocks and the genitals should be bathed and dried thoroughly.

Psychologic care is as important as physical care. The nurse must be patient and understanding because the child's movements constantly interfere with her giving care, and also because he is emotionally unstable and irritable. He should be allowed to help himself as much as the physician permits, since this gives him a feeling of independence. He needs both love and happiness in his contacts with his parents and nurses. The nurse should help the parents to give him these essentials.

Child-parent relations may have been strained by the child's behavior before his condition became so evident that he was taken to a physician. Some parents will feel guilty at having blamed him for clumsiness he could not help, and others will find it difficult to understand that his irritating behavior was and is due to his disease, and not under his control. They doubt whether his recovery will bring a return to good behavior. The nurse's understanding attitude toward their relations with the child will help them to see the situation objectively and to give the child the emotional support he badly needs.

The convalescent child may be taught at home or in a special school where the hours of study are short and the whole educational plan is adapted to his needs. During his convalescence play material appropriate to his needs should be provided. At first toys which exercise large muscles should be given, and then those which promote the use of small muscles. In this way the child will learn muscle control again.

The *prognosis* is good. There is spontaneous recovery in eight to ten weeks. Attacks may recur, but recovery eventually is complete. The child's progress may be gauged by observing the improvement in his handwriting. He is therefore asked to write his name daily. The disease is seldom fatal, but if the child dies, death is due to exhaustion or cardiac disease.

## Diabetes Mellitus

**Incidence and Pathology.** In diabetes mellitus the body is unable to metabolize carbohydrates, owing to insufficient production of insulin, an internal secretion of the pancreas. There is also abnormal metabolism of fat and protein. Approximately 5 per cent of all people with diabetes show the first symptoms in childhood. The disorder is not common among children, but when it occurs, it tends to be more serious than in later life. Heredity is important; the disease is inherited as a recessive characteristic.

Since there is a deficiency of insulin, or since its effect is inhibited, diabetic acidosis, coma and death may result. Hyperglycemia is produced, which, when it exceeds the normal threshold, causes glycosuria. Hyperglycemia initiates diuresis, and as a result excess glucose is excreted. In addition to glucose, electrolytes and water are lost from both the intracellular and extracellular compartments of the body.

Tissue breakdown is due in part to osmotic forces and in part to tissue catabolism because of the body's inability to use glucose for fuel. Protein and fat are oxidized more rapidly than is normal. Because of the increased rate of breakdown of fats, ketonuria results. Ketonuria, dehydration and kidney dysfunction result in acidosis.

Thus in uncontrolled diabetes body water, electrolytes and fixed base are lost, the plasma carbon dioxide content is lowered, acidosis develops, and glycogen stored in the muscles and liver is lost.

**Clinical Manifestations, Laboratory Studies and Diagnosis.** Diabetes may develop slowly or may first be recognized when the child is in coma. The onset in children is generally more rapid than in the adult, and the child is likely to be underweight at the onset. Obesity does not appear to be a factor in juvenile diabetes.

The *symptoms* are increased thirst and appetite, weight loss, polyuria (this may be the cause of bed wetting in children who had achieved night control of urination), possibly weakness and, over a period of time, pruritus, dry skin and excessive hairiness. In the nonacidotic stage the child will have glycosuria, possibly ketonuria, and hyperglycemia.

Nurses and all others responsible for the daily care of children should know the symptoms of *diabetic coma* or *acidosis*. Coma usually follows an infection in untreated diabetics who are not able to burn up carbohydrate and therefore utilize fat for energy. The symptoms are drowsiness, dry skin, cherry red lips and flushed cheeks, hyperpnea, acetone odor to the breath, abdominal pain, nausea and vomiting. When the child is in coma, he has Kussmaul breathing or severe hyperpnea, a rigid abdomen, rapid and weak pulse, lowered blood pressure and temperature and soft, sunken eyeballs.

*Laboratory studies* show a lowered carbon dioxide content of the blood and a shift of pH to the acid side. Albumin and casts may be present in the urine when the child has acidosis.

The *diagnosis* is based on the family history and that of the child's previous health, and on the clinical manifestations and laboratory studies. A fasting hyperglycemia with glycosuria is diagnostic of diabetes mellitus. Other conditions, however, may have to be ruled out. Whenever glycosuria is found, a blood sugar determination should be made. If the blood sugar level is more than 200 mg. per 100 ml., a diagnosis of diabetes mellitus is tentatively made. A glucose tolerance test may show prolonged, high levels of sugar in the blood, indicating that the body cannot burn carbohydrates. A high white blood cell count may be present with diabetic acidosis.

**Treatment.** Management of the preadolescent diabetic is usually not too difficult if the parents and the child understand the disease and his care. Management of the adolescent diabetic is more difficult because of his desire to rebel against the authority of his parents and the physician. If he is adequately treated, the diabetic child should be able to compete with his peers in physical, mental and social development.

Treatment includes a *diet* which supports normal growth and development and satisfies the child's appetite, and the administration of insulin in sufficient amount to maintain glycemic equilibrium. An important aspect of treatment is instruction of the child and his parents so that they can manage the treatment in the home. This requires acceptance by the child and his family of the fact that he is essentially a "normal" child.

Should diabetic acidosis develop, treatment involves close cooperation of the team members—physician, nurse and laboratory personnel. Laboratory examinations are needed to determine the blood sugar level and carbon dioxide-combining power or content, and urinalysis for sugar and acetone. Intravenous therapy is used. Electrolytes, carbohydrate and water are given with insulin. Vitamins may also be given. If the child is in severe acidosis, with a pH of less than 7.1 and a carbon dioxide measurement of less than 6 mEq. per liter, sodium bicarbonate may be given. Urine should be collected each hour in order to guide modification of the dosage of insulin and carbohydrates as therapy progresses. Warmth and comfort are essential for the child with acidosis. The nurse should observe for changes in color, type of respiration and degree of consciousness. Gastric aspiration may be carried out to relieve distention, to prevent pulmonary aspiration of vomitus and to hasten the time when the child can take fluids by mouth. Large doses of appropriate antibiotics may be given if infection is present. Oral feedings may be started when the child regains consciousness, usually after twelve to sixteen hours of parenteral therapy, and then carbohydrate and electrolyte mixtures are given. This dietary stage is followed with an adequate fluid diet. Small doses of insulin are given to cover the oral intake of carbohydrates; the amount is based on the findings of urinalysis for sugar. While taking oral feedings the child should be checked for symptoms of insulin shock or diabetic acidosis. An average diet may be given in a few days if the child shows no untoward symptoms.

Management after correction of the acidosis or of the child in whom diabetes was not adequately controlled requires the same teamwork that is necessary in the acute crisis, but nursing care becomes the center of the program. The child must be treated inlividually; each child needs a satisfactory diet and insulin dosage. The diet should be approximately that of a normal child and similar to the family's diet pattern. The specific requirements of the diet are that it supply caloric intake for activity and growth, sufficient protein intake for growth, and the required vitamins and minerals.

One of two types of diets may be ordered. (1) Quantities of food may be *measured*. Many parents find that children feel more secure when a definite dietary program is ordered and exactly followed. (2) The so-called *unrestricted* or *free diet*, which is that of a normal child. It is restricted only in that excesses, such as high carbohydrate intake, are avoided. On this diet the child feels as free as a normal child because he may eat practically whatever he wishes.

In general, the child is on a stabilized, measured diet only at the beginning of treatment. Upon his discharge from the hospital he and his parents should be given a list of foods which are exchangeable in planning his meals for the day. For such a diet gross household measures are adequate. They are not as rigid as in a weighed diet. Occasional deviations are not important. The child on such a diet should receive a satisfactory intake with adequate distribution of caloric intake at various meals. He should learn to manage his diet himself as he grows older.

The child should be stabilized on his diet and the amount of insulin he needs while he is in the hospital. Since the amount of exercise he takes changes his needs, for several days before his discharge he should take about the same amount of exercise as he will when he is at home. The diet should be so planned that his appetite is satisfied and his growth and development normal when leading the same kind of life his friends lead.

*Insulin* is a specially prepared extract of the pancreas. Injected into the body it enables the body to burn sugar. All juvenile diabetics need insulin. At present it is necessary to give it by subcutaneous injection. Although adult diabetics have profited from sulfonylureas, orally administered hypoglycemic agents, these do not at present provide a reliable replacement for insulin in the treatment of diabetic children.

Five types of insulin are used in the treatment of children. *Regular* or *unmodified insulin* affects the blood sugar in twenty to thirty minutes after injection, and the effect lasts from six to eight hours. *Protamine zinc insulin* affects the blood sugar in approximately an hour to three hours after injection, its influence lasting for twenty-four hours or more. *NPH insulin, globin insulin* and *Lente insulin* produce initial and long-maintained effects; the time in which these preparations of insulin are effective is between that of unmodified insulin and protamine zinc insulin. The physician generally orders a combination of unmodified insulin and another type which produces prolonged action. Both Lente insulin and NPH insulin can be given in the same syringe with unmodified insulin, but protamine zinc insulin cannot.

The dose of insulin is estimated on the basis of qualitative tests of the urine for sugar. Urine specimens should be collected at the following hours: (1) before breakfast, at 7 or 8 a.m., (2) before lunch, at 11:30 to 12 noon, (3) before the evening meal, at 5 to 6 p.m., and (4) before bedtime, at 7 to 9 p.m. If too large a dose of insulin, too little food or too much exercise is taken, insulin shock may result. With an even balance between the diet and the dosage of insulin the urine should be essentially sugar-free.

Several factors are important in varying the child's need for insulin. Adjustment must be made periodically in the relation of *diet* to insulin dosage. All children need *exercise*, but diabetics must take exercise that requires a relatively definite amount of energy expenditure. Exercise produces a lowering of the blood sugar level and may cause shock in children taking insulin. Only when the diet and exercise are standardized is it possible to give the requi-

Table 10.   Care of the Diabetic Child

---

### Symptoms of Insulin Shock and Diabetic Coma

| Insulin Shock (Due to overdose of insulin, reduction of diet or increase in exercise) | | Diabetic Coma (Acidosis) |
|---|---|---|
| Early manifestations: | Pallor<br>Weakness<br>Dizziness<br>Changes in disposition *<br>Sweating<br>Tremor<br>Sudden hunger<br>Dilated pupils | Changes in mental state (lethargic)*<br>Vomiting<br>Abdominal pain |
| Severe reactions: | Semiconsciousness<br>Later: convulsions, coma, death<br>Low blood sugar<br>Urine sugar-free<br>Acetone absent | Acetone odor on breath<br>Dehydration<br>Hyperpnea<br>Face flushed<br>Lips cherry red<br>Little perspiration<br>Blood sugar high, low carbon dioxide<br>Sugar and acetone present in urine |

\* The emotional reaction of the child is characteristic of him. He may cry, be hostile or appear happy.

The child and his parents should recognize the need for immediate medical assistance if symptoms of shock or acidosis occur. In case of shock the child should be given fruit juice or sugar. The child should carry a lump of sugar with him and, if he recognizes symptoms of shock, take the sugar. If the child becomes unconscious, he should be kept warm and receive immediate medical attention. When he is taken to a physician, glucose will be given intravenously. Recovery after treatment for shock is usually rapid.

---

*General Care*

1. Skin care to prevent infection
   a. Give frequent baths, at least every other day
   b. Provide inexpensive shoes which may be discarded when the child outgrows them
   c. Teach the child to report any break in the skin and treat it promptly

2. Maintenance of resistance to infection
   a. Dress the child appropriately according to the temperature, not the season of the year
   b. Keep the child away from anyone who has an upper respiratory tract infection or other infection
   c. Report infections promptly to the physician
   d. Immunize the child against common communicable diseases

3. Proper elimination

4. Regulation of exercise
   a. In the hospital keep him as busy as he would be at home
   b. At home encourage him to take moderate exercise regularly each day

5. Accuracy in saving of urine specimens
   a. Save and test a specimen of urine at prescribed hours. Parents and child can be taught to test urine specimens
   b. Be careful that the child does not dilute the urine to cover a break in adhering to his diet

6. Diet
   a. Let the child eat with other diabetics in the hospital, for he is then more likely to accept his diet
   b. Teach the child to keep to the diet ordered by the physician. Give the child the list of allowed exchanges of food if such is ordered
   c. Make adherence to the diet as easy as possible for the child by varying the diet as much as is permitted
   d. Teach the child to manage his own diet as early as possible

7. Administration of insulin
   a. Parents and child should learn the reason for and the procedure of administration of insulin

**Table 10.   Care of the Diabetic Child (continued)**

  b. Children 7 to 10 years of age can usually be taught to give insulin to themselves (even an intelligent 6-year-old can learn). The earlier the responsibility is given the child, the better it is for him
    (1) Make the explanation simple. After the nurse has explained the procedure initially, another child can assist him better than an adult can, perhaps because he has more time to spend on showing how and why each step is done
    (2) Let the child practice frequently under supervision
      (a) Use routine sites of injections: upper right arm, upper left arm, left thigh, right thigh (each extremity may be used for several weeks if injections are given ½ inch apart)
      (b) Check the dose measured by the child until his accuracy is proved
      (c) Pinch the skin, or teach the child to do so, when using a site on the thigh, because this minimizes the pain of injection
      (d) Do not give insulin too near the surface of the skin
8. Records
  a. The child should be taught to keep daily records of the insulin dose, diet, and urine test findings until he learns about his illness and it is under control
9. The child's part in his recovery
  a. Keep the child under supervision as long as necessary, but give him independence as soon as possible
  b. Get his cooperation in
    (1) Voluntary self-control in diet so that other children cannot tempt him
    (2) Taking regular exercise
    (3) Honest reporting if he transgresses against the physician's orders
    (4) Not fooling his parents with faked symptoms of insulin shock
    (5) Avoiding self-pity or exaggerating his handicap
  c. Guide the child to normal adolescence by understanding his aggressiveness, withdrawal or rebellion against restraint. Bring him, through understanding of his problem, to normal adulthood in which he can take his place in society

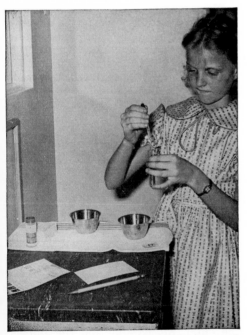

Figure 251.   This 11-year-old girl is responsible for testing her own urine specimens. She takes great pride in her accomplishment.

site amount of insulin. Changes in diet and in energy output make adjustment of the dose to the child's needs essential. This is difficult because of the difference in the child's activity on school days and on vacation days, and in wet and sunny weather. The child should always carry sugar with him and take it if he feels the symptoms of shock. If unusually strenuous activity is planned, insulin dosage must be reduced proportionally.

Since *infection* increases the need for insulin, the child may go into acidosis easily if he has an infection. During such periods additional amounts of insulin may be needed to prevent glycosuria. The amount is reduced during convalescence.

*Emotional disturbances* also increase the child's need for insulin. Diabetic children who are emotionally stable can be regulated more easily than can those who are easily upset.

**Nursing Care.**   An important part of the nursing care of the diabetic child is helping him and his parents to de-

**Figure 252.** Diabetes. *A*, This 11-year-old girl is learning how to prepare her dosage of insulin. Her mother, who has already learned the procedure, is interested in her progress. *B*, Having practiced the procedure, this child is now able to inject the insulin and thus to assume more responsibility for her own care.

velop positive attitudes toward his condition. Probably the central problem is to help them accept the fact that the child can be healthy and active if dietary rules are followed and insulin is given in adjustment to his needs. Their initial attitude is likely to be that restriction is necessary only when the child is sick. The parents and the child must learn that constant care is necessary. The nurse should listen to the parents when they express their feeling about the child's illness and try to reconcile both parents and child to maintaining the prescribed diet and dosage of insulin, together with regular exercise.

In the hospital the nurse must condition the child to self-control and make it easy for him, and instruct the mother in the need for, and the means of, helping the child conform to his regulated life. The child should have exercise *after* meals. All tempting but restricted food should be kept out of the way as far as possible. Nevertheless school children must learn to go without, while others eat, the foods they are denied. The diet should be made attractive. The child should understand that if he reports breaks in dietary rules, he will not be punished or scolded, but that unreported breaks may cause sudden sickness.

No attempt should be made to hide the fact that the child is a diabetic. He and those about him should know this so as to understand his restriction of diet and need for a regular life. But he should not be permitted to use illness as a defense against accepting the role of a well child. He should be encouraged to assume his share of family responsibilities. He should also participate on an equal basis with his peer group, not looking on his diabetes as a handicap.

Table 10 presents material which nurses will find useful in understanding the child's treatment in the hospital and care at home. If this information is given to parents, it supplements, but does not take the place of, individual instruction which the physicians, nurses and dietitians will give the parents and the child. Understanding the care given the child in the hospital not only brings about better cooperation between the child, his parents and the nurses, but also is the basis for the acceptance and following of the program for his care at home. The nurse should be thoroughly familiar with the information the table gives. Student nurses will find it an aid in learning the total care of the diabetic child and in teaching parents and children this care.

The teacher and school nurse should be aware of the child's illness and the manifestations of shock and coma so that they can help him in such emergencies. The school personnel, parents and the child must realize that readmission to the hospital will be necessary for evaluation and adjustment of the child's diet and insulin dosage.

**Complications, Course and Prognosis.** *Complications* are uncommon except in children who have been inadequately treated or have had the condition for a long time. The following may possibly result from diabetes: lack of development, stunted growth, amenorrhea and lack of development of secondary sex characteristics. Children may also suffer cataracts, gangrene and arteriosclerosis after the disease has been present for a period of years. Infections are common and heal more slowly than is normal in the poorly treated diabetic child. These include infections of the skin, respiratory tract and lower urinary tract. Dental caries is also common.

Complications which may occur as a result of insulin injections include atrophy of the subcutaneous fat and allergy to insulin.

The *course* and *prognosis* depend on the accuracy of control measures. Serious degenerative lesions appear in young adults who have had diabetes mellitus for ten to twenty years. These include arteriosclerosis with hypertension, nephropathy and retinal changes.

## Precocious Sexual Development

**Etiology and Treatment.** Precocious sexual development or precocious puberty can be diagnosed when secondary sexual characteristics such as breast development, menarche, pubic and axillary hair and enlargement of the genitals appear before the child is nine years of age (see Fig. 253).

Children undergoing precocious puberty may be divided into two groups: those with true precocious puberty with production of mature sperm or ova, and those with precocious pseudopuberty in which no sperm or ova are formed.

Most cases of *true precocious puberty*—with menstruation and ovulation in girls and the presence of sperm in the discharge of the organs of reproduction in boys—are due to a constitutional premature maturation of the endocrine control of the genital tissues. This occurs more commonly in girls than in boys. There are no obvious abnormalities which start the maturing effects of the pituitary gland prematurely. In some cases this condition appears to be hereditary.

Although the appearance of the child may be disturbing and embarrassing, other children eventually catch up with the preadolescent in development. No treatment is necessary. There is a decided spurt in physical growth when sexual development first appears. Early epiphysial closure of the long bones takes place, however; therefore the eventual height of these children tends to be below average on maturity. The physician will explain this condition to the parents and eventually to the child so that they and he may have the correct attitude toward this deviation. These children should be guarded against sexual abuses, which, in a girl, may lead to pregnancy.

A second type of true precocious puberty is due to a central nervous system infection such as encephalitis or a lesion which usually involves the hypothalamus or the floor of the third ventricle. Ovulation as well as menstruation occurs in this type. Usually other evidences of neurologic disturbances, such as convulsions or mental retardation, are also present in these children. Treatment should be directed to the cause itself. The prognosis depends upon the etiology.

*Precocious pseudopuberty*, the least common cause for precocious puberty, is due to a feminizing tumor of the ovary or the adrenal cortex. The physi-

**Figure 253.** Idiopathic precocious puberty. Girl aged 3 years, menstruating for one year. Note increased height, breast development, pubic hair growth. Her bone age was 8 plus years, and vaginal cytology was estrogenic. (From Robert B. Greenblatt, William E. Barfield, Edwin C. Jungck and Jorge Martinez Manautou: Pediat. Clin. North America, Vol. 5.)

cal changes are due, not to early activation of other endocrine glands, but to primary estrogen production. Treatment consists in surgery, depending upon the type of tumor and the presence of metastases. The prognosis depends upon the cause of the condition.

### Brain Tumor

**Etiology, Incidence, Clinical Manifestations and Types.** The majority of brain tumors in children are due to abnormal growth of cells already present in the brain; few are due to metastases from noncerebral neoplasms. Generally these tumors in children are located beneath the tentorium cerebri. (Most brain tumors in adults are located above it.)

The *incidence* of brain tumors among children is only one sixth that among adults. Tumors increase in incidence up to six years of age and then remain at a uniform level during the school period.

Most of the *symptoms* are due to increased intracranial pressure. Such symptoms include *vomiting,* usually in the morning, at first nonprojectile, but later projectile; *headache, diplopia* and *head enlargement,* if the tumor occurs before the sutures are firmly united; and *changes in mental awareness,* such as lethargy, drowsiness, stupor, coma and ultimately death. Changes in *vital signs* are important in diagnosing increased intracranial pressure. Convulsions are rare in infratentorial tumors, but may occur in some children having these lesions.

Other clinical manifestations depend on the type and location of the tumor.

Five types of tumors may be seen, as follows.

*Astrocytoma* may occur at any age, but the peak incidence is at eight years. The tumor is usually located in the cerebellum. The clinical manifestations differentiate this type of tumor from others. The onset is insidious, and the course is slow. Signs of focal disturbance or increase in intracranial pressure may occur. The child may have ataxia, hypotonia, diminished reflexes and nystagmus. Papilledema is present. Without operation the prognosis is poor. Total surgical removal with complete cure is possible.

*Medulloblastoma* is a fairly common type of tumor in children. The incidence is greatest during school age and reaches its highest point at five to six years. It is a highly malignant, rapidly developing tumor usually found in the cerebellum. Clinical manifestations are unsteadiness when the child walks, anorexia and vomiting, and headache, usually in the morning. Papilledema and ataxia are present. The child is drowsy, and nystagmus can be observed. Death usually results in less than a year.

*Ependymoma* is located in the fourth ventricle or in one of the lateral ventricles of the brain. Increased intracranial pressure and other manifestations are present, depending on the location of the tumor. The child will suffer from vomiting, headache, enlarged head and unsteady gait. Hydrocephalus may occur. The treatment is by internal compression and roentgen therapy.

*Craniopharyngioma* occurs in late childhood. The tumor is near the pituitary gland. There is pituitary or hypothalamic dysfunction. The most common hormonal disturbance observed is diabetes insipidus. The child may be stunted in growth and may have myxedema or delayed puberty. The cerebral disturbance results in defects of the visual fields. Later there may be memory or personality disturbances. There is evidence of increased intracranial pressure due to obstruction of the flow of cerebrospinal fluid. Headache and vomiting are noted. A roentgenogram of the skull reveals separated sutures.

Surgical removal of the entire tumor is usually impossible. Roentgen therapy may control for years a tumor which was not surgically removed.

*Brain stem gliomas* have a peak incidence among children about seven years old. The clinical manifestations are multiple cranial nerve palsies, ataxia of the trunk and little sensory loss, without indications of increased intracranial pressure. The course is slow, but the tumor is inoperable. Roentgen therapy may permit the child to survive for a while. Chemotherapy is being attempted.

**Diagnosis and Treatment.** Early *diagnosis* of brain tumor may be impossible because of its insidious beginning. The diagnosis is based on the history of symptoms of increased intracranial pressure and/or focal cerebral disturbances, and the findings in a physical examination. An electroencephalogram assists in locating superficial supratentorial tumors. A positive *Macewen's sign*

is associated with separation of the sutures. Roentgenograms may show splitting of the suture lines or calcification within the tumor. Ventriculograms and arteriograms help to localize the tumor. Lumbar puncture should not be done when increased intracranial pressure is present, because of the possibility of the medulla being pushed into the cervical spine.

The symptoms listed under the different types of tumors may also be found in children with encephalitis, brain abscess or some degenerative brain disease, and such conditions must be ruled out before a diagnosis of brain tumor is made unqualifiedly.

The *treatment* may be surgical or with deep radiation. In surgery as much of the tumor as possible is excised. Most brain tumors cannot be removed completely. Deep radiation may be of value in some cases. Even when complete cure is not possible, symptoms may be relieved and the child may be able to enjoy life for a variable time. Maintenance of his general nutrition and of his and his parents' morale and outlook about the condition are important.

**Nursing  Care.** *Emotional  Support.* Both the parents and the child should become familiar before operation with the nurse who will care for the child postoperatively. The relation should be one of mutual trust. The parents are naturally anxious. They as well as the child should be prepared for neurosurgery, for how the child will look postoperatively and for the treatment and procedures which will be necessary after operation. Conversation that would be anxiety-producing for the child should not be carried on where he can hear what is said, even though he appears to be unconscious. Parents need continued understanding and support from the nurse during the preoperative and postoperative periods.

*Preoperative Care and Observations.* Preoperative care consists in placing the child in a bed with crib sides or, if he is too large for a crib, side bars, because of the danger of his being confused or drowsy and falling out of bed.

Preoperatively the child should receive a nourishing diet. If he vomits, he can be refed, because usually he is not nauseated. Enemas are not given because of the danger of increasing the intracranial pressure.

Observations by the nurse in order to help the physician in localizing the tumor and appraising the increasing intracranial pressure are of the utmost importance. The nurse should listen to the complaints or comments of the older child and observe children of all ages. She should chart both complaints and observations fully and with the conditions under which they took place. Specifically she should note lowering of the pulse rate and change in its nature, gradual or sudden change in body temperature, decrease in the respiratory rate and change in the nature of respiration, especially irregular respiration, and any change in blood pressure, particularly a rise in the systolic pressure with widening pulse pressure.

The nurse should record vomiting, and indications of headache, lethargy and drowsiness. Any convulsions should be reported and recorded in full. (Seizure precautions should be followed—see page 380.) If possible, the nurse should ascertain whether there is limitation of the visual field or whether the child sees a double image of a single object. She should record the degree and situation of muscular weakness. Fecal and urinary incontinence or retention is routinely recorded. All complaints of pain and discomfort are noted.

The nurse should know where emergency equipment—such as oxygen, aspirator, sterile gloves, ventricular tap tray, emergency drugs and other supplies and equipment—are kept in case they are needed. Whenever the nurse is in doubt about the care of the child, she should call the supervisor or clinical instructor for instructions and explanations of the care he requires.

*Postoperative Care.* Postoperative care is exacting and requires both skill and experience in the nursing care of children undergoing brain surgery. Parenteral fluids are given postoperatively when the child cannot take fluids by mouth. Any difficulties with the intravenous setup should be reported at once. The rate of absorption of fluid should be noted carefully. Too rapid administration may produce a dangerous increase in the intracranial pressure. Mouth care is essential to prevent parotitis and monilia infection.

The child's position immediately postoperatively is lying flat on the unaffected side. After the danger of vomiting has passed and the child's nasopharynx no longer needs to be aspirated, his position should be changed frequently from side to back in order to prevent pressure areas and hypostatic pneumonia. For turning the child who has had surgery in the cerebellar area the nurse's movements should be slow and his body should be kept in a straight line; the position of the head should not be changed or turned. In moving the child the head, neck and shoulders should be well supported so that no twisting of these parts of the body occurs (see Fig. 254). Two nurses are needed to move the child of school age.

The patient should be kept clean and dry at all times. Back care is given frequently, and the area around pressure points is massaged. If paralysis or spasticity of the extremities occurs pillows or other types of support should be used. Foot drop must be prevented by adequate support.

The vital signs are taken as ordered by the physician—every fifteen minutes at first and then less frequently as the condition warrants—to determine indications of rising intracranial pressure

The nasopharynx is aspirated as necessary. The child is encouraged to breathe deeply at regular periods hourly or as ordered.

If shock occurs, warm blankets are applied. Emergency stimulants, intravenous fluids and oxygen should be kept on hand for immediate use. The foot of the bed is usually not raised because of the danger of increasing intracranial pressure. The nurse must be alert for, and immediately report urinary incontinence or retention.

Restraints should not be used unless

they are absolutely necessary, because the child may struggle against them and increase intracranial pressure. They should be used if the child pulls at his dressings, tries to dislodge the intravenous or gavage tube or in any way tries to injure himself. Elbow restraints, mitts for the hands or clove hitch restraints (see p. 168) may then be used.

If the head dressing becomes wet with drainage, the area is circled with gentian violet. If there is rapid enlargement of the stained area or if bright red blood appears on the dressing, the surgeon should be notified immediately. The nurse may reinforce the dressings with sterile pads held in place with a bandage. Meningitis may result from contamination of the surgical area.

Edema of the face, eyelids and brain may result from injury during operation. Because lacrimal secretion cannot circulate over the eyes when edema is present, the conjunctivae may become dry and infected. Warm saline irriga-

tions of the eyes, eye drops or the application of cold compresses to the swollen eyelids may be ordered to prevent this complication. Some physicians recommend that the eyelids be taped closed with small pieces of cellophane tape or covered with eye shields.

Hyperthermia may be caused by intracranial edema, by bleeding or by disturbance of the heat-regulating center. The temperature should be taken at least every half-hour when it is elevated. Methods to reduce fever include undressing the child and covering him with a sheet or only a diaper over the pubic area, reduction of room temperature, tepid sponge bath, cold water mattress, ice water enemas or small retention enemas containing aspirin. The body temperature usually is not brought down to normal, but it may be kept fairly low. If the child cannot swallow, gavage feedings may be given. If they are given, distention should be noted.

As soon as the child has ceased to vomit and shows signs of being able to

**Figure 254.** Suboccipital craniectomy dressings assist in keeping the head in correct alignment with the child's body even when the child is turned. *A*, Front view; *B*, back view.

**Figure 255.**   Legg-Perthes disease. Note the flattened head, dense epiphysis and wide femoral neck in contrast to the normal hip on the opposite side. (From G. A. Caldwell and H. D. Morris, in Ochsner and DeBakey: Christopher's Minor Surgery. 8th ed.)

swallow, small amounts of water may be given. Nourishing liquids and a soft diet are added gradually. Fluids and foods should not be encouraged too much because vomiting, which increases intracranial pressure, may result. Solid foods are given as soon as the child can tolerate them.

As the child recovers from operation he should be helped to gain greater independence in his own care. He should be given opportunities to play alone and with other children. Parents need assurance that he should continue to be given independence after discharge. They should also understand that the child needs continued medical supervision after discharge.

**Course and Prognosis.**   The *course* depends on the type of tumor involved. Illness may last from a few weeks to several years. The *prognosis* for living into adulthood is very poor.

### Legg-Calvé-Perthes Disease (Perthes's Disease, Coxa Plana)

**Etiology and Incidence.**   Perthes's disease is an aseptic necrosis of the head of the femur. The cause is unknown.

It is a self-limited disease occurring in children between five and ten years of age. The condition affects boys more frequently than girls, possibly as a result of trauma to the hip.

**Pathology, Clinical Manifestations, Treatment and Prognosis.**   The *pathology* may be divided into three stages, each lasting about nine months or a year. The first stage is an aseptic necrosis. Roentgen films show a relative opacity of the epiphysis. The bone becomes necrotic. The second stage is revascularization. On roentgen study the epiphysis is shown as fragmented and mottled. The third stage is reossification. Roentgen examination shows the head of the femur to be gradually re-forming.

If weight is placed on the leg, the head of the femur tends to become flattened and mushroom-shaped. Later in life degenerative changes occur because of discrepancies in shape between the acetabulum and the head of the femur.

The *clinical manifestations* are those of synovitis, i.e. a limp and pain in the hip. The pain is often referred to the knee. Muscle spasm is not commonly severe. Restriction of motion is usually only in relation to abduction and rotation.

The most important point in *treatment* is avoidance of weight bearing. Some physicians believe that the child should have complete rest and traction on the leg during the course of the disease. Others immobilize the hip by surgery, casts or braces to prevent the deformity resulting from weight bearing.

The younger the child at the onset of the condition, the more likely is he to retain a spherical than to acquire a deformed, flattened head of the femur. Complete recovery depends on when treatment was given and whether gross deformity of the hip occurred.

## EMOTIONAL DISTURBANCES

By the time the child is six years of age his personality is fairly well established. He should be free to gain further skill in the use of his body and mind and to develop both stronger inner controls and relations with children and adults outside his family. The child needs time to achieve these goals; during the same period he is making a good adjustment at school.

If the child shows behavior problems or emotional disturbances during the school years, his response usually resembles some adult reactions to difficulties. The child may present (1) neurotic symptoms such as nervousness, finger-sucking, nail-biting and fears, (2) conduct disorders (the problem child), (3) language disorders such as stuttering, and (4) psychosomatic illnesses such as anorexia, overeating, constipation, colitis and enuresis.

These disorders, serious in themselves, may also prevent the child from making a good adjustment at school. Failure in school may thus be due to emotional disturbance as well as to mental retardation. The child who is overanxious and tense cannot concentrate on learning even if he has the intellectual capacity to achieve.

The teacher and the school nurse should be aware of such problems as they arise. They should be able to work with parents and other team members in order to help the child.

## NEUROTIC SYMPTOMS

Physicians often find it difficult to differentiate between normal behavior and neurotic behavior of children. Some behavior, however, when it is consistent, must be classified as neurotic.

### Nervousness

**Etiology and Clinical Manifestations.** Nervousness is not to be considered a separate condition in itself, but represents a group of symptoms. Nervous children are physically and mentally restless, overexcitable, timid and easily fatigued.

The inciting cause of nervousness may be a continued heavy load of anxiety or stress, or severe acute or chronic illness. Some children become nervous because of parental pressure to achieve. Children may also be nervous because they feel inferior to others, are overstimulated at play or acquire anxiety from their parents.

The *manifestations* of nervousness are easily recognized. The child is tense and restless, the pulse and respiration rates are increased, the movements are jerky, and the child's responses are too rapid.

**Treatment and Prognosis.** *Treatment* may be given by a physician or a psychiatrist, depending upon the severity of the problem. The child should have adequate nutrition and sleep without excessive excitement, discipline or stimulation to achieve in either motor ability or school work. The nervous child needs support and a well planned routine. Sometimes such a child may need to be placed in a new environment away from an anxiety-producing home.

The *prognosis* depends upon the cause and the management of the child and his problems.

### Finger-Sucking

The average child gives up thumb- and finger-sucking by the time he is two years old; others relinquish it by five or six years of age. If a child continues past this time and into the school age, investigation should be made into the life of the child and his parents to find out the cause of his neurotic behavior. Punitive measures or those producing physical prevention of the sucking activity—e.g. splints on the arms and bandages on the fingers—or making the practice unpleasant—such as putting bad-tasting lotions on the thumb or fingers—should be avoided.

If a child stopped sucking his fingers at an early age and resumed the habit at seven or eight years, he probably met an unsolvable difficulty in his development and regressed to gain satisfaction. Such difficulties include the birth of a sibling, the mother's leaving home to work, the death of a loved grandparent or moving to a new home. The treatment is to learn and correct the child's attitude toward the traumatic event.

### Nail-Biting

Nail-biting is an indication of tension. In general, it is initially an outgrowth of the child's attempt to manicure his nails. If the parents resist his attempts to gain satisfaction by nail-biting too traumatically, a parent-child conflict is begun. Severe nail-biting becomes an attempt by the child to humiliate and annoy the parents. It is physically painful to the child; thus he punishes himself for his hostility against his parents. The child should be given a manicure set as soon as he is able to use it and praised for his well kept hands. He should be helped to express his hostile feelings so that he no longer needs to bite his nails. The child's self-confidence should be increased in the home situation.

Imitation may also be important in nail-biting. The child may be simply imitating a parent who has the same habit. The parent may accept the behavior in himself, but not in the child.

### Fears

Since children live in a real world, they must develop certain fears based on dangers that actually exist in that world. Such things as bonfires and sharp knives should arouse a degree of fear in children that they will be harmed unless they take necessary precautions.

Fear of the dark, one of childhood's most common fears, is due, however, to the fact that in the dark the child feels alone and deserted. The dark may be peopled for him with dangerous persons of his fantasy. Parents should assure such a child that they have not deserted him and that they do not fear the dark.

Crippling anxiety replaces fear when there is an unconscious distortion of reality. The distortion occurs because the real situation is equated with an unconscious conflict or an anxiety-charged previous experience. Usually the exact meaning of the previous experience is repressed.

If such anxiety persists in spite of the child's experience which should disprove it or of the passage of time which should weaken the fear, some symbolic significance is attached to what is feared, and professional help should be sought.

Children should not be exposed thoughtlessly to situations which generate anxiety. If they are exposed, they can handle the anxiety best if they have secure relations with their parents and can talk about their fears or act out their feelings in relation to the fear.

### CONDUCT DISORDERS (THE PROBLEM CHILD)

**Etiology, Types, Management and Prognosis.** The child whom the parents and teachers call a problem child is usually merely trying to solve a problem with his behavior. Such behavior may occur in any socio-economic group. It usually occurs because the child's basic emotional needs have not been met. The problem generally arises because his methods of expressing his distress are limited. Such children may steal, be truant from school, hurt smaller children, tell dirty stories or engage in sex play. Behavior may be, but is not always, directed toward those who, the child feels, are responsible for his problems.

In the management of this problem the psychiatrist first of all gains the child's confidence. He does not blame the child for his behavior. He encourages the child to tell his own story. *Treatment* must be extended in every phase of the child's life. It may require a team approach to the whole problem, including parents, physician, teacher, spiritual adviser, scout leader, social worker and nurse. The child also should be a partner in making the therapeutic plan. Treatment is usually directed at the parent-child relations and at the child's feelings of inferiority over a variety of problems.

The outlook is usually good if these children are given the understanding help which they need.

## LANGUAGE DISORDERS

**Etiology and Incidence.**   The cause of any language disorder is usually complex. The *incidence* of speech defects is greatest between the ages of four and eleven years. Boys are more frequently affected than girls.

**Types, Diagnosis and Management.** There are three types of speech disorders: functional disorders such as stuttering; defects due to anatomic malformations such as cleft palate (see p. 463) and cleft lip; and defects due to central nervous system lesions such as cerebral palsy (see p. 476). The whole child must be considered when the diagnosis is made and management is planned. The type of management depends on the basic problem causing the speech disorder.

**Figure 256.**   Children who are truant from school may engage in extremely dangerous activities. (H. Armstrong Roberts.)

## Stuttering

Stuttering is the most common functional speech disorder. The child is unable to speak freely because of incoordination and spasmodic action of the muscles involved in speech. Although there is some question about the etiology, there is increasing evidence that stuttering is a symptom of a profound emotional disturbance. Some experts believe that the emotional disturbance may be due to an enforced change of handedness. Before treatment can be planned the child's physical, intellectual and emotional status must be ascertained.

Management then consists in reducing the child's anxiety about his stuttering and treatment of any other problem found in the evaluation. The child should receive adequate health care and be helped to gain insight into, and understanding of, his disorder. Usually the services of a psychiatrist and a speech therapist are needed.

### PSYCHOSOMATIC ILLNESSES

**Etiology.** Psychosomatic illness is a physical disturbance that has a psychologic origin. There may also be an organic basis for such an illness, but the element of emotions enters into the etiology. Every child may have emotional reactions which interfere with his bodily functions. The degree of interference and the location of the problem vary with the individual child. In school children several psychosomatic illnesses arise in connection with the gastrointestinal tract, including anorexia, overeating, constipation and ulcerative colitis. Enuresis (see p. 664) and asthma (see p. 571) may also be classified as psychosomatic illnesses in children. The diagnosis and treatment of psychosomatic illnesses are the joint responsibilities of the physician and the psychiatrist.

## Anorexia Nervosa

The child who has anorexia nervosa seems to have a relentless drive toward self-destruction through starvation. Such a child at first deliberately refuses food, even though he has an excellent appetite. Anorexia nervosa occurs only if the child has some deep emotional problem. Among girls there is often an intense conflict between mother and daughter. The girl is likely to have many misconceptions about pregnancy and indulges in sexual fantasies. As the period of starvation is prolonged, real anorexia and self-induced vomiting of food directly after it has been eaten produce rapid weight loss and bodily changes due to food deprivation. The child may gain sympathy from the family because of these symptoms.

Treatment includes correcting any electrolyte imbalance and increasing the diet. The child is usually hospitalized. Psychiatric consultation should be obtained.

Anorexia nervosa is a chronic condition, and the ultimate prognosis is questionable even with adequate medical and psychiatric therapy.

## Overeating

Overeating which results in the child's becoming extremely obese is usually thought to be due to his need for love, which he equates with food. It may also be due, however, to his wanting to grow big in size or to other emotional factors in his life. Treatment of a child who overeats is generally difficult. Many times the services of both a physician and a psychiatrist are necessary to curb the child's desire for food.

## Constipation

Many cases of so-called constipation in children exist only in the minds of the parents. They feel that their child is constipated because he does not have evacuations as often as the parents think he should. Nevertheless children do have true constipation, and on occasion it is based on emotional factors.

There are two main causes of this sort of constipation. One occurs in children who show disgust at any form of dirt, especially excreta. These children, in the toddler and preschool ages, before control of elimination was definitely established, feared that their parents would punish them even if they defecated at socially approved times and places, and hence became afraid of *all* defecation. This early fear conditioned them to feel anxiety about defecation even after control was thoroughly established, with the result that they restrained the normal need to have bowel movements. The usual treatment for this sort of constipation is to add a small amount of bulk to the diet and to praise the child whenever he becomes dirty during play periods. The older child may have the hygienic aspect of regular evacuation explained to him.

The other kind of constipation is due to excessive early toilet training and results in the child's feeling that excreting is a hostile act against his parents. Such a child needs psychiatric help in order to uncover and remove his fear of his own emotional reactions.

## Chronic Ulcerative Colitis

**Etiology.** This is an inflammatory condition whose cause is unknown. Several theories have been advanced about the etiology; the most commonly accepted theory is that it is a psychosomatic illness.

**Pathology and Clinical Manifestations.** Part or all of the colon may be involved, as may be the ileum. The mucosa may be largely denuded, and multiple longitudinal ulcers may form a network over the colon. There may be fibrosis, and the colon may be decreased in size.

The onset may be insidious or acute. The most important symptom is frequent passage of small stools containing mucus, blood and pus. Diarrhea may occur on occasion. There is usually no fever, abdominal pain or vomiting, although these symptoms may occur during exacerbations of the condition. Hemorrhage from the bowel or rectal prolapse may be a complication. Emaciation, anemia, nutritional edema and vitamin deficiencies may also be present.

**Diagnosis and Treatment.** The *diagnosis* is made on the basis of the history, lack of causative organisms in the stools, and finding of ulceration and inflammation on proctoscopic examination. When the condition is prolonged, the colon becomes a smoothly outlined tube.

There is no specific *therapy*. The diet should be soft and bland with a low residue. Additional vitamins and minerals should be given. Blood transfusions may be given for anemia. Temporary relief may be achieved with one of the corticosteroids. Ileostomy or colectomy may be done. The most encouraging plan of therapy is that carried out jointly by the pediatrician and the psychiatrist. Emotional and en-

**Figure 257.** Ulcerative colitis. This preadolescent is retarded in growth and emaciated as a result of his chronic illness. His height is approximately 132.9 cm., or 52.3 inches. That of the average boy of 11½ years is 148.1 cm., or 58.3 inches.

vironmental stresses should be relieved.

**Course and Prognosis.** The chronic course is interrupted by periods of remission and exacerbations. The disease may continue for years. Death is usually caused by exhaustion.

### Enuresis

Enuresis, or wetting after the age when toilet training should have been completed, is basically due to a battle between the child's wish to please his parents and a desire to excrete where he pleases. Although these children are usually normal, they should have a physical examination to rule out such conditions as pyelitis or nocturnal epilepsy.

Enuresis has many causes. One of the most serious causes is a basic personality or character maladjustment. These children need psychiatric help for their basic emotional problem. Other kinds of enuresis may perhaps be due to jealousy of a new sibling, revenge enuresis because of lack of love from parents or a regressive neurosis. Treatment of these types consists in changing the parents' attitude toward the child so that they can give him more love. Treatment by restricting fluids before bedtime, with charts of achievement or by mechanical devices to waken the child may cure the enuresis, but will not cure the basic problem.

Additional causes of enuresis in the school child include retardation, lack of toilet training or a situational type in which the child's bedroom is too far from the bathroom. Treatment here is easier than for the child with a severe emotional problem.

### THERAPY

Parents may make mistakes, and the child may not be too much affected. Too many mistakes, however, will affect the child's behavior. Parents are too close to the situation to see what is really happening. They may be bothered by the child's behavior, but may not realize the basic problem involved. Sometimes a child's behavior is up-

setting to parents even though it is only a manifestation of his growth. All that such parents need is an explanation of the normal growth and development of a child. Usually no therapy is required.

Professional help may be needed, however, if the cause of the problem is deep-seated and not understood by the parents. Such help may be required if the child (1) is afraid to leave his level of development and advance toward maturity, (2) is not growing and developing according to the usual pattern of maturation, (3) is oversubmissive, overaggressive or not learning at a rate commensurate with his ability, (4) cannot deal with frustrations or challenges in a way that is socially acceptable for a child of his age or (5) shows behavior characteristics which are socially unacceptable.

**Sources and Types.** Outside help may be gained from the family physician, pediatrician, psychiatrist, parent study group, teachers or guidance counselors.

Parents often hesitate to seek help for emotionally disturbed children. They feel that they should know all the answers. A psychiatrist would want a detailed history of the parents' development and problems, as well as a history of the child. He would also want to know the relations between parents and other family members.

The psychiatrist uses the kind of therapy he considers best for the individual child. He may believe that the problem is typical for a child of this age and will help the parents handle the particular problem; he may believe that it is largely the parents' problem and recommend a change of environment for the child or secure help for the parents; or he may believe that it is largely the child's problem and ask to see him frequently in order to help him gain an understanding of his problem and see other ways to handle his needs.

Prolonged therapy may be necessary. At times during such therapy the child's behavior may seem to become worse in that he may act out impulses that previously were under control. Parents need the help of the psychiatrist to understand what is happening and know how to deal with the child's behavior. The psychiatrist does not divulge the material which the child gives him without the child's permission. This is difficult for the parents to understand, but it is essential that they accept this element in the counseling situation.

**Role of the Nurse.** Children with emotional illness are being admitted to hospitals much more frequently than they were in the past.

The nurse who cares for children having psychosomatic illnesses or emotional disturbances must be able to observe their behavior accurately and record what she hears, feels and sees. Such observations help those who are treating these children, as well as helping the nurses themselves in the care of the children.

Close cooperation with the therapist is essential. The therapist can help nurses to understand the meaning of the behavior they observe and help them provide the kind of nursing care these children need. Therapists are interested in the child's relations with his parents, his peers and other adults in the environment. They would also like to know his adjustment to the hospital situation, to school and to play activities.

Group conferences of all team members, including physicians, social workers, school teachers, play therapists, nurses, aides and other auxiliary personnel who have contact with these children, are necessary. They help everyone to understand the care of the child as well as the cause of his illness. Such conferences often also help the nurse to understand her own personality and thus improve her relations to the children under her care.

## CLINICAL SITUATIONS

Mr. and Mrs. Brodinsky brought seven-year-old Sydney to the hospital for treatment of cryptorchidism. His parents appeared extremely anxious during his admission. They related that he had been their only child since his two siblings had been killed in an automobile accident shortly before his birth. Mr. and Mrs. Brodinsky are obviously devoted to Sydney and grant his every wish.

1. Sydney seemed tense and restless during the afternoon prior to his operation. He asked many questions about his condition. In order to allay his fears, the nurse would
   a. Encourage other children to talk with him and provide suitable recreation for him, but ignore his questions.
   b. Encourage Sydney's parents to stay with him as long as they can, explain to the family that many little boys his age have operations, and turn the topic of conversation to their home life.
   c. Ask the anesthetist and the surgeon to talk with Sydney about his fears and give him adequate sedation when he appears to be anxious.
   d. Answer Sydney's questions about his operation as simply as she can, inform him that she will go to the operating room with him and that she will be waiting with his parents in his room when he returns.

2. The type of operation done for cryptorchidism is
   a. Orchidopexy.
   b. Fredet-Ramstedt.
   c. Cryptorchidectomy.
   d. Diverticulectomy.

3. When planning her care of Sydney after the operation, the nurse realizes that one of her major responsibilities is to
   a. Cleanse the incision and the tension mechanism several times a day with 70 per cent alcohol.
   b. Protect the tension mechanism so that it is not disturbed.
   c. Remove the tension mechanism so that the genitals may be thoroughly cleansed.
   d. Restrain the child's hands so that he cannot touch the tension mechanism.

4. Two days postoperatively Sydney asked his nurse to leave the night light on in his room after she had prepared him for bed. The nurse should
   a. Laugh at him and tell him big boys should not be afraid of the dark.
   b. Scold him because he obviously wants more attention than the other children.
   c. Turn the light off because the night supervisor has said that the unit should be darkened when the children are prepared for bed.
   d. Accept his fear and ask him to turn the light off when he feels that he can.

Marsha Dullin, a nine-year-old girl, has been admitted to the pediatric unit with a diagnosis of rheumatic fever. She lives with her parents, three brothers and two sisters in an apartment in a tenement house. Her father is a manual laborer and the family income is $60.00 per week. On admission Marsha's temperature was elevated, and she complained of joint pains.

5. When Marsha was admitted to the hos-

pital, the nurse found nits in her long blond hair, but she could see no pediculi. The physician ordered applications of DDT powder. The nurse removed the nits by

    a. Washing Marsha's hair daily with soap containing hexachlorophene.

    b. Sliding each nit off its hair shaft after applying DDT powder.

    c. Applying benzyl benzoate lotion and brushing the nits out of the hair.

    d. Combing her hair with a fine tooth comb dipped in hot vinegar.

6. Marsha had been ill at home only a brief time before her admission to the hospital. She is fortunate that her illness was diagnosed and treated early because

    a. Cardiac damage can be minimized or prevented.

    b. Manifestations of chorea can be prevented.

    c. Spread of this infection to her siblings is minimized.

    d. Large amounts of medications will not be necessary in her treatment.

7. The most important point in providing nursing care for Marsha during the acute phase of her illness is

    a. Maintaining contact with her parents.

    b. Physical and psychologic rest.

    c. A nutritious diet.

    d. Maintaining her interest in school.

8. The physician has ordered sodium salicylate for Marsha. The nurse should be aware that some of the toxic symptoms of this drug are

    a. Tinnitus and nausea.

    b. Dermatitis and blurred vision.

    c. Unconsciousness and acetone odor of the breath.

    d. Chills and an elevation of temperature.

9. Significant instructions which Marsha's mother will receive before the child is discharged will concern

    a. A high protein diet, adequate immunization and avoidance of contact with anyone having an upper respiratory tract infection.

    b. Routine immunizations, limited activity and adequate nutrition.

    c. Adequate nutrition, avoidance of contact with anyone having an upper respiratory tract infection and prophylactic medication.

    d. Limited activity, sodium salicylate and a high vitamin diet.

10. Marsha's one desire before the onset of rheumatic fever was to be a ballet dancer. Now that she may possibly have some cardiac involvement, the team in long-range planning for her rehabilitation would

    a. Avoid all reference to dancing in their discussions with her.

    b. Investigate Marsha's feelings about her future and help her to consider other career interests.

    c. Assure Marsha that a career in danc-

ing would be possible if she promised to take care of herself.

    d. Ignore her questions related to dancing because this problem can be discussed later.

Elaine Watson, an eleven-year-old child, was admitted to the pediatric unit four weeks ago in diabetic coma. Both her parents and her two older sisters have shown a deep interest in her condition. Elaine is in the sixth grade in school. Her teachers are proud of her level of achievement.

11. In the management of juvenile diabetics, which one of the following factors is considered the *least* important?

    a. Taking of regular daily exercise.

    b. Prompt treatment of all infections.

    c. Maintenance of emotional stability.

    d. Treatment of allergies.

12. In evaluating Elaine's ability to care for herself the nurse believes that

    a. Elaine is too young to give herself insulin.

    b. A visiting nurse should teach Elaine to give herself insulin after she is discharged.

    c. Elaine should be taught to give herself insulin while she is in the hospital.

    d. Elaine's mother should assume the responsibility for insulin administration until Elaine is an adolescent.

13. When Elaine returns to school, she should certainly remember to carry with her at all times

    a. A lump of sugar.

    b. A bag of salted nuts.

    c. Her insulin and a syringe.

    d. Sufficient money to telephone her mother in case she feels ill.

14. Mrs. Watson asks the nurse whether she believes that Elaine should join the Girl Scouts of America. Although the mother should make her own decision, the nurse could base her comments on her belief that

    a. If her closest friends are members of the troop, she should join regardless of whether she wants to or not.

    b. The leader will teach her many things a young girl should know.

    c. Elaine will meet many girls her own age who share her interests.

    d. If Elaine joins, she will probably lose interest in her school work.

15. Mrs. Watson is concerned because Elaine's friends have recently begun to use lipstick. Elaine has expressed a desire to use it also. The nurse believes that

    a. Mrs. Watson should forbid the use of lipstick for another year at least.

    b. Mrs. Watson should permit Elaine to use it, but that she should teach her to apply it correctly.

    c. Mrs. Watson should explain to Elaine that the use of lipstick at her age is not refined.

d. Mrs. Watson should degrade the mothers of Elaine's friends because they have permitted their daughters to use lipstick.

## GUIDES TO FURTHER STUDY

1. The children's clinic in your hospital does not have a playroom. Plan the room, including the furniture and the equipment (creative materials, toys, records and books) that would be needed. Indicate the personnel necessary. In your planning indicate your knowledge of safety factors for children of various ages who will be using the room.

2. Joseph Rank, a seven-year-old boy whose mother had warned him repeatedly about playing with matches, was burned when he fell into a pile of burning leaves. What might Joseph's feelings be about this accident? What initial reaction would you expect from his parents upon learning of this tragedy? How could you as a nurse help both the parents and the child to verbalize and work through these feelings?

3. Eight-year-old Rebecca Schwartz was recently admitted to the pediatric unit with a diagnosis of diabetes. She is the only child of older parents. Her father has a small grocery business of his own. Rebecca is in the third grade in school and has average scholastic ability. Discuss in seminar the guidance this child and her parents will need. Role-play with another student the process of teaching this child regulation of diet, testing of urine and administration of insulin. Discuss the principles of learning to be considered as well as the content to be presented.

4. Discuss with a school nurse in your community her total program in relation to prevention of disease, treatment of illness, rehabilitation of the handicapped and health education of children. Is her program based on the level of growth and development and understanding of the children in her school? Has she taken into consideration the cultural background and the socioeconomic level of these children and their families? What is the role of this nurse in relation to the children's parents? In your discussion of this question in seminar give specific illustrations to support your answers.

5. During your experience in the pediatric unit you have been caring for a school-age child with a diagnosis of ulcerative colitis. Incorporate in your plan of care the recommendations of his psychiatrist. Did your patient show any change in behavior as a result of your altered approach? Discuss any problems you had in attempting to carry out the recommendations of the therapist.

6. You are providing care for two eight-year-old boys whose oral fluid requirements are greater than normal. On the basis of your understanding of growth and development, suggest ways by which you could help these children to cooperate with you in meeting this particular need.

## TEACHING AIDS AND OTHER INFORMATION*

*American Cancer Society*
A Cancer Source Book for Nurses, Reprinted 1959.

*American Diabetes Association, Inc.*
Facts about Diabetes, 1956.

*American Heart Association, Inc.*
Dodds, M.: Have Fun . . . Get Well, 1957.
Heart Disease in Children, 1958.
Home Care of the Child with Rheumatic Fever, 1959.
If Your Child Has Rheumatic Fever, 1955.
What the Classroom Teacher Should Know and Do about Children with Heart Disease, 1955.

*Children's Medical Center, Boston, Mass.*
Rheumatic Fever and Rheumatic Heart Disease.

*Eli Lilly and Company*
A Pocket Reference for the Diabetic.
Diabetes Mellitus, Methods of Dietetic Management and The Use of Insulin Preparations.
Keith and Ellen Win a New Look on Life!

*E. R. Squibb and Sons*
A Handbook for Diabetics.

*John Hancock Mutual Life Insurance Company*
Diabetes.
Diversions for the Sick, 1954.

*Public Affairs Pamphlets*
Conklin, G., and Conklin, L.: Good News about Diabetes.
Taubenhaus, M.: Rheumatic Fever.

*Science Research Associates*
Josselyn, I. M.: Emotional Problems of Illness.

*U.S. Department of Health, Education, and Welfare.*
Stop Rheumatic Fever, 1955.
The Child with Rheumatic Fever, 1955.

## REFERENCES

Bakwin, H., and Bakwin, R. M.: Clinical Management of Behavior Disorders in Children. 2nd ed. Philadelphia, W. B. Saunders Company, 1960.
Birchfield, M. O.: Easier Said than Done. Am. J. Nursing, 59:1566, 1959.
Blom, G. E.: The Reactions of Hospitalized Children to Illness. Pediatrics, 22:590, 1958.
Brooks, M.: Constructive Play Experience for the Hospitalized Child. Journal of Nursery Education, 12:7, Winter, 1957.
Brownell, K. D.: A Program to Prevent Rheu-
*Complete addresses are given in the Appendix.

matic Fever Recurrence. Children, 6:92, 1959.

Calafiore, D. C.: Streptococcal Infections. Nursing Outlook, 7:712, 1959.

Corrie, R., and others: Comprehensive Care for the Rheumatic Heart Patient. Nursing World, 133:8, Feb., 1959.

Dimock, H. G.: The Child in Hospital. Philadelphia, F. A. Davis Company, 1960.

Fischer, A. E., and Horstmann, D. L.: Handbook for Diabetic Children. 3rd ed. New York, Grune & Stratton, Inc., 1960.

Greenblatt, R. B., and others: Gynecologic Aspects of Sexual Precocity. Pediat. Clin. North America, 5:71, 1958.

Harvie, F. H.: Pediatric Methods and Standards. 3rd ed. Philadelphia, Lea & Febiger, 1958.

Hodges, L. R.: Tumors of the Brain. Am. J. Nursing, 58:58, 1958.

Ingraham, F. D., and Matson, D. D.: Neurosurgery of Infancy and Childhood. Springfield, Ill., Charles C Thomas, 1954.

Kaye, R. K.: Summer Camp for Diabetic Children. Am. J. Nursing, 54:972, 1954.

Kuskin, L., and Siegel, M.: The Changing Pattern of Rheumatic Heart Disease. J. Pediat., 49:574, 1956.

Lammers, M. A.: Where Children Take Heart. Am. J. Nursing, 56:854, 1956.

Larson, C. B., and Gould M.: Calderwood's Orthopedic Nursing. 4th ed. St. Louis, C. V. Mosby Company, 1957.

Liebman, S.: Emotional Problems of Childhood. Philadelphia, J. B. Lippincott Company, 1958.

Martin, M. M.: A Teaching Center for Diabetics. Am. J. Nursing, 58:390, 1958.

Martin, M. M.: Diabetes Mellitus: A Handbook for Nurses. Philadelphia, W. B. Saunders Company, 1960.

Idem: The Diabetic at Home. Am. J. Nursing, 56:1294, 1956.

Miller, J. M.: Prophylaxis of Rheumatic Fever and Rheumatic Heart Disease. New England J. Med., 260:220, 1959.

Mustard, H. S., and Stebbins, E. L.: An Introduction to Public Health. 4th ed. New York, Macmillan Company, 1959.

Nelson, W. E. (editor): Textbook of Pediatrics.

7th ed. Philadelphia, W. B. Saunders Company, 1959.

Ochsner, A., and DeBakey, M. E. (editors): Christopher's Minor Surgery. 8th ed. Philadelphia, W. B. Saunders Company, 1959.

Paterson, D., and McCreary, J. F.: Pediatrics. Philadelphia, J. B. Lippincott Company, 1956.

Rauen, K. M.: Learning to Live with Diabetes. Am. J. Nursing, 59:1290, 1959.

Richmond, J. B., and Lustman, S. L.: Total Health—A Conceptual Visual Aid. J. Medical Education, 29:23, May, 1954.

Roessler, M.: Cardiac Health Records. Am. J. Nursing, 58:365, 1958.

Rosen, H. G.: Camping for the Emotionally Disturbed. Children, 6:86, 1959.

Rosenthal, H., and Rosenthal, J.: Diabetic Care in Pictures. 3rd ed. Philadelphia, J. B. Lippincott Company, 1960.

Rusk, H. A., and Taylor, E. J.: Rehabilitation Medicine. St. Louis, C. V. Mosby Company, 1958.

Schwarz, B. E., and Ruggieri, B. A.: Parent-Child Tensions. Philadelphia, J. B. Lippincott Company, 1958.

Silver, H. K., Kempe, C. H., and Bruyn, H. B.: Handbook of Pediatrics. 3rd ed. Los Altos, California, Lange Medical Publications, 1959.

Stewart, M.: Role of the Nurse in Pediatric Rehabilitation. Health News, 33:4, 1956.

Stollerman, G. H.: The Etiology and Prevention of Rheumatic Fever. Postgrad. Med., 25: 376, 1959.

Taylor, F. M.: One Type of Undisciplined Child: A Behavior Syndrome. Am. J. Nursing, 58:842, 1958.

Terry, F. J., and others: Principles and Technics of Rehabilitation Nursing. St. Louis, C. V. Mosby Company, 1957.

Thompson, R. M.: The Cardiac Child at Home. Nursing Outlook, 9:77, 1961.

Wallace, H. M., and Starr, H. M.: School Services for Handicapped Children in Urban Areas. Am. J. Pub. Health, 50:173, 1960.

Whittemore, R.: The Effectiveness of Oral Penicillin Prophylaxis of Rheumatic Fever. A.M.A. J. Dis. Child., 96:618, 1958.

# The Pubescent
# and the Adolescent

# Chapter 24

# The Normal Pubescent

# and the Normal Adolescent: Their

# Growth, Development and Care

ADOLESCENCE is unique to human beings. All other mammals achieve sexual maturity early, but man, with his long period of dependency, achieves sexual maturity much later. Thus the sexual function takes on certain features peculiar to man. This refers to the point that man is a social animal and in his highest state of maturity is able to find a balanced integration between his social part and his animal nature. Adolescence, then, is the period when the young person is struggling to find this balance within himself.

A host of possibilities enter into the success or failure of this struggle: genetic factors, health, family constitution and attitudes, economic level, the culture of the group to which the adolescent belongs and the various educational, recreational and vocational opportunities afforded him or her by society at local, state and national levels.

In order to differentiate the terms used in this chapter, the following definitions are given. The *prepuberty* or *prepubescent* period refers to the period of rapid physical growth when secondary sex characteristics appear. *Puberty* may be said to have occurred when the girl begins to menstruate and the boy to produce spermatozoa. *Menarche* refers more specifically to the time of the first menstrual period. *Adolescence* begins when the secondary sex characteristics appear and ends when somatic growth is completed and the individual is psychologically mature, capable of taking his place as a contributing mem-

**671**

ber of society. It is a period of conflict, stress and anxiety, as well as one of self-realization and accomplishment.

By about ten to twelve years of age the individual begins his or her last period of life before adulthood. Before that time the child should have developed a sense of trust in others, a sense of autonomy in that he is a human being with a mind and a will of his own, a sense of initiative in that he wants to learn to do what he sees others doing, and, during school age, a sense of duty, industry or accomplishment of real tasks which he can carry through to completion. The young person who approaches puberty and adolescence has two additional strides to make in his personality development. These can be termed a *sense of identity* and a *sense of intimacy*. Adolescence ends gradually with the beginning of adult life—about eighteen years in our culture. The termination of adolescence may be prolonged to the midtwenties or later because of social and economic factors.

Although the chronologic age of ten years may be given as the beginning of prepubescence and the chronologic age of eighteen years as the end of adolescence, few specific times when definite changes occur may be given during this period. As the youth grows older, the span of time in which a specific step in development occurs becomes wider. It is therefore possible to describe only the over-all changes in growth and development which occur during prepuberty, puberty and adolescence. Adolescence is basically a time when the individual battles for recognition of his adulthood, and yet at the same time desires unconsciously to remain a child.

Many young people at some time during these years reach a period of emotional crisis or change, with the outcome not easily assured. Such a crisis may lead to backtracking in development or to further growth and maturing. This crisis provides a new chance for the individual to resolve emotional problems which were not resolved before and have remained quiescent for a time.

# OVERVIEW OF EMOTIONAL AND SOCIAL DEVELOPMENT

## *PUBERTY*

The pubescent period may be considered a pause of two or three years between childhood and adolescence. It is basically the organic phenomenon of adolescence. It is a period of rapid physical change and personality growth when the individual achieves nearly his adult bodily stature. Girls begin their preadolescent growth spurt by about ten years and boys by about twelve years. Between twelve and thirteen years for girls and one or two years later for boys, they reach the end of puberty. Children who, during school years, resembled each other in body build now show definite indications of belonging to one or the other sex, of becoming taller, shorter, thinner or more obese than others.

The child during pubescence shows strides in his personality development as well as in physical growth. He becomes increasingly more adaptable, approaching his group of peers and problem situations at home and at school with greater confidence. He enjoys games that involve not only physical skill, but also team cooperation. Although there is a revival of love for the parent of the opposite sex, he argues with his parents frequently. He is able to assume increasing responsibility in what to him is reality. Parents may not have the same values that the child holds during this period. The parents may want him to assume greater responsibilities around the home, but he may feel that his responsibility lies in helping his friends win a game or in completing a project he has started.

The pubescent seems able to handle important emotional problems easily. If a parent, grandparent or sibling dies, the child may appear on the surface to adjust very well, turning rapidly to other activities in his environment. Later, however, he may have to face the problem again because it was not worked through satisfactorily; it was only hidden from his own as well as an observer's view.

Parents become aware that during pubescence the hostility which previously existed between boys and girls is gradually disappearing. There is an interest in "dating," in going to mixed parties, especially dances, and in talking about members of the opposite sex. Such activities do not really mean that the children have become emotionally mature. They merely indicate that the youngsters are trying to leave the period of childhood and to assume the pattern of behavior of the adolescent or adult group.

The child realizes that he is inadequate in these initial attempts to be grown up. He knows that he is not mature and that most of his activity still centers around school, friends, play and home. Unfortunately, many parents try to capitalize on this step in development and urge more rapid development of interest in the opposite

sex than the child is ready for. There may be reasons for parental pressure in this area, not the least of which is their wish that the child be popular with both sexes, that he be well accepted in his total peer group. Severe pressure of this sort usually does not achieve the positive goal that parents might wish.

On the whole, however, puberty is a period of comparative quiet for the child and for the adults in his environment. He seems now to be a relatively independent person. Parents can reason with him and come to some kind of solution for their problems. Both the school and society expect that he understands the mores of his group. Behavior such as lying and stealing, which were not punished too severely in earlier years because of the child's immaturity, are now unacceptable because the child is presumed to know what behavior society expects. Adults expect that the child during puberty has made a fairly

**Figure 258.** Pubescents enjoy attending mixed parties, especially dances. These 13-year-olds are practicing the newest dance steps and at the same time are learning to get along with each other. (H. Armstrong Roberts.)

adequate adjustment to the demands of reality in our society.

## ADOLESCENCE (THE SENSE OF IDENTITY AND THE SENSE OF INTIMACY)

The transition from childhood to adulthood is not a smooth one. Adolescence is a period of stress for young people and parents alike. The adolescent must learn who he is and must modify his conscience for his adult role in life. He now questions many of the beliefs that he held as certain and true. Besides this intellectual and emotional upheaval, his rapid body growth causes him anxiety, and the cultural pressures of today's world cause further stress to be added to his uncertainty.

Adolescents today are faced with many pressures which the older generation did not have. The rapid rate of social change, the ever-threatening presence of war, increase in the speed of travel and rapid technological progress impose problems unknown in previous generations.

Perhaps more important is the fact that adolescents today are faced with a problem of finding employment at a time when they seek independence from home. The child labor laws, which greatly restrict adolescents in terms of employment, have had beneficial effects, but have also made problems for the individual. This in turn makes for great problems for schools in that compulsory education laws become exceedingly difficult to administer in view of the increasing number of adolescents who are actually uneducable. This refers not only to mentally retarded children, but also to those having emotional difficulties.

The adolescent begins to wonder exactly who he is and what his role in society is to be.

Erikson has called the central problem of the early period of adolescence

**Figure 259.** This adolescent wonders who she is and what her role in society will be after graduation from high school. (H. Armstrong Roberts.)

the establishment of a *sense of identity*.

The adolescent wonders how he appears and will appear to others in the future. Does he fit what society expects him to be? This is really a question about the continuity of the individual, from early childhood to adult years.

Adolescents in primitive societies have an easier time defining their role than do those in our culture. They have initiation rites which symbolize to themselves and to others that they are young adults. In our society confirmation, or acceptance into the Church, is a ceremony that has similar meaning to the young person. Graduation from grade school or junior high school and the ceremonies of various youth organizations may mean the same thing to the adolescent who belongs to them. Although these ceremonies are important, they do not have the significance to the individual that initiation rites have in primitive societies.

Nevertheless, even though the rites in primitive societies do add a meas-

ure of security to the individual youth's life, they take away the freedom of choice which children of our culture have.

Since our society does not have rigid rules, mores, customs and taboos which govern the behavior of adolescents, they themselves must organize them. Patterns of dress, behavior or prejudice are set down by the group and tend to make the members feel worth while. Unfortunately, such limits on behavior tend to form groups from which many young people are excluded. Those who are excluded then have a much more difficult time in gaining a sense of security and of identity.

The young person in our society may be disturbed not only because he is not certain of himself, but also because he is not certain of who he is to become. There are so many choices to be made in growing up, so many opportunities ahead, that instead of being comforting, they are confusing.

The adolescent who is not able to

**Figure 260.**    Ceremonies and activities of young people's organizations help them to understand their role in our society. (H. Armstrong Roberts.)

**Figure 261.** Adolescents enjoy activities in which both sexes can participate. Only through close relations with members of the opposite sex can these young people begin to understand each other and thus form a basis for the future selection of a marital partner. (H. Armstrong Roberts.)

face himself and life squarely, who has a feeling of *self-diffusion,* may become delinquent, neurotic or psychotic. The outcome of the adolescent's struggle to establish his sense of identity is dependent largely on what his personality development was during childhood. The problem is further complicated in our society for the individual who belongs to a minority group.

The child whose personality development was not adequate may be helped during pubescence and the adolescent years through psychiatric therapy or helpful guidance of teachers and others. Less fortunate is the child whose security during his early years was based on the mores of a minority group. During adolescence the individual may decide to reject his past and try to become a true American middle-class citizen. This step may be too difficult, and he may falter and become delinquent. Although many professional persons are trying to find an answer for this problem, it has no easy solution.

Although the sense of identity is difficult to achieve, the young person must gain it in order to be saved from emotional turmoil. He must be able to find for himself a meaning to life; he must be able to see clearly that life has continuity for him individually. Probably never before in history has youth faced the difficulty that it faces today in a world of rapidly changing values and ideas, a world facing destruction at the same time that the youth is trying to save himself.

After the youth has developed a sense of identity during early adolescence he should be able to develop a *sense of intimacy* with himself and with persons of both sexes. If the youth is not certain of himself, he will not be able to form close ties of friendship or love with other people.

During the school period children are preoccupied with achieving a sense of identity with other members of their own sex. They imitate the activities of adults of their own sex. Although closer relations between boys and girls begin during pubescence, they are not intimate relations and serve only as settings for discussion of what they think and feel. During later adolescence these relations serve another purpose. They help to resolve the individual's preoccupation with the integration of the sexual function. They help one young person to unite with another. If the young person cannot do this because of his lack of a valued personality, he may become an isolate who keeps his relations with others on a cool, rigid, formal basis. If such a person rushes into an early marriage, it will probably fail because, lacking the ability to know himself, he is not able to know and love another.

During the time when the healthy adolescent is establishing his sense of intimacy he has a real struggle with sexual feelings. This new force drives the individual to his peers. In the healthy adolescent this does not lead to the sexual act, although some physical expressions of affection are common. Such an adolescent does not usually want to proceed with the sexual act, because this involves a feeling of loss of independence. Sexual promiscuity in adolescence is usually an attempt to find an infantile relation rather than a mature form of psychosexual development.

Unfortunately our culture places less emphasis on the young person's developing a sense of intimacy than it gives to his becoming independent and industrious. In our materialistic society the emphasis is often on success, not success in interpersonal relations, but success in the competitive world of work. For this reason many "successful" young people and adults have not developed the ability to understand the personality of others. They tend to be unhappy even though to the world they may appear to be highly successful.

### Problems of the Adolescent

The adolescent must face five important problems and find a solution to them if he is to gain a sense of identity and a sense of intimacy and to reach some degree of emotional maturity as an adult. These five problems are (1) integration of his personality for future responsibility, (2) emancipation from his parents and family, (3) creation of satisfactory relations with the opposite sex, (4) acceptance of a new body image after the rapid physical changes of this period, and (5) a decision about the vocation he will follow as an adult. If his development to puberty has been satisfactory, then these goals will not be too difficult, provided parents and other adults will give him the help and guidance he needs. All too frequently, however, much friction and misunderstanding between parents and their adolescent children exists, making the process of growing up more difficult than it might be.

**Integration of Personality.** By the time the child reaches adolescence he should already have made a beginning toward the integration of his personality. He should have some consistent ways of acting in certain situations. He should have a healthy way of meeting reality, of doing something constructive in problem situations. If he has not reached this point in development, he may enter adolescence shy, anxious and with a desire to retreat and isolate himself when a problem arises. He may avoid social contacts and responsibilities whenever possible. Such a person, without help, may complete adolescence poorly equipped to face life.

In order to achieve integration of personality the adolescent must participate in society as a whole, not only in relation to himself as an individual. He must be able to accept people—friends, and then later his wife, children, neighbors and those of cultures other than his own. He should refrain from being too critical of others and should try to see their point of view. He should take part in the life of the larger community. He must have a deep feeling of willingness to help others in order that he may achieve a feeling of social unity and thus gain social strength.

**The Adolescent and His Family.** Parents, teachers and other adults may not be as important to the adolescent as they were previously. He may be hostile to them and resent their authority. The adolescent is torn between his need for support and acceptance, to be dependent as a child, and his need for independence. He must defend himself against his unconscious love for the parent of the opposite sex and resolve his ambivalence toward the parent of the same sex. Although parents may consider the adolescent unmanageable and say that they cannot understand him, they should recognize his growing feelings of maturity and also his occasional need for help.

The adolescent, instead of wishing to be like the parent of the same sex, may attempt to be as different as possible. He may even ridicule his parents at home, but still evaluate them highly outside the home. Affection is turned from the parents to adults outside the family. This begins a series of brief "crushes" typical of adolescence. The adolescent loves the adult, desires to please him and identifies with him. The young adolescent thus makes some of the characteristics—a trait, a manner of speaking, a skill—of the adult a part of his own personality. Often the adult, whether a teacher, Scout leader, relative, minister, priest, rabbi, physician or someone in public life, never realizes the effect he has had upon these young people. Many times parents who do not wish their child to grow up resent the fact that another adult is imitated in this way.

On the other hand, such relations may be extremely helpful for the adolescent and his family. A trusted, respected adult outside the family can help the adolescent find himself and his role in life more easily than can the parent, who may be less objective. Such an adult can help the adolescent clarify his thinking, work out his solution and find more mature patterns of behavior. When an adolescent reaches this point, his behavior gradually becomes determined by his own judgment rather than by controls imposed from outside. His parents and friends become less frustrating, and his hostility toward them diminishes.

Some parents need as much help and understanding as their adolescents do. Having had stormy periods of adolescence themselves, they may have acute apprehension over the trials of their own children. If they do not get the help they need, they may be either too strict or too lenient in setting limits to their children's behavior. Neither of these extremes provides the help which youth needs at this crucial time. The adolescent needs acceptance and guidance as a growing individual. Only in this way can he discover his limitations and powers.

The adolescent's relations with his siblings may become exceedingly strained. This is especially true of a boy whose younger sister has already reached puberty and left him behind in growth. Yet both the brother and the sister should feel more confident about approaching the problems of adolescence, especially in adjusting to the opposite sex, because they have learned the acceptable patterns of behavior from each other.

In some families younger siblings may place an adolescent sister or brother in the role of a parent-substitute. This kind of identification is probably not harmful if it does not interfere too much with the adolescent's own development and social activities.

The battle for independence is fought in practically every family. The parents fight to maintain authority and prestige in the eyes of the young person, and the young person fights for liberty. The youth who fights such a battle should probably be less a source of worry than one who causes no conflict over his strivings to become independent. The latter will probably stay emotionally in childhood and not weather the storm of the adolescent period.

Adolescence is the ideal time for children to begin to have their own lives. Unfortunately parents often say that they want their children to mature, but block them at every turn. The greatest harm that parents can do is to expect the worst from their children, because then they will probably get it. If parents expect the best, children are more apt to live up to this expectation.

Emancipation from the family is difficult because both sides have their own problems. The adolescent is often reluctant to accept responsibility and fears criticism if he does accept it. At the same time that he needs to feel cared for he lacks a desire to cooperate with adults who could give him this feeling of security. Parents also usually unconsciously have their problems. They have great difficulty sharing the adolescent's love with others. They tend to underestimate the adolescent's strength to function away from them. They may desire to continue dominating the adolescent. They may say that they fear that he will be harmed if he leaves home. The mother often feels these problems to a greater degree than the father does, since she is left alone while he works.

Any activity of daily living may be the basis of conflict: the time of leaving or coming home, whether the car may be used, whether the adolescent may have a key to the house, the selection of clothes, and the like. The adolescent should gain emancipation slowly. Just as his parents should try to understand his role in this conflict, so he should attempt to understand their problems.

If parents and child build a good foundation during the first six years of life, these battles will not wreck the adolescent's life. Parents must let the youth develop his judgment and skills, tell him the truth and avoid attacking or ridiculing him.

There has been a tendency in recent years to be too permissive with adolescents, perhaps as a reaction to the former trend to handle all young people too rigidly. Some limits are still important. A tolerant parent does not have to condone completely everything the adolescent does. One of the most difficult problems parents face is the establishment of a relation that enables them to give their adolescent children the freedom they need while assuring their acceptance of guidance.

Eventually the adolescent's anxiety decreases, and his return to the more immature relation with his parents is no longer necessary. He is then able to have a mature, interdependent relation with them and others because his independence is more confidently maintained.

**The Adolescent and His Friends.** The young adolescent who becomes a group member is fortunate because then the whole group repudiates adult influence and tends to strengthen the individual's concept of his own capabilities. His ideas are dominated by the social and ethical codes of his friends in the group. Fads are important, whether they involve clothes or behavior. The adolescent must be accepted by his group to feel secure. He may not express his individuality beyond the limits imposed by the group.

As a result of mutual soul-searching by individual members of the group, standards concerning basic concepts of living are worked out. Attitudes about morality, ethics, religion and social customs are formulated and adopted by group members. The group thus plans how the individual member should behave and becomes an island of security in what seems to be a confused world.

As soon as an adult leader is introduced, this function of the group is lost. The young people are no longer fully able to develop themselves as individuals or to learn how to get along with their peers.

The child who does not reach puberty at the same time as others may have various emotional problems that are difficult for him to solve. He may find himself alienated from his peer group, yet not accepted by a younger or older group. Children who reach puberty late are especially at a disadvantage because feeling weak and less capable physically and physiologically causes their pride to be hurt.

Adolescents may develop a strong bond of friendship with just one or possibly two other adolescents of their own sex. This relation is based on similarities in interest, age and personality factors. Such friendships are important to personality development. These

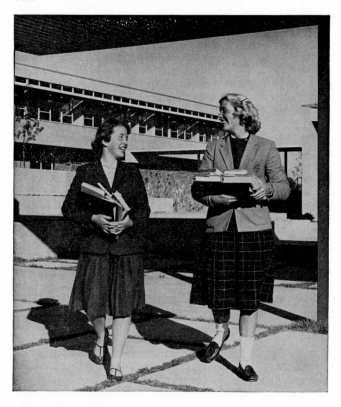

Figure 262. Close friendships are formed during adolescence. These friendships are characterized by a more mature understanding of each other's needs than was possible during earlier periods of development. (H. Armstrong Roberts.)

friends are devoted to each other and become inseparable. They have a relatively mature understanding and appreciation of each other's needs, reacting without the selfishness evident in earlier periods of development. Such friends share each other's ideas, deepest secrets, and troubles, and thus develop a sense of responsibility and loyalty to others that had not existed before. A great deal of whispering is evident in these friendships.

These relations help the young adolescent girl especially to break away from her attachment to her mother. Boys do not seem to have the intense friendship with other boys that girls have with other girls. Boys work out their feelings in horseplay, teasing and wrestling.

Gradually short-term attachments develop with members of the opposite sex which tend to break up these intense friendships with members of the same sex.

**Adjustment to the Opposite Sex.** When interest develops in the opposite sex, great secrecy surrounds it at first. When the boy sees a group of girls, he may perform acrobatics to attract their attention. He may say to himself and others that he was "just getting some exercise." The girls may giggle in response to attract the boy's attention.

Later, real interest and love affairs of a romantic nature develop. These are usually between a girl and a boy one or two years older than she because of the difference in physical maturation rates of the two sexes. These attachments are usually short-lived, but they do give those concerned some knowledge of the personality characteristics of the opposite sex which will help later when each is in a better position to fall in love.

To establish heterosexual relations the adolescent must rebel against and free himself from the forbidding infantile conscience. If he reduces his inner standards too rapidly, his anxiety becomes intolerable, and he tries even harder to control himself. Although he resents his parents' authority, the adolescent may at this time seek their control. He may also turn to religion or to the pursuit of intellectual interests to reduce his conflict. Ultimately his fear of his instincts will lessen, he will learn to control himself, and he will become able to enjoy pleasures which are needed for his growth.

Since marriage and parenthood lie just ahead for many adolescents, the two sexes must become accustomed to each other and learn to know each other well. Adolescents get practice in this by participation in dances, picnics, and the like. Physical expressions such as hand holding, kissing and embracing are normal functions of a person preparing for marriage.

In their efforts to develop an understanding of the other sex adolescents are often inhibited by adults. Parents are afraid that if young people are too much interested in the opposite sex,

they will marry too soon and be unable to finish their education or support themselves well. They are afraid of illegitimate pregnancy, disease, and disgrace to the family. The adolescent needs help from parents in accepting a masculine or feminine role and in understanding sex drives. Parents often do not remember that if good parent-child relations have existed, if the young person has been given adequate sex education and has been taught social responsibility and consideration for others, he will usually abide by his parents' wishes concerning sex behavior during adolescence. Young people should have an opportunity to mix with each other without anxiety and shame.

Many parents discourage young people from "going steady." They are afraid that the adolescents will be hurt when the friendship ends. Although the young people may be disappointed for a while, they have probably learned a great deal from their contact with each other, especially how to evaluate each

**Figure 263.** During later adolescence a young man and a young woman may single each other out from a large group of friends and prepare seriously for marriage. (H. Armstrong Roberts.)

other in terms of compatibility, which will be of great help when they select a marriage partner. Parents can give emotional support when such a relation ends. Actually, "going steady" helps young people to learn much more than they would gain from many short-lived, superficial relations.

If the child has had adequate sex education as he was growing up, if he was taught respect for others in these matters, and if he has had religious training on which he can base his decisions about his conduct, few problems are likely to arise during the adolescent years. Adolescents may need guidance, however, on specific problems that may arise in relation to their assuming an adult role. The adolescent must be helped to understand the moral and social customs that should govern his conduct in the matters of "dating" and sexual intercourse. He should be helped to find outlets for his interests that are socially acceptable.

Threatening the adolescent does more harm than good and may only serve to encourage the very behavior that adults have termed undesirable. The adolescent can thus rebel against adult authority and standards in a way that may be disastrous to him. Since the conduct of adolescents is controlled not only by what adults say, but also by what the group dictates, it is vitally important that the individual be a member of a group that upholds society's standards of conduct.

### Emotional Maturity

No one ever really becomes emotionally mature in all facets of his personality. There is always some development of the past that is incomplete, although the stages of development are the very cornerstones upon which a mature personality is built.

Theoretically, an emotionally and physically mature person is able to face reality, to use good judgment, to select a mate, to provide a home and to rear his children wisely. He should be able to meet responsibilities and get pleasure from activities participated in alone or with others. He should be able to balance responsibility and pleasure in a way that keeps him free from tension. Yet while he is master of himself and of his world, he should be humble, recognizing his own limitations as well as those of reality.

The mature person should be able to accept dependency of others and to be dependent himself when necessary. This capacity for mutual dependency is a crucial part of social living.

A mature person believes in himself and in others who love him and whom he loves. He is able to deal wisely with those who dislike him and whom he dislikes.

Toward this goal the adolescent must work. He must formulate a code of behavior and a philosophy of life that are his own. These must be based on his individual decisions, but both are influenced to a great degree by previous family life, by teaching in school and church, by all his contacts in his lifetime and by all the experiences he has lived through.

### OVERVIEW OF PHYSICAL DEVELOPMENT

During puberty and adolescence the young person not only makes great strides toward emotional maturity, but also reaches physical and physiologic maturity. Changes in physical appearance as a result of physical development may cause disturbances in emotional well-being.

### Puberty

Pubescence is associated with the child's reaching sexual maturity. During the year or two preceding puberty rapid changes occur in the rate of growth in weight and height, in body contours and in the physiology of the body as a result of maturation of the gonads and hormonal activity. These changes usually continue to puberty, which occurs by about twelve to thirteen years, with a range of eleven to fifteen years in girls and a year or two later for boys. Girls tend to develop more rapidly than boys and to maintain their lead until they reach adult maturity.

Physical changes in the boy include, in order of appearance, (1) increase in size of the genitals, (2) swelling of the breasts, (3) growth of pubic, axillary, facial and chest hair, (4) voice changes, and (5) production of spermatozoa. Boys grow rapidly in shoulder breadth from about the age of thirteen years.

Boys can become disturbed by nocturnal emissions, the loss of seminal fluid during sleep. If they have not been told that this is normal, they may regard it as a disease, or a punishment because of masturbation or thinking too much about sex. They may also believe that it is devitalizing to them. Nocturnal emissions are due to the activity of the sexual glands, and occasional release of spermatic fluid during sleep should cause no concern to boys. If they are not adequately prepared for this phenomenon, they ask either their father or their friends about it. Boys generally are able to talk more freely among themselves than girls are and therefore usually find a solution to this problem.

Changes in the girl, in order of appearance, include (1) increase in the transverse diameter of the pelvis, (2) development of the breasts, (3) change in the vaginal secretions, and (4) growth of pubic and axillary hair. The onset of menstruation occurs between the appearance of pubic hair and that of axillary hair. Girls begin to have broad hips from about the age of twelve years on.

Because of lack of adequate information, girls may have ambivalent feelings about menstruation. They may resent the fact that they cannot completely control all their bodily functions, and may therefore consider menstruation a burden.

Many parents do not adequately explain to girls the various changes in body contour indicative of puberty. Before puberty and adolescence the child should be well oriented as to the anatomic and functional differences between the sexes. The girl should have a clear conception of ovulation, fertilization, pregnancy and birth. She should certainly have been told about the process of menstruation before it occurs. Especially in discussing menstruation, adults are likely to pass on to their children the same beliefs and taboos which were told to them. They may say that the girl should rest or not participate in social activities during the menstrual period, thus implying that she is not well.

Menstruation is a normal physiologic phenomenon. There is no reason why women should curb their normal activities at this time. Menstruation is not debilitating. The blood loss is quickly made up. If mothers would only stress that menstruation is a normal phenomenon, young women would have fewer problems in relation to this process.

Other physical changes also occur in children of both sexes at adolescence. The sebaceous glands of the face, back and chest become more active. If the pores are too small, sebaceous material cannot escape, so that it collects beneath the skin and produces pimples or acne (see p. 693). Perspiration is increased. Vasomotor instability produces blushing.

Growth in height tends to decrease each year from birth, but with the onset of pubescence there is a rapid increase, and the child becomes tall. Gain in weight is proportionately greater than gain in height during early adolescence; therefore the adolescent appears to be stocky in appearance. This adolescent obesity has an important effect from both a physical and a psychologic standpoint.

There are differences in the rate of growth of various organ systems in the individual adolescent. The skeletal system often grows faster than its supporting muscles. This difference in growth rate tends to cause clumsiness and poor posture. Since large muscles may grow faster than small ones, the child is likely to lack coordination. His extremities, his hands and feet, may grow out of proportion to the rest of his body and cause more problems in coordination.

Since the heart and lungs usually grow more slowly than the rest of the body, the supply of oxygen may be inadequate, and the child may feel constantly tired.

The young girl or boy, and sometimes their parents, not realizing that this is just a stage every adolescent must go through, may feel inferior and socially embarrassed by these bodily changes. The youth may try to compensate for his supposed inferiority by ridiculing others, by trying to force his body to behave and to appear better by exercising and dieting, by attracting attention to himself by giggling and fidgetiness or by developing his intellect so that his physical appearance can be tolerated. Other pubescents may withdraw so that they cannot be compared with others. Parents should not scold or ridicule a child at this stage. Further growth will correct many of the problems. Instead, children should get from their parents reassurance and help to face the conflict between the image of themselves as they would like to be and as they are.

At puberty the child is flooded with new sensations and feelings which he cannot understand. This is one of the reasons why the youth may be alert and interested in everything for a time and then shortly after be bored, withdrawn and disinterested. By withdrawing, he is able to assimilate and digest the incoming sensations. This developmental phenomenon may occur about the time the child is thirteen years old. He may do poorly in school for about a year at this time. Parents and teachers can help him by being patient and by explaining to him that this is just a period in his growth. Certainly he should not be ridiculed at this time.

Motor behavior is influenced by the rapid changes taking place in the body. The young adolescent may appear awkward in his gross body movements because of his difficulty in adapting to these changes and because of his fear of ridicule, although he is actually gaining in strength and skill. As a result of rapid growth, pubescents may not have sufficient energy left for activity; therefore they may tire easily from their efforts.

Girls do not usually develop the gross motor ability that boys do. This may be partially due to the fact that girls have many interests other than sports.

When rapid physical changes and changes in motor skill occur, the pubescent may become intensely interested in his physical appearance. During preadolescence he created an image of what he would be like as an adult. If what he is becoming is unlike his previous image, he may become uncertain of himself and of his body. Parents should help the young adolescent to make a realistic appraisal of his appearance and to make the most of his outstanding qualities.

### Adolescence

After the pubescent years growth slows in rate, and the change in body proportions occurs more gradually. The adolescent must continue to live with organ systems and functional capacities of widely varying levels of maturity. Usually by fifteen to sixteen years the secondary sex characteristics have developed fully and adolescents are capable of reproduction. During the first year or longer of menstruation, periods are frequently missed or are irregular. Conception is unlikely until a year after periods have begun and usually does not occur until around the sixteenth year.

By this age the adolescent's motor abilities are similar to those of adults; thus adolescents can perform tasks which require muscular control and skill. Parents must guard against the adolescent's trying to live up to that part of his development which is most advanced, such as stature. They must try to help him set limits to his own behavior as a result of understanding the problems involved.

At the end of adolescence the young person appears physically like an adult. His head is approximately one eighth of his body length. When his wisdom teeth erupt, between eighteen and twenty-three years of age, he has his full set of thirty-two permanent teeth.

## SPECIFICS OF PHYSICAL, EMOTIONAL, SOCIAL AND MENTAL DEVELOPMENT

Pubescence and adolescence are best understood if they are considered a period of accelerated maturation and not a span of a certain number of years with specific steps in development to be accomplished each year. To subdivide this span of years is artificial, since development proceeds in individuals at varied rates. The rate of growth and development depends on all the factors mentioned throughout this text: heredity and constitutional make-up, racial and national characteristics, sex, environment—including prenatal envi-ronment—socio-economic status of the family, nutrition, climate, illness and injury, exercise, position in the family, intelligence, hormonal balance, and emotions.

## School

Adolescents as a group can do much more abstract thinking than they did when they were in the lower school grades. As their school subjects become more complex, there is a period of rapid increase in vocabulary and language development. Unfortunately, however, mental growth is not exactly correlated with increase in size. Parents and teachers should therefore not expect more mentally from a young person simply because of his rapid increase in physical size.

**Figure 264.**   After the pubescent years the rate of growth slows and changes in body proportions occur more gradually. These young people are 17 years of age and have nearly achieved their adult size. (H. Armstrong Roberts.)

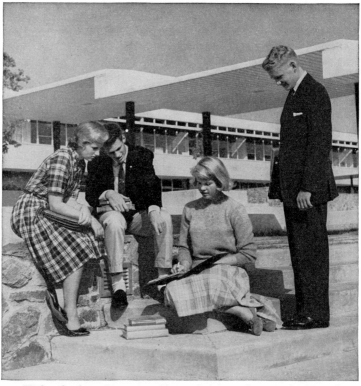

**Figure 265.** High school students are able to do more abstract thinking than they could when in elementary school. They involve themselves deeply in academic subjects that interest them. (H. Armstrong Roberts.)

Adolescents have some difficulties in adjustment to school. They may spend more time in extracurricular activities than in academic work. They may be so disturbed by the problems inherent in adolescence that they may not be able to concentrate long enough to study. The school, recognizing that such problems exist, should offer activities that will help them find answers to their problems and satisfy their social needs.

There is great variation in the degree of academic ability and interest of individual adolescents. A few excel in all areas, more excel in a few areas, and some excel in no areas. Often the degree of interest in school is based on the ultimate goal the adolescent has set for himself. If he needs further academic preparation leading to a professional role in the future, he will apply himself to his studies. If his goal is to be an unskilled laborer requiring no additional preparation, he may not see the necessity of achieving a level of excellence in his high school work.

Besides offering academic preparation for adult life, high school offers the adolescent opportunities in extracurricular activities for satisfying his needs for security, recognition and success for himself and his group. Adolescents should have opportunities to develop intellectual and physical skills and to satisfy their interests in areas such as crafts, music and art.

School programs should take into consideration the stage in development each child is going through. This is especially essential since the children in any one class may be prepubescent, pubescent or early adolescent, depending on their rate of growth.

Parents should continue to take an

interest in the school life of the adolescent. They should also invite him to some of the social activities of adults in the community. They may contribute to the development of youth by providing occupations which give adolescents a way to make money and an outlet for their energies. It has been said that high school activities such as sporting events, dances and parties are too expensive and that this is one reason why some children develop feelings of inferiority in their group and a desire to leave school before graduation. Adults in the community can help such children by providing opportunities for them to make their own money for these purposes.

Adults may also assist adolescents in their selection of a vocation by being willing to talk to groups about their own vocational choices.

### Play and Work

During pubescence and adolescence the sex of an individual makes more of a difference than ever in play and work interests.

Girls develop interests in social functions such as parties and dances, romance, housekeeping and child rearing responsibilities. They enjoy romantic motion pictures and television programs. They may spend hours making themselves more attractive, experimenting with hair styles, cosmetics and new clothes. They learn to cook, clean and sew. Their interests widen in such fields as art, poetry and music. They, as well as boys, may spend a long time talking on the telephone to someone they have just seen a short time before the telephone conversation began.

Boys are usually interested in competing and excelling in sports activities. They develop team loyalty and spirit. They are interested in mechanical things such as cars. Their acceptance in the group depends not so much on personal appearance as on their manliness, physical abilities and ability to complete a job.

Adolescents enjoy part-time work by which they can earn spending money for themselves. They may serve newspapers, mow lawns, shovel snow or care for young children. Although these activities have little relation in most cases to their ultimate work in life, the

**Figure 266.** The interests of adolescents vary. *A,* Some enjoy creating their own clothing. *B,* Some enjoy seemingly endless telephone conversations. (H. Armstrong Roberts.)

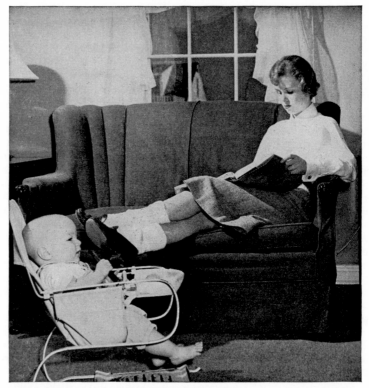

**Figure 267.**   Adolescents enjoy earning some, if not all, of their own spending money. (H. Armstrong Roberts.)

way they carry out their responsibilities gives some indication of their level of industry in whatever work they perform as adults. The adolescent thus learns to work with others, to cooperate even with those to whom he has no real personal attachment. He should find satisfaction in knowing that he has done a job well and that he can contribute in some way to society.

Adolescents gain great satisfaction from working for a worth-while cause. Feelings of altruism are well developed at this age, and the individual and the group can make valuable contributions to a worth-while effort.

### Choice of Vocation

Three types of vocation face the young person: the vocation of citizenship, the vocation which will make a living for himself and his family, and the vocation of parenthood. Parents should be honest with their children and tell them the problems involved in each type of vocation.

Probably the vocation which the adolescent believes is most immediately important is that of a career. The attitude among some groups that everyone will be taken care of, that adolescents need not worry about working, is an unhealthy one. The adolescent girl should probably prepare for both a career and marriage.

The adolescent should be guided in vocational preparation with consideration for his limitations and capacities. Simply that the father wanted to be a physician all his life is no reason why the son should be encouraged to study medicine. The young person can make his best contribution to society by doing something he is sincerely interested in. It is unfortunate if an adolescent's desires about his future must be changed because of his socio-economic status or level of intelligence. Guidance in vocational choice is essential if the young person is to avoid such a disappointment or is to make plans so that he can achieve his goal.

## CARE

The adolescent, after his attention has been turned to the opposite sex, becomes very much aware of how he appears to others. Parents are usually amazed at the change in the young person's behavior at this time. He becomes unusually clean, neat in dress and careful of grooming. Appearance is of the utmost importance socially. After this time parents need have little concern about the daily care of the adolescent, other than to see to it that he gets adequate rest and a balanced diet. Adolescents require about eight to nine hours of sleep a day. They require a higher caloric intake than ever before because of their rapid growth.

### Safety Education

Although much effort in the home, in schools and in youth organizations has gone into safety education for young people, the accident rate among adolescents continues to be distressingly high. In the teen-age group the greatest cause of accidents is motor vehicles. In an effort to reduce mortality and morbidity from this cause, many schools offer driver-training and safety programs for older children. Adolescents must learn to discipline themselves in order to become safe and courteous drivers, to save their own lives as well as those of others.

Other causes of accidental death important during the adolescent years are drowning and firearms. These kinds of accidents are largely preventable. Young people should learn to swim and should be taught to use firearms safely, if they are interested in using them at all.

To a degree adolescents must be safeguarded to prevent physical trauma

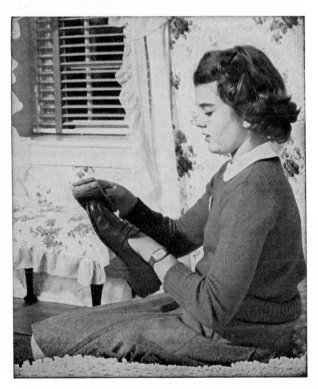

**Figure 268.** Adolescents become very much aware of their appearance. (H. Armstrong Roberts.)

when they want to do something beyond their physical endurance.

## NUTRITION

Adolescents must receive adequate nutrition, especially at the time of their greatest growth. Appetite usually poses no problem at this time. Adolescents are known for their propensity to raid the refrigerator.

Because of rapid growth the girl may need 2600 calories daily and the boy 3600 calories. Table 11 gives the nutritional requirements of adolescent boys and girls at different ages. The difference in nutritional requirements between the sexes is due largely to the difference in ultimate size and the fact that boys in general have a greater interest in physical activity than do girls.

As soon as interest in personal appearance develops, girls especially may resent the fact that they seem to be gaining too much weight. They may go on a diet which may be a danger to their health. Parents should supervise the adolescent's diet without being obvious about it. The adolescent may have practice in planning meals, in marketing and in balancing a day's meals and thereby learn the essentials of an adequate diet. This is especially important in order that the young woman may be in a state of adequate nutrition

when she is married and begins her childbearing period.

Both parents and school personnel should educate young people in the essentials of a good diet, because often adolescents tend to drink too many carbonated beverages and to eat too many cookies and candies. Since group consciousness is strong, at times a whole group must be helped toward an understanding of better eating habits. They should learn that only by eating a diet that includes meat and other protein foods, vegetables, fruits, whole grain cereals and milk will they achieve the health status in adulthood that is desired. The teenager's interest in his own health and appearance can be used to encourage wholesome food practices.

During this period approximately 15 per cent of the total calories should be derived from protein so as to maintain a positive nitrogen balance. This means that the adolescent should receive 75 to 100 gm. of protein a day. This may be obtained from milk, eggs, meat and cheese. He needs a quart of milk to provide 1.3 gm. of calcium. He also needs about 400 International units of vitamin D a day to absorb adequately and retain calcium in his body.

## HEALTH SUPERVISION

Adolescents in the past were cared for largely by pediatricians or general

*Table 11.   Recommended Daily Dietary Allowances for Pubescents and Adolescents*

|  | Boys | | Girls | |
|---|---|---|---|---|
|  | 13–15 Years | 16–19 Years | 13–15 Years | 16–19 Years |
| Calories | 3100 | 3600 | 2600 | 2400 |
| Protein | 85 gm. | 100 gm. | 80 gm. | 75 gm. |
| Calcium | 1.4 gm. | 1.4 gm. | 1.3 gm. | 1.3 gm. |
| Iron | 15 mg. | 15 mg. | 15 mg. | 15 mg. |
| Vitamin A | 5000 I.U. | 5000 I.U. | 5000 I.U. | 5000 I.U. |
| Thiamine | 1.6 mg. | 1.8 mg. | 1.3 mg. | 1.2 mg. |
| Riboflavin | 2.1 mg. | 2.5 mg. | 2.0 mg. | 1.9 mg. |
| Niacin equivalents | 21 mg. | 25 mg. | 17 mg. | 16 mg. |
| Ascorbid acid | 90 mg. | 100 mg. | 80 mg. | 80 mg. |
| Vitamin D | 400 I.U. | 400 I.U. | 400 I.U. | 400 I.U. |

From the Food and Nutrition Board, National Research Council: Recommended Daily Dietary Allowances (1958).

practitioners, neither of whom was basically interested in caring for persons of this age group. In recent years clinics for adolescents have been organized in several sections of this country. In these clinics all sorts of problems are seen and treated. They are general-practice clinics devoted to an age group instead of to a particular kind of illness or to a specific problem. Specialists' help is available if the adolescent needs it.

Usually youths between twelve and twenty-one years of age are offered help regardless of their complaint, whether emotional, physical, social or intellectual. A physician interested in the total adolescent and his problems sees the young person and establishes a close relation with him. The parents may be interviewed initially and as necessary, but the primary relation is between the physician and the adolescent. The adolescent is expected to take the responsibility for his own health.

The care these adolescents need usually involves four problem areas: concern for physical growth and development, concern about vigorous activity, concern with school and concern about emotional factors in their development. Physicians in these clinics also see illnesses common to young people (see Chap. 25). The focus in management of all these problems should be on the young person himself, not on the specific problem he presents.

Physicians trained in these clinics do not necessarily become specialists in the treatment of adolescents. They do, however, develop insights into the problems of this age group which will help them in their treatment of them, whether they are essentially pediatricians or internists.

Adolescents need someone to talk with about their problems. They also need measures to protect them against disease after their childhood immunizations have worn off. Adolescents who were immunized against diphtheria in childhood should be given the Schick test. If the result is positive, immunization should be repeated. This is especially important in girls, who, upon becoming pregnant, should be able to provide antibodies to protect their infants during the first months of life.

Vaccination for smallpox should be repeated every five years in order to prevent this disease. Protection against tetanus should be maintained by booster doses of tetanus toxoid about every three years after the initial immunization.

The adolescent also needs routine dental care in order that caries, which is prevalent during the second decade of life, may be treated. The adolescent, besides assuming responsibility for his own general medical care, should assume responsibility for his visits to the dentist.

Adolescents must develop a good attitude toward health so as to profit from factual information gained from various sources. Education about growth and development, ways to avoid accidents, nutrition, sex education and mental hygiene is of special interest to them.

## EFFECTS OF SEPARATION

The child during pubescence and the adolescent may be separated from their parents and home for long periods of time, with little problem, if their emotional development has been sound. Young adolescents may spend a few nights at the homes of friends under the supervision of their parents. They may go to camp in summer for several weeks at a time. Others may spend the school year at boarding schools some distance from home. Although homesickness may be a complaint at the beginning of a separation, even when the young person goes to college, activities in the new environment quickly seize upon his interest.

## TEACHING AIDS AND OTHER OTHER INFORMATION*

*Child Study Association of America*
  When Children Ask about Sex.
  *Complete addresses are given in the Appendix.

*Children's Medical Center, Boston, Mass.*
    Understanding Your Adolescent.

*John Hancock Mutual Life Insurance Company*
    When Your Child's in the Teens, 1955.

*National Dairy Council*
    Leverton, R. M.: A Girl and Her Figure.
    My Reflections.
    Who—Me?

*Personal Products Corporation*
    Growing up and Liking It, 1956.
    Also other educational materials on menstrual hygiene.

*Public Affairs Pamphlets*
    Duvall, E. M.: Keeping up with Teen-Agers.
    Kirkendall, L. A.: Too Young to Marry?
    Landis, P. H.: Coming of Age: Problems of Teen-Agers.
    Osborne, E.: How to Teach Your Child about Work.

*Science Research Associates, Inc.*
    English, O. S., and Finch, S. M.: Emotional Problems of Growing Up.
    Kirkendall, L. A.: Helping Children Understand Sex.
    Neisser, E. G.: When Children Start Dating.

*U.S. Department of Health, Education, and Welfare*
    A Healthy Personality for Your Child, 1952.
    The Adolescent in Your Family, 1955.

## REFERENCES

Baruch, D. W.: New Ways in Sex Education. New York, McGraw-Hill Book Company, Inc., 1959.

Breckenridge, M. E., and Vincent, E. L.: Child Development. 4th ed. Philadelphia, W. B. Saunders Company, 1960.

Bueker, K.: Adolescents Need Attention. Am. J. Nursing, 60:372, 1960.

Cooper, L. F., Barber, E. M., Mitchell, H. S., and Rynbergen, H. J.: Nutrition in Health and Disease. 13th ed. Philadelphia, J. B. Lippincott Company, 1958.

Douvan, E. M.: Independence and Identity in Adolescence. Children, 4:186, 1957.

Erikson, E. H.: Childhood and Society. New York, W. W. Norton and Co., 1950.

Gallagher, J. R.: Medical Care of the Adolescent. New York, Appleton-Century-Crofts, Inc., 1960.

Gesell, A., Ilg, F. L., and Ames, L. B.: Youth: The Years from Ten to Sixteen. New York, Harper and Brothers, 1956.

Grout, R. E.: Health Teaching in Schools. 3rd ed. Philadelphia, W. B. Saunders Co., 1958.

Horn, D.: Modifying Smoking Habits in High School Students. Children, 7:63, 1960.

Hurlock, E. B.: Child Development. 3rd ed. New York, McGraw-Hill Book Company, Inc., 1956.

Jersild, A. T.: Psychology of Adolescence. New York, Macmillan Company, 1957.

Josselyn, I. M.: Psychological Changes in Adolescence. Children, 6:43, 1959.

Landis, B. Y.: Religion and Youth; in E. Ginzberg (editor): The Nation's Children. 2. Development and Education. New York, Columbia University Press, 1960, p. 186.

Lerrigo, M. O., and Southard, H.: Learning about Love. New York, E. P. Dutton & Co., Inc., 1956.

Idem: Sex Facts and Attitudes. New York, E. P. Dutton & Co., Inc., 1956.

Idem: What's Happening to Me? New York, E. P. Dutton & Co., Inc., 1956.

Markoff, S.: Youth and Work. Children, 4:61, 1957.

Miller, E. F.: Adolescence on the Road to Womanhood. Nursing Outlook, 8:505, 1960.

Nelson, W. E. (editor): Textbook of Pediatrics. 7th ed. Philadelphia, W. B. Saunders Company, 1959.

Paterson, D., and McCreary, J. F.: Pediatrics. Philadelphia, J. B. Lippincott Company, 1956.

Recommended Dietary Allowances. Revised 1958. Washington, D.C., National Academy of Sciences, National Research Council.

Schlesinger, A. M.: Adolescence . . . Time of Weal or Time of Woe? Nursing Outlook, 8:496, 1960.

Shultz, G. D.: It's Time You Knew. Philadelphia, J. B. Lippincott Company, 1955.

Stone, L. J., and Church, J.: Childhood and Adolescence. New York, Random House, Inc., 1957.

Watson, E. H., and Lowery, G. H.: Growth and Development of Children. 3rd ed. Chicago, Year Book Publishers, Inc., 1958.

Witmer, H. L., and Kotinsky, R.: Personality in the Making: The Fact-Finding Report of the Midcentury White House Conference on Children and Youth. New York, Harper and Brothers, 1952.

Wright, S. P.: Youth Participation in Community Affairs. Children, 6:140, 1959.

# Chapter 25

# Problems of Pubescence

# and Adolescence Related to the

# Process of Growth and Development

MANY of the symptoms of physical distress complained of by pubescents and adolescents are the manifestations of normal physical and physiologic changes occurring in their bodies and of inner emotional turmoils they are experiencing. Treatment of these problems often requires the close cooperation of the patient, his parents, physician, teacher, counselor and the school, infirmary or public health nurse.

These problems cannot be clearly divided into physical or emotional groups, since each may be caused by a mixture of both.

## Acne Vulgaris

Acne vulgaris is an inflammatory condition of the skin which occurs in and around sebaceous glands during adolescence especially, because of changes in the skin at this period. During adolescence the sebaceous glands become overactive. Not all the material formed can be eliminated to the skin surface. The glands become dilated, the pores become darkened from dirt accumulation, and bacteria thrive in the retained material.

**Incidence and Clinical Manifestations.** Acne occurs in both sexes so commonly that it can almost be called a normal manifestation of sexual development. At first blackheads or comedones form. These are followed by superficial and deep papules. If no treatment is given, pustules and cysts are apt to form which later produce disfiguring scars.

The areas most commonly affected are the forehead, chin and cheeks. The back, shoulders and chest may also be

**693**

**Figure 269.** Acne vulgaris. *A,* Comedones are the first evidence of acne in a preadolescent. *B,* Moderately severe acne, with comedones, papules, and pustules. *C,* The formation of cysts is a complication. (Lewis: Practical Dermatology. 2nd ed.)

involved. Itching may or may not be present. Acne may lead to the youth's withdrawal from social contact and ultimately to emotional problems.

**Treatment and Prognosis.** Acne vulgaris should be treated as early as possible by the following measures.

The general health should be im-proved through dietary management, provision of adequate sleep and ade-quate cleanliness. Chocolate and espe-cially foods with a high carbohydrate or fat content should be eliminated.

For local therapy (*a*) cleanse the skin frequently with a coarse wash-cloth, soap and hot water to remove bacteria and dirt. Soaps which contain hexachlorophene tend to reduce the severity of the lesions. (b) At bedtime a lotion such as lotio alba with 3 per cent sulfur may be applied. (c) Several proprietary cosmetic preparations which contain sulfur compounds are available. If the skin is oily, 70 per cent alcohol or acetone may be applied before these preparations to encourage drying. These preparations may prevent emotional upset in the adolescent by covering disfiguring lesions. (d) Vitamin A may also be ordered during the winter months. (e) Natural sunlight or ultraviolet light may help if mild erythema and desquamation occur. (f) If the foregoing treatment does not succeed, roentgen therapy may be tried. (g) If deep scarring occurs, dermabrasion may be used to reduce the depth of the scars.

Acne vulgaris is usually relieved as adolescence is completed.

### Postural Defects

The erect posture of the adult is usually attained during adolescence. There may be a period, however, during pubescence and early adolescence when posture is poor. There may be three reasons for this. Physically, since the bony structure of the body develops more rapidly than the muscles, the child may appear clumsy and have poor posture. Another reason may be the emotional reaction of the youth who suddenly finds himself much taller than his peers. Since he does not want to appear different from them, he slumps so that he can be more nearly their size. Both boys and girls may have this difficulty. In addition, some girls may resent their developing breasts, and slump to hide this manifestation of their sexual development.

Treatment of the problem of faulty posture may need to be of two types. If the cause is slow growth of muscles, a period of waiting until strength is gained may be all that is required. If faulty posture is due to embarrassment over rapid growth or sexual development, the problem should be discussed realistically with the adolescent. Ridicule, shaming or threatening should never be used.

### Fatigue

Pubescents and adolescents frequently complain of being tired. They may be tired because of extremely rapid physical growth, overactivity, lack of sleep, faulty nutrition, anemia or an emotional problem. If the degree of fatigue seems excessive or if fatigue is prolonged, the underlying cause should be found and corrected.

### Anemia

Before puberty the hemoglobin level is the same for both sexes. After puberty the level in girls is approximately 2 gm. below the level in boys. Although the incidence of anemia is less than it was in the past, hypochromic anemia may occur and may be the cause of fatigue and fainting in this age group.

### Obesity

Incidence. Obesity is a generalized and excessive accumulation of fat in

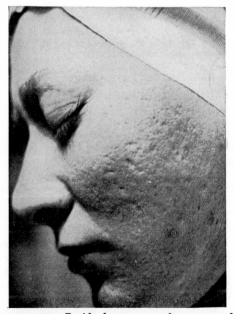

Figure 270.  Residual scars are often a sequel to acne. (Lewis: Practical Dermatology. 2nd ed.)

**Figure 271.** Throughout the period of physical growth the child, the pubescent and the adolescent need furniture that encourages them to maintain correct posture.

subcutaneous tissues. It is relatively common during pubescence and adolescence. It occurs in both sexes. It is more frequent in the lower socio-economic classes. Children with moderate obesity in the pubescent years usually require no treatment, since this may be considered normal.

**Etiology, Clinical Manifestations and Diagnosis.** The amount of food needed by any person is determined by the energy needed for basal metabolism, growth and activity. The amount of food an adolescent requires and the amount he takes are influenced by a number of factors. Among the common causes of obesity are overeating with inactivity; hereditary, familial or racial factors; and emotional difficulties. An unhappy, withdrawn adolescent may develop an excessive appetite in order to try to escape from a difficult environment. Often the obesity makes the problem even more difficult, however. In other cases some overprotective mothers may force food upon their children. The children continue in a dependent state upon their mothers and are likely to turn to eating as a comforting device for any deprivation.

Obesity due to endocrine problems such as hypothyroidism is rare. Hyperadrenocorticism, which results in Cushing's syndrome, also rarely produces obesity.

Intracranial lesions may cause obesity as in Froelich's syndrome, but this too is rare.

The *clinical manifestations* are many. Obese adolescents are usually taller than the average for their age. The adolescent's appearance is a better criterion by which to judge obesity than is an arbitrary standard for normal and excess weight. These adolescents are usually inactive. Their facial features often appear fine or small. There may be collections of adipose tissue in the breast region, and they may have pendulous abdomens with striae. The external genitals of boys may seem small, but this is only because the genitals are buried in pubic fat.

The upper arms and the thighs may appear obese. These adolescents are often very clumsy and unable to take part successfully in competitive games. Slipping of the epiphysis of the head of the femur may occur. Flat feet and knock knees are common.

Emotional disturbances are also common.

In making a *diagnosis* of the cause of obesity, the possibility of endocrine or other physical disturbance must be excluded. The diet must be recorded to determine whether overeating is really present. Many of these adolescents eat normally at meals, but overeat between meals. An evaluation of the emotional status must be made.

**Treatment and Prognosis.** The cooperation of the adolescent and his family in the treatment of obesity is essential. If the cause is dietary, the diet should be reduced. Often the diet of the entire family must be adjusted. The diet should be based on the nutritional needs, but the caloric intake may be reduced to 1000 to 1200 calories for pubescents or for adolescents 10 to 14 years of age. The protein content should be high, and the fat and carbohydrate content low. The diet should contain as much bulk as possible. Vitamin concentrates, especially those containing vitamin D, for growth may also be given. Since adolescents often desire a midafternoon or an evening snack, these should be calculated in the diet. The energy output should be increased through exercise. The objective is burning of body fat to provide energy. A weight loss of 1 or 2 pounds a week is desirable.

Emotional problems should be managed, and the child should be helped to make a more adequate adjustment in his home, school and community. School personnel can often be of value in helping the child to form better relations with his peers. Psychotherapy may be necessary along with drug therapy.

The *prognosis* depends on the extent of cooperation among parents, child and physician. If even the best treatment ordered is not followed, there will be no weight reduction.

## Menstrual Irregularities

Menstruation occurs, on the average, at thirteen years of age, although the range is from eleven to fifteen years at onset. Since the cycles at first are anovulatory, irregularity in menstrual periods or a prolonged or scanty flow may be expected. If these symptoms continue to the second year, evaluation of the problem should be made. It is true that the normal cycle is more closely related to the general health status of the girl than to hormonal activity. If the girl is malnourished or obese, problems may be expected. Another frequent cause of menstrual difficulty during adolescence may be overactivity or underactivity. Constipation may likewise be a factor. Improvement of diet and general hygiene are usually sufficient treatment.

Some young adolescents who are emotionally disturbed, who may be striving too hard to achieve at school or who may be socially insecure may also have menstrual difficulties.

Less commonly, disturbance in thyroid functioning or organic lesions of the reproductive system may cause problems. Any young woman who continues to have difficulties despite an improvement in her general well-being should have a basal metabolic rate determination and a gynecologic examination done.

## Hyperthyroidism

The basal metabolic rate generally decreases from early infancy to the end of the growth period. There is a relative increase, however, during the period of rapid growth preceding puberty. This temporarily elevated metabolic rate probably is related to the hyperthyroidism noted at this age.

Treatment includes a high caloric diet, reduction in school schedule and activity, and administration of iodine. This type of hyperthyroidism disappears when sexual maturity is reached.

Hyperthyroidism or exophthalmic goiter with excessive liberation of thyroid hormone is uncommon in children or adolescents.

## Minor Neuroses

Mildly neurotic symptoms are present in many adolescents. These are usually short-lived and may result from some stress or challenge the youth has had. They persist only if he finds that the symptoms bring rewards from others in his environment.

The adolescent may show symptoms of tension over unpopularity, poor athletic ability or poor school work. Failure to participate in recreational activities or to gain a degree of independence from his parents, guilt about masturbation, fear of sexual development and fear of being unsuccessful may cause neurotic manifestations.

The parents and the adolescent may complain specifically that he has insomnia, nightmares, headaches, difficulty in concentration, and gastrointestinal or menstrual problems.

Treatment of these mild neuroses consists in helping the adolescent to appreciate the basic cause of the problem. The physician should have good rapport with the parents and with the adolescent so that they will accept his plan of treatment and cooperate with him. The family physician or the pediatrician can usually treat these young people successfully. If there is a question of a deeper difficulty, however, consultation with a psychiatrist should be sought.

## REFERENCES

Baird, J. W.: Acne. A New Approach to an Old Problem. J. Pediat., 52:152, 1958.

Bruch, H.: Psychological Aspects of Obesity in Adolescence. Am. J. Pub. Health, 48:1349, 1958.

Cormia, F. E.: Acne Vulgaris. Am. J. Nursing, 57:198, 1957.

Eberlein, W. R., Bongiovanni, A. M., and Jones, I. T.: Obesity in Childhood. Pediat. Clin. North America, 4:949, 1957.

Gallagher, J. R.: A Clinic for Adolescents. Children, 1:165, 1954.

Idem: Adolescents Have Special Health Problems. The Child, 15:29, Aug., 1950.

Idem: Medical Care of the Adolescent. New York, Appleton-Century-Crofts, Inc., 1960.

Howorth, M. B.: Posture in Adolescents and Adults, Am. J. Nursing, 56:34, 1956.

Huffman, J. W., and Wieczorowski, E.: Gynecology of Children and Adolescents. Pediatrics, 22:395, 1958.

James, K. W., and Tisserand, J. B.: Treatment of Acne Vulgaris. GP, 18:130, 1958.

Krehl, W. A.: Skin Disease and Nutritional Therapy. J. Am. Dietetic A., 35:923, 1959.

Lewis, G. M.: Practical Dermatology. 2nd ed. Philadelphia, W. B. Saunders Company, 1959.

Lowrey, G. H.: Obesity in the Adolescent. Am. J. Pub. Health, 48:1354, 1958.

McGloin, E.: How to Help Teen-Agers with Acne. R. N., 22:40, Jan., 1959.

Nelson, W. E. (editor): Textbook of Pediatrics. 7th ed. Philadelphia, W. B. Saunders Company, 1959.

Paterson, D., and McCreary, J. F.: Pediatrics. Philadelphia, J. B. Lippincott Company, 1956.

Pillsbury, D. M., Shelley, W. B., and Kligman, A. M.: Dermatology. Philadelphia, W. B. Saunders Company, 1956.

Rattner, H.: Acne—The Situation at Present. Postgrad. Med., 25:446, 1959.

Silver, H. K., Kempe, C. H., and Bruyn, H. B.: Handbook of Pediatrics. 3rd ed. Los Altos, California, Lange Medical Publications, 1959.

Sulzberger, M. B., and Witten, V. H.: The Management of Acne Today. M. Clin. North America, 43:887, 1959.

# Chapter 26

# Conditions of the Adolescent

## EFFECT OF ILLNESS ON ADOLESCENTS

SERIOUS or prolonged illness during childhood may have negative effects on the personality of the adolescent unless special care has been taken to prevent this from happening. Illness or accident may interfere with the child's sense of trust that his own body or the outside world is really dependable. Illness or accident may prove to the child that he is loved only when he is not well. Prolonged illness may lead the child whose sense of autonomy is not fully developed into overdependency on others. Illness may also in later years so curb the development of a sense of initiative or a sense of industry that the adolescent is unable to gain satisfaction from seeking the answers to questions or from starting or completing a project. Malnutrition occurring alone or in relation to a disease may result in apathy and listlessness.

Adolescence is difficult enough for normal young people, but more so for the handicapped person. Accepting his sex role, finding himself, emancipating himself from his family and selecting a career are difficult. The social aspects of his handicap are much greater during adolescence than they were earlier. If he did not accept the reality of his handicap earlier, he may be emotionally disturbed about it in adolescence.

The effects of a handicap such as impaired hearing, blindness, cardiac disease, diabetes or cerebral palsy tend to make children of all ages overdependent on adults and to warp their personality development in several ways. These and other conditions tend to limit both their social contacts with other children and their ability to relieve their pent-up emotions through physical activity, and to cause various degrees of rejection in themselves, their parents and peers. The adolescent, because of his feelings of guilt about his illness or handicap, may develop feelings of mistrust, self-doubt and inferiority. He may either give up in the battle for healthy personality development or may seek to punish others for his failure.

On the other hand, if handicapped or chronically ill children have been given the opportunity to master themselves

**699**

and their environment within the limits of reality, to become independent, they will probably succeed in the battle of life. They must be given the opportunity to try; if they fail, they must be helped in their effort so that they can achieve success. If the adolescent cannot achieve success in the use of his legs, for instance, he can be helped to achieve by using his head or hands. Many people in our society, even so-called normal people, have limitations which only they know. They have been able to use what they have to such advantage that the world is unaware of their handicap. They have developed a sense of security in their achievements with the help of their parents and other adults. Both they and their parents, facing the handicap realistically together, have been able to build a parent-child relation which many normal children and parents might envy.

Illness during adolescence may have disastrous effects. During illness the young person is unable to discover the kind of person he really is or what his role in the future will be, much less develop the sense of intimacy which is important to his later adjustment.

## HOSPITAL CARE OF THE ILL ADOLESCENT

Hospitals in the past were not organized to care specifically for adolescents. Adolescents were admitted to either an adult or a pediatric unit. Internists admitted them to adult units. Pediatricians, when they did not discharge their patients at adolescence, admitted them to pediatric units. It is now believed that adolescents need a continuing relation with their physicians until they reach maturity and find their place in the world.

In either the adult or the pediatric unit adolescents were likely to feel uncomfortable and out of place because no one seemed to be especially interested in them. In recent years adolescent units have been opened in hospitals. In these units adolescents are comfortable with others in their own age group. Physicians and nurses are also likely to give more understanding care to their patients because they enjoy working with them.

### Role of the Nurse in Caring for Adolescents

The student nurse who herself has not had too many years' experience in being an adult may find working with adolescents a difficult matter if she does not understand them and does not remember her professional role in working with them. The nurse, whatever her age, must help the adolescent to feel that he is important. The adolescent patient should be properly introduced to others and asked his opinions on matters that concern him.

The nurse must understand that adolescents are frequently unpredictable, that they may be emotionally unstable and torn between their desires to be dependent and independent. She must also remember their great need for security, to love and be loved, to be an accepted group member and to be approved. Sometimes these very needs make it difficult for them to verbalize their anxieties and feelings about illness and hospitalization to her. In addition, their language may be such that adults may not be able to understand the real meaning of what they say.

The nurse must be able to detect hostility and rejection in this group of patients. When these feelings are evident, she must often alter her approach completely in order to gain cooperation from them. She must remember not to argue with them, to avoid giving orders to them and to let them be as independent as possible. She should trust them and treat them as if they were grown up.

If the nurse is aware of a problem concerning an adolescent's acceptance of his newly developing body, she may be of great help to him at the time of a physical examination or when she carries out treatments. If she recognizes the fears characteristic of this phase of growth, she will sense the meaning behind some of his seemingly purposeless questions. She can help him by explaining that fears of this sort are common among adolescents and are understandable to her. They need assurance that they are normal males or females. For a nurse to say to a pubescent girl, "Your genitalia must be abnormal, because I cannot locate the meatus," during a catheterization is inexcusable.

Adolescent girls are interested in making themselves as attractive as possible. Lipstick and other cosmetics are important to them. The nurse must understand that helping a young girl comb her hair in an attractive way, even though she is immobilized in a cast, is an important part of nursing care.

When adolescents are grouped together in one unit or part of a unit, the boys and girls have separate rooms and separate lavatories. These patients will form their own social group, much as they would if they were in their own communities. The nurse must be aware of the structure of such a group, its leader and its followers. She can do much to influence the group if she can convince the leader of the value of her ideas.

In such a situation the nurse must also remember the emotional development of the persons involved. One of the greatest fears of adolescents is that of losing control of themselves in front of their peers. The nurse can see to it that this does not happen by handling them in a firm but fair manner. If a boy or a girl, but particularly a boy, is to face a painful treatment, it might be better to remove him from the group so that he can express his feelings openly rather than have him cry in the presence of others and be humiliated.

The young nurse may feel that simply because the patient is older than a child he should understand that whatever is done is for his good, and she may fail to explain treatments to him. The adolescent, who is keenly interested in himself, his body and his illness, needs detailed explanations frequently. In giving such explanations the nurse must be willing to answer questions and to offer reassurance just as she did to younger children.

The adolescent should be helped to continue with his school work, even though he is hospitalized, so that he can join his group at school when he is discharged. The teenager's mind must be occupied with recreational interests when he is not doing school work. He will enjoy watching television, listening to the radio or helping with the care of younger children.

The physician and the nurse can help the adolescent by keeping the school teacher in the hospital and the school nurse in the community informed of the adolescent's disability and thereby help them to gain insight into his physical and psychologic needs in relation to his illness. They can also interpret to members of the community the fact that his basic needs are like those of normal adolescents.

## ILLNESS DURING ADOLESCENCE

The fact that children grow rapidly, physically and emotionally, during adolescence makes them particularly vulnerable to certain illnesses which may result in significant effects on the developmental process. Accidents, however, are the principal cause of death. The death rate from illness in this age group is relatively low. Although tuberculosis was at one time a leading cause of death, its incidence has been reduced in recent years. It is still true, however, that adolescents seem more susceptible than persons in other age groups to this disease.

### Tuberculosis

Tuberculosis is a worldwide disease. Although its incidence has decreased in the more advanced countries, it is still prevalent in underdeveloped countries. The methods used to control tuberculosis in this country have brought excellent results, but they cannot be applied with equal success in other areas. Each country must find methods which can be utilized successfully with its own people in the areas of educational programs, better standards of living,

**Figure 272.** Calcified tuberculous focus (right arrow) and calcified tracheobronchial lymph node (left arrow) in a young girl. (R. H. High and W. E. Nelson in Nelson: Textbook of Pediatrics. 7th ed.)

ways to diagnose the condition earlier and the best methods of treatment. The World Health Organization is working to help countries to bring this infection under control.

**Incidence.** Tuberculosis during adolescence was once a real menace in this country. The fact that adolescent girls seem to be more susceptible at an earlier age than boys may be related to their earlier age of maturation. Negro girls seem to be more susceptible than white girls, probably because the environment in which they live is often a contributing factor. The incidence is high in slum areas where overcrowding and poor health conditions are prevalent. There is also a higher incidence in areas with periods of flood or famine.

Early discovery and improved methods of treatment provide these young people with a good chance of cure.

**Etiology and Epidemiology.** Tuberculosis is caused by an acid-fast bacillus, *Mycobacterium tuberculosis*. Disease in human beings is produced by organisms causing either the bovine or the human form of the disease. An individual may contract tuberculosis by drinking contaminated milk, although this method of infection has been almost completely eliminated in this country, owing to the practice of killing diseased cattle, forbidding the sale of contaminated milk, pasteurization of milk and testing milk handlers for tuberculosis.

The bacillus enters the body through the respiratory or the gastrointestinal tract. It is spread today chiefly by droplet infection or by direct contact with infected human beings. Entrance into the body may also take place by ingestion.

Children most frequently contract tuberculosis from an infected adult in the home. This is the reason why newborn infants should be removed from mothers who have the disease; the mothers cannot then contaminate the children by breathing or coughing on them during the process of feeding or caring for them. Older children and adolescents may contract the disease in their own homes or in the homes of friends or from close contact with their peer groups. Children of any age may put contaminated objects into their mouths. The unhygienic practice of sharing taffies, candy, or drinking or eating utensils may cause spread of the disease.

**Predisposing Factors, Types of Infection and Pathology.** Chronic illness, fatigue or undernutrition may predispose to tuberculosis.

A *primary infection* occurs when the tubercle bacillus enters the body, usually in the tissues of the lungs. Individual resistance and the number of organisms entering the body determine the extent of the disease. The reaction of the invaded tissue is basically one of inflammation and repair with later calcification, which may be noted on an x-ray film. The primary focus usually heals spontaneously.

The primary (Ghon) complex includes the initial lesion and lesions in the regional lymph nodes. The disease process may extend to other parts of the lung and to the gastrointestinal tract because of ingestion of infected sputum. In some cases the organisms may produce symptoms of mild pneumonia. The organisms may enter the lymph nodes, lymph vessels and the blood vessels. Foci of infection then occur in various organs and in serous membranes.

When widespread infection occurs, the child is said to have *miliary tuberculosis*. This type generally occurs in the infant or very young child. Its onset is usually acute, with an irregular fever, rales in the chest, possibly an enlarged spleen, distended abdomen, prostration, dyspnea, cough and cyanosis. The mortality rate in past years was very high, but has been reduced through the use of newer drugs.

If the disease affects the meninges, *tuberculous meningitis* may result. Tuberculosis of the mesenteric or cervical lymph nodes, peritoneum, bones and joints may also occur. The bones most frequently involved include the head of the femur (*tuberculous coxitis*), fingers and toes (*tuberculous dactylitis*) and vertebrae (*tuberculous spondylitis* or *Pott's disease*).

If the child's resistance is good, healing of a primary lesion and calcification may take place. Later, because of lowered resistance, the latent lesion may again become active.

*Secondary infections* usually occur during adolescence or early in adult life either from the original focus or from reinfection. They differ from the primary type because of the allergic response of the body. Reinfection is a much more destructive process than the primary lesion. Secondary infection may include extensive inflammatory reaction with tissue destruction and cavitation. Healing in secondary infections is largely by means of scar tissue or fibrosis. The pulmonary lesion in a secondary infection is likely to be in the apex of the lung.

**Clinical Manifestations and Diagnosis.** In primary tuberculosis the *manifestations* of a pulmonary lesion may or may not be evident. The child may complain of malaise, fatigue and anorexia and have a weight loss and be irritable. If tuberculosis is suspected, but no symptoms are evident, the *diagnosis* may be made with a tuberculin test and an x-ray film of the chest.

The clinical manifestations of *secondary* tuberculosis may resemble those of infected adults. The disease may become chronic, progressive pulmonary tuberculosis with symptoms of cough

**Figure 273.** Miliary tuberculosis of the lungs in a white boy 3 years of age. His mother had pulmonary tuberculosis. The physical findings were fine, crackling rales throughout both lungs. Death occurred shortly after this roentgenogram was taken. The tuberculin reaction was positive. (R. H. High and W. E. Nelson in Nelson: Textbook of Pediatrics, 7th ed.)

and expectoration, fever, hemoptysis, weight loss and night sweats.

For diagnostic testing two types of tuberculin are available: old tuberculin (O.T.) and purified protein derivative (P.P.D.). The tests used in the diagnosis of tuberculosis are the Mantoux test and the patch test of Vollmer.

*Mantoux Test.* About six weeks after infection of a tuberculin-negative person the presence of allergy or hypersensitivity to tuberculoprotein may be observed by a positive skin test reaction to tuberculin. A known amount of tuberculin is injected intracutaneously. This is a most accurate test. The test should be read in forty-eight hours. In a positive reaction an area of at least 5 mm. in diameter with erythema and definite induration occurs.

*Vollmer Patch Test.* In this test no injection is necessary. Filter paper containing old tuberculin is attached with adhesive to the skin. The skin is cleansed with ether or acetone and permitted to dry before the filter paper is applied. In forty-eight hours the patch is removed. The test is read ninety-six hours after the patch was applied. A reddened, indurated area or vesiculation indicates a positive reaction. A false reading may be made if the patch becomes loosened before the time of removal. The main advantage of this test is the ease of administration.

*Meaning of Reactions.* A positive tuberculin reaction is usually evidence that the person has been infected with the tubercle bacillus and is allergic or hypersensitive to its protein. It does not necessarily mean that the person tested has an active lesion at the time of testing. The size of the skin reaction indicates that the test is positive or negative.

A negative reaction, if the dose has been carried to 1.0 mg. (O.T.), eliminates the possibility of tuberculosis. False negatives may occur because of impotent tuberculin or hyperpyrexia.

Tuberculin tests should be done every two years on children from one year of age until the test becomes positive. This would help in locating their source of infection.

Every child who shows a positive reaction to tuberculin should have a physical examination, have his temperature checked, and have a chest roentgenogram, blood cell count and sedimentation rate made. Contacts, whether parents, grandparents, siblings or friends, should be located and checked for tuberculosis.

A positive diagnosis of tuberculosis can be made if the tubercle bacillus is found in the gastric contents or sputum. Young children seldom expectorate. Since sputum is swallowed, examination of the stomach contents obtained by gastric aspiration is of value.

Before breakfast a lavage tube is passed. After a few cubic centimeters of water have been injected a sample of the stomach contents is withdrawn by means of a syringe. The sediment in the return is examined for the tubercle bacillus by culture or guinea pig inoculation, or both. The test should be repeated three times before the result is considered to be negative.

**Treatment and Nursing Care.** Whether the child or adolescent is given care at home or in a hospital depends on the total situation. If someone in the patient's environment is infected, the patient should be removed from continued contact with this source of infection.

The plan of care should be based on the total situation. The patient should have mental and physical rest. A daily schedule to which he adheres is necessary. Too much activity must be avoided. He must be kept out of school for his own sake and for the safety of other pupils. Adequate health supervision is essential.

The emotional attitude of the child and his family should be optimistic. The child should be isolated from close contact with other family members to prevent the spread of infection. This is not only for their protection from tuberculosis, but also for his protection from exposure to other infections which would tend further to drain his bodily resources. Measles is especially dangerous for a child with tuberculosis.

The patient requires an adequate diet, high in protein, calcium and vitamins, particularly B, C and D. Feeding should not be forced, but the child should be encouraged to eat sufficient food. Fresh air and sunshine may aid in his recovery and add to his sense of well-being.

The patient resumes his usual activities gradually as the lesion heals. He should be encouraged to do whatever he can for himself in order to prevent invalidism. He should be encouraged to plan with his parents and counselor for the future. The adolescent and even the older grade school child should be a member of the health team which plans for his care and rehabilitation. This team also includes his parents, physician, social worker, public school teacher or visiting teacher, and nurse. Even during convalescence the child should be helped to keep in contact with his friends. A telephone near his bed and an active correspondence with relatives and friends are of great value in helping him to feel that he is still a part of his group and will return to them.

Several drugs have been used successfully in the treatment of tuberculosis, although there is no one specific drug which will cure the disease. Prolonged treatment, from six months to a year, is usually necessary.

Streptomycin is given intramuscularly. Long-term treatment may be complicated by damage to the eighth cranial nerve resulting in deafness. Streptomycin should not be used alone against tuberculosis, since streptomycin-resistant organisms rapidly emerge. Another tuberculostatic agent should be given concurrently.

Isoniazid (INH) has a low degree of toxicity, can control progressive lesions and is effective in preventing hematogenous dissemination. It may be given orally or parenterally.

Para-aminosalicylic acid (PAS) is given orally. It is not as effective as either streptomycin or isoniazid. The usual toxic reaction is gastric irritation. PAS is valuable because it inhibits the development of resistance by the bacilli to both streptomycin and isoniazid.

These drugs in various combinations have reduced the length of tuberculous infection and also certain secondary forms of the infection.

Other drugs which may be used include Promin, Promizole, kanamycin, neomycin and viomycin. Whether cortisone and corticotropin therapy is used depends on the type of lesion present.

Surgical treatment of tuberculous lesions is rarely indicated in children. Treatments to put the lung at rest include pneumothorax, pneumoperitoneum or phrenic crush.

**Prognosis and Methods of Control.** In general the mortality rate is higher in infancy and adolescence and lower in the span of years comprising childhood.

The primary lesion, usually benign, may become an extensive infection. The younger the child, the greater is the danger. During adolescence, however, there is an increased risk of development of chronic, progressive pulmonary tuberculosis, either from the primary focus or from reinfection. With secondary lesions the prognosis depends on the severity of the lesion, sex, age and environment of the child.

The only effective means to prevent tuberculosis is to avoid contact with infected persons. Widespread education of the public is essential. They should be helped to understand the disease and the value of early diagnosis and treatment. Communities should organize tuberculin-testing and case-finding programs and also public health programs for control of this disease. These programs should include treatment of infectious patients, case-finding, examination of contacts, supervision of inactive cases, x-ray screening and measures to improve community health. Mobile x-ray units are used to locate patients who appear healthy, but are capable of spreading tuberculosis to others.

Ways to develop artificial immunity against tuberculosis have been attempted. Vaccination with BCG (bacillus of Calmette and Guérin) has been used. This vaccine may be given intradermally. The actual period of resistance to infection after the use of BCG is not known. Because BCG vaccine changes nonreactors to tuberculin tests

**Figure 274.** Scoliosis in a young girl, showing the tilt of the pelvis and shoulder and the deformity of the chest. (C. C. Chapple and J. R. Moore, in W. E. Nelson: Textbook of Pediatrics. 7th ed.)

into reactors, tests subsequent to its administration are of no value.

### Scoliosis

**Incidence and Types.** Scoliosis is an S-shaped lateral curvature usually associated with rotation of the spine. Scoliosis is most frequent between the ages of twelve and sixteen years, a period of rapid growth.

There are two *types* of scoliosis: correctable or functional scoliosis and fixed or structural scoliosis. Correctable or *functional* scoliosis is usually caused by poor posture. It is seen especially in young persons who sit slumped over desks. Such persons can correct their scoliosis by bending toward the side of the curvature. If faulty posture is not corrected, structural changes may occur, and curvature is then not fully correctable.

The deformity of fixed or *structural* scoliosis is due to changes in the shape of the vertebrae or thorax. The patient cannot correct the deformity by bending.

The type of structural scoliosis most frequently seen is idiopathic and is usually found in young girls. Other causes may be congenital deformities (fusion of the ribs or vertebrae, hemivertebrae), infections of the vertebrae such as occur in Pott's disease caused by tuberculous infection, or paralytic diseases such as poliomyelitis.

**Clinical Manifestations and Diagnosis.** *Clinical manifestations* usually occur during periods of spinal growth such as at pubescence. The child or adolescent has no pain until the later stages of the disease. One shoulder is elevated, one hip may be prominent, or the spinal curve itself may be obvious.

The *diagnosis* is made on physical examination. An x-ray picture of the entire spine is taken with the patient in a standing position. Roentgenograms may also be taken with the patient bending as far as possible to the right and to the left.

**Treatment.** The child should receive a well balanced diet high in animal proteins. Postural curves with no structural changes may be corrected by improving sitting habits and general health, by getting more rest and by doing appropriate exercises. The physiotherapist may teach the child exercises to correct the condition. The child can be appealed to through his desire to improve his appearance. If the scoliosis is not caused merely by faulty posture, the primary condition must be corrected before structural changes occur in the vertebrae.

Bracing is used to prevent the degree of curvature from increasing. A plaster cast with wedging may be used to obtain maximal correction. The scoliosis turnbuckle plaster jacket including the head and leg is designed in such a way that it can be cut at the apex of the primary curve and wedged to overcome the deformity. Application of such a cast is exhausting to the patient. In a few days the cast is cut, and the turnbuckle is placed on the side of the concavity. The turnbuckle is turned each day. The wedge-shaped opening on one side becomes smaller, and the opening on the side where the turnbuckle is becomes larger. When maximal correction has been obtained, a window is cut in the back of the cast through which operation is done. The primary deforming curve is then fused.

A newer device is the Risser localizer jacket. This is a lightweight cast in which the patient can walk. It is removed for operation, but must be reapplied afterwards. Spinal fusion may be done after maximum growth has occurred. For extensive surgery, fusion may have to be done in more than one stage.

**Nursing Care.** The nurse assists with therapeutic exercises designed to promote realignment of the body. Since these patients tire easily, periods of exercise should be alternated with periods of rest. Rest positions may be specified by the physician or physiotherapist and can be as valuable as exercises. The physiotherapist, the nurse, the parents and the patient must work closely together.

The young patient in a thick, heavy Risser type of turnbuckle cast or lighter cast requires comprehensive nursing care.

Skin care is important. The nurse must observe and explore the skin with her fingers for pressure areas, especially over the ribs. She must check for the cause of all complaints of pain or discomfort. All exposed edges of the cast must be covered with large adhesive petals (see p. 237), or stockinet should be pulled over the edges of the cast and securely fastened to the cast. The exposed skin should be rubbed frequently. Slight padding may be used to allay discomfort from pressure by the cast, but too much padding may cause extra pressure. The cast around the buttocks and genitals must be protected with waterproof material. The skin should be cleansed thoroughly after soiling.

After spinal fusion, immobilization in casts or braces may be continued for six to twelve months. If a tibial graft has been taken, the limb should be handled carefully for at least eight weeks until healing has taken place.

Comprehensive nursing care is planned to meet the patient's needs during the long-term treatment of scoliosis. The patient may be cared for at home and taken to the outpatient department before and after hospitalization. The orthopedist, the physiotherapist and the nurse must work closely together. Crippled children's services in many states provide physiotherapy follow-up in the home. The child should continue exercises for months or years.

The public health nurse should give the child encouragement. An adolescent girl may not want to wear a brace because she is "too tired" or thinks it ruins her appearance. Parents should be warned of such complaints and be given support in insisting that the physician's orders be carried out for the girl's future welfare.

Early recognition and treatment are vitally important to prevent serious deformity. The school nurse or public health nurse should make observations on the posture of children. The tendency to postpone treatment while waiting to see whether the adolescent will outgrow the condition is dangerous.

### Slipped Femoral Epiphysis

**Etiology and Incidence.** Epiphysial closure, which marks the completion of skeletal growth, also coincides with the attainment of sexual maturity. This is related more to physiologic than to chronologic age. This fact of development is especially important in the occurrence of slipped epiphysis, which is one of the outstanding osseous disturbances of adolescence. Exactly why this condition occurs is not known, but trauma may be a factor.

The phase of maximum growth is, on the average, for girls twelve years and for boys between fourteen and fifteen years. Usually the adolescent in whom slipped femoral epiphysis occurs is tall and heavy, but not fat. Such a person needs larger than average amounts of calcium and vitamin D during the pre-adolescent growth spurt.

**Clinical Manifestations, Diagnosis and Treatment.** In the early stages signs and symptoms of synovitis are present. Pain in the hip causes the child to limp (the pain is sometimes referred to the knee). The symptoms are similar to those in Legg-Perthes disease in school children. The onset is insidious. The condition is frequently bilateral.

The *diagnosis* is based on roentgen examination, which shows that the femoral capital epiphysis has slipped posteriorly and inferiorly on a lateral view. The neck of the femur assumes a horseneck appearance. Early diagnosis and treatment are essential.

The main objective of *treatment* is to arrest slipping by internal fixation with a cast, followed by avoidance of weight bearing by use of crutches until healing occurs. In severe cases osteotomy or other operative procedures may be necessary.

### Malignant Tumors of Bone

The most frequent primary malignant bone tumors are osteosarcoma and Ewing's tumor. These occur most often between ten and twenty years of age and in boys more often than in girls.

The etiology of such tumors is unknown, but heredity may be a factor.

Roentgenographic features resemble those of non-neoplastic lesions of bone. Careful diagnosis must be made on the bases of roentgenographic examinations and surgical biopsy.

### Osteosarcoma (Osteogenic Sarcoma)

**Clinical Manifestations, Diagnosis, Treatment and Prognosis.** Osteosarcoma occurs more frequently than Ewing's tumor and usually involves the metaphysial end of a long bone—the lower end of the femur or the upper end of the tibia or humerus. It may also occur in other locations. The *clinical manifestations* are pain and swelling of the affected part. The *diagnosis* is made on roentgenographic examination, which

reveals destruction of bone and new bone formation. The only *treatment* is amputation of the affected extremity. The neoplasm may involve the medullary cavity, the cortex and the adjoining soft tissue. The sarcoma commonly metastasizes to the lungs, although other organs may be involved. The mortality rate is high.

**Nursing care** is similar to that of patients having Ewing's tumors.

### Ewing's Tumor

**Clinical Manifestations, Diagnosis, Treatment, Nursing Care and Prognosis.** Ewing's tumor usually involves the shaft of a long bone. It may also involve the flat bones and ribs. The *clinical manifestations* are similar to those of osteosarcoma. Fever and leukocytosis may also be present. Usually at the time of diagnosis only one bone is involved, but other bones become affected. The *diagnosis* is made on roentgenographic examination. *Treatment* is unsatisfactory. The neoplasm usually responds at first to roentgen therapy, but few young people are cured. Amputation is the only other treatment used.

When a nurse sees an adolescent with the symptoms of a malignant tumor of the bone, she should suggest a medical examination, without alarming him or his parents by telling them that she suspects a tumor of the bone.

As the disease progresses, the patient will become anemic and look pale and tired. The optimism the patient shows at the onset of the condition changes to depression. The parents, visitors and nurses should try to provide emotional support in helping the patient to face the probable outcome of the disease.

Since a pathologic fracture may occur at or near the site of the tumor, the nurse should be gentle with the extremity when making the bed or bathing the patient. If he is ambulatory, he should be protected from falling. Such fractures may be painless; therefore the nurse must observe carefully for evidence of fracture if the patient falls or otherwise sustains any trauma which could result in a fracture of the diseased bone.

The diet should be high in protein and vitamins to counteract the progressive anemia.

The nurse should observe for indications of lung involvement such as pain in the chest, coughing, and expectoration of blood, and report her findings immediately. As with osteogenic sarcoma, metastases to the lungs occur frequently.

## Failure of Sexual Development

Delayed puberty, like precocious puberty, may occur in both sexes. Parents may be much concerned when puberty is delayed in their son or daughter. The child may also be much concerned, since prolonged delay usually means that friends have outgrown him or her physically and emotionally.

### Delayed Puberty in the Female

**Etiology, Clinical Manifestations and Treatment.** In primary hypogonadism there is ovarian agenesis or destruction. This may be due to surgical removal or destruction by roentgen therapy. Secondary hypogonadism may be due to destruction of or defect in the pituitary gland or in hypothalamic connections with the pituitary gland or to a severe systemic disease causing secondary pituitary deficiency, such as hypothyroidism (cretinism) (see p. 369), uncontrolled diabetes (see p. 647), fibrocystic disease (see p. 352) or tuberculosis (see p. 701).

At the normal age of puberty *clinical manifestations* become evident. There is failure of body hair growth and of the characteristic breast development. The genitalia remain infantile, and menstruation does not occur. There is retarded physical growth, and the epiphyses are late in closing. If the hypothalamus has been severely affected by a tumor, obesity may be seen occasionally in addition to sexual infantilism. This combination of clinical manifestations is termed *Froehlich's syndrome.*

*Treatment* for primary hypogonadism consists in administration of stilbestrol after the child has reached the age of puberty. Intermittent therapy with stilbestrol is continued indefinitely. Artificial menses occur without ovulation. These women are therefore sterile. There are positive psychologic benefits from therapy in addition to the fact that premature senility from lack of estrogen is prevented. In secondary hypogonadism the treatment of the underlying disorder may bring about normal sexual development.

### Delayed Puberty in the Male

**Etiology, Clinical Manifestations, Treatment and Prognosis.** Failure of sexual development in the male is known as *eunuchoidism.* If the testes are missing or have been destroyed, there is no abnormality until puberty, when the genitals fail to enlarge, pubic hair is sparse or absent, the voice remains childlike, and epiphysial closure is slow. The 17-ketosteroid excretion is usually low. The *treatment* is by substitution therapy with testosterone given orally or intramuscularly. Prolonged effects may be obtained if pellets are implanted subcutaneously. Masculinization occurs with therapy, but the youths are sterile.

### Venereal Diseases: Syphilis and Gonorrhea

Venereal disease is present to an alarming degree among the adolescent group, especially in those from fifteen to nineteen years. These adolescents are from all socio-economic groups. They engage in sexual intercourse because they are lonely or want status, not because they have a deep relation with their partners. Since adolescents are prone to worry about their bodies, their concern over subsequent venereal disease often prompts them to seek treatment. Some may not seek treatment, however, for fear that their behavior will become known.

Treatment must be undertaken by a large health team if success is to be achieved. Many of the aspects of adult treatment and control apply equally to adolescents, though special problems are present in the younger group.

The two most common venereal diseases are syphilis and gonorrhea. These diseases follow the adult pattern in adolescents. The medical aspects will not be discussed here, since they have already been discussed (see pp. 164, 554).

Both diseases are contracted through sexual promiscuity. The mouth, face, neck, genitals and anus may be the primary site of a chancre. The important problems in relation to adolescents are treatment of the disease, case-finding, and prevention by the health team. Early case-finding is especially important if the young girl is pregnant, in order that treatment may be completed before delivery of the infant.

Both diseases are treated with penicillin. Although the mortality rates from these diseases have decreased as a result of treatment, the infections persist and are being seen increasingly in the adolescent group. The social problem, a violation of sexual mores, is perhaps a greater problem than the morbidity.

The fact that adolescents turn to such an extent to promiscuous heterosexual relations may be a reflection of social maladjustment. Other indications of the same problem include increasing illegitimate parenthood, juvenile delinquency and emotional problems.

Several members of the health team must work together to help control the problem of venereal disease: (a) the parents, who have contributed to the adolescent's forming a philosophy of life and his concept of other people, and have given approval to his selection of friends. Often it is the friends who initially lead the adolescent into this behavior. (b) The teacher, who helps to build proper attitudes toward these diseases through counseling, can disseminate information about venereal disease and can help to guide troubled adolescents to appropriate sources for help. (c) The clergyman, who appreciates the fact that religious motives have a great effect on the degree of inhibition exercised in subordinating unacceptable sexual expression, is an important team member. Apparently, the more active adolescents are in religion, the less they engage in promiscuity. (d) The social worker, working with nurses in helping these adolescents, can help the nurse appreciate the probable causes of such antisocial behavior and what disease means to the individual patient. (e) The family physician can teach his young patients about venereal disease, treat and report cases and locate their contacts. (f) The venereal disease investigator is a trained interviewer who interviews patients with an aim to locating contacts.

**Role of the Nurse.** The nurse cannot fully understand her own role without appreciating the roles of other members of the health team. One of her most important roles is assisting other members of the health team in case-finding.

The school nurse should be aware of signs and symptoms of venereal disease as she is of other communicable diseases in students. The school nurse should be able to evaluate complaints and refer such adolescents to the physician. She should keep adequate health records on all students so that she knows their individual problems. She must have a nonjudgmental attitude about these diseases. The school nurse may also function as a teacher of health and as a counselor for the students on matters of this sort.

The hospital nurse works in conjunction with the school nurse. Although syphilis and gonorrhea are usually treated on an outpatient basis, the nurse caring for adolescent patients in the hospital units must remember that because the incubation period of syphilis is about three weeks and of gonorrhea about five days, some adolescents recently admitted may manifest symptoms during the early part of a hospitalization period.

The primary chancre of syphilis and the pustular discharge of gonorrhea are highly infectious. Isolation technique to protect other patients as well as personnel is thus necessary in the care of such patients.

The treatment of choice is penicillin. If the patient has gonorrhea, penicillin is given for a few days. If the patient has syphilis, penicillin is given for about two weeks. The nurse must observe for signs of untoward reaction to the drug during the course of therapy.

The clinic or office nurse can encourage the adolescent to return regularly for therapy. The nurse must know the diagnostic and therapeutic measures so that she can interpret these to the patients and reassure them. Adolescents want answers to their questions, especially those in relation to their own bodies. Such a nurse can also be active in case-finding.

The public health nurse can do a great deal in controlling venereal disease among adolescents by knowing her families well, by guidance, by case-finding and by helping infected persons understand their responsibility in controlling the spread of infection to others.

The only way to control venereal disease in the adolescent group is by a multidisciplinary approach. The nurse should understand her responsibility as a cooperating member of the health team in order to reduce the incidence of this social tragedy of youth.

## Severe Psychoneuroses

Adolescents may reveal manifestations of more severe neuroses similar to those seen in adults. They may show symptoms of severe depression, hysteria, anxiety or withdrawal. The patient usually shows a mixture of these symptoms. Older adolescents may become anxious and show a deep concern about their physical health. Although this may be an extension of their normal concern about their health, they resist reassurance from their physician. They may also evidence highly organized compulsions and phobias. The physician and the nurse may need guidance from a psychiatrist in the care of such patients.

## Juvenile Delinquency

**Incidence and Etiology.** A delinquent is one who does not behave in accordance with standards set by his society or community. Basically, delinquent behavior is antisocial, aggressive behavior usually due to anxiety and frustrations. Juvenile delinquency in the United States has increased for more than ten consecutive years.

There is usually a combination of causative factors in any one problem of delinquency.

*Delinquency Due to Force of Circumstances.* An example of this kind of delinquency is stealing so that the adolescent can have necessities—e.g. food. Spending money such as his friends have appears to many adolescents as a necessity. He may steal so that he can remain in the group. This sort of child is essentially normal and dislikes stealing from others. He needs the help of the sociologist, the educator and the economist.

*Delinquency Due to Poor Home and Community Environment.* The adolescent whose insecurity at home, in his community and in society is very great

**Figure 275.** Juvenile delinquency is still rising. Increases in police arrests of young people and juvenile court delinquency cases were much greater than the increase in the number of adolescents between 10 and 17 years during the 5- to 10-year period before 1957. (Interdepartmental Committee on Children and Youth, Golden Anniversary White House Conference on Children and Youth: Children in a Changing World.)

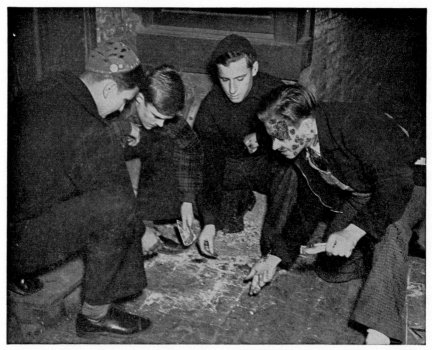

**Figure 276.** These adolescents are members of a gang in a large urban area. They gain status from belonging to the gang and emotional support from other gang members. (H. Armstrong Roberts.)

may become delinquent. As a child he may have felt rejection or lack of understanding. As an adolescent he may engage in criminal activity such as robbery, sex orgies, addiction to narcotics or alcohol, and even apparently unmotivated murder. Actually, when he gets into trouble with the law, he harms his parents more than he does himself, because he gains a stronger position in his peer group by his delinquencies. He is thus likely to do anything the gang says so as not to be rejected by them. Treatment may be very difficult, since the basis of the insecurity is in the home and the community. Treatment lies in education and helping these adolescents to accept the mores of a new group.

A child who has been brought up according to one set of mores and then is transplanted to another may be considered normal in his original society, but delinquent in the new one. In other words, the child who has been reared in a poor neighborhood may not be termed a delinquent when he steals an apple from a fruit stand, because this is fairly normal behavior. If he moves to a better neighborhood and steals fruit from a store, he is apprehended and held as a delinquent. The treatment again lies in education and helping the youth to accept the mores of his new group.

*Delinquency Due to Mental Retardation.* A mentally retarded adolescent depends on other persons for emotional support and therefore is easily led by them. He is not able to distinguish clearly what property does not belong to him or what will happen to him as a result of asocial acts. Often he has not been able to develop a conscience, so that he does not know right from wrong. Since he probably has not received adequate love, he may develop an aggressive reaction pattern. He may be used by intelligent delinquents and many times is the one who is caught by the authorities. He needs protection, training and supervision.

*Delinquency Due to Neurosis.* Some adolescents become delinquent because they have a need to be punished, since they feel guilty over something in the past. They carry out delinquent acts in order to be punished.

*Delinquency Due to Character Disorder.* Delinquents may have character disorders which result in behavior similar to that of adults who have psychopathic personalities. These adolescents seem to have weak characters. They cannot learn from experience. They cannot establish meaningful relations even with those persons who try to help them with their problems. They cannot control their desire to do exactly what they want without regard for the consequences to others or the long-term consequences to themselves. They may require institutionalization and treatment in order to protect society from their acts. Many such delinquents could have been recognized in early childhood and given adequate treatment. Unfortunately, too often they are not given help until they come in conflict with the law, and then only if the court has facilities for treatment other than confinement in the outdated home for delinquents. Such institutions often have no psychiatrist or counselor, or so few in proportion to the number of inmates that individual treatment of only a small number of selected patients is possible.

*Delinquency Due to Emotional Disturbances* (*Psychoses*). Emotionally disturbed or psychotic adolescents may become delinquent. Their behavior would be normal if the world of reality were like their world of delusions. This kind of delinquency is relatively rare in adolescence, but when it does occur, psychiatric treatment is necessary.

**Treatment, Prevention and Role of the Nurse.** If the delinquent adolescent is to be given adequate *treatment*, emphasis must be placed on the total individual in his home and community and on the reasons why he committed the delinquent act. Emphasis should not be on the act alone.

The delinquent adolescent can best be managed by personnel in the juvenile courts instead of the adult courts. The objectives of juvenile courts are basically diagnostic, protective and educational. After a study of the total individual has been made management is planned on the basis of his fundamental problem and what is best for him and for society.

Many suggestions for *prevention* have been made: more and better schools, playgrounds and recreational facilities and better housing. Authorities have also recommended that more attention be paid to children of minority groups (see p. 676) and to their economic and social status in their communities. The basic problem confronting all growing children in our society must be better understood if delinquency is to be prevented. If the living situation could be stabilized for all children, there would probably be less delinquency.

Broadly, prevention lies not only in relation to individual delinquents, but also in relation to the causative factors operating in communities which lead adolescents into asocial acts. The sociologist, the educator, the economist, the psychologist and the psychiatrist must make efforts to alter customs and mores which our culture seems to have outgrown. Any preventive effort must combine the skills of many disciplines if it is to be successful.

The nurse may be called upon to care for delinquent adolescents. She must recognize that her patient is first of all an individual and must accept him as such without emphasis on his asocial acts. She must make accurate observations of his behavior, provide him with support and work closely with other members of the health team in his treatment.

The nurse must also use her professional insights in working with others in the community to help prevent the formation of personality traits which lead to delinquency.

### Schizophrenic Reactions

**Incidence and Etiology.** Although schizophrenic reactions are not too common in children, they are the most important kind of mental illness seen during the adolescent years.

There are several theories about the *etiology* of schizophrenic reactions. No one cause has been proved. It is not certain to what extent heredity is a factor. There may also be a basic neurologic defect in schizophrenics. Environmental stresses may cause a defect in interpersonal relations. The schizophrenic has never in his life felt accepted by others or gained satisfaction from what he attempted to do. Usually, as a child he received too little love and affection. Too much was expected of him, and too little happiness or reward was given in return.

**Clinical Manifestations and Diagnosis.** The onset may seem acute, but personality changes have probably been going on for months or years. The following behavior may be shown. (*a*) Rigidity in adjustment to various persons or situations in the environment. The child cannot tolerate any kind of life other than his own. He abides by his rituals in his daily life and cannot change them quickly. (*b*) He begins to draw a curtain between himself and others. He becomes reserved and seems to have only brief periods of contact with reality. His personality becomes disorganized to a degree. (*c*) There is a split between the meaning of the act itself and his response to it. He may laugh when a tragedy occurs. He appears odd in his behavior. (*d*) He becomes careless, untidy and tardy and finally is satisfied just to sit alone. At last he retreats into his own world because the world of reality is intolerable. Delusions and hallucinations occur. Speech becomes irregular and illogical.

Mental illness is difficult to *diagnose* in adolescence because normal children and adolescents at one time or another in the developmental process may show similar manifestations of behavior. It is the degree to which abnormal behavior occurs that is important in making a diagnosis.

**Treatment, Nursing Care and Prognosis.** Psychiatric *treatment* should be given as promptly as possible. Individual care, to be effective, must be given by accepting, warm adults who give the young person their undivided attention. The adolescent must be provided with love, acceptance and praise for his efforts in order to compensate for his previous deprivations. His physical condition should be improved. He should be released from educational and social pressures and frustrations. Institutional care should be provided as necessary.

Before the age of twelve years it is difficult to be certain of the *prognosis*. Even with therapy and institutional care the prognosis has been poor. In recent years some success has been achieved with intensive patient therapy. Cure occurs rarely, but a satisfactory social adjustment can be made. More and more work is being done so that treatment of these adolescents can be more successful.

**Figure 277.** The schizophrenic prefers to sit alone, to withdraw from the world of reality to a world of his own making. (H. Armstrong Roberts.)

## CLINICAL SITUATIONS

Mrs. Horter brought her fourteen-year-old daughter, Barbara, to the adolescent clinic because she had "pimples on her face" which she persisted in picking. After an examination of the lesions the physician made the diagnosis of acne vulgaris. Barbara is a well developed and attractive adolescent whose menarche occurred when she was twelve years of age. Both Barbara and her mother appeared to be alert and interested in the activities of the clinic.

1. Acne vulgaris is caused primarily by
   a. The erratic diet of the adolescent.
   b. Changes in the skin during adolescence.
   c. Irritation of the skin due to the habit of picking the face.
   d. Allergy to foods containing chocolate.

2. Several weeks later the nurse, who had previously established a good relation with Barbara, met her in the clinic and commented on the improvement of her acne. During the conversation Barbara said, "I'm glad my mother didn't come with me today. She's always telling me what to do, and when I refuse to do what she says, she threatens to tell my father." In response to this expression of feeling the nurse would answer
   a. "Your mother did seem to be a domineering type of woman. Perhaps if you do what she says, she won't bother you so much."
   b. "If you would act your age, your mother wouldn't have to tell you what to do."
   c. "Why don't you talk to your father about this situation and see how he feels about your mother?"
   d. "Your mother may be having difficulty in remembering that you are almost grown up now. Perhaps if you would talk with her about this problem, you both would understand each other better."

3. Mrs. Horter confides in the nurse her deep concern because she has observed Barbara daydreaming on occasion. Some of the mothers of Barbara's friends are equally disturbed about this behavior in their adolescents. The nurse should realize in order to answer this comment that
   a. Adolescents daydream because they want to evade doing their homework or helping with the housework.
   b. They are showing early indications of becoming schizophrenics and should be examined by their physicians as soon as possible.
   c. They need time to formulate their philosophies of life, to learn to know themselves and to plan for their futures.
   d. They are growing rapidly and are too fatigued to engage in activities such as sports.

Fifteen-year-old Carmella Nignari has been admitted to the hospital with a diagnosis of pulmonary tuberculosis. Her father is a guard at a local warehouse, and her mother before Carmella's hospitalization worked as a waitress in the evenings and over the weekends to supplement the family income. When her mother worked, Carmella had cared for the six younger siblings. Now her mother must stay home from work to assume this responsibility.

4. As a result of Carmella's illness all the other members of her family had tuberculin tests and chest x-rays to determine whether they also had the infection. The infant and toddler were examined thoroughly to determine the presence of
   a. Miliary tuberculosis.
   b. Pott's disease.
   c. Tuberculosis of the cervical lymph nodes.
   d. Tuberculous dactylitis.

5. A positive reaction to a tuberculin skin test indicates that the individual
   a. Has an active lesion of pulmonary tuberculosis.
   b. Has never had tuberculosis or come in contact with the disease.
   c. Has been infected with the *Mycobacterium tuberculosis* and is hypersensitive to its protein.
   d. Has not been infected with the disease, but is allergic to the *Mycobacterium tuberculosis*.

6. Carmella is concerned about her health and asks many questions about her condition. The nurse would
   a. Ask the physician to talk with her about each question she asks.
   b. Explain that worrying about her health is harmful for her. Assure her that the physician knows how to care for persons having tuberculosis.
   c. Ignore most of her questions because Carmella only wants attention.
   d. Answer her questions to the best of her ability and refer those which she cannot answer to the physician.

7. Carmella asked why she could not be treated with only one kind of medication. To answer her question the nurse would need to know that streptomycin should not be used alone in the treatment of tuberculosis because
   a. Streptomycin - resistant organisms emerge rapidly.
   b. The eighth cranial nerve may be damaged.
   c. The drug is not very effective against the *Mycobacterium tuberculosis*.
   d. Treatment with more than one drug hastens recovery.

8. The nurse who cared for Carmella had had a negative reaction to the Mantoux test when she entered the school of nursing. The physician had recommended that she be protected against the Mycobacterium tuberculosis by
   a. Bacillus of Calmette and Guérin vaccine.
   b. Plague vaccine.
   c. Salk vaccine.
   d. Pertussis vaccine.

## GUIDES TO FURTHER STUDY

1. Observe a group of adolescents in high school, a recreation center or a neighborhood meeting place. Describe the general activity of the members of the group. Were any adolescents paired off in couples? What activity, if any, were the ones doing who did not mix with the others? Observe their posture when sitting and standing. Observe their manner of dress and their grooming. Compare your observations with your knowledge of the normal behavior patterns of adolescents.

2. What is your understanding of the function of a clinic for adolescents? How many adolescent clinics have been organized in your state or community?

3. A thirteen-year-old delinquent has been admitted to the pediatric unit with a diagnosis of tuberculosis. What would be your approach to this adolescent and his parents? What would be your role and responsibility as a member of the health team in providing care for this young person? Investigate the agencies in your community which could assist in his rehabilitation.

4. What are the most recent statistics in your state on the causes of mortality in the adolescent age group? What preventive measures could be taken to reduce these tragedies?

5. What rehabilitative services are available for physically and mentally handicapped adolescents in your hospital, your community and your state? Evaluate these services to determine whether they are adequately meeting the need.

6. What facilities are available in your state for the care of adolescents having a diagnosis of schizophrenia? Are these facilities adequately meeting the need?

7. Select the three experiences which were most disturbing to you in providing care for children. Select the three experiences which were most satisfying to you in providing care for children. State for each incident the age of the patient, his diagnosis and a description of the situation. Analyze each of these incidents to determine why they were disturbing or satisfying to you and discuss them in seminar.

## TEACHING AIDS AND OTHER INFORMATION*

*American Cancer Society*
  A Cancer Source Book for Nurses. Reprinted 1959.

*Community Service Society of New York*
  Tuberculosis, 1956.

*John Hancock Mutual Life Insurance Company*
  About Tuberculosis.

*National Tuberculosis Association*
  Children with Special Health Problems.
  Safer Ways in Nursing.

*Complete addresses are given in the Appendix.

*Public Affairs Pamphlets*
  Barnouw, E., and Clark, E. G.: Syphilis: The Invader.
  Polier, J. W.: Back to What Woodshed?
  Puner, H. W.: Children in Court.

*U.S. Department of Health, Education, and Welfare*
  A Look at Juvenile Delinquency, 1960.
  Coordination of the National Effort for Dealing with Juvenile Delinquency, Governmental Responsibility, 1960.
  Delinquency and the Adolescent Crisis, 1960.
  Delinquency Prevention: The Size of the Problem, 1960.
  Family Courts—An Urgent Need, 1960.
  Health Services and Juvenile Delinquency. A Report on a Conference on the Role of Health Services in Preventing Dissocial Behavior, 1955.
  Identifying Potential Delinquents, 1960.
  State Agencies and Juvenile Delinquency, 1960.
  The Children's Bureau and Juvenile Delinquency, 1960.

## REFERENCES

American Academy of Pediatrics: Care of Children in Hospitals. Evanston, Illinois, American Academy of Pediatrics, 1960.

Bakwin, H., and Bakwin, R. M.: Clinical Management of Behavior Disorders in Children. 2nd ed. Philadelphia, W. B. Saunders Company, 1960.

Bower, A. G., Pilant, E. B., and Craft, N. B.: Communicable Diseases. 8th ed. Philadelphia, W. B. Saunders Company, 1958.

Bruce, S. J.: Adolescence, Delinquent or Distressed? Nursing Outlook, 8:499, 1960.

Cady, L. L.: Nursing in Tuberculosis. 2nd ed. Philadelphia, W. B. Saunders Company, 1961.

Caloz, R.: The Birth of the Bacillus Calmette Guerin. World Health Organization, World Health, 13:26, Jan.-Feb., 1960.

Chwast, J.: Value Conflicts in Treating Delinquents. Children, 6:95, 1959.

Clise, M. H.: Disturbed Children Are Disturbing Children. Nursing Outlook, 5:638, 1957.

Craig, L. P.: Reaching Delinquents through Cottage Committees. Children, 6:129, 1959.

Cromwell, G. E.: The Teenager and Venereal Disease. Am. J. Nursing, 59:1738, 1959.

Daniels, L.: Pediatrics and Delinquency. Children, 6:113, 1959.

Daubenmire, M. J., Pierce, L. M., and Weaver, B. R.: Adolescence in the Hospital. Nursing Outlook, 8:502, 1960.

Erickson, E. H.: Youth and The Life Cycle. Children, 7:43, 1960.

Falstein, E. I., and Sutton, H. A.: Childhood Schizophrenia. Am. J. Nursing, 58:666, 1958.

Feldmann, F.: How to Use the Tuberculin Test. Am. J. Nursing, 59:856, 1959.

Idem: The Practical Value of the Tuberculin Test. Pediatrics, 21:319, 1958.

Finch, S. M.: Fundamentals of Child Psychiatry. New York, W. W. Norton Co., 1960.

Freeman, R. B.: Public Health Nursing Practice. 2nd ed. Philadelphia, W. B. Saunders Company, 1957.

Gibson, F. J., and Taylor, R. M.: Selective Case-finding in Tuberculosis. Nursing Outlook, 7:641, 1959.

Greenwald, W. F.: Scoliosis. Am. J. Nursing, 59:817, 1959.

Greenwich, J. F.: A New Look for the Youngster with Scoliosis. Am. J. Nursing, 59:814, 1959.

Hawken, P.: Needed: Security and Love. Am. J. Nursing, 58:103, 1958.

Hetherington, H. W., and Eshleman, F. W.: Tuberculosis: Prevention and Control. 4th ed. New York, G. P. Putnam's Sons, 1958.

Krapp, E. E., and Gibbens, T.: Who Are They? World Health Organization, World Health, 13:28, May-June, 1960.

Kvaraceus, W. C.: Assessing Efforts to Prevent Delinquency. Children, 6:150, 1959.

Lane, H.: No Child Is Born to Be Delinquent. Childhood Education, 32:355, Apr., 1956.

Langer, M. F.: Parent Groups in Total Family Therapy. Children, 6:69, 1959.

Larson, C. B., and Gould, M.: Calderwood's Orthopedic Nursing. 4th ed. St. Louis, C. V. Mosby Company, 1957.

Liebman, S.: Emotional Problems of Childhood. Philadelphia, J. B. Lippincott Company, 1958.

MacIver, R. M.: Juvenile Delinquency; in E. Ginzberg (editor): The Nation's Children. 3. Problems and Prospects. New York, Columbia University Press, 1960, p. 103.

Nelson, W. E. (editor): Textbook of Pediatrics. 7th ed. Philadelphia, W. B. Saunders Company, 1959.

Paterson, D., and McCreary, J. F.: Pediatrics. Philadelphia, J. B. Lippincott Company, 1956.

Robinson, A. M.: Communicating with Schizophrenic Patients. Am. J. Nursing, 60:1120, 1960.

Robinson, S. M.: Juvenile Delinquency. New York, Holt, Rinehart and Winston, 1960.

Schwarz, B. E., and Ruggieri, B. A.: Parent-Child Tensions. Philadelphia, J. B. Lippincott Company, 1958.

Silver, H. K., Kempe, C. H., and Bruyn, H. B.: Handbook of Pediatrics. 3rd ed. Los Altos, California, Lange Medical Publications, 1959.

Spahn, C. H.: Tuberculosis or Coccidioidomycosis? Nursing Outlook, 8:25, 1960.

Steiner, L. R.: Understanding Juvenile Delinquency. Philadelphia, Chilton Co., 1960.

Strecker, E. A.: Their Mothers' Sons. Philadelphia, J. B. Lippincott Company, 1951.

Strecker, E. A., and Lathbury, V. T.: Their Mothers' Daughters. Philadelphia, J. B. Lippincott Company, 1956.

Top, F. H.: Communicable and Infectious Diseases. 4th ed. St. Louis, C. V. Mosby Company, 1960.

Tuberculosis Nursing Advisory Service, National League for Nursing: Nurses' Participation in Tuberculin and Other Skin Testing Programs. Nursing Outlook, 8:201, 1960.

Weiss, M.: Chemotherapy and Tuberculosis. Am. J. Nursing, 59:1711, 1959.

# Appendix

# Addresses for Sources of Materials

# Listed at the Ends of Chapters

Abbott Laboratories: 14th Street and Sheridan Rd., North Chicago, Ill.

American Academy of Pediatrics: 1801 Hinman Ave., Evanston, Ill.

American Cancer Society, Inc.: 521 W. 57th St., New York 19, N. Y.

American Dental Association: 222 E. Superior St., Chicago 11, Ill.

American Diabetes Association, Inc.: 1 East 45th St., New York 17, N. Y.

American Heart Association, Inc.: 44 E. 23rd St., New York 10, N. Y.

American Medical Association: 535 N. Dearborn St., Chicago 10, Ill.

American Public Health Association, Inc.: 1790 Broadway, New York 19, N. Y.

Bureau of Publications, Teachers College, Columbia University: 525 W. 120th St., New York 27, N. Y.

Child Study Association of America, Inc.: 9 E. 89th St., New York 28, N. Y.

Community Service Society of New York, Division of Family Services, Public Health Nursing: 105 E. 22nd St., New York 10, N. Y.

Eli Lilly and Co.: Indianapolis 6, Ind.

Equitable Life Assurance Society of the United States: 393 Seventh Ave., New York 1, N. Y.

E. R. Squibb and Sons: 745 Fifth Ave., New York 22, N. Y.

F. A. Davis Company: 1914–16 Cherry St., Philadelphia 3, Pa.

Federal Association for Epilepsy, Inc.: 1729 F. St., N. W., Washington 6, D.C.

Golden Anniversary White House Conference on Children and Youth, Inc.: 330 Independence Ave., S. W., Washington 25, D.C.

Hart Publishing Company, Inc.: 74 5th Ave., New York 11, N. Y.

H. J. Heinz Company: Pittsburgh 30, Pa.

John Hancock Mutual Life Insurance Company: Boston, Mass.

Mead Johnson and Company: Evansville 21, Ind.

Mental Health Division, Dept. of National Health and Welfare: Ottawa, Canada.

National Association for Mental Health: 10 Columbus Circle, New York 19, N.Y.

National Association for Retarded Children, Inc.: 386 Park Ave. S, New York 16, N. Y.

National Dairy Council: 111 North Canal St., Chicago 6, Ill.

National Education Association of the United States: 1201 Sixteenth St., N.W., Washington 6, D.C.

National Paint, Varnish and Lacquer Association, Inc.: 1500 Rhode Island Avenue, N.W., Washington 5, D.C.

National Society for the Prevention of Blindness: 1790 Broadway, New York 19, N. Y.

National Tuberculosis Association: 1790 Broadway, New York 19, N.Y.

Personal Products Corporation: Milltown, N. J.

Public Affairs Committee, Inc.: 22 East 38th St., New York 16, N. Y.

Ross Laboratories: Columbus 16, Ohio.

Science Research Associates, Inc.: 259 E. Erie St., Chicago 11, Ill.

State of Illinois, Department of Public Welfare: Springfield, Ill.

The Children's Medical Center, Department of Public Relations: 300 Longwood Ave., Boston 15, Mass.

U.S. Department of Health, Education, and Welfare, Social Security Administration, Children's Bureau: U.S. Government Printing Office, Division of Public Documents, Washington 25, D.C.

Wonder Books Inc. (Grosset and Dunlap, Inc.): 1107 Broadway, New York 10, N. Y.

# Index

Rehabilitation, 635. See also *Habilitation.*
after burns, 629
of school child, 635–6
Relaxation, problems of, in cerebral palsy, 478, 479
Religious education for preschool child, 505–507
Renal. See *Kidneys.*
Reserpine in glomerulonephritis, 552
Resilience, physiologic, of newborn, 83–4
Resolution in pneumonia, 447
Respiration, artificial, 185
in laryngotracheobronchitis, 445
control, 298
difficult, in premature infant, 143–4
in newborn, 84–5
establishment and maintenance, 97–9
in premature infant, initiation, 145
maintenance, 147–8
muscles of, 298
problems of, in cerebral palsy, 478
Respiratory conditions in newborn, 184–8
in infant, 298–308
Respiratory distress in newborn, 105
Respiratory tract. See also *Lungs; Nose;* etc.
in newborn, 89
infections, 622–3
in premature infants, 152
mortality due to, 33, 34
of infant, 298
Rest, bed, in rheumatic fever, 640
for preschool child in hospital, 538
in nasopharyngitis, 300
Restraint, abdominal, 225
after brain surgery, 656, 657
ankle, 225
clove hitch, 168, 169
elbow, 200
extremity, 225
in infantile eczema, 375, 376
mummy, 150
safety measures, 48
Retardation, mental, delinquency due to, 712
Reticulocytes, 361
Retrolental fibroplasia, 153–4
Retropharyngeal abscess, 436–7
Revolution, Industrial, child care during, 4
Rh incompatibility, hemolytic disease of newborn due to, 160–61
Rhagades in congenital syphilis, 165
Rheumatic fever, 636–45
Aschoff bodies, 637
Rhinitis, allergic, 573
vs. nasopharyngitis, 300
in congenital syphilis, 164
Riboflavin. See also *Vitamin B.*
requirements, for adolescent, 690
for infants, 280
for preschool child, 530
for school children, 614
for toddlers, 427
Rickets, 345–7
in premature infant, tendency for, 144
Rickettsia rickettsii, 548
Rigidity, 476
Ringworm, 623
of feet, 624
of scalp, 623
of skin, 623

Risser localizer jacket in scoliosis, 707
Risus sardonicus, 194, 550
Ritualistic behavior in toddler, 404–405
Rocky Mountain spotted fever, 548, 549
Roentgen therapy, in acne vulgaris, 695
in leukemia, 563
Romance, family, in preschool child, 498–9
Room, delivery. See *Delivery room.*
furnishings, for newborn, 136
Rooming-in, 77–9
disadvantages, 78
Rooting reflex, 92
Rosary, rachitic, 346
scorbutic, 351
Roundworm infection. See *Ascariasis.*
Rubella, 544, 545
maternal, effort on fetus, 173
Rubeola. See *Measles.*
Rule of Nines in burns, 627
Rules for drug dosage, 61
Rumination, 135, 324

SABER shin in congenital syphilis, 164
Saddle nose in congenital syphilis, 164
Safety, education, for adolescents, 689–90
factors, in selection of toys for toddlers, 417
measures, for infants, 278–9
for preschool child, 526–7
for school child, 610–11
for toddlers, 420–25
in pediatric unit, 48–9
parent-nurse learning, 422–5
pins, safety measures, 48, 49
St. Louis encephalitis, 542
St. Vitus's dance. See *Chorea, Sydenham's.*
Salicylates in rheumatic fever, 639
Saline soaks in infantile eczema, 376
Salt solution in poisoning, 457
Sarcoma, osteogenic. See *Osteosarcoma.*
Scabies, 626
Scalp, ringworm, 623
Scaphocephaly, 383
Scarlatina. See *Scarlet fever.*
Scarlet fever, 548, 549
Dick test, 540, 549
Schick test for diphtheria, 540, 543
Schizophrenia, childhood. See *Autism.*
Schizophrenic reactions, 713–14
Schoenlein-Henoch syndrome. See *Purpura, anaphylactoid.*
School, 601–604
adolescent and, 685–7
age, health problems during, 613
child, 12, 587–668
bathing, 610
care, 610–11
conditions, requiring immediate or short-term care, 618–34
requiring long-term care, 635–68
cruelty, 593
development, 6 years, 594–6
7 years, 596–7
8 years, 597–8
9 years, 598
10 years, 598–99
10–12 years, 599–601
dressing, 610